DEDICATION

To the contributors to this and past editions, who took time to share their knowledge, insight, and humor for the benefit of students.

and

To Dr. William Ganong, a beloved teacher and an early believer in the power of *First Aid*.

CONTENTS

CONTRIBUTING AUTHORS

FERAS AKBIK
Medical Scientist Training Program
Yale University

DEEPALI DHAR
Yale School of Medicine
Class of 2012

JONATHAN FU
Yale School of Medicine
Class of 2012

JEFFREY S. FUTTERLEIB
Yale School of Medicine
Class of 2012

CLAYTON HALDEMAN
Yale School of Medicine
Class of 2012

JOHN HSI-EN HO
Yale School of Medicine
Class of 2012

ESTHER S. LEE
Yale School of Medicine
Class of 2012

BABITA PANIGRAHI
Yale School of Medicine
Class of 2012

RANY WOO
Yale School of Medicine
Class of 2012

CATHERINE YANG
Yale School of Medicine
Class of 2012

WEB CONTRIBUTORS

JOSEPH A. SANFORD, MD
Resident in Anesthesiology
University of Arkansas for Medical Sciences
Web 2.0 Editor

KEISHA BARWISE
Universidad Iberoamericana
Class of 2009

JAYSSON BROOKS
Loma Linda University
Class of 2011

STEVE COHEN, PA-C
University of Sint Eustatius
Class of 2013

MICHAEL L. STERN
Albany Medical Center
Class of 2011

FACULTY REVIEWERS

DIANA M. ANTONIUCCI, MD, MAS

Assistant Clinical Professor
University of California, San Francisco

LINDA S. COSTANZO, PhD

Professor of Physiology
Virginia Commonwealth University

STUART D. FLYNN, MD

Dean, College of Medicine
University of Arizona (Phoenix)

RYAN HALL, MD

Assistant Professor, Department of Psychiatry
University of Central Florida
Affiliate and Assistant Professor, Department of Psychiatry
University of South Florida
Adjunct Professor
Barry University

RAJESH JARI, MD, MSC

International Pain Fellow, Department of Physical Medicine and
   Rehabilitation
Temple University

BERTRAM KATZUNG, MD, PhD

Professor Emeritus
University of California, San Francisco

WARREN LEVINSON, MD, PhD

Professor of Microbiology and Immunology
University of California, San Francisco

PETER MARKS, MD, PhD

Associate Professor of Internal Medicine
Yale University

ANDREA OECKINGHAUS, PhD

Postdoctoral Research Scientist, Department of Microbiology and
   Immunology
Columbia University

DANIEL RUBIN, MD

Assistant Professor of Medicine, Section of Endocrinology
Temple University

SANJIV J. SHAH, MD

Assistant Professor of Medicine
Division of Cardiology, Department of Medicine
Northwestern University Feinberg School of Medicine

STEPHEN F. THUNG, MD

Assistant Professor, Department of Obstetrics, Gynecology, and
   Reproductive Sciences
Yale University

ADAM WEINSTEIN, MD

Assistant Professor, Department of Pediatrics/Pediatric Nephrology
Dartmouth Medical Center

With this edition of *First Aid for the USMLE Step 1*, we continue our commitment to providing students with the most useful and up-to-date preparation guide for the USMLE Step 1. This edition represents a major revision in many ways and includes:

- A revised and updated exam preparation guide for the USMLE Step 1. Includes detailed analysis as well as study and test-taking strategies for the FRED v2 format.
- Revisions and new material based on student experience with the 2010 administrations of the computerized USMLE Step 1.
- Revised USMLE advice for international medical graduates, osteopathic medical students, podiatry students, and students with disabilities.
- More than 1100 frequently tested facts and useful mnemonics, including hundreds of new or revised entries in reorganized sections.
- A high-yield collection of nearly 200 glossy photos similar to those appearing on the USMLE Step 1 exam.
- An updated guide to hundreds of recommended USMLE Step 1 review resources, based on a nationwide survey of randomly selected third-year medical students.
- Bonus Step 1 high-yield facts, cases, video lectures, corrections, and updates exclusively at our blog at **www.firstaidteam.com.**

The improvements in this edition would not have been possible without the help of the hundreds of students and faculty members who contributed their feedback and suggestions. We invite students and faculty to continue sharing their thoughts and ideas to help us improve *First Aid for the USMLE Step 1.* (See How to Contribute, p. xv.)

Louisville	Tao Le
Los Angeles	Vikas Bhushan
New Haven	Juliana Tolles
Providence	Jeffrey Hofmann

ACKNOWLEDGMENTS

This has been a collaborative project from the start. We gratefully acknowledge the thoughtful comments, corrections, and advice of the many hundreds of medical students, international medical graduates, and faculty who have supported the authors in the continuing development of *First Aid for the USMLE Step 1.*

Thanks to our faculty reviewers Dr. Susan Baserga, Dr. Janine Evans, Dr. Fred Gorelick, Dr. Christian Merlo, Dr. Shanta Kapadia, and Dr. Dhasakumar S. Navaratnam. For help on the web team, thanks to Nicki Zevola. For support and encouragement throughout the process, we are grateful to Thao Pham and Jonathan Kirsch, Esq. Thanks to Selina Franklin and Louise Petersen for organizing and supporting the project. Thanks to our publisher, McGraw-Hill, for the valuable assistance of its staff. For enthusiasm, support, and commitment for this ongoing and ever-challenging project, thanks to our editor, Catherine Johnson.

For editorial support, an enormous thanks to Andrea Fellows and Carol Ayres. A special thanks to Rainbow Graphics, especially David Hommel and Susan Cooper, for remarkable editorial and production work.

For submitting contributions and corrections, thanks to Dan Abenroth, Bayan Aghdasi, Nina Akbar, Amin Akhlaghi, Yassar Alamri, Sean Alemi, Kelvin Allenson, Nathon Allred, Hina Ansar, David Anstey, Adisa Aphaithoonsert, Amran Asadi, Arneh Babakhani, Nima Baradaran, Kevin Barley, Irving Basanez, Jessica Bear, Tamara Berger, Grishma Bharucha, Mario Bialostozky, Adam Bied, Frank Bittner, Jeff Boatright, Hein Bogers, Jonathan Bonchak, William Bowen, Ben Burris, Roberto Calix, Zac Camann, Michael Caposole, Michael Carlton, Luis Cayamcela, Shruti Chandra, Angel Chang, Teena Charalel, Rohan Chaubey, Noe Chavez, Yucui Chen, Yixiao Chen, Kevin Chen, Edwin Chen, Nelson Chiu, Clara Choo, Karen Chopra, Daniel Churgin, Lauren Ciminello, Christine Clavell, Crysta Clemente, Eve Cohen, Ohmar Coughlin, Cory Criss, Carla Cruz, Julia Curtis, Laura D' Addese, Nicholas D'Aloisio, Riva Das, Ilka Decker, Jose Delgado, Amanda Deming, Robert Desimone, Gemmie Devera, Patrick Do, Epameinondas Dogeas, Emily Donelan, Tina Dong, Maia Dorsett, Zvi Dubin, Ross Dunbar, Chris Duncan, Rafael Eduardo, Kristen Ehrenberger, Panuch Eiamprapaporn, John Ekladous, Khalid Elkady, Ross England, Amy Eppstein, Kevin Evans, Chizoba Ezepue, David Faleck, Joshua Farhadian, Saul Feierstein, Joshua Feuerstein, Yale Fillingham, Clark Fisher, Kathryn Fong, Alex Foyshteter, Erin Fuchs, Niral Gandhi, Robert Gemignani, Lee Gerson, Kenn Ghaffarian, Meridith Gilliam, Ryan Gindi, Christopher Goiney, Sari Goldman, Bernard Goldwasser, Victor Gonzalez, Michael Gottlieb, Amit Goya, Samita Goyal, Stephen Gregory, Senthil Gunasekaran, Bryce Haac, Jennifer Hadley, Rimoun Hakim, Tiffany Hall, Lauren Hamlin-Douglas, Stephen Harmon, Sarah Haseltine, Ken He, Daniel Hendry, Elise Henning, Mara Holcom, Maura Holcomb, Avinash Honasoge, Jamael Hoosain, Kathleen Hurley, Omer Iftikhar, Benjamin Illum, Omar Imam, Mohamad Imam, Erik Interval, Arya Iranmanesh, Naomi Izmailova, Parisa Javedani, Michael Jenkins, Brianna Jewel, Cali Johnson, Dejah Judelson, Ryan Kachur, Steven Kane, Adiyta Karnik, Shwetha Katta, Alyn Kelley, Mona Kessas, Victor Kha, Ali Khalil, Shaheen Khan, Harry Khlon, Isaac Kim, Heather Klavan, Annie Ko, Richard Koff, Patrick Koo, Brenden Kootsey, Petro Kostandy, Erik Kramer, Jacob Krazanowski, Karen Kumar, Shelby Kunishima, Waleed Kurtom, Wai Yim Lam, Kam Lam, Jenny Lam, David Landis, Kevin Lee, James Lee, Jessica Lee, Ana Liang, Michael Lin, Kyle Lineberry, Peter Liou, Jon Liu, Erqi Liu, Joyce Liu, Maureen Looby, Jose Lopez, Erika Lundgrin, Namutebi Lwanga, Shalin Maheshwari, Angel Maldonado, Alex Maley, Stuart Marcotte, Michael Markiewicz, Danielle Martin, Alex Mathai, David Matlock, Kristina Medhus, Amar Mehta, Visha

Mehta, James Melotek, Leo Menashe, Sherif Mikhail, Lindsey Miller, Eliza Miller, Daniel Mindlin, Lina Miyakawa, Jeremy Moore, Syed Moosavi, Jonathan Morris, Joseph Mulvey, Adel Naji, Anna Nam, Anita Namutebi, Mark Neahring, Igor Nestrasil, Paul Neubarer, Julius Nga, To Dung Nguyen, Quyen Nguyen, Daniel Nimmo, Zorawar Noor, Uchenna Nwosu, Oluwatosin Ogunjemilusi, Brenda Oiyemhonlan, Alana Otto, Sobia Ozair, Tejal Pandya, Tajinder Parhar, Josh Parker, Shama Patel, Keval Patel, Devi Patel, Anand Patel, Sagar Patel, Jay Patel, Jeffrey Peck, Ryan Pedigo, Monica Peng, Marlene Maria Perez Mateo, Garrett Perrin, William Pientka, Salvador Plasencia, Tess Pollinger, Katherine Poruk, Bipin Rajendran, Sandhya Ravichandrian, Vineet Reddy, Aurora Reese, Arthur Richard, Ted Ritchie, Carlos Rivas, Brandon Roberts, Jose Rodriguez, Zach Rogers, Gisela Rosario, KC Rosburg, Ryan Ross, Evangiline Roxas, Galen Royce-Nagel, Mike Rozell, Faysal Saab, Hemal Sampat, Fares Samra, Ulises García Sánchez, Matt Sanders, Timothy Schmidt, Robin Schroeder, Adam Schwabauer, Brandon Scott, Josh Segal, Satbeer Sembhi, Monica Serrano, Ankit Shah, Ashish Shah, Jay Shah, Dan Short, Roni Shouval, Rachael Shulte, Jasleen Sikka, Sunpreet Singh, Sophia Siu, Travis Sizemore, Clark Sleeth, Jake Smith, Timothy Sommerville, Sundeep Srikakulam, Reb ekah Stalter, Bryan Stanistreet, Jehu Strange, Shasha Strul, Zhifei Sun, Jeremy Sutton, Aslam Syed1, Nicholas Szrama, Sajal Tanna, Branden Tarlow, Christopher Tarolli, Brent Tatsuno, Siddarth Thakur, Lisa To, Viviana Torres, Thanh Tran, Tung Minh Tran, Michelle Trani, David Turer, Chau Uong, John Vance, John Velasquez, Krishanthan Vigneswaran, Clementine Vo, Earl Walker, Jennfier Wan, Siu-Hin Wan, Tian Wang, Daniel Wang, Adam Was, Emily Rose Wenrich, Odette Williams, Alexander Willis, Blake Windsor, Daniel Wiznia, Katherine Wu, Ami Yamamoto, Mu Yang, Siamak Yasmeh, Nitin Yerram, Angelina Yogarajah, Sun Yoo, Christine Yoo, Lucia Young, Deena Yousef, Michelle Yu, Joyce Yuan, Yanmin Zang, JD Zipkin, and Michelle Zubair

For submitting book reviews, thank you to Shloka Ananthanarayanan, Melissa Appio, Arpit Arora, Violeta Ashby, RichardByrne, MichaelCarreras, Carmen Castilla, Julia Chen, Lucy Chen, Silas Chiu, William Chong, Hector Colon, Nicholas Costa, Naznin Daginawala, Anthony DeCicco, Gerald Dekker, Swati Dhanireddy, Caroline Dias, Katerina Dukleska, Stephen Dunay, Yonatan Faiwiszewski, Max Falkoff, David Glazer, Evan Grant, Kevin Gurcharran, Peter Hahn, Eugene Han, Amanda Hong, Jeffrey Hsu, Linda Huang, Ibrahim Hussain, Briana Jackson, Paul Johnson, Ashley Jones, Sagar Kadakia, Janelle Kalir, Stacey Kallem, Alexis Kearney, Kevin Koo, Vivian Ku, Neha Kumar, Gregory Kuzmik, Eliza Lamin, Shani Lampley, Kathleen Lee, Aron Legler, Rachel Lentz, Kiran Mahmood, Miriam Makola, Mithra Maneyapanda, Isis Martinez-Hernandez, Arun Mathew, Richard May, Kantha Medepalli, Kapil Mehrotra, Rachel Meyer, Luke Misquitta, Justin Morton, Jonathan Mosser, Alfredo Ok, Amit Padaki, Andrew Park, Alopi Patel, Punam Patel, Smruti Patel, Michael Peluso, June Peng, Rebecca Pfaff, Omesh Qasba, Patricia Richardson, Talia Rosenberg, Alyssa Santos, Melissa Schneiderman, Gregory Serrao, Radhika Shah, Amit Sharma, Rishi Sharma, Jeff Shrensel, Daniel Simmons, Whitney Smith, Fiona Somers, Resha Soni, David Swope Jr., Benjamin Taylor, Christopher Tran, Chiachien Wang, Chase Warren, Brent Wolford, Vincent Wong, Mona Wood, Yinfei Xu, and Annie Yang

Thanks to Kristopher Jones, Kristina Panizzi, and Peter Anderson of the Department of Pathology, University of Alabama at Birmingham, for use of images from the Pathology Education Instructional Resource Digital Library (http://peir.net), and to Vishal Pall, Vipal Soni, and Dhanashree Rajderkar for their contributions to the High-Yield Image section.

Finally, thanks to Ted Hon, one of the founding authors of this book, for his vision in developing this guide on the computer, and to Chirag Amin for his enormous contributions as an editor and author over many editions.

Louisville	Tao Le
Los Angeles	Vikas Bhushan
New Haven	Juliana Tolles
Providence	Jeffrey Hofmann

HOW TO CONTRIBUTE

This version of *First Aid for the USMLE Step 1* incorporates hundreds of contributions and changes suggested by faculty and student reviewers. We invite you to participate in this process. We also offer **paid internships** in medical education and publishing ranging from three months to one year. Please send us your suggestions for:

- Study and test-taking strategies for the new computerized USMLE Step 1
- New facts, mnemonics, diagrams, and illustrations
- High-yield topics that may reappear on future Step 1 exams
- Personal ratings and comments on review books that you have examined

For each entry incorporated into the next edition, you will receive a **$10 gift certificate** per entry from the author group, as well as personal acknowledgment in the next edition. Diagrams, tables, partial entries, updates, corrections, and study hints are also appreciated, and significant contributions will be compensated at the discretion of the authors. Also let us know about material in this edition that you feel is low yield and should be deleted.

The preferred way to submit entries, suggestions, or corrections is via our blog:

www.firstaidteam.com

Alternatively, you can e-mail us at: firstaidteam@yahoo.com. Otherwise, please send entries, neatly written or typed or on disk (Microsoft Word), to:

First Aid Team
914 N. Dixie Avenue
Suite 100
Elizabethtown, KY 42701

Contributions received by June 15, 2011, receive priority consideration for the 2012 edition of *First Aid for the USMLE Step 1*. We thank you for taking the time to share your experience and apologize in advance that we cannot individually respond to all contributors as we receive hundreds of contributions each year.

NOTE TO CONTRIBUTORS

All contributions become property of the authors and are subject to editing and reviewing. Please verify all data and spellings carefully. In the event that similar or duplicate entries are received, only the first entry received will be used. Include a reference to a standard textbook to facilitate verification of the fact. Please follow the style, punctuation, and format of this edition if possible.

The First Aid author team is pleased to offer part-time and full-time paid internships in medical education and publishing to motivated medical students and physicians. Internships may range from a few months (e.g., a summer) up to a full year. Participants will have an opportunity to author, edit, and earn academic credit on a wide variety of projects, including the popular *First Aid* series. English writing/editing experience, familiarity with Microsoft Word, and Internet access are required. Go to our blog at www.firstaidteam.com to apply for an internship or e-mail us at firstaidteam@yahoo.com. A sample of your work or a proposal of a specific project is helpful.

HOW TO USE THIS BOOK

Medical students who have used previous editions of this guide have given us feedback on how best to make use of the book.

It is recommended that you begin using this book as early as possible when learning the basic medical sciences. You can use Section IV to select first-year course review books and Internet resources and then use those books for review while taking your medical school classes.

Use different parts of the book at different stages in your preparation for the USMLE Step 1. Before you begin to study for the USMLE Step 1, we suggest that you read Section I: Guide to Efficient Exam Preparation and Section IV: Top-Rated Review Resources. **If you are an international medical graduate student, an osteopathic medical student, a podiatry student, or a student with a disability,** refer to the appropriate Section I supplement for additional advice. Devise a study plan and decide what resources to buy. We strongly recommend that you invest in at least one or two top-rated review books in each subject.

First Aid is not a comprehensive review book, and it is not a panacea that can compensate for not studying during the first two years of medical school. Scanning Sections II and III will give you an initial idea of the diverse range of topics covered on the USMLE Step 1.

As you study each discipline, **use the corresponding high-yield-fact section in *First Aid for the USMLE Step 1* as a means of consolidating the material and testing yourself** to see if you have covered some of the frequently tested items. Work with the book to integrate important facts into your fund of knowledge. Using *First Aid for the USMLE Step 1* as a review can serve as both a self-test of your knowledge and a repetition of important facts to learn. High-yield topics and vignettes are abstracted from recent exams to help guide your preparation.

To **broaden** your learning strategy, you can **integrate** your *First Aid* study with *First Aid Cases for the USMLE Step 1* and *First Aid Q&A for the USMLE Step 1*. *First Aid Cases* and *First Aid Q&A* are organized to match *First Aid for the USMLE Step 1* **chapter for chapter.** After reviewing a discipline or organ system chapter within *First Aid*, you can **review cases** on the same topics and then **test your knowledge** in the corresponding chapters of *First Aid Cases* and *First Aid Q&A*. If you want a **deeper review** of the high-yield topics, then you should consider adding *First Aid for the Basic Sciences: General Principles* and *Organ Systems* to your study plan.

Return to Sections II and III frequently during your preparation and fill your short-term memory with remaining high-yield facts a few days before the USMLE Step 1. The book can serve as a useful way of retaining key associations and keeping high-yield facts fresh in your memory just prior to the examination. Reviewing the book immediately after the exam is probably the best way to **help us improve the book in the next edition.** Decide what was truly high and low yield and **send in your comments or your entire annotated book.**

First Aid Checklist for the USMLE Step 1

This is an example of how you might use the information in Section I to prepare for the USMLE Step 1. Refer to corresponding topics in Section I for more details.

Years Prior

☐ Select top-rated review books as study guides for first-year medical school courses.

Months Prior

☐ Review computer test format and registration information.

☐ Register six months in advance. Carefully verify name and address printed on scheduling permit. Call Prometric for test date ASAP.

☐ Define goals for the USMLE Step 1 (e.g., comfortably pass, beat the mean, ace the test).

☐ Set up a realistic timeline for study. Cover less crammable subjects first. Review subject-by-subject emphasis and clinical vignette format.

☐ Simulate the USMLE Step 1 to pinpoint strengths and weaknesses in knowledge and test-taking skills.

☐ Evaluate and choose study methods and materials (e.g., review books, practice tests, software).

☐ Ask for advice from those who have recently taken the USMLE Step 1.

Weeks Prior

☐ Simulate the USMLE Step 1 again. Assess how close you are to your goal.

☐ Pinpoint remaining weaknesses. Stay healthy (exercise, sleep).

☐ Verify information on admission ticket (e.g., location, date).

One Week Prior

☐ Remember comfort measures (loose clothing, earplugs, etc.).

☐ Work out test site logistics such as location, transportation, parking, and lunch.

☐ Call Prometric and confirm your exam appointment.

One Day Prior

☐ Relax.

☐ Lightly review short-term material if necessary. Skim high-yield facts.

☐ Get a good night's sleep.

☐ Make sure the name printed on your photo ID appears EXACTLY the same as the name printed on your scheduling permit.

Day of Exam

☐ Relax. Eat breakfast. Minimize bathroom breaks during the exam by avoiding excessive morning caffeine.

☐ Analyze and make adjustments in test-taking technique. You are allowed to review notes/study material during breaks on exam day.

After the Exam

☐ Celebrate, regardless.

☐ Send feedback to us on our blog at **www.firstaidteam.com**.

Guide to Efficient Exam Preparation

▶ **INTRODUCTION**

Relax.

This section is intended to make your exam preparation easier, not harder. Our goal is to reduce your level of anxiety and help you make the most of your efforts by helping you understand more about the United States Medical Licensing Examination, Step 1 (USMLE Step 1). As a medical student, you are no doubt familiar with taking standardized examinations and quickly absorbing large amounts of material. When you first confront the USMLE Step 1, however, you may find it all too easy to become sidetracked and not achieve your goal of studying with maximal effectiveness. Common mistakes that students make when studying for Step 1 include the following:

- Not understanding how scoring is performed or what your score means
- Starting *First Aid* too late
- Starting to study too late
- Using inefficient or inappropriate study methods
- Buying the wrong books or buying more books than you can ever use
- Buying only one publisher's review series for all subjects
- Not using practice examinations to maximum benefit
- Not using review books along with your classes
- Not analyzing and improving your test-taking strategies
- Getting bogged down by reviewing difficult topics excessively
- Studying material that is rarely tested on the USMLE Step 1
- Failing to master certain high-yield subjects owing to overconfidence
- Using *First Aid* as your sole study resource

In this section, we offer advice to help you avoid these pitfalls and be more productive in your studies.

▶ **USMLE STEP 1—THE BASICS**

The USMLE Step 1 is the first of three examinations that you must pass in order to become a licensed physician in the United States. The USMLE is a joint endeavor of the National Board of Medical Examiners (NBME) and the Federation of State Medical Boards (FSMB). The USMLE serves as the single examination system for U.S. medical students and international medical graduates (IMGs) seeking medical licensure in the United States.

The CBT format of Step 1 is simply a computerized version of the former paper exam.

How Is the Computer-Based Test (CBT) Structured?

The CBT Step 1 exam consists of seven question "blocks" of 46 questions each (see Figure 1) for a total of 322 questions, timed at 60 minutes per block. A short 11-question survey follows the last question block. The computer begins the survey with a prompt to proceed to the next block of questions.

FIGURE 1. Schematic of CBT Exam.

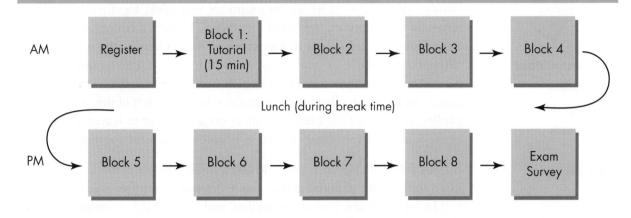

Once an examinee finishes a particular question block on the CBT, he or she must click on a screen icon to continue to the next block. Examinees **cannot** go back and change their answers to questions from any previously completed block. However, changing answers is allowed **within** a block of questions as long as time permits—**unless** the questions are part of a sequential-item test set (see What Is the CBT Like?).

What Is the CBT Like?

Given the unique environment of the CBT, it's important that you become familiar ahead of time with what your test-day conditions will be like. In fact, familiarizing yourself with the testing interface before the exam can add 15 minutes to your break time! This is because the 15-minute tutorial offered on exam day may be skipped if you are already familiar with the exam procedures and the testing interface. The 15 minutes is then added to your allotted break time (should you choose to skip the tutorial). Examinees may familiarize themselves with the CBT format by taking the 150 practice questions available online or by signing up for a practice session at a test center (for details, see What Does the CBT Format Mean to Me?).

Skip the tutorial and add 15 minutes to your break time!

For security reasons, examinees are not allowed to bring any personal electronic equipment into the testing area. This includes both digital and analog watches, cellular telephones, and electronic paging devices. Food and beverages are also prohibited. The testing centers are monitored by audio and video surveillance equipment. However, most testing centers allot each examinee a small locker outside the testing area in which he or she can store snacks, beverages, and personal items.

In May 2009, the USMLE began transitioning from the FRED v1 computer-based format to FRED v2. FRED v2 is similar to FRED v1 but has several additional features. These include highlight and strikeout functions for text, searchable lab values, and a calculator function. The USMLE advises examinees to familiarize themselves with both versions, information on which can be downloaded from www.usmle.org.

Test illustrations include:

- *Gross photos*
- *Histology slides*
- *Radiographs*
- *EMs*
- *Line drawings*

Familiarize yourself with the commonly tested normal laboratory values.

Ctrl-Alt-Delete are the keys of death during the exam. Don't touch them!

The typical question screen in FRED consists of a question followed by a number of choices on which an examinee can click, together with several navigational buttons on the top of the screen. There is a countdown timer on the upper left-hand corner of the screen as well. There is also a button that allows the examinee to mark a question for review. If a given question happens to be longer than the screen (which occurs very rarely), a scroll bar will appear on the right, allowing the examinee to see the rest of the question. Regardless of whether the examinee clicks on the answer or leaves it blank, he or she must click the "Next" button to advance to the next question.

In May 2008, the USMLE began to add a small number of media clips to the exam in the form of audio and/or video. No more than five media questions will be found on any given examination, and the USMLE orientation materials now include several practice questions in these new formats.

In 2009, USMLE introduced a sequential-item test format for some questions. This format will be indicated in the numbering of questions at the left-hand side of the screen. Questions in a sequential set must be completed in order. After an examinee answers the first question, he or she will be given the option to proceed to the next item but will be warned that his or her answer to the first question will be locked. **After proceeding, examinees will not be able to change the answer selected for that question.** The question stem and the answer chosen will be available to the examinee as he or she answers the next question in the sequence. No more than five sets of sequential questions will be found in any given examination.

Some Step 1 questions may also contain figures or color illustrations. These are typically situated to the right of the question. Although the contrast and brightness of the screen can be adjusted, there are no other ways to manipulate the picture (e.g., there is no zooming or panning). During the exam tutorial, however, examinees are given an opportunity to ensure that both the audio headphones and the volume are functioning properly.

The examinee can call up a window displaying normal lab values. In order to do so, he or she must click the "Lab" icon on the top part of the screen. Afterward, the examinee will have the option to choose between "Blood," "Cerebrospinal," "Hematologic," or "Sweat and Urine." The normal-values screen may obscure the question if it is expanded. The examinee may have to scroll down to search for the needed laboratory values.

FRED allows the examinee to see a running list of questions on the left part of the screen at all times. The new software also permits examinees to highlight or cross out information by using their mouse. Finally, there is an "Annotate" icon on the top part of the screen that allows students to write notes to themselves for review at a later time. Examinees need to be careful with all of these new features, because failure to do so can cost valuable time!

What Does the CBT Format Mean to Me?

The significance of the CBT to you depends on the requirements of your school and your level of computer knowledge. If you hate computers and freak out at the mere sight of one, you might want to confront your fears as soon as possible. Spend some time playing with a Windows-based system and pointing and clicking icons or buttons with a mouse. These are the absolute basics, and you won't want to waste valuable exam time figuring them out on test day. Your test taking will proceed by pointing and clicking, essentially without the use of the keyboard.

For those who feel they might benefit, the USMLE offers an opportunity to take a simulated test, or "CBT Practice Session at a Prometric center." Students are eligible to register for this three-and-one-half-hour practice session after they have received their scheduling permit.

The same USMLE Step 1 sample test items (150 questions) available on the USMLE Web site, www.usmle.org, are used at these sessions. **No new items will be presented.** The session is divided into three one-hour blocks of 50 test items each and costs about $42. Students receive a printed percent-correct score after completing the session. No explanations of questions are provided.

You may register for a practice session online at www.usmle.org. A separate scheduling permit is issued for the practice session. Students should allow two weeks for receipt of this permit.

How Do I Register to Take the Exam?

Prometric test centers offer Step 1 on a year-round basis, except for the first two weeks in January and major holidays. The exam is given every day except Sunday at most centers. Some schools administer the exam on their own campuses.

You can apply for Step 1 at the NBME Web site. This application allows applicants to select one of 12 overlapping three-month blocks in which to be tested (e.g., April–May–June, June–July–August). The application also includes a photo ID form that must be certified by an official at your medical school to verify your enrollment. After the NBME processes your application, it will send you a scheduling permit.

The scheduling permit you receive from the NBME will contain your USMLE identification number, the eligibility period in which you may take the exam, and two additional numbers. The first of these is known as your "scheduling number." You must have this number in order to make your exam appointment with Prometric. The second number is known as the "candidate identification number," or CIN. Examinees must enter their CINs at the Prometric workstation in order to access their exams. Prometric has no access to the codes. **Do not lose your permit!** You will not be allowed to take the boards unless you present this permit along with an unexpired, government-issued photo identification that includes your signature (such as a

Keyboard shortcuts:
A–E–Letter choices.
Enter or spacebar–Move to
  next question.
Esc–Exit pop-up Lab and
  Exhibit windows.
Alt-T–Countdown timers for
  current session and overall
  test.

Test scheduling is done on a "first-come, first-served" basis. It's important to call and schedule an exam date as soon as you receive your scheduling permit.

Testing centers are closed on major holidays and during the first two weeks of January.

driver's license or passport). Make sure the name on your photo ID exactly matches the name that appears on your scheduling permit.

Once you receive your scheduling permit, you may call Prometric's toll-free number to arrange a time to take the exam. Although requests for taking the exam may be completed more than six months before the test date, examinees will not receive their scheduling permits earlier than six months before the eligibility period. The eligibility period is the three-month period you have chosen to take the exam. Most medical students choose the April–June or June–August period. Because exams are scheduled on a "first-come, first-served" basis, it is recommended that you telephone Prometric as soon as you receive your permit. After you've scheduled your exam, it's a good idea to confirm your exam appointment with Prometric at least one week before your test date. Prometric does not provide written confirmation of exam date, time, or location. Be sure to read the *2011 USMLE Bulletin of Information* for further details.

What If I Need to Reschedule the Exam?

You can change your test date and/or center by contacting Prometric at 1-800-MED-EXAM (1-800-633-3926) or www.prometric.com. Make sure to have your CIN when rescheduling. If you are rescheduling by phone, you must speak with a Prometric representative; leaving a voice-mail message will not suffice. To avoid a rescheduling fee, you will need to request a change before noon EST at least five business days before your appointment. Please note that your rescheduled test date must fall within your assigned three-month eligibility period.

When Should I Register for the Exam?

Register six months in advance for seating and scheduling preference.

Although there are no deadlines for registering for Step 1, you should plan to register at least six months ahead of your desired test date. This will guarantee that you will get either your test center of choice or one within a 50-mile radius of your first choice. For most U.S. medical students, the desired testing window is in June, since most medical school curricula for the second year end in May or June. Thus, U.S. medical students should plan to register before January in anticipation of a June test date. The timing of the exam is more flexible for IMGs, as it is related only to when they finish exam preparation.

Choose your three-month eligibility period wisely. If you need to reschedule outside your initial three-month period, you must submit a new application along with another application fee.

Where Can I Take the Exam?

Your testing location is arranged with Prometric when you call for your test date (after you receive your scheduling permit). For a list of Prometric locations nearest you, visit www.prometric.com.

How Long Will I Have to Wait Before I Get My Scores?

The USMLE reports scores three to six weeks after the examinee's test date. Examinees will be notified via e-mail when their scores are available. By following the online instructions, examinees will be able to view, download, and print their score report. Additional information about score timetables and accessibility is available on the official USMLE Web site.

What About Time?

Time is of special interest on the CBT exam. Here's a breakdown of the exam schedule:

15 minutes	Tutorial (skip if familiar)
7 hours	60-minute question blocks
45 minutes	Break time (includes time for lunch)

Be careful to watch the clock on your break time.

The computer will keep track of how much time has elapsed on the exam. However, the computer will show you only how much time you have remaining in a given block. Therefore, it is up to you to determine if you are pacing yourself properly (at a rate of approximately one question per 78 seconds).

Gain extra break time by skipping the tutorial or finishing a block early.

The computer will **not** warn you if you are spending more than your allotted time for a break. You should therefore budget your time so that you can take a short break when you need one and have time to eat. You must be especially careful not to spend too much time in between blocks (you should keep track of how much time elapses from the time you finish a block of questions to the time you start the next block). After you finish one question block, you'll need to click the mouse to proceed to the next block of questions.

Forty-five minutes is the minimum break time for the day. You can gain extra break time (but not time for the question blocks) by skipping the tutorial or by finishing a block ahead of the allotted time.

If I Freak Out and Leave, What Happens to My Score?

Your scheduling permit shows a CIN that you will enter onto your computer screen to start your exam. Entering the CIN is the same as breaking the seal on a test book, and you are considered to have started the exam when you do so. However, no score will be reported if you do not complete the exam. In fact, if you leave at any time from the start of the test to the last block, no score will be reported. The fact that you started but did not complete the exam, however, will appear on your USMLE score transcript.

The exam ends when all question blocks have been completed or when their time has expired. As you leave the testing center, you will receive a printed test-completion notice to document your completion of the exam. To receive an official score, you must finish the entire exam.

What Types of Questions Are Asked?

One-best-answer items are the only multiple-choice format on the exam. Most questions consist of a clinical scenario or a direct question followed by a list of five or more options. You are required to select the one best answer among the options given. There are no "except," "not," or matching questions on the exam. A number of options may be partially correct, in which case you must select the option that best answers the question or completes the statement. Additionally, keep in mind that experimental questions may appear on the exam (see Difficult Questions, p. 20).

How Is the Test Scored?

Each Step 1 examinee receives an electronic score report that includes the examinee's pass/fail status, two test scores, and a graphic depiction of the examinee's performance by discipline and organ system or subject area. The actual organ system profiles reported may depend on the statistical characteristics of a given administration of the examination.

The NBME provides two overall test scores based on the total number of items answered correctly on the examination (see Figure 2). The first score, the three-digit score, is reported as a scaled score in which the mean is 221 and the standard deviation is approximately 23. The second score scale, the two-digit score, defines 75 as the minimum passing score (equivalent to a score of 188 on the first scale). A score of 82 is equivalent to a score of 200 on the three-digit score scale. To minimize confusion, we refer to scores using the three-digit scale.

FIGURE 2. 2010 Scoring Scales for the USMLE Step 1.

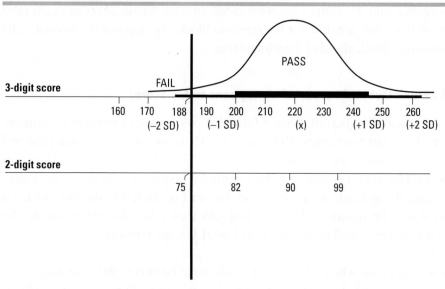

A score of **188** or higher is required to pass Step 1 as of 2010. Passing Step 1 is estimated to correspond to answering 60–70% of questions correctly. The NBME may adjust the minimum passing score in the future, so please check the USMLE Web site or Firstaidteam.com for updates (see Table 1).

According to the USMLE, medical schools receive a listing of total scores and pass/fail results plus group summaries by discipline and organ system. Students can withhold their scores from their medical school if they wish. Official USMLE transcripts, which can be sent on request to residency programs, include only total scores, not performance profiles.

Consult the USMLE Web site or your medical school for the most current and accurate information regarding the examination.

Passing the CBT Step 1 is estimated to correspond to answering 60–70% of the questions correctly.

What Does My Score Mean?

For students, the most important point with the Step 1 score is passing versus failing. Passing essentially means, "Hey, you're on your way to becoming a fully licensed doc."

Beyond that, the main point of having a quantitative score is to give you a sense of how you've done aside from the fact that you've passed the exam.

TABLE 1. Passing Rates for the 2008–2009 USMLE Step 1.

	2008		2009	
	No. Tested	% Passing	No. Tested	% Passing
Allopathic 1st takers	17,494	94%	18,003	94%
Repeaters	1,361	61%	1,496	65%
Allopathic total	18,855	92%	19,499	92%
Osteopathic 1st takers	1,605	81%	1,808	81%
Repeaters	56	46%	55	49%
Osteopathic total	1,661	80%	1,863	80%
Total U.S./Canadian	**20,516**	**91%**	**21,362**	**91%**
IMG 1st takers	14,889	73%	14,055	73%
Repeaters	5,534	37%	4,881	36%
IMG total	20,423	63%	18,936	63%
Total Step 1 examinees	**40,939**	**77%**	**40,298**	**78%**

The two-digit or three-digit score gauges how well you have performed with respect to the content of the exam.

Since the content of the exam is what drives the score, the profile of the exam is what remains relatively constant over the years. That is to say that each exam profile includes a certain number of "very hard" questions along with "medium" and "easy" ones. The questions vary, but the profile of the exam doesn't change substantially. This ensures that someone who scored 200 on the boards yesterday has achieved a level of knowledge comparable to that of a person who scored 200 four years ago.

Official NBME/USMLE Resources

We strongly encourage students to use the free materials provided by the testing agencies (see p. 22) and to study in detail the following NBME resources, all of which are available at the USMLE Web site, www.usmle.org:

Practice questions may be easier than the actual exam.

- *USMLE Step 1 2011 Computer-based Content and Sample Test Questions* (information given free to all examinees)
- *2011 USMLE Bulletin of Information* (information given free to all examinees)
- Comprehensive Basic Science Self-Assessment

The *USMLE Step 1 2011 Computer-based Content and Sample Test Questions* contains approximately 150 questions that are similar in format and content to the questions on the actual USMLE Step 1 exam. This practice test offers one of the best means of assessing your test-taking skills. However, it does not contain enough questions to simulate the full length of the examination, and its content represents a limited sampling of the basic science material that may be covered on Step 1. Moreover, most students felt that the questions on the actual 2010 exam were more challenging than those contained in that year's sample questions. Others, however, reported that they had encountered a few near-duplicates of these sample questions on the actual Step 1 exam. Presumably, these are "experimental" questions, but who knows? So the bottom line is, know these questions!

The extremely detailed *Step 1 Content Outline* provided by the USMLE has not proved useful for students studying for the exam. The USMLE even states that ". . . the content outline is not intended as a guide for curriculum development or as a study guide."[1] We concur with this assessment.

The *2011 USMLE Bulletin of Information* contains detailed procedural and policy information regarding the CBT, including descriptions of all three Steps, scoring of the exams, reporting of scores to medical schools and residency programs, procedures for score rechecks and other inquiries, policies for irregular behavior, and test dates.

The NBME also offers the Comprehensive Basic Science Self-Assessment (CBSSA), which tests users on topics covered during basic science courses in a format similar to that of the USMLE Step 1 examination. Students who prepared for the examination using this Web-based tool reported that they found the format and content highly indicative of questions tested on the Step 1 examination. In addition, the CBSSA is a fair predictor of USMLE performance (see Table 2).

The CBSSA exists in two forms: a standard-paced and a self-paced format, both of which consist of four sections of 50 questions each (for a total of 200 multiple-choice items). The standard-paced format allows the user up to one hour to complete each section, reflecting the time limits of the actual exam. By contrast, the self-paced format places a four-hour time limit on answering the multiple-choice questions. Keep in mind that this bank of questions is available only on the Web. The NBME requires that users log on, register, and start the test within 30 days of registration. Once the assessment has begun, users are required to complete the sections within 20 days. Following completion of the questions, the CBSSA will provide a performance profile indicating each user's relative strengths and weaknesses, much like the report profile for the USMLE Step 1 exam. However, keep in mind that this self-assessment does **not** provide the user with a list of correct answers. Table 2 provides an approximate correlation of scores between the CBSSA and the USMLE. Feedback from the self-assessment takes the form of a performance profile and nothing more. The NBME charges $45 for this service, which is payable by credit card or money order. For more information regarding the CBSSA, please visit the NBME's Web site at www.nbme.org and click on the link labeled "NBME Self-Assessment Services."

▶ DEFINING YOUR GOAL

It is useful to define your own personal performance goal when approaching the USMLE Step 1. Your style and intensity of preparation can then be matched to your goal. Your goal may depend on your school's requirements, your specialty choice, your grades to date, and your personal assessment of the test's importance. Do your best to define your goals early so that you can prepare accordingly.

Certain highly competitive residency programs, such as those in plastic surgery and orthopedic surgery, have acknowledged their use of Step 1 scores in the selection process. In such residency programs, greater emphasis may be placed on attaining a high score, so students who seek to enter these programs may wish to consider aiming for a very high score on the Step 1 exam (see Figure 3). At the same time, your Step 1 score is only one of a number of factors that are assessed when you apply for residency. Indeed, many residency programs value other criteria more highly than a high score on Step 1. Fourth-year medical students who have recently completed the residency application process can be a valuable resource in this regard.

TABLE 2. CBSSA to USMLE Score Comparison.

CBSSA SCORE	APPROXIMATE USMLE STEP 1 SCORE
200	< 136
250	148
300	163
350	178
400	192
450	206
500	219
550	230
600	240
650	248
700	256
750	261
800	> 265

Fourth-year medical students have the best feel for how Step 1 scores factor into the residency application process.

Some competitive residency programs place more weight on Step 1 scores in their selection process.

FIGURE 3. Median USMLE Step 1 Score for Matched U.S. Seniors.[a]

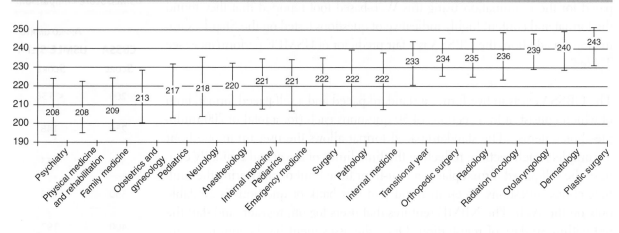

a Vertical lines show interquartile range. Source: www.nrmp.org.

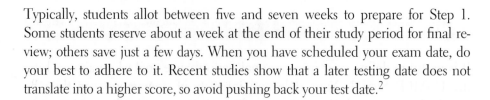

▶ **TIMELINE FOR STUDY**

Make a Schedule

Time management is key. Customize your schedule to your goals and available time.

After you have defined your goals, map out a study schedule that is consistent with your objectives, your vacation time, and the difficulty of your ongoing coursework (see Figure 4). Determine whether you want to spread out your study time or concentrate it into 14-hour study days in the final weeks. Then factor in your own history in preparing for standardized examinations (e.g., SAT, MCAT).

Typically, students allot between five and seven weeks to prepare for Step 1. Some students reserve about a week at the end of their study period for final review; others save just a few days. When you have scheduled your exam date, do your best to adhere to it. Recent studies show that a later testing date does not translate into a higher score, so avoid pushing back your test date.[2]

Another important consideration is when you will study each subject. Some subjects lend themselves to cramming, whereas others demand a substantial long-term commitment. The "crammable" subjects for Step 1 are those for which concise yet relatively complete review books are available. (See Section IV for highly rated review and sample examination materials.) Behavioral science and physiology are two subjects with concise review books. Three subjects with longer but quite comprehensive review books are microbiology, pharmacology, and biochemistry. Thus, these subjects could be covered toward the end of your schedule, whereas other subjects (anatomy and pathology) require a longer time commitment and could be studied earlier. Many students prefer using a "systems-based" approach (e.g., GI, renal, cardiovascular) to integrate the material across basic science subjects. See Section III to study anatomy, pathology, physiology, and pharmacology facts by organ system.

Make your schedule realistic, and set achievable goals. Many students make the mistake of studying at a level of detail that requires too much time for a compre-

FIGURE 4. Typical Timeline for the USMLE Step 1.

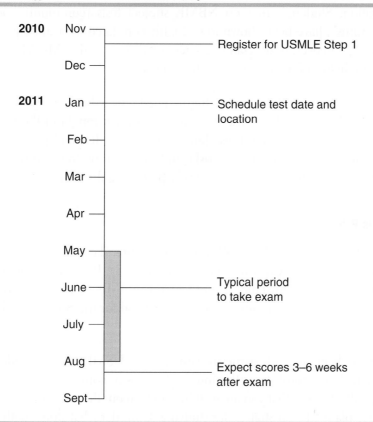

hensive review—reading *Gray's Anatomy* in a couple of days is not a realistic goal! Revise your schedule regularly on the basis of your actual progress. Be careful not to lose focus. Beware of feelings of inadequacy when comparing study schedules and progress with your peers. **Avoid students who stress you out.** Focus on a few top-rated resources that suit your learning style—not on some obscure books your friends may pass down to you. Accept the fact that you cannot learn it all.

You will need time for uninterrupted and focused study. Plan your personal affairs to minimize crisis situations near the date of the test. Allot an adequate number of breaks in your study schedule to avoid burnout. Maintain a healthy lifestyle with proper diet, exercise, and sleep.

Year(s) Prior

Although you may be tempted to rely solely on cramming in the weeks and months before the test, you should not have to do so. The knowledge you gained during your first two years of medical school and even during your un-

"Crammable" subjects should be covered later and less crammable subjects earlier.

Avoid burnout. Maintain proper diet, exercise, and sleep habits.

Buy review books early (first year) and use while studying for courses.

dergraduate years should provide the groundwork on which to base your test preparation. Student scores on NBME subject tests (commonly known as "shelf exams") have been shown to be highly correlated with subsequent Step 1 scores.[3] Moreover, undergraduate science GPAs as well as MCAT scores are strong predictors of performance on the Step 1 exam.[4]

We also recommend that you buy highly rated review books early in your first year of medical school and use them as you study throughout the two years. When Step 1 comes along, these books will be familiar and personalized to the way in which you learn. It is risky and intimidating to use unfamiliar review books in the final two or three weeks preceding the exam.

Months Prior

Review test dates and the application procedure. Testing for the USMLE Step 1 is done on a year-round basis (see Table 3). If you have any disabilities or "special circumstances," contact the NBME as early as possible to discuss test accommodations (see p. 44, First Aid for the Student with a Disability).

Simulate the USMLE Step 1 under "real" conditions before beginning your studies.

Before you begin to study earnestly, simulate the USMLE Step 1 under "real" conditions to pinpoint strengths and weaknesses in your knowledge and test-taking skills. Be sure that you are well informed about the examination and that you have planned your strategy for studying. Consider what study methods you will use, the study materials you will need, and how you will obtain your materials. Plan ahead. Get advice from third- and fourth-year medical students who have recently taken the USMLE Step 1. There might be strengths and weaknesses in your school's curriculum that you should take into account in deciding where to focus your efforts. You might also choose to share books, notes, and study hints with classmates. That is how this book began.

Three Weeks Prior

Two to four weeks before the examination is a good time to resimulate the USMLE Step 1. You may want to do this earlier depending on the progress of

TABLE 3. 2009 USMLE Exams.

STEP	FOCUS	NO. OF QUESTIONS/ NO. OF QUESTION BLOCKS	TEST SCHEDULE/ LENGTH OF CBT EXAM	PASSING SCORE
Step 1	Basic mechanisms and principles	322/7	One day (eight hours)	188
Step 2 CK	Clinical diagnosis and disease pathogenesis	368/8	One day (nine hours)	189
Step 3	Clinical management	480/11	Two days (16 hours)	187

your review, but be sure not to do it later, when there will be little time to remedy defects in your knowledge or test-taking skills. Make use of remaining good-quality sample USMLE test questions, and try to simulate the computerized test conditions so that you can adequately assess your test performance. Recognize, too, that time pressure is increasing as more and more questions are framed as clinical vignettes. Most sample exam questions are shorter than the real thing. Focus on reviewing the high-yield facts, your own notes, clinical images, and very short review books.

In the final two weeks, focus on review and endurance. Avoid unfamiliar material. Stay confident!

One Week Prior

Make sure you have your CIN (found on your scheduling permit) as well as other items necessary for the day of the examination, including a driver's license or another form of photo identification with your signature (make sure the name on your ID **exactly** matches that on your scheduling permit). Confirm the Prometric testing center location and test time. Work out how you will get to the testing center and what parking and traffic problems you might encounter. If possible, visit the testing site to get a better idea of the testing conditions you will face. Determine what you will do for lunch. Make sure you have everything you need to ensure that you will be comfortable and alert at the test site.

Confirm your testing date at least one week in advance.

One Day Prior

Try your best to relax and rest the night before the test. Double-check your admissions and test-taking materials as well as the comfort measures discussed earlier so that you will not have to deal with such details on the morning of the exam. Do not study any new material. If you do feel compelled to study, quickly review short-term-memory material (e.g., Rapid Review) before going to sleep. However, do not quiz yourself, as you may risk becoming flustered and confused. Remember that regardless of how hard you have studied, you cannot know everything. There will be things on the exam that you have never even seen before, so do not panic. Do not underestimate your abilities.

Many students report difficulty sleeping the night prior to the exam. This is often exacerbated by going to bed much earlier than usual. Do whatever it takes to ensure a good night's sleep (e.g., massage, exercise, warm milk). Do not change your daily routine prior to the exam. Exam day is not the day for a caffeine-withdrawal headache.

No notes, books, calculators, pagers, recording devices, or watches of any kind are allowed in the testing area.

Morning of the Exam

On the morning of the Step 1 exam, wake up at your regular time and eat a normal breakfast. Make sure you have your scheduling permit admission ticket, test-taking materials, and comfort measures as discussed earlier. Wear loose, comfortable clothing. Plan for a variable temperature in the testing center. Arrive at the test site 30 minutes before the time designated on the admission

Arrive at the testing center 30 minutes before your scheduled exam time. If you arrive more than half an hour late, you will not be allowed to take the test.

Some students recommend reviewing certain "theme" topics that tend to recur throughout the exam.

ticket; however, do not come too early, as doing so may intensify your anxiety. When you arrive at the test site, the proctor should give you a USMLE information sheet that will explain critical factors such as the proper use of break time. The USMLE uses the Biometric Identity Management System (BIMS) at some test center locations. BIMS converts a fingerprint, taken on test day, to a digital image used for identification of examinees during the testing process. Seating may be assigned, but ask to be reseated if necessary; you need to be seated in an area that will allow you to remain comfortable and to concentrate. Get to know your testing station, especially if you have never been in a Prometric testing center before. Listen to your proctors regarding any changes in instructions or testing procedures that may apply to your test site.

Finally, remember that it is natural (and even beneficial) to be a little nervous. Focus on being mentally clear and alert. Avoid panic. Avoid panic. Avoid panic. When you are asked to begin the exam, take a deep breath, focus on the screen, and then begin. Keep an eye on the timer. Take advantage of breaks between blocks to stretch and relax for a moment.

After the Test

After you have completed the exam, be sure to have fun and relax regardless of how you may feel. Taking the test is an achievement in itself. Remember, you are much more likely to have passed than not. Enjoy the free time you have before your clerkships. Expect to experience some "reentry" phenomena as you try to regain a real life. Once you have recovered sufficiently from the test (or from partying), we invite you to send us your feedback, corrections, and suggestions for entries, facts, mnemonics, strategies, resource ratings, and the like (see p. xv, How to Contribute). Sharing your experience will benefit fellow medical students and IMGs.

▶ IF YOU THINK YOU FAILED

If you pass Step 1, you are not allowed to retake the exam in an attempt to raise your score.

After the test, many examinees feel that they have failed, and most are at the very least unsure of their pass/fail status. There are several sensible steps you can take to plan for the future in the event that you do not achieve a passing score. First, save and organize all your study materials, including review books, practice tests, and notes. Familiarize yourself with the reapplication procedures for Step 1, including application deadlines and upcoming test dates. The CBT format allows an examinee who has failed the exam to retake it no earlier than the first day of the month after 60 days have elapsed since the last test date. Examinees will, however, be allowed to take the Step 1 exam no more than four times within a 12-month period should they repeatedly fail.

The performance profiles on the back of the USMLE Step 1 score report provide valuable feedback concerning your relative strengths and weaknesses. Study these profiles closely. Set up a study timeline to strengthen gaps in your knowledge as well as to maintain and improve what you already know. Do not neglect high-yield subjects. It is normal to feel somewhat anxious about retaking the test—but if anxiety becomes a problem, seek appropriate counseling.

Fifty-two percent of the NBME-registered first-time takers who failed the June 1998 Step 1 repeated the exam in October 1998. The overall pass rate for that group in October was 60%. Eighty-five percent of those scoring near the old pass/fail mark of 176 (173–176) in June 1998 passed in October. However, 1999 pass rates varied widely depending on initial score (see Table 4, which reflects the most current data available at the time of publishing).

Although the NBME allows an unlimited number of attempts to pass Step 1, the NBME recommends that licensing authorities allow a maximum of six attempts for each Step examination.[5] Again, review your school's policy regarding retakes.

TABLE 4. Pass Rates for USMLE Step 1 Repeaters, 1999.

INITIAL SCORE	% PASS
176–178	83
173–175	74
170–172	71
165–169	64
160–164	54
150–159	31
< 150	0
Overall	**67**

▶ **IF YOU FAILED**

Even if you came out of the exam room feeling that you failed, seeing that failing grade can be traumatic, and it is natural to feel upset. Different people react in different ways: For some it is a stimulus to buckle down and study harder; for others it may "take the wind out of their sails" for a few days; and for still others it may lead to a reassessment of individual goals and abilities. In some instances, however, failure may trigger weeks or months of sadness, feelings of hopelessness, social withdrawal, and inability to concentrate—in other words, true clinical depression. If you think you are depressed, please seek help.

Near the failure threshold, each three-digit scale point is equivalent to about 1.5 questions answered correctly.[6]

▶ **STUDY MATERIALS**

Quality and Cost Considerations

Although an ever-increasing number of review books and software are now available on the market, the quality of such material is highly variable. Some common problems are as follows:

- Certain review books are too detailed to allow for review in a reasonable amount of time or cover subtopics that are not emphasized on the exam.
- Many sample question books were originally written years ago and have not been adequately updated to reflect recent trends.
- Many sample question books use poorly written questions or contain factual errors in their explanations.
- Explanations for sample questions vary in quality.

Basic Science Review Books

In selecting review books, be sure to weigh different opinions against each other, read the reviews and ratings in Section IV of this guide, examine the books closely in the bookstore, and choose carefully. You are investing not only money but also your limited study time. Do not worry about finding the "perfect" book, as many subjects simply do not have one, and different students prefer different styles.

If a given review book is not working for you, stop using it no matter how highly rated it may be or how much it costs.

There are two types of review books: those that are stand-alone titles and those that are part of a series. Books in a series generally have the same style, and you must decide if that style works for you. However, a given style is not optimal for every subject. For example, charts and diagrams may be the best approach for physiology and biochemistry, whereas tables and outlines may be preferable for microbiology.

You should also find out which books are up to date. Some new editions represent major improvements, whereas others contain only cursory changes. Take into consideration how a book reflects the format of the USMLE Step 1.

Practice Tests

Taking practice tests provides valuable information about potential strengths and weaknesses in your fund of knowledge and test-taking skills. Some students use practice examinations simply as a means of breaking up the monotony of studying and adding variety to their study schedule, whereas other students rely almost solely on practice tests. Your best preview of the computerized exam can be found in the practice exams on the USMLE Web site. Some students also recommend using computerized test simulation programs. In addition, students report that many current practice-exam books have questions that are, on average, shorter and less clinically oriented than those on the current USMLE Step 1.

Most practice exams are shorter and less clinical than the real thing.

After taking a practice test, try to identify concepts and areas of weakness, not just the facts that you missed. Do not panic if you miss a lot of questions on a practice examination; instead, use the experience you have gained to motivate your study and prioritize those areas in which you need the most work. Use quality practice examinations to improve your test-taking skills. Analyze your ability to pace yourself.

Use practice tests to identify concepts and areas of weakness, not just facts that you missed.

Clinical Review Books

Keep your eye out for more clinically oriented review books; purchase them early and begin to use them. A number of students are turning to Step 2 books, pathophysiology books, and case-based reviews to prepare for the clinical vignettes. Examples of such books include:

- *First Aid for the Wards* (McGraw-Hill)
- *First Aid Clerkship* series (McGraw-Hill)

- *Blueprints* clinical series (Lippincott Williams & Wilkins)
- *PreTest Physical Diagnosis* (McGraw-Hill)
- *Washington Manual* (Lippincott Williams & Wilkins)
- Various USMLE Step 2 review books

Texts, Syllabi, and Notes

Limit your use of texts and syllabi for Step 1 review. Many textbooks are too detailed for high-yield review and include material that is generally not tested on the USMLE Step 1 (e.g., drug dosages, complex chemical structures). Syllabi, although familiar, are inconsistent and frequently reflect the emphasis of individual faculty, which often does not correspond to that of the USMLE Step 1. Syllabi also tend to be less organized than top-rated books and generally contain fewer diagrams and study questions.

▶ TEST-TAKING STRATEGIES

Your test performance will be influenced by both your fund of knowledge and your test-taking skills. You can strengthen your performance by considering each of these factors. Test-taking skills and strategies should be developed and perfected well in advance of the test date so that you can concentrate on the test itself. We suggest that you try the following strategies to see if they might work for you.

Practice and perfect test-taking skills and strategies well before the test date.

Pacing

You have seven hours to complete 322 questions. Note that each one-hour block contains 46 questions. This works out to about 78 seconds per question. NBME officials note that time was not an issue for most takers of the CBT field test. However, pacing errors have in the past been detrimental to the performance of even highly prepared examinees. The bottom line is to keep one eye on the clock at all times!

Time management is an important skill for exam success.

Dealing with Each Question

There are several established techniques for efficiently approaching multiple-choice questions; see what works for you. One technique begins with identifying each question as easy, workable, or impossible. Your goal should be to answer all easy questions, resolve all workable questions in a reasonable amount of time, and make quick and intelligent guesses on all impossible questions. Most students read the stem, think of the answer, and turn immediately to the choices. A second technique is to first skim the answer choices and the last sentence of the question and then read through the passage quickly, extracting only relevant information to answer the question. Try a variety of techniques on practice exams and see what works best for you.

Do not dwell excessively on questions that you are on the verge of "figuring out." Make your best guess and move on.

Difficult Questions

Because of the exam's clinical emphasis, you may find that many of the questions on the Step 1 exam appear workable but take more time than is available to you. It can be tempting to dwell on such questions because you feel you are on the verge of "figuring it out," but resist this temptation and budget your time. Answer difficult questions with your best guess, mark them for review, and come back to them only if you have time after you have completed the rest of the questions in the block. This will keep you from inadvertently leaving any questions blank in your efforts to "beat the clock."

Another reason for not dwelling too long on any one question is that certain questions may be **experimental** or may be **incorrectly phrased**. Moreover, not all questions are scored. Some questions serve as "embedded pretest items" that do not count toward your overall score. In fact, anywhere from 10% to 20% of exam questions have been designated as experimental on past exams.

Remember that some questions may be experimental.

Guessing

There is **no penalty** for wrong answers. Thus, no test block should be left with unanswered questions. A hunch is probably better than a random guess. If you have to guess, we suggest selecting an answer you recognize over one with which you are totally unfamiliar.

Changing Your Answer

Your first hunch is not always correct.

The conventional wisdom is not to change answers that you have already marked unless there is a convincing and logical reason to do so—in other words, go with your "first hunch." However, studies show that if you change your answer, you are twice as likely to change it from an incorrect answer to a correct one than vice versa. So if you have a strong "second hunch," go for it!

Fourth-Quarter Effect (Avoiding Burnout)

Do not terminate a question block too early. Carefully review your answers if possible.

Pacing and endurance are important. Practice helps develop both. Fewer and fewer examinees are leaving the examination session early. Use any extra time you might have at the end of each block to return to marked questions or to recheck your answers; you cannot add the extra time to any remaining blocks of questions or to your break time. Do not be too casual in your review or you may overlook serious mistakes. Remember your goals, and keep in mind the effort you have devoted to studying compared with the small additional effort you will need to maintain focus and concentration throughout the examination. Never give up. If you begin to feel frustrated, try taking a 30-second breather.

► CLINICAL VIGNETTE STRATEGIES

In recent years, the USMLE Step 1 has become increasingly clinically oriented. This change mirrors the trend in medical education toward introducing students to clinical problem solving during the basic science years. The increasing clinical emphasis on Step 1 may be challenging to those students who attend schools with a more traditional curriculum.

Be prepared to read fast and think on your feet!

What Is a Clinical Vignette?

A clinical vignette is a short (usually paragraph-long) description of a patient, including demographics, presenting symptoms, signs, and other information concerning the patient. Sometimes this paragraph is followed by a brief listing of important physical findings and/or laboratory results. The task of assimilating all this information and answering the associated question in the span of one minute can be intimidating. So be prepared to read quickly and think on your feet. Remember that the question is often indirectly asking something you already know.

Practice questions that include case histories or descriptive vignettes are critical for Step 1 preparation.

Strategy

Remember that Step 1 vignettes usually describe diseases or disorders in their most classic presentation. So look for buzzwords or cardinal signs (e.g., malar rash for SLE or nuchal rigidity for meningitis) in the narrative history. Be aware, however, that the question may contain classic signs and symptoms instead of mere buzzwords. Sometimes the data from labs and the physical exam will help you confirm or reject possible diagnoses, thereby helping you rule answer choices in or out. In some cases, they will be a dead giveaway for the diagnosis.

Step 1 vignettes usually describe diseases or disorders in their most classic presentation.

Making a diagnosis from the history and data is often not the final answer. Not infrequently, the diagnosis is divulged at the end of the vignette, after you have just struggled through the narrative to come up with a diagnosis of your own. The question might then ask about a related aspect of the diagnosed disease.

One strategy that many students suggest is to skim the questions and answer choices before reading a vignette, especially if the vignette is lengthy. This focuses your attention on the relevant information and reduces the time spent on that vignette. Sometimes you may not need much of the information in the vignette to answer the question.

Sometimes making a diagnosis is not necessary at all.

■ **National Board of Medical Examiners (NBME)**
Department of Licensing Examination Services
3750 Market Street
Philadelphia, PA 19104-3102
(215) 590-9700
Fax: (215) 590-9457
E-mail: webmail@nbme.org
www.nbme.org

■ **Educational Commission for Foreign Medical Graduates (ECFMG)**
3624 Market Street
Philadelphia, PA 19104-2685
(215) 386-5900
Fax: (215) 386-9196
E-mail: info@ecfmg.org
www.ecfmg.org

■ **Federation of State Medical Boards (FSMB)**
P.O. Box 619850
Dallas, TX 75261-9850
(817) 868-4000
Fax: (817) 868-4099
E-mail: usmle@fsmb.org
www.fsmb.org

■ **USMLE Secretariat**
3750 Market Street
Philadelphia, PA 19104-3190
(215) 590-9700
E-mail: webmail@nbme.org
www.usmle.org

▶ REFERENCES

1. United States Medical Licensing Examination. Step 1 Content Description Online. Available at: http://www.usmle.org/Examinations/step1/step1_content.html. Accessed August 22, 2010.

2. Pohl, Charles A., Robeson, Mary R., Hojat, Mohammadreza, and Veloski, J. Jon, "Sooner or Later? USMLE Step 1 Performance and Test Administration Date at the End of the Second Year," *Academic Medicine*, 2002, Vol. 77, No. 10, pp. S17–S19.

3. Holtman, Matthew C., Swanson, David B., Ripkey, Douglas R., and Case, Susan M., "Using Basic Science Subject Tests to Identify Students at Risk for Failing Step 1," *Academic Medicine*, 2001, Vol. 76, No. 10, pp. S48–S51.

4. Basco, William T., Jr., Way, David P., Gilbert, Gregory E., and Hudson, Andy, "Undergraduate Institutional MCAT Scores as Predictors of USMLE Step 1 Performance," *Academic Medicine*, 2002, Vol. 77, No. 10, pp. S13–S16.

5. United States Medical Licensing Examination. 2009 USMLE Bulletin—Eligibility. Available at: http://www.usmle.org/general_information/bulletin/2009/eligibility.html. Accessed August 22, 2010.

6. O'Donnell, M. J., Obenshain, S. Scott, and Erdmann, James B., "I: Background Essential to the Proper Use of Results of Step 1 and Step 2 of the USMLE," *Academic Medicine*, October 1993, Vol. 68, No. 10, pp. 734–739.

NOTES

Special Situations

"International medical graduate" (IMG) is the term now used to describe any student or graduate of a non-U.S., non-Canadian, non–Puerto Rican medical school, regardless of whether he or she is a U.S. citizen. The old term "foreign medical graduate" (FMG) was replaced because it was misleading when applied to U.S. citizens attending medical schools outside the United States.

The IMG's Steps to Licensure in the United States

If you are an IMG, you must go through the following steps (not necessarily in this order) to become licensed to practice in the United States. You must complete these steps even if you are already a practicing physician and have completed a residency program in your own country.

- Complete the basic sciences program of your medical school (equivalent to the first two years of U.S. medical school).
- Take the USMLE Step 1. You can do this while still in school or after graduating, but in either case your medical school must certify that you completed the basic sciences portion of your school's curriculum before taking the USMLE Step 1.
- Complete the clinical clerkship program of your medical school (equivalent to the third and fourth years of U.S. medical school).
- Take the USMLE Step 2 Clinical Knowledge (CK) exam. If you are still in medical school, you must have completed two years of school.
- Take the Step 2 Clinical Skills (CS) exam.
- Graduate with your medical degree.
- Send the ECFMG a copy of your degree and transcript, which will be verified with your medical school.
- Obtain an ECFMG certificate. To do this, candidates must accomplish the following:
  - Graduate from a medical school that is listed in the International Medical Education Directory (IMED). The list can be accessed at www.ecfmg.org.
  - Pass Step 1, the Step 2 CK, and the Step 2 CS within a seven-year period.
  - Have your medical credentials verified by the ECFMG.
- The standard certificate is usually sent two weeks after all the above requirements have been fulfilled. You must have a valid certificate before entering an accredited residency program, although you may begin the application process before you receive your certification.
- Apply for residency positions in your field of interest, either directly or through the Electronic Residency Application Service (ERAS) and the National Residency Matching Program, or NRMP ("the Match"). To be entered into the Match, you need to have passed all the examinations necessary for ECFMG certification (i.e., Step 1, the Step 2 CK, and the Step 2 CS) by the rank order list deadline (usually in late February before the Match). If you do not pass these exams by the deadline, you will be withdrawn from the Match.

More detailed information can be found in the ECFMG Information Booklet, *available at www.ecfmg.org/ pubshome.html.*

Applicants may apply online for the USMLE Step 2 CK or Step 2 CS or request an extension of the USMLE eligibility period at www. ecfmg.org/usmle/ index.html or www.ecfmg.org/ usmle/ step2cs/index.html.

- Obtain a visa that will allow you to enter and work in the United States if you are not already a U.S. citizen or a green-card holder (permanent resident).

- If required for IMGs by the state in which your residency is located, obtain an educational/training/limited medical license. Your residency program may assist you with this application. Note that medical licensing is the prerogative of each individual state, not of the federal government, and that states vary with respect to their laws about licensing (although all 50 states recognize the USMLE).

- In order to begin your residency program, make sure your scores are valid.

- Once you have the ECFMG certification, take the USMLE Step 3 during your residency, and then obtain a full medical license. Once you have a license in any state, you are permitted to practice in federal institutions such as VA hospitals and Indian Health Service facilities in any state. This can open the door to "moonlighting" opportunities and possibilities for an H1B visa application. For details on individual state rules, write to the licensing board in the state in question or contact the FSMB.

- Complete your residency and then take the appropriate specialty board exams in order to become board certified (e.g., in internal medicine or surgery). If you already have a specialty certification in your home country (e.g., in surgery or cardiology), some specialty boards may grant you six months' or one year's credit toward your total residency time.

- Currently, many residency programs are accepting applications through ERAS. For more information, see *First Aid for the Match* or contact:

  ECFMG/ERAS Program
  3624 Market Street
  Philadelphia, PA 19104-2685 USA
  (215) 386-5900
  e-mail: eras-support@ecfmg.org
  www.ecfmg.org/eras

The USMLE and the IMG

The USMLE is a series of standardized exams that give IMGs a level playing field. It is the same exam series taken by U.S. graduates even though it is administered by the ECFMG rather than by the NBME. This means that passing marks for IMGs for Step 1, the Step 2 CK, and the Step 2 CS are determined by a statistical process that is based on the scores of U.S. medical students. For example, to pass Step 1, you will probably have to score higher than the bottom 8–10% of U.S. and Canadian graduates.

Timing of the USMLE

For an IMG, the timing of a complete application is critical. It is extremely important that you send in your application early if you are to garner the maximum number of interview calls. A rough guide would be to complete all exam requirements by August of the year in which you wish to apply. This would translate into sending both your score sheets and your ECFMG certificate with your application.

In terms of USMLE exam order, arguments can be made for taking the Step 1 or the Step 2 CK exam first. For example, you may consider taking the Step 2 CK exam first if you have just graduated from medical school and the clinical topics are still fresh in your mind. However, keep in mind that there is substantial overlap between Step 1 and Step 2 CK topics in areas such as pharmacology, pathophysiology, and biostatistics. You might therefore consider taking the Step 1 and Step 2 CK exams close together to take advantage of this overlap in your test preparation.

USMLE Step 1 and the IMG

What Is the USMLE Step 1? It is a computerized test of the basic medical sciences that consists of 322 multiple-choice questions divided into seven question blocks.

Content. Step 1 includes test items in the following content areas:

- Anatomy
- Behavioral sciences
- Biochemistry
- Microbiology and immunology
- Pathology
- Pharmacology
- Physiology
- Interdisciplinary topics such as nutrition, genetics, and aging

Significance of the Test. Step 1 is required for the ECFMG certificate as well as for registration for the Step 2 CS. Since most U.S. graduates apply to residency with their Step 1 scores only, it may be the only objective tool available with which to compare IMGs with U.S. graduates.

Official Web Sites. www.usmle.org and www.ecfmg.org/usmle.

Eligibility. Both students and graduates from medical schools that are listed in IMED are eligible to take the test. Students must have completed at least two years of medical school by the beginning of the eligibility period selected.

Eligibility Period. A three-month period of your choice.

Fee. The fee for Step 1 is $740 plus an international test delivery surcharge (if you choose a testing region other than the United States or Canada).

Retaking the Exam. In the event that you failed the test, you can apply to retake the exam. You cannot take Step 1 more than four times in any 12-month period. You cannot retake the exam if you passed. The minimum score to pass the exam is 75 on a two-digit scale. To pass, you must answer roughly 60–70% of the questions correctly.

Statistics. In 2008, only 73% of ECFMG examinees passed Step 1 on their first attempt, compared with 94% of those from the United States and Canada. Of note, 1994–1995 data showed that USFMGs (U.S. citizens attending non-U.S. medical schools) performed 0.4 SD lower than IMGs (non-U.S. citizens attending non-U.S. medical schools). Although their overall scores were lower, USFMGs performed better than IMGs on behavioral sciences. In general, students from non-U.S. medical schools perform worst in behavioral science and biochemistry (1.9 and 1.5 SDs below U.S. students) and comparatively better in gross anatomy and pathology (0.7 and 0.9 SD below U.S. students). Although derived from data collected in 1994–1995, these data may help you focus your studying efforts.

Tips. Although few if any students feel totally prepared to take Step 1, IMGs in particular require serious study and preparation in order to reach their full potential on this exam. It is also imperative that IMGs do their best on Step 1, as a poor score on Step 1 is a distinct disadvantage in applying for most residencies. Remember that if you pass Step 1, you cannot retake it in an attempt to improve your score. Your goal should thus be to beat the mean, because you can then assert with confidence that you have done better than average for U.S. students. Good Step 1 scores will also lend credibility to your residency application and help you get into highly competitive specialties such as radiology, orthopedics, and dermatology.

Commercial Review Courses. Do commercial review courses help improve your scores? Reports vary, and such courses can be expensive. Many IMGs decide to try Step 1 on their own and then consider a review course only if they fail. Just keep in mind that many states require that you pass Step 1 within three attempts. (For more information on review courses, see Section IV.)

USMLE Step 2 CK and the IMG

What Is the Step 2 CK? It is a computerized test of the clinical sciences consisting of 368 multiple-choice questions divided into eight blocks. It can be taken at Prometric centers in the United States and several other countries.

Content. The Step 2 CK includes test items in the following content areas:

- Internal medicine
- Obstetrics and gynecology
- Pediatrics
- Preventive medicine
- Psychiatry
- Surgery
- Other areas relevant to the provision of care under supervision

Significance of the Test. The Step 2 CK is required for the ECFMG certificate. It reflects the level of clinical knowledge of the applicant. It tests clinical subjects, primarily internal medicine. Other areas that are tested are surgery, obstetrics and gynecology, pediatrics, orthopedics, psychiatry, ENT, ophthalmology, and medical ethics.

Official Web Sites. www.usmle.org and www.ecfmg.org/usmle.

Eligibility. Students and graduates from medical schools that are listed in IMED are eligible to take the Step 2 CK. Students must have completed at least two years of medical school. This means that students must have completed the basic medical science component of the medical school curriculum by the beginning of the eligibility period selected.

Eligibility Period. A three-month period of your choice.

Fee. The fee for the Step 2 CK is $740 plus an international test delivery surcharge (if you choose a testing region other than the United States or Canada).

Retaking the Exam. In the event that you fail the Step 2 CK, you can apply to take the exam again. You cannot take Step 2 CK more than four times within a 12-month period. You cannot retake the exam if you passed.

Statistics. In 2008–2009, 83% of ECFMG candidates passed the Step 2 CK on their first attempt, compared with 96% of U.S. and Canadian candidates.

Tips. It's better to take the Step 2 CK after your internal medicine rotation because most of the questions on the exam give clinical scenarios and ask you to make medical diagnoses and clinical decisions. In addition, because this is a clinical sciences exam, cultural and geographic considerations play a greater role than is the case with Step 1. For example, if your medical education gave you ample exposure to malaria, brucellosis, and malnutrition but little to alcohol withdrawal, child abuse, and cholesterol screening, you must work to familiarize yourself with topics that are more heavily emphasized in U.S. medicine. You must also have a basic understanding of the legal and social aspects of U.S. medicine, because you will be asked questions about communicating with and advising patients.

USMLE Step 2 CS and the IMG

What Is the Step 2 CS? The Step 2 CS is a test of clinical and communication skills administered as a one-day, eight-hour exam. It includes 10 to 12 encounters with standardized patients (15 minutes each, with 10 minutes to write a note after each encounter). Test results are valid indefinitely.

Content. The Step 2 CS tests the ability to communicate in English as well as interpersonal skills, data-gathering skills, the ability to perform a physical exam, and the ability to formulate a brief note, a differential diagnosis, and a list of diagnostic tests. The areas that are covered in the exam are as follows:

- Internal medicine
- Surgery
- Obstetrics and gynecology
- Pediatrics
- Psychiatry
- Family medicine

Unlike the USMLE Step 1, Step 2 CK, or Step 3, there are no numerical grades for the Step 2 CS—it's simply either a "pass" or a "fail." To pass, a candidate must attain a passing performance in **each** of the following three components:

- Integrated Clinical Encounter (ICE): includes Data Gathering, Physical Exam, and the Patient Note
- Spoken English Proficiency (SEP)
- Communication and Interpersonal Skills (CIS)

According to the NBME, the most common component that IMGs fail on the Step 2 CS is the CIS component.

Significance of the Test. The Step 2 CS is required for the ECFMG certificate. It has eliminated the Test of English as a Foreign Language (TOEFL) as a requirement for ECFMG certification.

Official Web Site. www.ecfmg.org/usmle/step2cs.

Eligibility. Students must have completed at least two years of medical school in order to take the test. That means students must have completed the basic medical science component of the medical school curriculum at the time they apply for the exam.

Fee. The fee for the Step 2 CS is $1295.

Scheduling. You must schedule the Step 2 CS within **four months** of the date indicated on your notification of registration. You must take the exam within 12 months of the date indicated on your notification of registration. It is generally advisable to take the Step 2 CS as soon as possible in the year before your Match, as often the results either come in late or arrive too late to allow you to retake the test and pass it before the Match.

Retaking the Exam. There is no limit to the number of attempts you can make to pass the Step 2 CS. However, you cannot take the exam more than three times in a 12-month period.

Test Site Locations. The Step 2 CS is currently administered at the following five locations:

- Philadelphia, PA
- Atlanta, GA
- Los Angeles, CA
- Chicago, IL
- Houston, TX

For more information about the Step 2 CS exam, please refer to *First Aid for the Step 2 CS*.

USMLE Step 3 and the IMG

What Is the USMLE Step 3? It is a two-day computerized test in clinical medicine consisting of 480 multiple-choice questions and nine computer-based case simulations (CCS). The exam aims at testing your knowledge and its application to patient care and clinical decision making (i.e., this exam tests if you can safely practice medicine independently and without supervision).

Significance of the Test. Taking Step 3 before residency is critical for IMGs seeking an H1B visa and is also a bonus that can be added to the residency application. Step 3 is also required to obtain a full medical license in the United States and can be taken during residency for this purpose.

Official Web Site. www.usmle.org.

Fee. The fee for Step 3 is $705 in all states except Iowa ($755), South Dakota ($855), and Vermont ($740).

Eligibility. Most states require that applicants have completed one, two, or three years of postgraduate training (residency) before they apply for Step 3 and permanent state licensure. The exceptions are the 13 states mentioned below, which allow IMGs to take Step 3 at the beginning of or even before residency. So if you don't fulfill the prerequisites to taking Step 3 in your state of choice, simply use the name of one of the 13 states in your Step 3 application. You can take the exam in any state you choose regardless of the state that you mentioned on your application. Once you pass Step 3, it will be recognized by all states. Basic eligibility requirements for the USMLE Step 3 are as follows:

- Obtaining an MD or DO degree (or its equivalent) by the application deadline.
- Obtaining an ECFMG certificate if you are a graduate of a foreign medical school or are successfully completing a "fifth pathway" program (at a date no later than the application deadline).
- Meeting the requirements imposed by the individual state licensing authority to which you are applying to take Step 3. Please refer to www.fsmb.org for more information.

The following states do not have postgraduate training as an eligibility requirement to apply for Step 3:

- Arkansas
- California
- Connecticut
- Florida
- Louisiana
- Maryland
- Nebraska*
- New York
- South Dakota
- Texas
- Utah*
- Washington
- West Virginia

* Requires that IMGs obtain a "valid indefinite" ECFMG certificate.

The Step 3 exam is not available outside the United States. Applications can be found online at www.fsmb.org and must be submitted to the FSMB.

Residencies and the IMG

In the residency Match, the number of U.S.-citizen IMG applications has grown for the past few years, while the percentage accepted has been stable (see Table 5). More information about residency programs can be obtained at www.ama-assn.org.

The Match and the IMG

Given the growing number of IMG candidates with strong applications, you should bear in mind that good USMLE scores are not the only way to gain a competitive edge. However, USMLE Step 1 and Step 2 CK scores continue

TABLE 5. IMGs in the Match.

APPLICANTS	2008	2009	2010
U.S.-citizen IMGs	2,969	3,390	3,695
% U.S.-citizen IMGs accepted	52	48	47
Non-U.S.-citizen IMGs	7,335	7,484	7,246
% non-U.S.-citizen IMGs accepted	42	42	40
U.S. graduates (non-IMGs)	15,242	15,638	16,070
% U.S. graduates accepted	94	93	93

to be used as the initial screening mechanism when candidates are being considered for interviews.

Based on accumulated IMG Match experiences over recent years, here are a few pointers to help IMGs maximize their chances for a residency interview:

- **Apply early.** Programs offer a limited number of interviews and often select candidates on a first-come, first-served basis. Because of this, you should aim to complete the entire process of applying for the ERAS token, registering with the Association of American Medical Colleges (AAMC), mailing necessary documents to ERAS, and completing the ERAS application before September (see Figure 5). Community programs usually send out interview offers earlier than do university and university-affiliated programs.
- **U.S. clinical experience helps.** Externships and observerships in a U.S. hospital setting have emerged as an important credential on an IMG application. Externships are like short-term medical school internships and offer hands-on clinical experience. Observerships, also called "shadowing," involve following a physician and observing how he or she manages patients. Externships are considered superior to observerships, but having either of them is always better than having none. Some programs require students to have participated in an externship or observership before ap-

FIGURE 5. IMG Timeline for Application.

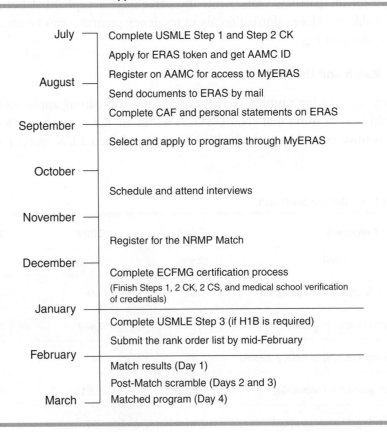

July	Complete USMLE Step 1 and Step 2 CK
	Apply for ERAS token and get AAMC ID
	Register on AAMC for access to MyERAS
August	Send documents to ERAS by mail
	Complete CAF and personal statements on ERAS
September	Select and apply to programs through MyERAS
October	
	Schedule and attend interviews
November	
	Register for the NRMP Match
December	Complete ECFMG certification process
	(Finish Steps 1, 2 CK, 2 CS, and medical school verification of credentials)
January	Complete USMLE Step 3 (if H1B is required)
	Submit the rank order list by mid-February
February	Match results (Day 1)
	Post-Match scramble (Days 2 and 3)
March	Matched program (Day 4)

plying. It is best to gain such an experience before or at the time you apply to various programs so that you can mention it on your ERAS application. If such an experience or opportunity comes up after you apply, be sure to inform the programs accordingly.

- **Clinical research helps.** University programs are attracted to candidates who show a strong interest in clinical research and academics. They may even relax their application criteria for individuals with unique backgrounds and strong research experience. Publications in well-known journals are an added bonus.

- **Time the Step 2 CS well.** ECFMG has published the new Step 2 CS score-reporting schedule for the years 2010–2011 at http://ecfmg.org/announce.htm#reportsched. Most program directors would like to see a passing score on the Step 1, Step 2 CK, and Step 2 CS exams before they rank an IMG on their rank order list in mid-February. There have been many instances in which candidates have relinquished a position on the rank order list—and have thus lost a potential match—either because of delayed CS results or because they have been unable to retake the exam on time following a failure. It is difficult to predict a result on the Step 2 CS, since the grading process is not very transparent. Therefore, it is advisable to take the Step 2 CS as early as possible in the application year.

- **U.S. letters of recommendation help.** Letters of recommendation from clinicians practicing in the United States carry more weight than recommendations from home countries.

- **Step up the Step 3.** If H1B visa sponsorship is desired, aim to have Step 3 results by January of the Match year. In addition to the visa advantage you will gain, an early and good Step 3 score may benefit IMGs who have been away from clinical medicine for a while as well as those who have low scores on Step 1 and the Step 2 CK.

- **Verify medical credentials in a timely manner.** Do not overlook the medical school credential verification process. The ECFMG certificate arrives only after credentials have been verified and after you have passed Step 1, the Step 2 CK, and the Step 2 CS, so you should keep track of the process and check with the ECFMG from time to time about your status.

- **Schedule interviews with pre-Matches in mind.** Schedule interviews with your favorite programs first. This will leave you better prepared to make a decision in the event that you are offered a pre-Match position.

Resources for the IMG

- **ECFMG**
  3624 Market Street
  Philadelphia, PA 19104-2685
  (215) 386-5900
  Fax: (215) 386-9196
  www.ecfmg.org

The ECFMG telephone number is answered only between 9:00 A.M. and 12:30 P.M. and between 1:30 P.M. and 5:00 P.M. Monday through Friday EST. The ECFMG often takes a long time to answer the phone, which is frequently busy at peak times of the year, and then gives you a long voice-mail message—so it is better to write or fax early than to rely on a last-minute phone call. Do not contact the NBME, as all IMG exam matters are conducted by the ECFMG. The ECFMG also publishes an information booklet on ECFMG certification and the USMLE program, which gives details on the dates and locations of forthcoming USMLE and English tests for IMGs together with application forms. It is free of charge and is also available from the public affairs offices of U.S. embassies and consulates worldwide as well as from Overseas Educational Advisory Centers. You may order single copies of the handbook by calling (215) 386-5900, preferably on weekends or between 6 P.M. and 6 A.M. Philadelphia time, or by faxing to (215) 386-9196. Requests for multiple copies must be made by fax or mail on organizational letterhead. The full text of the booklet is also available on the ECFMG's Web site at www.ecfmg.org.

- **FSMB**
  400 Fuller Wiser Road, Suite 300
  Euless, TX 76039
  (817) 868-4000
  Fax: (817) 868-4099
  www.fsmb.org

  The FSMB has a number of publications available, including free policy documents. To obtain these publications, print and mail the order form on the Web site listed above. Alternatively, write to Federation Publications at the above address. All orders must be prepaid with a personal check drawn on a U.S. bank, a cashier's check, or a money order payable to the FSMB. Foreign orders must be accompanied by an international money order or the equivalent, payable in U.S. dollars through a U.S. bank or a U.S. affiliate of a foreign bank. For Step 3 inquiries, the telephone number is (817) 868-4041. You may e-mail the FSMB at usmle@fsmb.org or write to Examination Services at the address above.

- The AMA has dedicated a portion of its Web site to information on IMG demographics, residencies, immigration, and the like. This information can be found at www.ama-assn.org/ama/pub/about-ama/our-people/member-groups-sections/international-medical-graduates.shtml.

Other resources that may be useful and of interest to IMGs include the following:

- *The International Medical Graduate's Guide to US Medicine and Residency Training*, by Patrick C. Alquire, Gerald P. Whelan, and Vijay Rajput (2009; ISBN 9781934465080).
- *The International Medical Graduate's Best Hope*, by Franck Belibi and Suzanne Belibi (2009; ISBN 9780979877308).

What Is the COMLEX-USA Level 1?

The National Board of Osteopathic Medical Examiners (NBOME) administers the Comprehensive Osteopathic Medical Licensing Examination, or COMLEX-USA. Like the USMLE, the COMLEX-USA is administered over three levels. Currently, the COMLEX-USA sequence is accepted for licensure in all 50 states.

The COMLEX-USA series assesses osteopathic medical knowledge and clinical skills using clinical presentations and physician tasks. A description of the COMLEX-USA Written Examination Blueprints for each level, which outline the various clinical presentations and physician tasks that examinees will encounter, is given on the NBOME Web site. Another stated goal of the COMLEX-USA Level 1 is to create a more primary care–oriented exam that integrates osteopathic principles into clinical situations.

To be eligible to take the COMLEX-USA Level 1, you must have satisfactorily completed at least one-half of your sophomore year in an American Osteopathic Association (AOA)–approved medical school. In addition, you must obtain verification that you are in good standing at your medical school via approval of your dean. Applications may be downloaded from the NBOME Web site.

For all three levels of the COMLEX-USA, raw scores are converted to a percentile score and a score ranging from 5 to 800. For Levels 1 and 2, a score of 400 is required to pass; for Level 3, a score of 350 is needed. COMLEX-USA scores are usually mailed eight weeks after the test date. The mean score is always 500.

If you pass a COMLEX-USA examination, you are not allowed to retake it to improve your grade. If you fail, there is no specific limit to the number of times you can retake it in order to pass. Level 2 and 3 exams must be passed in sequential order within seven years of passing Level 1.

What Is the Structure of the COMLEX-USA Level 1?

The COMLEX-USA Level 1 is a computer-based examination consisting of 400 questions over an eight-hour period in a single day. Most of the questions are in one-best-answer format, but a small number are matching-type questions. Some one-best-answer questions are bundled together around a common question stem that usually takes the form of a clinical scenario. New question formats may gradually be introduced, but candidates will be notified if this occurs.

Questions are grouped into eight sections of 50 questions each in a manner similar to the USMLE. Reviewing and changing answers may be done only in the current section. A "review page" is presented for each block in order to advise test takers of questions completed, questions marked for further review, and incomplete questions for which no answer has been given.

Students are allowed to take a 10-minute break at the end of two sections. Students who do not take this 10-minute break and continue to section 3 can apply the 10 minutes toward their test time. Similarly, after section 4, students are given a 40-minute lunch break and another 10-minute break after section 6. More information about the computer-based COMLEX-USA examinations can be obtained from www.nbome.org.

What Is the Difference Between the USMLE and the COMLEX-USA?

According to the NBOME, the COMLEX-USA Level 1 focuses broadly on the following categories, with osteopathic principles and practices integrated into each section:

- Health promotion and disease prevention
- The history and physical
- Diagnostic technologies
- Management
- Scientific understanding of mechanisms
- Health care delivery

Although the COMLEX-USA and the USMLE are similar in scope, content, and emphasis, some differences are worth noting. For example, the COMLEX-USA Level 1 tests osteopathic principles in addition to basic science materials but does not emphasize lab techniques. In addition, although both exams often require that you apply and integrate knowledge over several areas of basic science to answer a given question, many students who took both tests reported that the questions differed somewhat in style. Students reported, for example, that USMLE questions generally required that the test taker reason and draw from the information given (often a two-step process), whereas those on the COMLEX-USA exam tended to be more straightforward. Furthermore, USMLE questions were on average found to be considerably longer than those on the COMLEX-USA.

Students also commented that the COMLEX-USA utilized "buzzwords," although limited in their use (e.g., "rose spots" in typhoid fever), whereas the USMLE avoided buzzwords in favor of descriptions of clinical findings or symptoms (e.g., rose-colored papules on the abdomen rather than rose spots). Finally, USMLE appeared to have more photographs than did the COMLEX-USA. In general, the overall impression was that the USMLE was a more "thought-provoking" exam, while the COMLEX-USA was more of a "knowledge-based" exam.

Who Should Take Both the USMLE and the COMLEX-USA?

Aside from facing the COMLEX-USA Level 1, you must decide if you will also take the USMLE Step 1. We recommend that you consider taking both the USMLE and the COMLEX-USA under the following circumstances:

- **If you are applying to allopathic residencies.** Although there is growing acceptance of COMLEX-USA certification on the part of allopathic residencies, some allopathic programs prefer or even require passage of the USMLE Step 1. These include many academic programs, programs in competitive specialties (e.g., orthopedics, ophthalmology, or dermatology), and programs in competitive geographic areas (such as California). Fourth-year doctor of osteopathy (DO) students who have already matched may be a good source of information about which programs and specialties look for USMLE scores. It is also a good idea to contact program directors at the institutions you are interested in to ask about their policy regarding the COMLEX-USA versus the USMLE.
- **If you are unsure about your postgraduate training plans.** Successful passage of both the COMLEX-USA Level 1 and the USMLE Step 1 is certain to provide you with the greatest possible range of options when you are applying for internship and residency training.

The clinical coursework that some DO students receive during the summer of their third year (as opposed to their starting clerkships) is considered helpful in integrating basic science knowledge for the COMLEX-USA or the USMLE.

In addition, the COMLEX-USA Level 1 has in recent years placed increasing emphasis on questions related to primary care medicine and prevention. Having a strong background in family or primary care medicine can help test takers when they face questions on prevention.

How Do I Prepare for the COMLEX-USA Level 1?

Student experience suggests that you should start studying for the COMLEX-USA four to six months before the test is given, as an early start will allow you to spend up to a month on each subject. The recommendations made in Section I regarding study and testing methods, strategies, and resources, as well as the books suggested in Section IV for the USMLE Step 1, hold true for the COMLEX-USA as well.

Another important source of information is in the *Examination Guidelines and Sample Exam*, a booklet that discusses the breakdown of each subject while also providing sample questions and corresponding answers. Many students, however, felt that this breakdown provided only a general guideline and was not representative of the level of difficulty of the actual COMLEX-USA. The sample questions did not provide examples of clinical vignettes, which made up approximately 25% of the exam. You will receive this publication with registration materials for the COMLEX-USA Level 1, but you can also receive a copy and additional information by writing:

NBOME
8765 W. Higgins Road, Suite 200
Chicago, IL 60631-4174
(773) 714-0622
Fax: (773) 714-0631

or by visiting the NBOME Web page at www.nbome.org.

The NBOME developed the Comprehensive Osteopathic Medical Self-Assessment Examination (COMSAE) series to fill the need for self-assessment on the part of osteopathic medical students. Many students take the COMSAE exam before the COMLEX-USA in addition to using test-bank questions and board review books. Students can purchase a copy of this exam at www.nbome.org/comsae.asp.

In recent years, students have reported an emphasis in certain areas. For example:

- There was an increased emphasis on upper limb anatomy/brachial plexus.
- Specific topics were repeatedly tested on the exam. These included cardio-vascular physiology and pathology, acid-base physiology, diabetes, benign prostatic hyperplasia, sexually transmitted diseases, measles, and rubella. Thyroid and adrenal function, neurology (head injury), specific drug treatments for bacterial infection, migraines/cluster headaches, and drug mechanisms also received heavy emphasis.
- Behavioral science questions were based on psychiatry.
- High-yield osteopathic manipulative technique (OMT) topics included an emphasis on the sympathetic and parasympathetic innervations of viscera and nerve roots, rib mechanics/diagnosis, and basic craniosacral theory. Students who spend time reviewing basic anatomy, studying nerve and dermatome innervations, and understanding how to perform basic OMT techniques (e.g., muscle energy or counterstrain) can improve their scores.

The COMLEX-USA Level 1 also includes multimedia-based questions. Such questions test the student's ability to perform a good physical exam and to elicit various physical diagnostic signs (e.g., Murphy's sign).

Since topics that were repeatedly tested appeared in all four booklets, students found it useful to review them in between the two test days. It is important to understand that the topics emphasized on the current exam may not be stressed on future exams. However, some topics are heavily tested each year, so it may be beneficial to have a solid foundation in the above-mentioned topics.

The National Board of Podiatric Medical Examiners (NBPME) tests are designed to assess whether a candidate possesses the knowledge required to practice as a minimally competent entry-level podiatrist. The NBPME examinations are used as part of the licensing process governing the practice of podiatric medicine. The NBPME exam is recognized by all 50 states and the District of Columbia, the U.S. Army, the U.S. Navy, and the Canadian provinces of Alberta, British Columbia, and Ontario. Individual states use the examination scores differently; therefore, doctor of podiatric medicine (DPM) candidates should refer to the *NBPME Bulletin of Information: 2011 Examinations*.

The NBPME Part I is generally taken after the completion of the second year of podiatric medical education. Unlike the USMLE Step 1, there is no behavioral science section, nor is biomechanics tested. The exam samples seven basic science disciplines: general anatomy (10%); lower extremity anatomy (22%); biochemistry (10%); physiology (12%); medical microbiology and immunology (15%); pathology (15%); and pharmacology (16%). A detailed outline of topics and subtopics covered on the exam can be found in the *NBPME Bulletin of Information*, available on the NBPME Web site.

Your NBPME Appointment

In early spring, your college registrar will have you fill out an application for the NBPME Part I. After your application and registration fees are received, you will be mailed the *NBPME Bulletin of Information: 2011 Examinations*. The exam will be offered at an independent location in each city with a podiatric medical school (New York, Philadelphia, Miami, Cleveland, Chicago, Des Moines, Phoenix, and San Francisco). You may take the exam at any of these locations regardless of which school you attend. However, you must designate on your application which testing location you desire. Specific instructions about exam dates and registration deadlines can be found in the *NBPME Bulletin*.

Exam Format

The NBPME Part I is a written exam consisting of 205 questions. The test consists entirely of multiple-choice questions with four answer choices. Examinees have three hours in which to take the exam and are given scratch paper and a calculator, both of which must be turned in at the end of the exam. Some questions on the exam will be "trial questions." These questions are evaluated as future board questions but are not counted in your score.

Interpreting Your Score

Three to four weeks following the exam date, test takers will receive their scores by mail. NBPME scores are reported as pass/fail, with a scaled score of at least 75 needed to pass. Eighty-five percent of first-time test takers pass the

NBPME Part I. Failing candidates receive a report with one score between 55 and 74 in addition to diagnostic messages intended to help identify strengths or weaknesses in specific content areas. If you fail the NBPME Part I, you must retake the entire examination at a later date. There is no limit to the number of times you can retake the exam.

Preparation for the NBPME Part I

Students suggest that you begin studying for the NBPME Part I at least three months prior to the test date. The suggestions made in Section I regarding study and testing methods for the USMLE Step 1 can be applied to the NBPME as well. This book should, however, be used as a supplement and not as the sole source of information. Keep in mind that you need only a passing score. Neither you nor your school or future residency will ever see your actual numerical score. Competing with colleagues should not be an issue, and study groups are beneficial to many.

A potential study method that helps many students is to copy the outline of the material to be tested from the *NBPME Bulletin.* Check off each topic during your study, because doing so will ensure that you have engaged each topic. If you are pressed for time, prioritize subjects on the basis of their weight on the exam. Approximately 22% of the NBPME Part I focuses on lower extremity anatomy. In this area, students should rely on the notes and material that they received from their class. Remember, lower extremity anatomy is the podiatric physician's specialty—so everything about it is important. Do not forget to study osteology. Keep your old tests and look through old lower extremity class exams, since each of the podiatric colleges submits questions from its own exams. This strategy will give you an understanding of the types of questions that may be asked. On the NBPME Part I, you will see some of the same classic lower extremity anatomy questions you were tested on in school.

The NBPME, like the USMLE, requires that you apply and integrate knowledge over several areas of basic science in order to answer exam questions. Students report that many questions emphasize clinical presentations; however, the facts in this book are very useful in helping students recall the various diseases and organisms. DPM candidates should expand on the high-yield pharmacology section and study antifungal drugs and treatments for *Pseudomonas*, methicillin-resistant *S. aureus*, candidiasis, and erythrasma. The high-yield section focusing on pathology is very useful; however, additional emphasis on diabetes mellitus and all its secondary manifestations, particularly peripheral neuropathy, should not be overlooked. Students should also focus on renal physiology and drug elimination, the biochemistry of gout, and neurophysiology, all of which have been noted to be important topics on the NBPME Part I exam.

A sample set of questions is found in the *NBPME Bulletin of Information: 2011 Examinations.* These samples are similar in difficulty to actual board questions. If you do not receive an *NBPME Bulletin* or if you have any questions regarding registration, fees, test centers, authorization forms, or score reports, please contact your college registrar or:

NBPME
P.O. Box 510
Bellefonte, PA 16823
(814) 357-0487
E-mail: NBPMEOfc@aol.com

or visit the NBPME Web page at www.nbpme.info.

The USMLE provides accommodations for students with documented disabilities. The basis for such accommodations is the Americans with Disabilities Act (ADA) of 1990. The ADA defines a disability as "a significant limitation in one or more major life activities." This includes both "observable/physical" disabilities (e.g., blindness, hearing loss, narcolepsy) and "hidden/mental disabilities" (e.g., attention-deficit hyperactivity disorder, chronic fatigue syndrome, learning disabilities).

To provide appropriate support, the administrators of the USMLE must be informed of both the nature and the severity of an examinee's disability. Such documentation is required for an examinee to receive testing accommodations. Accommodations include extra time on tests, low-stimulation environments, extra or extended breaks, and zoom text.

Who Can Apply for Accommodations?

Students or graduates of a school in the United States or Canada that is accredited by the Liaison Committee on Medical Education (LCME) or the AOA may apply for test accommodations directly from the NBME. Requests are granted only if they meet the ADA definition of a disability. If you are a disabled student or a disabled graduate of a foreign medical school, you must contact the ECFMG (see below).

Who Is Not Eligible for Accommodations?

Individuals who do not meet the ADA definition of disabled are not eligible for test accommodations. Difficulties not eligible for test accommodations include test anxiety, slow reading without an identified underlying cognitive deficit, English as a second language, and learning difficulties that have not been diagnosed as a medically recognized disability.

Understanding the Need for Documentation

Although most learning-disabled medical students are all too familiar with the often exhausting process of providing documentation of their disability, you should realize that **applying for USMLE accommodation is different from these previous experiences.** This is because the NBME determines whether an individual is disabled solely on the basis of the guidelines set by the ADA. Previous accommodation does not in itself justify provision of an accommodation, so be sure to review the NBME guidelines carefully.

Getting the Information

The first step in applying for USMLE special accommodations is to contact the NBME and obtain a guidelines and questionnaire booklet. This can be obtained by calling or writing to:

Testing Coordinator
Office of Test Accommodations
National Board of Medical Examiners
3750 Market Street
Philadelphia, PA 19104-3102
(215) 590-9509

Internet access to this information is also available at www.nbme.org. This information is also relevant for IMGs, since the information is the same as that sent by the ECFMG.

Foreign graduates should contact the ECFMG to obtain information on special accommodations by calling or writing to:

ECFMG
3624 Market Street
Philadelphia, PA 19104-2685
(215) 386-5900

When you get this information, take some time to read it carefully. The guidelines are clear and explicit about what you need to do to obtain accommodations.

NOTES

High-Yield General Principles

"There comes a time when for every addition of knowledge you forget something that you knew before. It is of the highest importance, therefore, not to have useless facts elbowing out the useful ones."
— Sir Arthur Conan Doyle, *A Study in Scarlet*

"Never regard study as a duty, but as the enviable opportunity to learn."
—Albert Einstein

"Live as if you were to die tomorrow. Learn as if you were to live forever."
—Gandhi

▶ Behavioral Science

▶ Biochemistry

▶ Embryology

▶ Microbiology

▶ Immunology

▶ Pathology

▶ Pharmacology

The 2011 edition of *First Aid for the USMLE Step 1* contains a revised and expanded database of basic science material that student authors and faculty have identified as high yield for board reviews. The information is presented in a partially organ-based format. Hence, Section II is devoted to pathology, the foundational principles of behavioral science, biochemistry, embryology, microbiology and immunology, and pharmacology. Section III focuses on organ systems, with subsections covering the embryology, anatomy and histology, physiology, pathology, and pharmacology relevant to each. Each subsection is then divided into smaller topic areas containing related facts. Individual facts are generally presented in a three-column format, with the **Title** of the fact in the first column, the **Description** of the fact in the second column, and the **Mnemonic** or **Special Note** in the third column. Some facts do not have a mnemonic and are presented in a two-column format. Others are presented in list or tabular form in order to emphasize key associations.

The database structure used in Sections II and III is useful for reviewing material already learned. These sections are **not** ideal for learning complex or highly conceptual material for the first time. At the beginning of each subsection, we list supplementary high-yield clinical vignettes and topics that have appeared on recent exams in order to help focus your review.

The database of high-yield facts is not comprehensive. Use it to complement your core study material and not as your primary study source. The facts and notes have been condensed and edited to emphasize the essential material, and as a result each entry is "incomplete." Work with the material, add your own notes and mnemonics, and recognize that not all memory techniques work for all students.

We update the database of high-yield facts annually to keep current with new trends in boards content as well as to expand our database of information. However, we must note that inevitably many other very high yield entries and topics are not yet included in our database.

We actively encourage medical students and faculty to submit entries and mnemonics so that we may enhance the database for future students. We also solicit recommendations of alternate tools for study that may be useful in preparing for the examination, such as diagrams, charts, and computer-based tutorials (see How to Contribute, p. xv).

Disclaimer

The entries in this section reflect student opinions of what is high yield. Owing to the diverse sources of material, no attempt has been made to trace or reference the origins of entries individually. We have regarded mnemonics as essentially in the public domain. All errors and omissions will gladly be corrected if brought to the attention of the authors, either through the publisher or directly by e-mail.

Behavioral Science

"It's psychosomatic. You need a lobotomy. I'll get a saw."
　　　　　　　　　　—Calvin, "Calvin & Hobbes"

▶ Epidemiology/
　Biostatistics

▶ Ethics

▶ Development

▶ Physiology

A heterogeneous mix of epidemiology, biostatistics, ethics, psychology, sociology, and more falls under the heading of behavioral science. Many medical students do not study this discipline diligently because the material is felt to be easy or a matter of common sense. In our opinion, this is a missed opportunity.

Behavioral science questions may seem less concrete than questions from other disciplines, requiring an awareness of the social aspects of medicine. For example: If a patient does or says something, what should you do or say in response? These so-called "quote" questions now constitute much of the behavioral science section. Medical ethics and medical law are also appearing with increasing frequency. In addition, the key aspects of the doctor-patient relationship (e.g., communication skills, open-ended questions, facilitation, silence) are high yield, as are biostatistics and epidemiology. Make sure you can apply biostatistical concepts such as specificity and predictive values in a problem-solving format.

HIGH-YIELD PRINCIPLES

BEHAVIORAL SCIENCE

Types of studies

Study type	Design	Measures/example
Case-control study Observational and retrospective	Compares a group of people with disease to a group without. Looks for prior exposure or risk factor. Asks, "What happened?"	**Odds ratio** (OR). "Patients with COPD had higher odds of a history of smoking than those without COPD."
Cohort study Observational and prospective	Compares a group with a given exposure or risk factor to a group without. Looks to see if exposure ↑ the likelihood of disease. Asks, "What will happen?"	**Relative risk** (RR). "Smokers had a higher risk of developing COPD than did nonsmokers."
Cross-sectional study Observational	Collects data from a group of people to assess frequency of disease (and related risk factors) at a particular point in time. Asks, "What is happening?"	**Disease prevalence.** Can show risk factor association with disease, but does not establish causality.

Case control ←——————|——————→ Cohort

Cross-sectional

Twin concordance study	Compares the frequency with which both monozygotic twins or both dizygotic twins develop a disease.	Measures heritability.
Adoption study	Compares siblings raised by biologic vs. adoptive parents.	Measures heritability and influence of environmental factors.

Clinical trial	Experimental study involving humans. Compares therapeutic benefits of 2 or more treatments, or of treatment and placebo. Highest-quality study when randomized, controlled, and double-blinded (i.e., neither patient nor doctor knows if the patient is in the treatment or control group).	
	Study sample	**Purpose**
Phase I	Small number of patients, usually healthy volunteers.	Assesses safety, toxicity, and pharmacokinetics.
Phase II	Small number of patients with disease of interest.	Assesses treatment efficacy, optimal dosing, and adverse effects.
Phase III	Large number of patients randomly assigned either to the treatment under investigation or to the best available treatment (or placebo).	Compares the new treatment to the current standard of care.
Phase IV	Postmarketing surveillance trial of patients after approval.	Detects rare or long-term adverse effects.

Meta-analysis	Pools data from several studies to come to an overall conclusion. Achieves greater statistical power and integrates results of similar studies. Highest echelon of clinical evidence.	May be limited by quality of individual studies or bias in study selection.

| **Evaluation of diagnostic tests** | Uses 2 × 2 table comparing test results with the actual presence of disease. TP = true positive; FP = false positive; TN = true negative; FN = false negative. | |

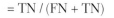

Disease

		⊕	⊖
Test	⊕	TP	FP
	⊖	FN	TN

| Sensitivity | Proportion of all people with disease who test positive, or the ability of a test to detect a disease when it is present.

 Value approaching 1 is desirable for ruling **out** disease and indicates a low false-negative rate. Used for screening in diseases with low prevalence. | $= \text{TP} / (\text{TP} + \text{FN})$
 $= 1 - \text{false-negative rate}$
 SNOUT = **SeN**sitivity rules **OUT**.
 If 100% sensitivity, $\text{TP} / (\text{TP} + \text{FN}) = 1$, $\text{FN} = 0$, and all negatives must be TNs. |

| Specificity | Proportion of all people without disease who test negative, or the ability of a test to indicate non-disease when disease is not present.

 Value approaching 1 is desirable for ruling **in** disease and indicates a low false-positive rate. Used as a confirmatory test after a positive screening test.

 Example: HIV testing. Screen with ELISA (sensitive, high false-positive rate, low threshold); confirm with Western blot (specific, high false-negative rate, high threshold). | $= \text{TN} / (\text{TN} + \text{FP})$
 $= 1 - \text{false-positive rate}$
 SPIN = **SP**ecificity rules **IN**.
 If 100% specificity, $\text{TN} / (\text{TN} + \text{FP}) = 1$, $\text{FP} = 0$, and all positives must be TPs. |

| Positive predictive value (PPV) | Proportion of positive test results that are true positive. Probability that person actually has the disease given a positive test result.
 (Note: If the prevalence of a disease in a population is low, even tests with high specificity or high sensitivity will have low positive predictive values!) | $= \text{TP} / (\text{TP} + \text{FP})$ |

| Negative predictive value (NPV) | Proportion of negative test results that are true negative. Probability that person actually is disease free given a negative test result. | $= \text{TN} / (\text{FN} + \text{TN})$ |

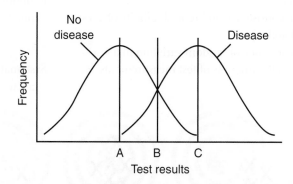

A = 100% sensitivity
B = most accurate
C = 100% specificity

(Adapted, with permission, from McPhee SJ et al. *Current Medical Diagnosis & Treatment*, 47th ed. New York: McGraw-Hill, 2007: Fig. 43-3.)

Prevalence vs. incidence

$$\text{Point prevalence} = \frac{\text{total cases in population at a given time}}{\text{total population at a given time}}$$

$$\text{Incidence} = \frac{\begin{array}{c}\text{new cases in population}\\\text{over a given time period}\end{array}}{\begin{array}{c}\text{total population at risk}\\\text{during that time period}\end{array}}$$

Incidence is new **incidents**.

Prevalence $\cong$ incidence $\times$ disease duration.
Prevalence > incidence for chronic diseases (e.g., diabetes).
Prevalence = incidence for acute disease (e.g., common cold).

When calculating incidence, don't forget that people currently with the disease, or those previously positive for it, are not considered at risk.

Odds ratio vs. relative risk

Odds ratio (OR) for case-control studies	Odds of having disease in exposed group divided by odds of having disease in unexposed group. Approximates relative risk if prevalence of disease is not too high.	
Relative risk (RR) for cohort studies	Relative probability of getting a disease in the exposed group compared to the unexposed group. Calculated as percent with disease in exposed group divided by percent with disease in unexposed group.	
Attributable risk	The difference in risk between exposed and unexposed groups, or the proportion of disease occurrences that are attributable to the exposure (e.g., smoking causes one-third of cases of pneumonia).	
Absolute risk reduction	The reduction in risk associated with a treatment as compared to a placebo.	
Number needed to treat	1/absolute risk reduction.	
Number needed to harm	1/attributable risk.	

$$\text{Odds ratio} = \frac{a/b}{c/d} = \frac{ad}{bc}$$

$$\text{Relative risk} = \frac{a/(a+b)}{c/(c+d)}$$

$$\text{Attributable risk} = \frac{a}{a+b} - \frac{c}{c+d}$$

Disease

		$\oplus$	$\ominus$
Risk factor	$\oplus$	a	b
	$\ominus$	c	d

Precision vs. accuracy

Precision is:
1. The consistency and reproducibility of a test (reliability)
2. The absence of random variation in a test

Accuracy is the trueness of test measurements (validity).

Random error—reduced precision in a test.

Systematic error—reduced accuracy in a test.

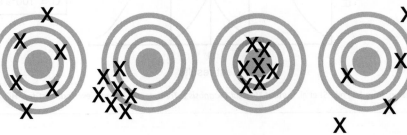

| Accurate | Precise | Accurate and precise | Not accurate, not precise |

Bias	Occurs when 1 outcome is systematically favored over another. Systematic errors.	Ways to reduce bias:

Occurs when 1 outcome is systematically favored over another. Systematic errors.

1. **Selection bias**—nonrandom assignment to study group (e.g., Berkson's bias)
2. **Recall bias**—knowledge of presence of disorder alters recall by subjects
3. **Sampling bias**—subjects are not representative relative to general population; therefore, results are not generalizable
4. **Late-look bias**—information gathered at an inappropriate time—e.g., using a survey to study a fatal disease (only those patients still alive will be able to answer survey)
5. **Procedure bias**—subjects in different groups are not treated the same—e.g., more attention is paid to treatment group, stimulating greater compliance
6. **Confounding bias**—occurs with 2 closely associated factors; the effect of 1 factor distorts or confuses the effect of the other
7. **Lead-time bias**—early detection confused with ↑ survival; seen with improved screening (natural history of disease is not changed, but early detection makes it seem as though survival ↑)
8. **Pygmalion effect**—occurs when a researcher's belief in the efficacy of a treatment changes the outcome of that treatment
9. **Hawthorne effect**—occurs when the group being studied changes its behavior owing to the knowledge of being studied

Ways to reduce bias:
1. Blind studies (double blind is better)
2. Placebo responses
3. Crossover studies (each subject acts as own control)
4. Randomization

Statistical distribution

Terms that describe statistical distributions:

Normal ≈ Gaussian ≈ bell-shaped (mean = median = mode).

Bimodal is simply 2 humps (2 modal peaks).

Positive skew—mean > median > mode. Asymmetry with tail on right.

Negative skew—mean < median < mode. Asymmetry with tail on left.

Mode is least affected by outliers in the sample.

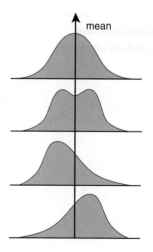

Statistical hypotheses

Null (H_0) Hypothesis of no difference (e.g., there is no association between the disease and the risk factor in the population).

Alternative (H_1) Hypothesis that there is some difference (e.g., there is some association between the disease and the risk factor in the population).

	Reality	
	H_1	H_0
Study results H_1	Power $(1 - \beta)$	α
Study results H_0	β	

Error types

Type I error (α) Stating that there **is** an effect or difference when none exists (to mistakenly accept the experimental hypothesis and reject the null hypothesis). p = probability of making a type I error. p is judged against a preset level of significance (usually < .05). "False-positive error."

If $p < .05$, then there is less than a 5% chance that the data will show something that is not really there.

α = you "saw" a difference that did not exist—for example, convicting an innocent man.

Type II error (β) Stating that there **is not** an effect or difference when one exists (to fail to reject the null hypothesis when in fact H_0 is false). β is the probability of making a type II error. "False-negative error."

β = you did not "see" a difference that does exist— for example, setting a guilty man free.

Power (1 – β) Probability of rejecting null hypothesis when it is in fact false, or the likelihood of finding a difference if one in fact exists. It depends on:
1. Total number of end points experienced by population
2. Difference in compliance between treatment groups (differences in the mean values between groups)
3. Size of expected effect

If you ↑ sample size, you ↑ power. There is power in numbers.

Power = $1 - \beta$.

Standard deviation vs. standard error

n = sample size.
σ = standard deviation.
SEM = standard error of the mean.
SEM = $\sigma/\sqrt{n}$.
Therefore, SEM < σ and SEM decreases as n increases.

Normal (Gaussian) distribution:

Confidence interval	Range of values in which a specified probability of the means of repeated samples would be expected to fall. CI = confidence interval. CI = range from [mean – Z(SEM)] to [mean + Z(SEM)]. The 95% CI (corresponding to $p = .05$) is often used. For the 95% CI, Z = 1.96.	If the 95% CI for a mean difference between 2 variables includes 0, then there is no significant difference and H_0 is not rejected. If the 95% CI for odds ratio or relative risk includes 1, H_0 is not rejected. If the CI between 2 groups overlaps, then these groups are not significantly different.
t-test vs. ANOVA vs. χ^2	t-test checks difference between the **means** of 2 groups. ANOVA checks difference between the means of 3 or more groups. χ^2 (chi-square) test checks difference between 2 or more percentages or proportions of categorical outcomes (not mean values).	Mr. **T** is **mean**. **ANOVA** = **AN**alysis **O**f **VA**riance of 3 or more variables. χ^2 = compare percentages (%) or proportions.
Correlation coefficient (r)	r is always between −1 and +1. The closer the absolute value of r is to 1, the stronger the correlation between the 2 variables. Coefficient of determination = r^2 (value that is usually reported).	
Disease prevention	1°—prevent disease occurrence (e.g., HPV vaccination). 2°—early detection of disease (e.g., Pap smear). 3°—reduce disability from disease (e.g., chemotherapy).	**PDR:** **P**revent **D**etect **R**educe disability

Reportable diseases	Only some infectious diseases are reportable in all states, including AIDS, chickenpox, gonorrhea, hepatitis A and B, measles, mumps, rubella, salmonella, shigella, syphilis, and TB.	Hep, Hep, Hep, Hooray, the **SSSMMART Chick** is **Gone**!
	Other diseases (including HIV) vary by state.	Hep A
		Hep B
		Hep C
		HIV
		Salmonella
		Shigella
		Syphilis
		Measles
		Mumps
		AIDS
		Rubella
		Tuberculosis
		Chickenpox
		Gonorrhea

Leading causes of death in the United States by age

Infants	Congenital anomalies, sudden infant death syndrome, respiratory distress syndrome.
Age 1–14	Injuries, cancer, congenital anomalies, homicide, heart disease.
Age 15–24	Injuries, homicide, suicide.
Age 25–64	Cancer, heart disease, injuries.
Age 65+	Heart disease, cancer, stroke.

Medicare and Medicaid	Medicare and Medicaid—federal programs that originated from amendments to the Social Security Act.	MedicarE is for Elderly. MedicaiD is for Destitute.
	Medicare is available to patients > 65 years of age, < 65 with certain disabilities, and those with ESRD.	
	Medicare parts:	
	Part A = inpatient care in hospitals, skilled nursing, hospice, and home health care.	
	Part B = outpatient care, doctors' services, PT/OT.	
	Part C = combination of A & B.	
	Part D = stand-alone prescription drug coverage.	
	Medicaid is federal and state health assistance for people with very low income.	

Core ethical principles

Autonomy	Obligation to respect patients as individuals and to honor their preferences in medical care.
Beneficence	Physicians have a special ethical (fiduciary) duty to act in the patient's best interest. May conflict with autonomy. If the patient can make an informed decision, ultimately the patient has the right to decide.
Nonmaleficence	"Do no harm." However, if the benefits of an intervention outweigh the risks, a patient may make an informed decision to proceed (most surgeries fall into this category).
Justice	To treat persons fairly.

Informed consent

Legally requires:
1. Discussion of pertinent information
2. Patient's agreement to the plan of care
3. Freedom from coercion

Patients must understand the risks, benefits, and alternatives, which include no intervention.

Exceptions to informed consent

1. Patient lacks decision-making capacity or is legally incompetent
2. Implied consent in an emergency
3. Therapeutic privilege—withholding information when disclosure would severely harm the patient or undermine informed decision-making capacity
4. Waiver—patient waives the right of informed consent

Consent for minors

A minor is any person < 18 years of age. Parental consent must be obtained unless minor is emancipated (e.g., is married, is self-supporting, has children, or is in military). However, parental consent is **not** required in emergency situations; when prescribing contraceptives; or in treatment involving STDs, medical care during pregnancy, or the management of drug addiction.

Decision-making capacity

1. Patient makes and communicates a choice
2. Patient is informed
3. Decision remains stable over time
4. Decision is consistent with patient's values and goals
5. Decision is not a result of delusions or hallucinations

The patient's family cannot require that a doctor withhold information from the patient.

Advance directives

Instructions given by a patient in anticipation of the need for a medical decision.

Oral advance directive—incapacitated patient's prior oral statements commonly used as guide. Problems arise from variance in interpretation. If patient was informed, directive is specific, patient made a choice, and decision was repeated over time, the oral directive is more valid.

Living will (written advance directive)—describes treatments the patient wishes to receive or not receive if he/she becomes incapacitated and cannot communicate about treatment decisions. Usually, patient directs physician to withhold or withdraw life-sustaining treatment if he/she develops a terminal disease or enters a persistent vegetative state.

Durable power of attorney—patient designates a surrogate to make medical decisions in the event that he/she loses decision-making capacity. Patient may also specify decisions in clinical situations. Surrogate retains power unless revoked by patient. More flexible than a living will.

Confidentiality	Confidentiality respects patient privacy and autonomy. Disclosing information to family and friends should be guided by what the patient would want. The patient may waive the right to confidentiality (e.g., insurance companies).

Exceptions to confidentiality	1. Potential harm to others is serious
	2. Likelihood of harm to self is great
	3. No alternative means exist to warn or to protect those at risk
	4. Physicians can take steps to prevent harm
	Examples include:
	1. Infectious diseases—physicians may have a duty to warn public officials and identifiable people at risk
	2. The Tarasoff decision—law requiring physician to directly inform and protect potential victim from harm; may involve breach of confidentiality
	3. Child and/or elder abuse
	4. Impaired automobile drivers
	5. Suicidal/homicidal patients

Malpractice	Civil suit under negligence requires:	The **4 D's.**
	1. Physician had a duty to the patient (**D**uty)	Unlike a criminal suit, in which the burden of proof is "beyond a reasonable doubt," the burden of proof in a malpractice suit is "more likely than not."
	2. Physician breached that duty (**D**ereliction)	
	3. Patient suffers harm (**D**amage)	
	4. The breach of the duty was what caused the harm (**D**irect)	
	The most common factor leading to litigation is poor communication between physician and patient.	

Ethical situations

Situation	Appropriate response
Patient is noncompliant.	Attempt to identify the patient's reason for noncompliance; determine patient's willingness to change harmful behavior or undergo a necessary procedure; do not attempt to coerce the patient into complying or refer the patient to another physician.
Patient continues to smoke, believing that cigarettes are good for him.	Ask how the patient feels about his/her smoking. Offer advice on cessation if the patient seems willing to make an effort to quit.
Patient desires an unnecessary procedure.	Attempt to understand why the patient wants the procedure. Do not refuse to see the patient or refer him/her to another physician. Address the underlying concerns. Avoid performing unnecessary procedures.
Patient has difficulty taking medications.	Provide written instructions; attempt to simplify treatment regimens.
Family members ask for information about patient's prognosis.	Avoid discussing issues with relatives without the permission of the patient.
A child wishes to know more about his illness.	Ask what the parents have told the child about his/her illness. Parents of a child decide what information can be relayed about the illness.
A 17-year-old girl is pregnant and requests an abortion.	Many states require parental notification or consent for minors for an abortion. Unless she is at medical risk, do not advise a patient to have an abortion regardless of her age or the condition of the fetus.
A 15-year-old girl is pregnant and wants to keep the child. Her parents want you to tell her to give the child up for adoption.	The patient retains the right to make decisions regarding her child, even if her parents disagree. Provide information to the teenager about the practical issues of caring for a baby. Discuss the options, if requested. Encourage discussion between the teenager and her parents to reach the best decision.
A terminally ill patient requests physician assistance in ending his life.	In the overwhelming majority of states, refuse involvement in any form of physician-assisted suicide. Physicians may, however, prescribe medically appropriate analgesics that coincidentally shorten the patient's life.
Patient is suicidal.	Assess the seriousness of the threat; if it is serious, suggest that the patient remain in the hospital voluntarily; patient can be hospitalized involuntarily if he/she refuses.
Patient states that he finds you attractive.	Ask direct, closed-ended questions and use a chaperone if necessary. Romantic relationships with patients are **never** appropriate. Never say, "There can be no relationship while you are a patient," because it implies that a relationship may be possible if the individual is no longer a patient.
A middle-aged married woman who had a mastectomy says she feels "ugly" when she undresses at night.	Find out why the patient feels this way. Do not offer falsely reassuring statements (e.g., "You still look good.").
Patient is angry about the amount of time he spent in the waiting room.	Acknowledge the patient's anger, but do not take a patient's anger personally. Apologize for any inconvenience. Stay away from efforts to explain the delay.
Patient is upset with the way he was treated by another doctor.	Suggest that the patient speak directly to that physician regarding his concerns. If the problem is with a member of the office staff, tell the patient you will speak to that individual.
A drug company offers a "referral fee" for every patient a physician enrolls in a study.	Eligible patients who may benefit from the study may be enrolled, but it is never acceptable for a physician to receive compensation from a drug company.

Apgar score	Assessment of newborn health via a 10-point scale evaluated at 1 minute and 5 minutes.		
	0 points	**1 point**	**2 points**
Appearance	Blue	Trunk pink	All pink
Pulse	0	< 100/min	> 100/min
Grimace	None	Grimace	Grimace + cough
Activity	Limp	Some	Active
Respiration	None	Irregular	Regular

Low birth weight	Defined as < 2500 g. Associated with greater incidence of physical and emotional problems. Caused by prematurity or intrauterine growth retardation. Complications include infections, respiratory distress syndrome, necrotizing enterocolitis, intraventricular hemorrhage, and persistent fetal circulation.

Early developmental milestones

Approximate age	Motor milestone	Cognitive/social milestone
Infant		
Birth–3 mo	Rooting reflex	Orients to voice
3 mo	Holds head up, Moro reflex disappears	Social smile
7–9 mo	Sits alone, crawls	Stranger anxiety
15 mo	Walks, Babinski disappears	Few words, separation anxiety
Toddler		
12–24 mo	Climbs stairs; stacks 3 blocks at 1 year, 6 blocks at 2 years (number of blocks stacked = age in years × 3)	Object permanence; 200 words and 2-word sentences at age 2
24–36 mo		Core gender identity, parallel play
Preschool		
30–36 mo	Stacks 9 blocks	Toilet training ("**pee** at age **3**")
3 yrs	Rides tricycle (rides **3**-cycle at age **3**); copies line or circle drawing	900 words and complete sentences
4 yrs	Simple drawings (stick figure), hops on 1 foot	Cooperative play, imaginary friends, grooms self, brushes teeth, buttons and zips

Tanner stages of sexual development	1. Childhood
	2. Pubic hair appears (adrenarche); breasts enlarge
	3. Pubic hair darkens and becomes curly; penis size/length ↑
	4. Penis width ↑, darker scrotal skin, development of glans, raised areolae
	5. Adult; areolae are no longer raised

Changes in the elderly	1. Sexual changes:
	   Men—slower erection/ejaculation, longer refractory period
	   Women—vaginal shortening, thinning, and dryness
	2. Sleep patterns— ↓ REM, slow-wave sleep; ↑ latency and awakenings
	3. ↓ incidence of psychiatric disorders
	4. ↑ suicide rate (males 65–74 years of age have the highest suicide rate in the United States)
	5. ↓ vision, hearing, immune response, bladder control
	6. ↓ renal, pulmonary, GI function
	7. ↓ muscle mass, ↑ fat
		Sexual interest does not ↓.
		Intelligence does not ↓.

Grief	Normal bereavement characterized by shock, denial, guilt, and somatic symptoms. Can last up to 2 months. May experience illusions. Pathologic grief includes excessively intense grief; prolonged grief lasting > 2 months; or grief that is delayed, inhibited, or denied. May experience depressive symptoms, delusions, and hallucinations.	
Kübler-Ross grief stages	Denial, Anger, Bargaining, Grieving (depression), Acceptance. Stages do not necessarily occur in this order, and > 1 stage can be present at once.	Death Arrives Bringing Grave Adjustments.

▶ BEHAVIORAL SCIENCE–PHYSIOLOGY

Stress effects	Stress induces production of free fatty acids, 17-OH corticosteroids (immunosuppression), lipids, cholesterol, catecholamines; affects water absorption, muscular tonicity, gastrocolic reflex, and mucosal circulation.	
Sexual dysfunction	Differential diagnosis includes: 1. Drugs (e.g., antihypertensives, neuroleptics, SSRIs, ethanol) 2. Diseases (e.g., depression, diabetes) 3. Psychological (e.g., performance anxiety)	
Body-mass index (BMI)	BMI is a measure of weight adjusted for height. $$BMI = \frac{\text{weight in kg}}{(\text{height in meters})^2}$$	< 18.5 underweight; 18.5–24.9 normal; 25.0–29.9 overweight; > 30.0 obese; > 40.0 morbidly obese.

Sleep stages

Stage (% of total sleep time in young adults)	Description	EEG waveform
	Awake (eyes open), alert, active mental concentration	Beta (highest frequency, lowest amplitude)
	Awake (eyes closed)	Alpha
1 (5%)	Light sleep	Theta
2 (45%)	Deeper sleep; bruxism	Sleep spindles and K complexes
3–4 (25%)	Deepest, non-REM sleep; sleepwalking; night terrors; bedwetting (slow-wave sleep)	Delta (lowest frequency, highest amplitude)
REM (25%)	Dreaming, loss of motor tone, possibly a memory processing function, erections, ↑ brain O_2 use	Beta
		At night, **BATS** Drink **B**lood.

1. Serotonergic predominance of raphe nucleus key to initiating sleep
2. NE reduces REM sleep
3. Extraocular movements during REM due to activity of PPRF (paramedian pontine reticular formation/conjugate gaze center)
4. REM sleep having the same EEG pattern as while awake and alert has spawned the terms "paradoxical sleep" and "desynchronized sleep"
5. Imipramine is used to treat enuresis because it ↓ stage 4 sleep
6. Alcohol, benzodiazepines, and barbiturates are associated with reduced REM and delta sleep
7. Benzodiazepines are useful for night terrors and sleepwalking

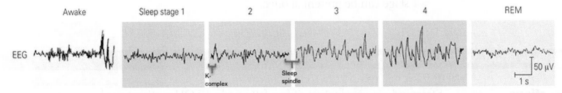

(Adapted, with permission, from Barrett KE et al. *Gonong's Review of Medical Physiology*, 23rd ed. New York: McGraw-Hill, 2010, Fig 15–7.)

REM sleep	↑ and variable pulse, REM, ↑ and variable blood pressure, penile/clitoral tumescence. Occurs every 90 minutes; duration ↑ through the night. ACh is the principal neurotransmitter involved in REM sleep.	REM sleep is like sex: ↑ pulse, penile/clitoral tumescence, ↓ with age.
Sleep patterns of depressed patients	Patients with depression typically have the following changes in their sleep stages: 1. ↓ slow-wave sleep 2. ↓ REM latency 3. ↑ REM early in sleep cycle 4. ↑ total REM sleep 5. Repeated nighttime awakenings 6. Early-morning awakening (important screening question)	

Narcolepsy	Disordered regulation of sleep-wake cycles; primary characteristic is excessive daytime sleepiness. May include hypnagogic (just before sleep) or hypnopompic (just before awakening) hallucinations. The patient's nocturnal and narcoleptic sleep episodes start off with REM sleep. **Cataplexy** (loss of all muscle tone following a strong emotional stimulus) in some patients. Strong genetic component. Treat with stimulants (e.g., amphetamines, modafinil) and sodium oxybate (GHB).
Circadian rhythm	Driven by suprachiasmatic nucleus (SCN) of hypothalamus; controls ACTH, prolactin, melatonin, nocturnal NE release. SCN → NE release → pineal gland → melatonin. SCN is regulated by environment (i.e., light).
Sleep terror disorder	Periods of terror with screaming in the middle of the night; most common in children; occurs during slow-wave sleep; no memory of arousal.

NOTES

Biochemistry

"Biochemistry is the study of carbon compounds that crawl."
—Mike Adams

"We think we have found the basic mechanism by which life comes from life."
—Francis H. C. Crick

▶ Molecular

▶ Cellular

▶ Laboratory Techniques

▶ Genetics

▶ Nutrition

▶ Metabolism

This high-yield material includes molecular biology, genetics, cell biology, and principles of metabolism (especially vitamins, cofactors, minerals, and single-enzyme-deficiency diseases). When studying metabolic pathways, emphasize important regulatory steps and enzyme deficiencies that result in disease, as well as reactions targeted by pharmacologic interventions. For example, understanding the defect in Lesch-Nyhan syndrome and its clinical consequences is higher yield than memorizing every intermediate in the purine salvage pathway. Do not spend time on hard-core organic chemistry, mechanisms, and physical chemistry. Detailed chemical structures are infrequently tested; however, many structures have been included here to help students learn reactions and the important enzymes involved. Familiarity with the biochemical techniques that have medical relevance—such as enzyme-linked immunosorbent assay (ELISA), immunoelectrophoresis, Southern blotting, and PCR—is useful. Beware if you placed out of your medical school's biochemistry class, for the emphasis of the test differs from that of many undergraduate courses. Review the related biochemistry when studying pharmacology or genetic diseases as a way to reinforce and integrate the material.

Chromatin structure

DNA exists in the condensed, chromatin form in order to fit into the nucleus. Negatively charged DNA loops twice around positively charged histone octamer (2 sets of H2A, H2B, H3, and H4) to form nucleosome "bead." Octamer subunits consist primarily of lysine and arginine amino acids (postively charged). H1 ties nucleosome beads together in a string.

In mitosis, DNA condenses to form mitotic chromosomes.

Think of "**beads on a string.**"

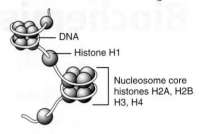

H1 is the only histone that is not in the nucleosome core.

HeteroChromatin = Highly Condensed.

Eu = true, "truly transcribed."

Heterochromatin — Condensed, transcriptionally inactive, sterically inaccessible.

Euchromatin — Less condensed, transcriptionally active, sterically accessible.

Nucleotides

Purines (**A, G**)—2 rings.
Pyrimidines (**C, T, U**)—1 ring.
Guanine has a ketone. Thymine has a methyl.
  Deamination of cytosine makes uracil.

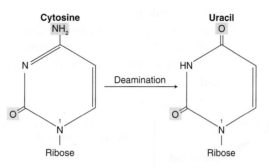

Uracil found in RNA; thymine in DNA.
G-C bond (3 H-bonds) stronger than A-T bond
  (2 H-bonds). ↑ G-C content → ↑ melting
  temperature.

PURe As Gold: **PUR**ines.
CUT the **PY** (pie):
  PYrimidines.

THYmine has a me**THY**l.

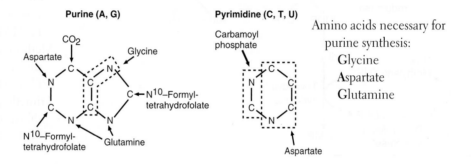

Amino acids necessary for
  purine synthesis:
    Glycine
    Aspartate
    Glutamine

Nucleoside = base + ribose.
Nucleotides = base + ribose + phosphate; linked by
  3'-5' phosphodiester bond.

De novo pyrimidine and purine synthesis

Purines are made from IMP precursor.

Pyrimidines are made from orotate precursor, with PRPP added later.

Ribonucleotides are synthesized first and are converted to deoxyribonucleotides by ribonucleotide reductase.

Carbamoyl phosphate is involved in 2 metabolic pathways: de novo pyrimidine synthesis and the urea cycle. Ornithine transcarbamoylase deficiency (urea cycle) leads to an accumulation of carbamoyl phosphate, which is then converted to orotic acid.

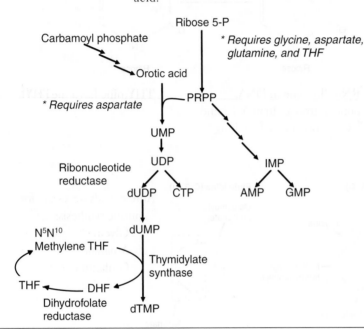

Various antineoplastic and antibiotic drugs function by interfering with nucleotide synthesis.

Hydroxyurea inhibits ribonucleotide reductase.

6-mercaptopurine (6-MP) blocks de novo purine synthesis.

5-fluorouracil (5-FU) inhibits thymidylate synthase (↓ dTMP).

Methotrexate (MTX) inhibits dihydrofolate reductase (↓ dTMP).

Trimethoprim inhibits bacterial dihydrofolate reductase (↓ dTMP).

Orotic aciduria

Inability to convert orotic acid to UMP (de novo pyrimidine synthesis pathway) due to defect in either orotic acid phosphoribosyltransferase or orotidine 5′-phosphate decarboxylase. Autosomal recessive.

Findings: ↑ orotic acid in urine, megaloblastic anemia (does not improve with administration of vitamin B_{12} or folic acid), failure to thrive. No hyperammonemia (vs. OTC deficiency—↑ orotic acid with hyperammonemia).

Treatment: oral uridine administration.

Purine salvage deficiencies

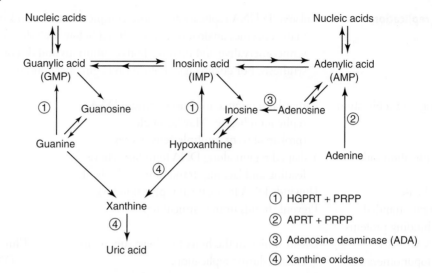

① HGPRT + PRPP
② APRT + PRPP
③ Adenosine deaminase (ADA)
④ Xanthine oxidase

Adenosine deaminase deficiency	Excess ATP and dATP imbalances nucleotide pool via feedback inhibition of ribonucleotide reductase → prevents DNA synthesis and thus ↓ lymphocyte count. One of the major causes of SCID.	**SCID**—severe combined immunodeficiency disease. **SCID** happens to **kids** (e.g., "bubble boy"). 1st disease to be treated by experimental human gene therapy.
Lesch-Nyhan syndrome	Defective purine salvage owing to absence of **HGPRT**, which converts hypoxanthine to IMP and guanine to GMP. Results in excess uric acid production. Findings: retardation, self-mutilation, aggression, hyperuricemia, gout, choreoathetosis.	X-linked recessive. **H**e's **G**ot **P**urine **R**ecovery **T**rouble.

Genetic code features

		Exceptions
Unambiguous	Each codon specifies only 1 amino acid.	
Degenerate/ redundant	More than 1 codon may code for the same amino acid.	Methionine encoded by only 1 codon (AUG).
Commaless, nonoverlapping	Read from a fixed starting point as a continuous sequence of bases.	Some viruses.
Universal	Genetic code is conserved throughout evolution.	Mitochondria, archaebacteria, *Mycoplasma*, and some yeasts.

Mutations in DNA

Silent	Same aa, often base change in 3rd position of codon (tRNA wobble).	Severity of damage: nonsense > missense > silent.
Missense	Changed aa (conservative—new aa is similar in chemical structure).	
Nonsense	Change resulting in early **stop** codon.	**Stop** the **nonsense!**
Frame shift	Change resulting in misreading of all nucleotides downstream, usually resulting in a truncated, nonfunctional protein.	

HIGH-YIELD PRINCIPLES

BIOCHEMISTRY

DNA replication   Eukaryotic DNA replication is more complex than the prokaryotic process but uses many enzymes analogous to those listed below. In both cases, DNA replication is semiconservative and involves both continuous and discontinuous (Okazaki fragment) synthesis. For eukaryotes, replication begins at a consensus sequence of base pairs.

Origin of replication	Particular sequence in genome where DNA replication begins. May be single (prokaryotes) or multiple (eukaryotes).	
Replication fork	Y-shaped region along DNA template where leading and lagging strands are synthesized.	
Helicase	Unwinds DNA template at replication fork.	
Single-stranded binding proteins	Prevent strands from reannealing.	
DNA topoisomerases	Create a nick in the helix to relieve supercoils created during replication.	**Fluoroquinolones**—inhibit DNA gyrase (specific prokaryotic topoisomerase).
Primase	Makes an RNA primer on which DNA polymerase III can initiate replication.	
DNA polymerase III	Prokaryotic only. Elongates leading strand by adding deoxynucleotides to the 3′ end. Elongates lagging strand until it reaches primer of preceding fragment. 3′ → 5′ exonuclease activity "proofreads" each added nucleotide.	DNA polymerase III has 5′ → 3′ synthesis and proofreads with 3′ → 5′ exonuclease.
DNA polymerase I	Prokaryotic only. Degrades RNA primer and fills in the gap with DNA.	DNA polymerase I excises RNA primer with 5′ → 3′ exonuclease.
DNA ligase	Seals.	

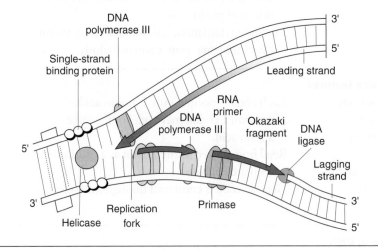

DNA repair

Single strand

Nucleotide excision repair	Specific endonucleases release the oligonucleotide-containing damaged bases; DNA polymerase and ligase fill and reseal the gap, respectively.	Mutated in **xeroderma pigmentosum** (dry skin with melanoma and other cancers, "children of the night"), which prevents repair of thymidine dimers.
Base excision repair	Specific glycosylases recognize and remove damaged bases, AP endonuclease cuts DNA at apyrimidinic site, empty sugar is removed, and the gap is filled and resealed.	
Mismatch repair	Unmethylated, newly synthesized string is recognized, mismatched nucleotides are removed, and the gap is filled and resealed.	Mutated in **hereditary nonpolyposis colorectal cancer** (HNPCC).

Double strand

Nonhomologous end joining	Brings together 2 ends of DNA fragments. No requirement for homology.	

DNA/RNA/protein synthesis direction	DNA and RNA are both synthesized 5′ → 3′. Remember that the 5′ of the incoming nucleotide bears the triphosphate (energy source for bond). The triphosphate bond is the target of the 3′ hydroxyl attack. Drugs blocking DNA replication often have modified 3′ OH, preventing addition of the next nucleotide (aka "chain termination").	mRNA is read 5′ to 3′. Protein synthesis is N to C.

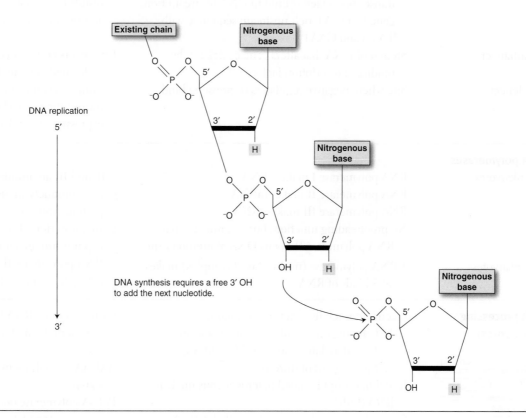

DNA replication

5′

3′

DNA synthesis requires a free 3′ OH to add the next nucleotide.

Types of RNA

rRNA is the most abundant type.
mRNA is the longest type.
tRNA is the smallest type.

Rampant, **M**assive, **T**iny.

Start and stop codons

mRNA start codons	AUG (or rarely GUG).	**AUG** in**AUG**urates protein synthesis.
Eukaryotes	Codes for methionine, which may be removed before translation is completed.	
Prokaryotes	Codes for formyl-methionine (f-Met).	
mRNA stop codons	UGA, UAA, UAG.	UGA = U Go Away.
		UAA = U Are Away.
		UAG = U Are Gone.

Functional organization of the gene

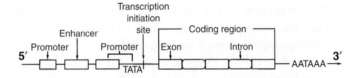

Regulation of gene expression

Promoter	Site where RNA polymerase and multiple other transcription factors bind to DNA upstream from gene locus (AT-rich upstream sequence with TATA and CAAT boxes).	Promoter mutation commonly results in dramatic ↓ in amount of gene transcribed.
Enhancer	Stretch of DNA that alters gene expression by binding transcription factors.	Enhancers and silencers may be located close to, far from, or even within (in an intron) the gene whose expression it regulates.
Silencer	Site where negative regulators (repressors) bind.	

RNA polymerases

Eukaryotes	RNA polymerase I makes **r**RNA. RNA polymerase II makes **m**RNA. RNA polymerase III makes **t**RNA. No proofreading function, but can initiate chains. RNA polymerase II opens DNA at promoter site.	I, II, and III are numbered as their products are used in protein synthesis. α-amanitin (found in death cap mushrooms) inhibits RNA polymerase II. Causes liver failure if ingested.
Prokaryotes	1 RNA polymerase (multisubunit complex) makes all 3 kinds of RNA.	

RNA processing (eukaryotes)

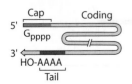

Occurs in nucleus. After transcription:
1. Capping on 5′ end (7-methylguanosine)
2. Polyadenylation on 3′ end (≈ 200 A's)
3. Splicing out of introns

Initial transcript is called heterogeneous nuclear RNA (hnRNA).

Capped and tailed transcript is called mRNA.

Only processed RNA is transported out of the nucleus.

AAUAAA = polyadenylation signal.

Poly-A polymerase does not require a template.

Splicing of pre-mRNA

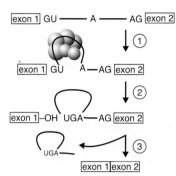

Pre-mRNA splicing occurs in eukaryotes.

1—Primary transcript combines with snRNPs and other proteins to form spliceosome.

2—Lariat-shaped (looped) intermediate is generated.

3—Lariat is released to remove intron precisely and join 2 exons.

Patients with lupus make antibodies to spliceosomal snRNPs.

Introns vs. exons

Exons contain the actual genetic information coding for protein.

Introns are intervening noncoding segments of DNA.

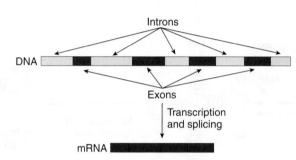

INtrons are **IN**tervening sequences and stay **IN** the nucleus, whereas **EX**ons **EX**it and are **EX**pressed.

Different exons can be combined by **alternative splicing** to make unique proteins in different tissues (e.g., β-thalassemia mutations).

tRNA

Structure | 75–90 nucleotides, 2° structure, cloverleaf form, anticodon end is opposite 3′ aminoacyl end. All tRNAs, both eukaryotic and prokaryotic, have CCA at 3′ end along with a high percentage of chemically modified bases. The amino acid is covalently bound to the 3′ end of the tRNA.

Charging | Aminoacyl-tRNA synthetase (1 per aa, "matchmaker," uses ATP) scrutinizes aa before and after it binds to tRNA. If incorrect, bond is hydrolyzed. The aa-tRNA bond has energy for formation of peptide bond. A mischarged tRNA reads usual codon but inserts wrong amino acid. | Aminoacyl-tRNA synthetase and binding of charged tRNA to the codon are responsible for accuracy of amino acid selection. **Tetracyclines** bind 30S subunit, preventing attachment of aminoacyl-tRNA.

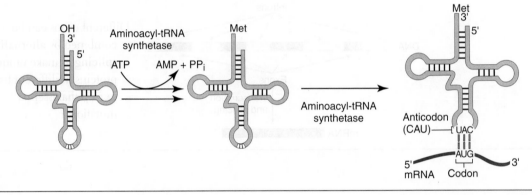

tRNA wobble | Accurate base pairing is required only in the first 2 nucleotide positions of an mRNA codon, so codons differing in the 3rd "wobble" position may code for the same tRNA/amino acid (due to degeneracy of genetic code).

Protein synthesis

Initiation	Activated by GTP hydrolysis, initiation factors (eIFs) help assemble the 40S ribosomal subunit with the initiator tRNA and are released when the mRNA and the ribosomal subunit assemble with the complex.	Eukaryotes: 40S + 60S → 80S (Even). PrOkaryotes: 30S + 50S → 70S (Odd). ATP—tRNA Activation (charging). GTP—tRNA Gripping and Going places (translocation).
Elongation	1. Aminoacyl-tRNA binds to A site (except for initiator methionine) 2. Ribosomal rRNA (aka "ribozyme") catalyzes peptide bond formation, transfers growing polypeptide to amino acid in A site 3. Ribosome advances 3 nucleotides toward 3′ end of RNA, moving peptidyl RNA to P site (translocation)	Think of "going APE": A site = incoming Aminoacyl tRNA. P site = accommodates growing Peptide. E site = holds Empty tRNA as it Exits.
Termination	Stop codon is recognized by release factor, and completed protein is released from ribosome.	Many antibiotics act as protein synthesis inhibitors. **Aminoglycosides** inhibit formation of the initiation complex and cause misreading of mRNA. **Chloramphenicol** inhibits 50S peptidyltransferase. **Macrolides** and **clindamycin** bind 50S, blocking translocation.

Ribosome

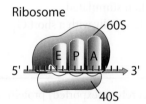

Posttranslational modifications

Trimming	Removal of N- or C-terminal propeptides from zymogens to generate mature proteins.
Covalent alterations	Phosphorylation, glycosylation, and hydroxylation.
Proteasomal degradation	Attachment of ubiquitin to defective proteins to tag them for breakdown.

Cell cycle phases

Checkpoints control transitions between phases of cell cycle. This process is regulated by cyclins, CDKs, and tumor suppressors. Mitosis (shortest phase): prophase-metaphase-anaphase-telophase. G_1 and G_0 are of variable duration.

Regulation of cell cycle

CDKs	Cyclin-dependent kinases; constitutive and inactive.	G = Gap or Growth.
Cyclins	Regulatory proteins that control cell cycle events; phase specific; activate CDKs.	S = Synthesis.
Cyclin-CDK complexes	Must be both activated and inactivated for cell cycle to progress.	
Tumor suppressors	Rb and p53 normally inhibit G_1-to-S progression; mutations in these genes result in unrestrained growth.	

Cell types

Permanent	Remain in G_0, regenerate from stem cells.	Neurons, skeletal and cardiac muscle, RBCs.
Stable (quiescent)	Enter G_1 from G_0 when stimulated.	Hepatocytes, lymphocytes.
Labile	Never go to G_0, divide rapidly with a short G_1.	Bone marrow, gut epithelium, skin, hair follicles.

Rough endoplasmic reticulum (RER)

Site of synthesis of secretory (exported) proteins and of N-linked oligosaccharide addition to many proteins.

Nissl bodies (RER in neurons)—synthesize enzymes (e.g., ChAT) and peptide neurotransmitters.

Free ribosomes—unattached to any membrane; site of synthesis of cytosolic and organellar proteins.

Mucus-secreting goblet cells of the small intestine and antibody-secreting plasma cells are rich in RER.

Smooth endoplasmic reticulum (SER)

Site of steroid synthesis and detoxification of drugs and poisons.

Liver hepatocytes and steroid hormone–producing cells of the adrenal cortex are rich in SER.

Golgi apparatus

1. Distribution center of proteins and lipids from ER to the plasma membrane, lysosomes, and secretory vesicles
2. Modifies N-oligosaccharides on asparagine
3. Adds O-oligosaccharides to serine and threonine residues
4. Addition of mannose-6-phosphate to specific lysosomal proteins → targets the protein to the lysosome
5. Proteoglycan assembly from core proteins
6. Sulfation of sugars in proteoglycans and of selected tyrosine on proteins

Vesicular trafficking proteins:
COPI: retrograde, Golgi → ER.
COPII: anterograde, RER → cis-Golgi.
Clathrin: trans-Golgi → lysosomes, plasma membrane → endosomes (receptor-mediated endocytosis).

I-cell disease (inclusion cell disease)—inherited lysosomal storage disorder; failure of addition of mannose-6-phosphate to lysosome proteins (enzymes are secreted outside the cell instead of being targeted to the lysosome). Results in coarse facial features, clouded corneas, restricted joint movement, and high plasma levels of lysosomal enzymes. Often fatal in childhood.

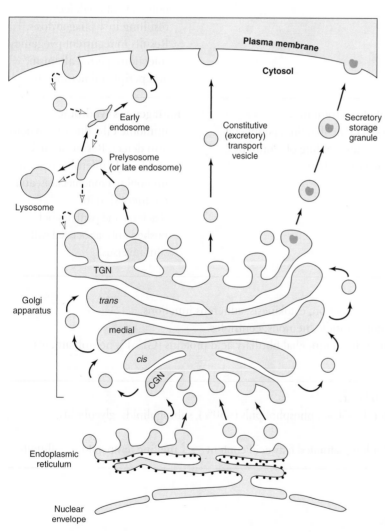

(Reproduced, with permission, from Murray RK et al. *Harper's Illustrated Biochemistry*, 27th ed. New York: McGraw-Hill, 2005: Fig. 45-2.)

Microtubule

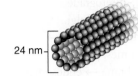

24 nm

Cylindrical structure composed of a helical array of polymerized dimers of α- and β-tubulin. Each dimer has 2 GTP bound. Incorporated into flagella, cilia, mitotic spindles. Grows slowly, collapses quickly. Also involved in slow axoplasmic transport in neurons.

Molecular motor proteins—transport cellular cargo toward opposite ends of microtubule tracks.

    Dynein = retrograde to microtubule (+ → –).

    Kinesin = anterograde to microtubule (– → +).

Drugs that act on microtubules:
1. Mebendazole/thiabendazole (antihelminthic)
2. Griseofulvin (antifungal)
3. Vincristine/vinblastine (anti-cancer)
4. Paclitaxel (anti–breast cancer)
5. Colchicine (anti-gout)

Chédiak-Higashi syndrome —microtubule polymerization defect resulting in ↓ phagocytosis. Results in recurrent pyogenic infections, partial albinism, and peripheral neuropathy.

Cilia structure

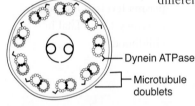

Dynein ATPase

Microtubule doublets

9 + 2 arrangement of microtubules.

Axonemal dynein—ATPase that links peripheral 9 doublets and causes bending of cilium by differential sliding of doublets.

Kartagener's syndrome— immotile cilia due to a dynein arm defect. Results in male and female infertility (sperm immotile), bronchiectasis, and recurrent sinusitis (bacteria and particles not pushed out); associated with situs inversus.

Cytoskeletal elements

Actin and myosin — Microvilli, muscle contraction, cytokinesis, adherens junctions.

Microtubule — Cilia, flagella, mitotic spindle, neurons, centrioles.

Intermediate filaments — Vimentin, desmin, cytokeratin, glial fibrillary acid proteins (GFAP), neurofilaments.

Plasma membrane composition

Asymmetric lipid bilayer.

Contains cholesterol (~50%), phospholipids (~50%), sphingolipids, glycolipids, and proteins.

High cholesterol or long saturated fatty acid content → ↑ melting temperature, ↓ fluidity.

Immunohistochemical stains

Stain	Cell type
Vimentin	Connective tissue
Desmin	Muscle
Cytokeratin	Epithelial cells
GFAP	Neuroglia
Neurofilaments	Neurons

Sodium pump

Na$^+$-K$^+$ ATPase is located in the plasma membrane with ATP site on cytoplasmic side. For each ATP consumed, 3 Na$^+$ go out and 2 K$^+$ come in. During cycle, pump is phosphorylated.

Ouabain inhibits by binding to K$^+$ site.
Cardiac glycosides (digoxin and digitoxin) directly inhibit the Na$^+$-K$^+$ ATPase, which leads to indirect inhibition of Na$^+$/Ca^{2+} exchange. ↑ [Ca^{2+}]$_i$ → ↑ cardiac contractility.

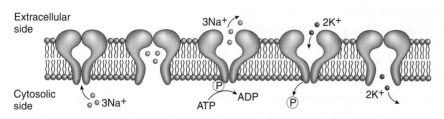

Extracellular side

3Na$^+$ 2K$^+$

Cytosolic side   3Na$^+$ ATP   ADP   P   2K$^+$

Collagen

Most abundant protein in the human body. Extensively modified.
Organizes and strengthens extracellular matrix.
Type I (90%)—**B**one, **S**kin, **T**endon, dentin, fascia, cornea, late wound repair.
Type II—**C**artilage (including hyaline), vitreous body, nucleus pulposus.
Type III (**R**eticulin)—skin, blood vessels, uterus, fetal tissue, granulation tissue.
Type IV—**B**asement membrane or basal lamina.

Be (**S**o **T**otally) **C**ool, **R**ead **B**ooks.

Type I: BONE.

Type II: car**TWO**lage.

Type IV: Under the **floor** (basement membrane).

Collagen synthesis and structure

Inside fibroblasts

1. Synthesis (RER)

Translation of collagen α chains (**preprocollagen**)— usually Gly-X-Y polypeptide (X and Y are proline, hydroxyproline, or hydroxylysine).

2. Hydroxylation (ER)

Hydroxylation of specific proline and lysine residues (requires **vitamin C**).

3. Glycosylation (ER)

Glycosylation of pro-α-chain lysine residues and formation of **procollagen** (triple helix of 3 collagen α chains).

4. Exocytosis

Exocytosis of procollagen into extracellular space.

Outside fibroblasts

5. Proteolytic processing

Cleavage of terminal regions of procollagen transforms it into insoluble **tropocollagen.**

6. Cross-linking

Reinforcement of many staggered tropocollagen molecules by covalent lysine-hydroxylysine cross-linkage (by lysyl oxidase) to make **collagen fibrils.**

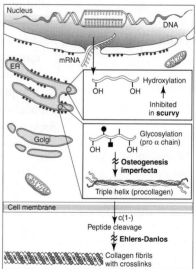

Nucleus   DNA
mRNA
ER
Hydroxylation
OH   OH
Inhibited in **scurvy**
Glycosylation (pro α chain)
OH   OH
Osteogenesis imperfecta
Triple helix (procollagen)
Golgi
Cell membrane
c(1-)
Peptide cleavage
Ehlers-Danlos
Collagen fibrils with crosslinks

Ehlers-Danlos syndrome	Faulty collagen synthesis causing: 1. Hyperextensible skin 2. Tendency to bleed (easy bruising) 3. Hypermobile joints 6 types. Inheritance and severity vary. Can be autosomal dominant or recessive. May be associated with joint dislocation, berry aneurysms, organ rupture.	**Type III** collagen is most frequently affected.

Osteogenesis imperfecta	Genetic bone disorder (brittle bone disease) caused by a variety of gene defects.
	Most common form is autosomal dominant with abnormal type I collagen, causing:
	   1. **Multiple fractures** with minimal trauma; may occur during the birth process
	   2. **Blue sclerae** due to the translucency of the connective tissue over the choroid
	   3. Hearing loss (abnormal middle ear bones)
	   4. Dental imperfections due to lack of dentin
		May be confused with child abuse.
		Type II is fatal in utero or in the neonatal period.
		Incidence is 1:10,000 (see Image 90).

Alport's syndrome	Due to a variety of gene defects resulting in abnormal type IV collagen. Most common form is X-linked recessive. Characterized by progressive hereditary nephritis and deafness. May be associated with ocular disturbances.	Type IV collagen is an important structural component of the basement membrane of the kidney, ears, and eyes.
Elastin	Stretchy protein within lungs, large arteries, elastic ligaments, vocal cords, ligamenta flava (connect vertebrae → relaxed and stretched conformations). Rich in proline and glycine, nonglycosylated forms. Tropoelastin with fibrillin scaffolding. Broken down by elastase, which is normally inhibited by α_1-antitrypsin.	**Marfan's syndrome**—caused by a defect in fibrillin. **Emphysema**—can be caused by α_1-antitrypsin deficiency, resulting in excess elastase activity.

Polymerase chain reaction (PCR)	Molecular biology laboratory procedure used to amplify a desired fragment of DNA. Steps:

1. Denaturation—DNA is denatured by heating to generate 2 separate strands
2. Annealing—during cooling, excess premade DNA primers anneal to a specific sequence on each strand to be amplified
3. Elongation—heat-stable DNA polymerase replicates the DNA sequence following each primer

These steps are repeated multiple times for DNA sequence amplification.

Agarose gel electrophoresis—used for size separation of PCR products (smaller molecules travel further); compared against DNA ladder.

Blotting procedures

Southern blot	A **DNA** sample is electrophoresed on a gel and then transferred to a filter. The filter is then soaked in a denaturant and subsequently exposed to a radiolabeled DNA probe that recognizes and anneals to its complementary strand. The resulting double-stranded labeled piece of DNA is visualized when the filter is exposed to film.	**SNoW DRoP:** Southern = **D**NA Northern = **R**NA Western = **P**rotein
Northern blot	Similar technique, except that Northern blotting involves radiolabeled DNA probe binding to sample **RNA.**	
Western blot	Sample protein is separated via gel electrophoresis and transferred to a filter. Labeled antibody is used to bind to relevant **protein.**	

Microarrays	Thousands of nucleic acid sequences are arranged in grids on glass or silicon. DNA or RNA probes are hybridized to the chip, and a scanner detects the relative amounts of complementary binding.

Used to profile gene expression levels of thousands of genes simultaneously to study certain diseases and treatments. Able to detect single nucleotide polymorphisms (SNPs) for a variety of applications including genotyping, forensic analysis, predisposition to disease, cancer mutations, and genetic linkage analysis.

Enzyme-linked immunosorbent assay (ELISA)

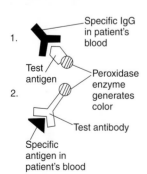

1. Specific IgG in patient's blood
   Test antigen
   Peroxidase enzyme generates color
2. Test antibody
   Specific antigen in patient's blood

A rapid immunologic technique testing for **antigen-antibody** reactivity.

Patient's blood sample is probed with either

1. Test antigen (coupled to color-generating enzyme)—to see if immune system recognizes it; or
2. Test antibody (coupled to color-generating enzyme)—to see if a certain antigen is present

If the target substance is present in the sample, the test solution will have an intense color reaction, indicating a positive test result.

Used in many laboratories to determine whether a particular antibody (e.g., anti-HIV) is present in a patient's blood sample. Both the sensitivity and the specificity of ELISA approach 100%, but both false-positive and false-negative results do occur.

Fluorescence in situ hybridization (FISH)	Fluorescent DNA or RNA probe binds to specific gene site of interest. Used for specific localization of genes and direct visualization of anomalies (e.g., microdeletions) at molecular level (when deletion is too small to be visualized by karyotype). Fluorescence = gene is present; no fluorescence = gene has been deleted.
Cloning methods	Cloning is the production of a recombinant DNA molecule that is self-perpetuating. 1. DNA fragments are inserted into bacterial plasmids that contain antibiotic resistance genes. These plasmids can be selected for by using media containing the antibiotic, and amplified. 2. Restriction enzymes cleave DNA at 4- to 6-bp palindromic sequences, allowing for insertion of a fragment into a plasmid. 3. Tissue mRNA is isolated and exposed to reverse transcriptase, forming a cDNA (lacks introns) library.

Gene expression modifications

Transgenic strategies in mice involve:
1. Random insertion of gene into mouse genome (constitutive)
2. Targeted insertion or deletion of gene through homologous recombination with mouse gene (conditional)

Cre-lox system—Can inducibly manipulate genes at specific developmental points using an antibiotic-controlled promoter (e.g., to study a gene whose deletion causes embryonic death).

RNAi—dsRNA is synthesized that is complementary to the mRNA sequence of interest. When transfected into human cells, dsRNA separates and promotes degradation of target mRNA, knocking down gene expression.

Knock-out = removing a gene.
Knock-in = inserting a gene.

Karyotyping	A process in which metaphase chromosomes are stained, ordered, and numbered according to morphology, size, arm-length ratio, and banding pattern. Can be performed on a sample of blood, bone marrow, amniotic fluid, or placental tissue. Used to diagnose chromosomal imbalances (e.g., autosomal trisomies, sex chromosome disorders).

Genetic terms

Term	Definition	Example
Codominance	Neither of 2 alleles is dominant.	Blood groups (A, B, AB).
Variable expression	Nature and severity of phenotype vary from 1 individual to another.	2 patients with neurofibromatosis type 1 (NF1) may have varying disease severity.
Incomplete penetrance	Not all individuals with a mutant genotype show the mutant phenotype.	–
Pleiotropy	1 gene has > 1 effect on an individual's phenotype.	PKU causes many seemingly unrelated symptoms ranging from mental retardation to hair/ skin changes.
Imprinting	Differences in phenotype depend on whether the mutation is of maternal or paternal origin.	Prader-Willi and Angelman's syndromes.
Anticipation	Severity of disease worsens or age of onset of disease is earlier in succeeding generations.	Huntington's disease.
Loss of heterozygosity	If a patient inherits or develops a mutation in a tumor suppressor gene, the complementary allele must be deleted/mutated before cancer develops. This is not true of oncogenes.	Retinoblastoma.
Dominant negative mutation	Exerts a **dominant effect.** A heterozygote produces a nonfunctional altered protein that also prevents the normal gene product from functioning.	Mutation of Tx factor in its allosteric site. Nonfunctioning mutant can still bind DNA, preventing wild-type Tx factor from binding.
Linkage disequilibrium	Tendency for certain alleles at 2 linked loci to occur together more often than expected by chance. Measured in a population, not in a family, and often varies in different populations.	–
Mosaicism	Occurs when cells in the body have different genetic makeup. Can be a germ-line mosaic, which may produce disease that is not carried by parent's somatic cells.	Lyonization—random X inactivation in females.
Locus heterogeneity	Mutations at different loci can produce the same phenotype.	Marfan's syndrome, MEN 2B, and homocystinuria; all cause marfanoid habitus. Albinism.
Heteroplasmy	Presence of both normal and mutated **mtDNA,** resulting in variable expression in **mitochondrial** inherited disease.	–
Uniparental disomy	Offspring receives 2 copies of a chromosome from 1 parent and no copies from the other parent.	–

Hardy-Weinberg population genetics	If a population is in Hardy-Weinberg equilibrium and p and q are separate alleles, then: Disease prevalence: $p^2 + 2pq + q^2 = 1$ Allele prevalence: $p + q = 1$ $2pq$ = heterozygote prevalence. The prevalence of an X-linked recessive disease in males = q and in females = q^2.	Hardy-Weinberg law assumes: 1. No mutation occurring at the locus 2. No selection for any of the genotypes at the locus 3. Completely random mating 4. No migration
Imprinting	At a single locus, only 1 allele is active; the other is inactive (imprinted/inactivated by methylation). Deletion of the active allele → disease.	Both syndromes due to inactivation or deletion of genes on chromosome 15. Can also occur as a result of uniparental disomy.
Prader-Willi syndrome	Deletion of normally active **P**aternal allele.	Mental retardation, hyperphagia, obesity, hypogonadism, hypotonia.
AngelMan's syndrome	Deletion of normally active **M**aternal allele.	Mental retardation, seizures, ataxia, inappropriate laughter ("happy puppet").

Modes of inheritance

Autosomal dominant

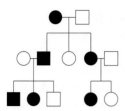

Often due to defects in structural genes. Many generations, both male and female, affected.

Often pleiotropic and, in many cases, present clinically after puberty. Family history crucial to diagnosis.

Autosomal recessive

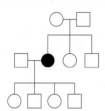

25% of offspring from 2 carrier parents are affected. Often due to enzyme deficiencies. Usually seen in only 1 generation.

Commonly more severe than dominant disorders; patients often present in childhood.

X-linked recessive

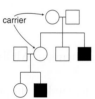

carrier

Sons of heterozygous mothers have a 50% chance of being affected. No male-to-male transmission.

Commonly more severe in males. Heterozygous females may be affected.

X-linked dominant

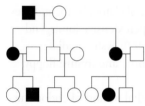

Transmitted through both parents. Either male or female offspring of the affected mother may be affected, while **all** female offspring of the affected father are diseased.

Hypophosphatemic rickets— formerly known as vitamin D–resistant rickets. Inherited disorder resulting in ↑ phosphate wasting at proximal tubule. Results in rickets-like presentation.

Mitochondrial inheritance

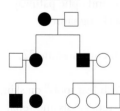

Transmitted only through mother. All offspring of affected females may show signs of disease.

Variable expression in population due to heteroplasmy.

Mitochondrial myopathies, Leber's hereditary optic neuropathy— degeneration of retinal ganglion cells and axons. Leads to acute loss of central vision.

Autosomal-dominant diseases

Achondroplasia	Cell-signaling defect of fibroblast growth factor (FGF) receptor 3. Results in dwarfism; short limbs, but head and trunk are normal size. Associated with advanced paternal age.
Autosomal-dominant polycystic kidney disease (ADPKD)	Formerly known as adult polycystic kidney disease. **Always bilateral,** massive enlargement of kidneys due to multiple large cysts. Patients present with flank pain, hematuria, hypertension, progressive renal failure. 90% of cases are due to mutation in *APKD1* (chromosome **16; 16** letters in "polycystic kidney"). Associated with polycystic liver disease, **berry aneurysms,** mitral valve prolapse. Infantile form is recessive.
Familial adenomatous polyposis	Colon becomes covered with adenomatous polyps after puberty. Progresses to colon cancer unless resected. Deletion on chromosome **5 (*APC* gene); 5** letters in "polyp."
Familial hypercholesterolemia (hyperlipidemia type IIA)	Elevated LDL due to defective or absent LDL receptor. Heterozygotes (1:500) have cholesterol ≈ 300 mg/dL. Homozygotes (very rare) have cholesterol ≈ 700+ mg/dL, severe atherosclerotic disease early in life, and tendon xanthomas (classically in the Achilles tendon); MI may develop before age 20.
Hereditary hemorrhagic telangiectasia (Osler-Weber-Rendu syndrome)	Inherited disorder of blood vessels. Findings: telangiectasia, recurrent epistaxis, skin discolorations, arteriovenous malformations (AVMs).
Hereditary spherocytosis	Spheroid erythrocytes due to spectrin or ankyrin defect; hemolytic anemia; ↑ MCHC. Splenectomy is curative.
Huntington's disease	Findings: depression, progressive dementia, choreiform movements, caudate atrophy, and ↓ levels of GABA and ACh in the brain. Symptoms manifest in affected individuals between the ages of 20 and 50. Gene located on chromosome **4;** trinucleotide repeat disorder: $(CAG)_n$. "Hunting **4** food."
Marfan's syndrome	Fibrillin gene mutation → connective tissue disorder affecting skeleton, heart, and eyes. Findings: tall with long extremities, pectus excavatum, hyperextensive joints, and long, tapering fingers and toes (arachnodactyly; see Image 99); cystic medial necrosis of aorta → aortic incompetence and dissecting aortic aneurysms; floppy mitral valve. Subluxation of lenses.
Multiple endocrine neoplasias (MEN)	Several distinct syndromes (1, 2A, 2B) characterized by familial tumors of endocrine glands, including those of the pancreas, parathyroid, pituitary, thyroid, and adrenal medulla. MEN 2A and 2B are associated with *ret* gene.
Neurofibromatosis type 1 (von Recklinghausen's disease)	Findings: café-au-lait spots, neural tumors, Lisch nodules (pigmented iris hamartomas). Also marked by skeletal disorders (e.g., scoliosis) and optic pathway gliomas. On long arm of chromosome **17; 17** letters in von Recklinghausen.
Neurofibromatosis type 2	Bilateral acoustic schwannomas, juvenile cataracts. *NF2* gene on chromosome **22;** type **2 = 22.**
Tuberous sclerosis	Findings: facial lesions (adenoma sebaceum), hypopigmented "ash leaf spots" on skin, cortical and retinal hamartomas, seizures, mental retardation, renal cysts and renal angiomyolipomas, cardiac rhabdomyomas, ↑ incidence of astrocytomas. Incomplete penetrance, variable presentation.
von Hippel–Lindau disease	Findings: hemangioblastomas of retina/cerebellum/medulla; about half of affected individuals develop multiple bilateral renal cell carcinomas and other tumors. Associated with deletion of *VHL* gene (tumor suppressor) on chromosome 3 (3p). Results in constitutive expression of HIF (transcription factor) and activation of angiogenic growth factors. Von Hippel–Lindau = **3** words for chromosome **3.**

Autosomal-recessive diseases	Albinism, ARPKD (formerly known as infantile polycystic kidney disease), cystic fibrosis, glycogen storage diseases, hemochromatosis, mucopolysaccharidoses (except Hunter's), phenylketonuria, sickle cell anemias, sphingolipidoses (except Fabry's), thalassemias.	
Cystic fibrosis	Autosomal-recessive defect in **CFTR gene** on chromosome 7, commonly deletion of Phe 508. CFTR channel actively secretes Cl^- in lungs and GI tract and actively reabsorbs Cl^- from sweat. Defective Cl^- channel → secretion of abnormally thick mucus that plugs lungs, pancreas, and liver → recurrent pulmonary infections (*Pseudomonas* species and *S. aureus*), chronic bronchitis, bronchiectasis, pancreatic insufficiency (malabsorption and steatorrhea), meconium ileus in newborns. Mutation causes abnormal protein folding, resulting in degradation of channel before reaching cell surface.	Infertility in males due to bilateral absence of vas deferens. Fat-soluble vitamin deficiencies (A, D, E, K). Can present as failure to thrive in infancy. Most common lethal genetic disease of Caucasians. ↑ concentration of Cl^- ions in sweat test is diagnostic. Treatment: N-acetylcysteine to loosen mucous plugs (cleaves disulfide bonds within mucous glycoproteins).
X-linked recessive disorders	Bruton's agammaglobulinemia, Wiskott-Aldrich syndrome, Fabry's disease, G6PD deficiency, Ocular albinism, Lesch-Nyhan syndrome, Duchenne's (and Becker's) muscular dystrophy, Hunter's Syndrome, Hemophilia A and B. Female carriers are rarely affected due to random inactivation of an X chromosome in each cell.	Be Wise, Fool's **GOLD** Heeds Silly Hope.
Muscular dystrophies		
Duchenne's	X-linked frame-shift mutation → deletion of dystrophin gene → accelerated muscle breakdown. Weakness begins in pelvic girdle muscles and progresses superiorly. Pseudohypertrophy of calf muscles due to fibrofatty replacement of muscle; cardiac myopathy. Use of Gowers' maneuver, requiring assistance of the upper extremities to stand up, is characteristic. Onset before 5 years of age.	Duchenne's = Deleted Dystrophin. Dystrophin gene (**DMD**) is the longest known human gene → ↑ rate of spontaneous mutation. Dystrophin helps anchor muscle fibers, primarily in skeletal and cardiac muscle.
Becker's	X-linked mutated dystrophin gene. Less severe than Duchenne's. Onset in adolescence or early adulthood.	Diagnose muscular dystrophies by ↑ CPK and muscle biopsy.
Fragile X syndrome	X-linked defect affecting the methylation and expression of the **FMR1 gene**. Associated with chromosomal breakage. The 2nd most common cause of genetic mental retardation (after Down syndrome). Findings: macro-orchidism (enlarged testes), long face with a large jaw, large everted ears, autism, mitral valve prolapse.	Trinucleotide repeat disorder $(CGG)_n$. Fragile **X** = e**X**tra-large testes, jaw, ears.

Trinucleotide repeat expansion diseases	Huntington's disease, myotonic dystrophy, Friedreich's ataxia, fragile **X** syndrome. Huntington's disease = $(CAG)_n$. MyoTonic dystrophy = $(CTG)_n$. FraGile X syndrome = $(CGG)_n$. Friedreich's ataxia = $(GAA)_n$.	**Try** (trinucleotide) **hunting** for **my fried** eggs (**X**). May show genetic anticipation (disease severity ↑ and age of onset ↓ in successive generations; germline expansion in females).

Autosomal trisomies

Down syndrome (trisomy 21), 1:700	Findings: mental retardation, **flat facies**, prominent **epicanthal folds, simian crease** (see Image 100), gap between 1st 2 toes, duodenal atresia, congenital heart disease (most commonly septum primum–type ASD). Associated with ↑ risk of ALL and Alzheimer's disease (> 35 years of age). 95% of cases due to meiotic nondisjunction of homologous chromosomes (associated with advanced maternal age; from 1:1500 in women < 20 to 1:25 in women > 45). 4% of cases due to robertsonian translocation. 1% of cases due to Down mosaicism (no maternal association).	Drinking age (21). Most common chromosomal disorder and most common cause of congenital mental retardation. Results of pregnancy quad screen: ↓ α-fetoprotein, ↑ β-hCG, ↓ estriol, ↑ inhibin A. Ultrasound shows ↑ nuchal translucency.
Edwards' syndrome (trisomy 18), 1:8000	Findings: severe mental retardation, rocker-bottom feet, **micrognathia** (small jaw), low-set ears, **clenched hands**, prominent occiput, congenital heart disease. Death usually occurs within 1 year of birth.	Election age (18). Most common trisomy resulting in live birth after Down syndrome.
Patau's syndrome (trisomy 13), 1:15,000	Findings: severe mental retardation, rocker-bottom feet, microphthalmia, microcephaly, **cleft lip/ Palate, holoProsencephaly, Polydactyly,** congenital heart disease. Death usually occurs within 1 year of birth.	Puberty (13).

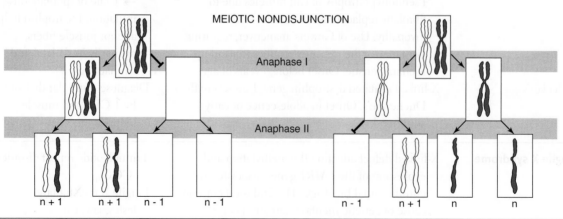

MEIOTIC NONDISJUNCTION

Robertsonian translocation	Nonreciprocal chromosomal translocation that commonly involves chromosome pairs 13, 14, 15, 21, and 22. One of the most common types of translocation. Occurs when the long arms of 2 acrocentric chromosomes (chromosomes with centromeres near their ends) fuse at the centromere and the 2 short arms are lost. Balanced translocations normally do not cause any abnormal phenotype. Unbalanced translocations can result in miscarriage, stillbirth, and chromosomal imbalance (e.g., Down syndrome, Patau's syndrome).	
Cri-du-chat syndrome	Congenital microdeletion of short arm of chromosome 5 (46,XX or XY, 5p–). Findings: microcephaly, moderate to severe mental retardation, high-pitched crying/mewing, epicanthal folds, cardiac abnormalities.	*Cri du chat* = cry of the cat.
Williams syndrome	Congenital microdeletion of long arm of chromosome 7 (deleted region includes elastin gene). Findings: distinctive "elfin" facies, mental retardation, hypercalcemia ($\uparrow$ sensitivity to vitamin D), well-developed verbal skills, extreme friendliness with strangers, cardiovascular problems.	
22q11 deletion syndromes	Variable presentation, including **C**left palate, **A**bnormal facies, **T**hymic aplasia → T-cell deficiency, **C**ardiac defects, **H**ypocalcemia 2° to parathyroid aplasia, due to microdeletion at chromosome 22q11. **DiGeorge syndrome**—thymic, parathyroid, and cardiac defects. **Velocardiofacial syndrome**—palate, facial, and cardiac defects.	CATCH-22. Due to aberrant development of 3rd and 4th branchial pouches.

Vitamins

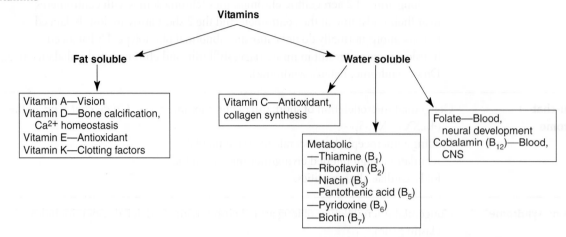

Vitamins: fat soluble	A, D, E, K. Absorption dependent on gut (ileum) and pancreas. Toxicity more common than for water-soluble vitamins, because these accumulate in fat.	Malabsorption syndromes (steatorrhea), such as cystic fibrosis and sprue, or mineral oil intake can cause fat-soluble vitamin deficiencies.
Vitamins: water soluble	B_1 (thiamine: TPP) B_2 (riboflavin: FAD, FMN) B_3 (niacin: NAD^+) B_5 (pantothenic acid: CoA) B_6 (pyridoxine: PLP) B_{12} (cobalamin) C (ascorbic acid) Biotin Folate	All wash out easily from body except B_{12} and folate (stored in liver). B-complex deficiencies often result in dermatitis, glossitis, and diarrhea.

Vitamin A (retinol)

Function	Antioxidant; constituent of visual pigments (retinal); essential for normal differentiation of epithelial cells into specialized tissue (pancreatic cells, mucus-secreting cells). Used to treat measles.	**Retinol** is vitamin **A**, so think **Retin-A** (used topically for wrinkles and acne). Found in liver and leafy vegetables.
Deficiency	Night blindness, dry skin.	
Excess	Arthralgias, fatigue, headaches, skin changes, sore throat, alopecia. Teratogenic (cleft palate, cardiac abnormalities), so a pregnancy test must be done before isotretinoin is prescribed for severe acne.	

Vitamin B$_1$ (thiamine)

Function	In thiamine pyrophosphate (TPP), a cofactor for several enzymes: 1. Pyruvate dehydrogenase (glycolysis) 2. α-ketoglutarate dehydrogenase (TCA cycle) 3. Transketolase (HMP shunt) 4. Branched-chain AA dehydrogenase	Spell beriberi as **Ber1Ber1**. Wernicke-Korsakoff—confusion, ophthalmoplegia, ataxia + confabulation, personality change, memory loss (permanent). Damage to medial dorsal nucleus of thalamus, mamillary bodies. Dry beriberi—polyneuritis, symmetrical muscle wasting. Wet beriberi—high-output cardiac failure (dilated cardiomyopathy), edema.
Deficiency	Impaired glucose breakdown → ATP depletion (glucose infusion can worsen); highly aerobic tissues (brain and heart) are affected first. Wernicke-Korsakoff syndrome and beriberi. Seen in malnutrition as well as alcoholism (2° to malnutrition and malabsorption).	

Vitamin B$_2$ (riboflavin)

Function	Cofactor in oxidation and reduction (e.g., FADH$_2$).	**FAD** and **FMN** are derived from ribo**Flavin** (B$_2$ = 2 ATP).
Deficiency	Cheilosis (inflammation of lips, scaling and fissures at the corners of the mouth), Corneal vascularization.	The **2 C's.**

Vitamin B$_3$ (niacin)

Function	Constituent of NAD$^+$, NADP$^+$ (used in redox reactions). Derived from tryptophan. Synthesis requires vitamin B$_6$.	**NAD** derived from **N**iacin (B$_3$ = 3 ATP).
Deficiency	Glossitis. Severe deficiency leads to pellagra, which can be caused by Hartnup disease (↓ tryptophan absorption), malignant carcinoid syndrome (↑ tryptophan metabolism), and INH (↓ vitamin B$_6$).	The **3 D's:** of pellagra: **D**iarrhea, **D**ermatitis, **D**ementia.
Excess	Facial flushing (due to pharmacologic doses for treatment of hyperlipidemia).	

Vitamin B$_5$ (pantothenate)

Function	Essential component of CoA (a cofactor for acyl transfers) and fatty acid synthase.	Pantothen-**A** is in Co-**A**.
Deficiency	Dermatitis, enteritis, alopecia, adrenal insufficiency.	

Vitamin B$_6$ (pyridoxine)

Function	Converted to pyridoxal phosphate, a cofactor used in transamination (e.g., ALT and AST), decarboxylation reactions, glycogen phosphorylase, cystathionine synthesis, and heme synthesis. Required for the synthesis of niacin from tryptophan.
Deficiency	Convulsions, hyperirritability, peripheral neuropathy (deficiency inducible by INH and oral contraceptives), sideroblastic anemias.

Vitamin B$_{12}$ (cobalamin)

Function	Cofactor for homocysteine methyltransferase (transfers CH$_3$ groups as methylcobalamin) and methylmalonyl-CoA mutase.	Found in animal products. Synthesized only by microorganisms. Very large reserve pool (several years) stored primarily in the liver. Deficiency is usually caused by malabsorption (sprue, enteritis, *Diphyllobothrium latum*), lack of intrinsic factor (pernicious anemia, gastric bypass surgery), or absence of terminal ileum (Crohn's disease).
Deficiency	Macrocytic, megaloblastic anemia, hypersegmented PMNs, neurologic symptoms (paresthesias, subacute combined degeneration) due to abnormal myelin. Prolonged deficiency leads to irreversible nervous system damage.	Use Schilling test to detect the etiology of the deficiency.

$$\text{Homocysteine + N-methyl THF} \xrightarrow{\text{B}_{12}} \text{Methionine + THF}$$

$$\text{Methylmalonyl-CoA} \xrightarrow{\text{B}_{12}} \text{Succinyl-CoA}$$

Folic acid

Function	Converted to tetrahydrofolate (THF), a coenzyme for 1-carbon transfer/methylation reactions. Important for the synthesis of nitrogenous bases in DNA and RNA.	**FOL**ate from **FOL**iage. Small reserve pool stored primarily in the liver. Eat green leaves.
Deficiency	Macrocytic, megaloblastic anemia; no neurologic symptoms (as opposed to vitamin B$_{12}$ deficiency). Most common vitamin deficiency in the United States. Seen in alcoholism and pregnancy.	Deficiency can be caused by several drugs (e.g., phenytoin, sulfonamides, MTX). Supplemental folic acid in early pregnancy reduces neural tube defects.

S-adenosyl-methionine

	ATP + methionine → **SAM**. SAM transfers methyl units. Regeneration of methionine (and thus SAM) is dependent on vitamin B$_{12}$ and folate.	**SAM** the methyl donor man. Required for the conversion of NE to epinephrine.

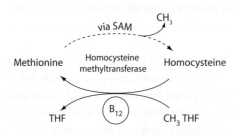

Biotin

Function	Cofactor for carboxylation enzymes (which add a 1-carbon group):	"**AVID**in in egg whites **AVID**ly binds biotin."
	1. Pyruvate carboxylase: Pyruvate (3C) → oxaloacetate (4C)	
	2. Acetyl-CoA carboxylase: Acetyl-CoA (2C) → malonyl-CoA (3C)	
	3. Propionyl-CoA carboxylase: Propionyl-CoA (3C) → methylmalonyl-CoA (4C)	
Deficiency	Relatively rare. Dermatitis, alopecia, enteritis. Caused by antibiotic use or excessive ingestion of raw eggs.	

Vitamin C (ascorbic acid)

Function	Antioxidant. Also:	Found in fruits and vegetables.
	1. Facilitates iron absorption by keeping iron in Fe^{2+} reduced state (more absorbable)	
	2. Necessary for hydroxylation of proline and lysine in collagen synthesis	
	3. Necessary for dopamine β-hydroxylase, which converts dopamine to NE	
Deficiency	Scurvy—swollen gums, bruising, hemarthrosis, anemia, poor wound healing. Weakened immune response.	British sailors carried limes to prevent scurvy (origin of the word "limey").

Vitamin D

	D_2 = ergocalciferol—ingested from plants. D_3 = cholecalciferol—consumed in milk, formed in sun-exposed skin. 25-OH D_3 = storage form. $1,25\text{-}(OH)_2\ D_3$ (calcitriol) = active form.	Drinking milk (fortified with vitamin D) is good for bones.
Function	↑ intestinal absorption of calcium and phosphate, ↑ bone resorption.	
Deficiency	Rickets in children (bending bones), osteomalacia in adults (soft bones), hypocalcemic tetany. Breast milk has ↓ vitamin D (supplement in dark-skinned patients).	
Excess	Hypercalcemia, hypercalciuria, loss of appetite, stupor. Seen in sarcoidosis (↑ activation of vitamin D by epithelioid macrophages).	

Vitamin E

Function	Antioxidant (protects erythrocytes and membranes from free-radical damage).	E is for Erythrocytes.
Deficiency	↑ fragility of erythrocytes (hemolytic anemia), muscle weakness, posterior column and spinocerebellar tract demyelination.	

Vitamin K

Function	Catalyzes γ-carboxylation of glutamic acid residues on various proteins concerned with blood clotting. Synthesized by intestinal flora.	**K** for **K**oagulation. Necessary for the synthesis of clotting factors II, VII, IX, X, and protein C and S. Warfarin—vitamin K antagonist.
Deficiency	Neonatal hemorrhage with ↑ PT and ↑ aPTT but normal bleeding time (neonates have sterile intestines and are unable to synthesize vitamin K). Can also occur after prolonged use of broad-spectrum antibiotics.	Neonates are given vitamin K injection at birth to prevent hemorrhage.

Zinc

Function	Essential for the activity of 100+ enzymes. Important in the formation of zinc fingers (transcription factor motif).
Deficiency	Delayed wound healing, hypogonadism, ↓ adult hair (axillary, facial, pubic), dysgeusia, anosmia. May predispose to alcoholic cirrhosis.

Ethanol metabolism

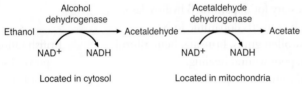

NAD$^+$ is the limiting reagent.
Alcohol dehydrogenase operates via zero-order kinetics.

Fomepizole—inhibits alcohol dehydrogenase and is an antidote for methanol or ethylene glycol poisoning.
Disulfiram (Antabuse)—inhibits acetaldehyde dehydrogenase (acetaldehyde accumulates, contributing to hangover symptoms).

Ethanol hypoglycemia

Ethanol metabolism ↑ NADH/NAD$^+$ ratio in liver, causing diversion of pyruvate to lactate and OAA to malate, thereby inhibiting gluconeogenesis and stimulating fatty acid synthesis. Leads to hypoglycemia and hepatic fatty change (hepatocellular steatosis) seen in chronic alcoholics.

NADH   NAD$^+$

1. Pyruvate ────────→ lactate

NADH   NAD$^+$

2. Oxaloacetate ────────→ malate

Kwashiorkor vs. marasmus

Kwashiorkor—protein malnutrition resulting in skin lesions, edema, liver malfunction (fatty change due to ↓ apolipoprotein synthesis). Clinical picture is small child with swollen belly.
Marasmus—energy malnutrition resulting in tissue and muscle wasting, loss of subcutaneous fat, and variable edema.

Kwashiorkor results from a protein-deficient **MEAL**:
Malnutrition
Edema
Anemia
Liver (fatty)
Marasmus results in
Muscle wasting.

Metabolism sites

Mitochondria	Fatty acid oxidation (β-oxidation), acetyl-CoA production, TCA cycle, oxidative phosphorylation.
Cytoplasm	Glycolysis, fatty acid synthesis, HMP shunt, protein synthesis (RER), steroid synthesis (SER).
Both	Heme synthesis, Urea cycle, Gluconeogenesis. HUGs take **two.**

Enzyme terminology

An enzyme's name often describes its function. For example, glucokinase is an enzyme that catalyzes the phosphorylation of glucose using a molecule of ATP. The following are commonly used enzyme descriptors:

1. Kinase—uses ATP to add high-energy phosphate group onto substrate (e.g., phosphofructokinase)
2. Phosphorylase—adds inorganic phosphate onto substrate without using ATP (e.g., glycogen phosphorylase)
3. Phosphatase—removes phosphate group from substrate (e.g., fructose-1,6-bisphosphatase)
4. Dehydrogenase—oxidizes substrate (e.g., pyruvate dehydrogenase)
5. Carboxylase—adds 1 carbon with the help of biotin (e.g., pyruvate carboxylase)

Rate-determining enzymes of metabolic processes

Process	Enzyme
Glycolysis	Phosphofructokinase-1 (PFK-1)
Gluconeogenesis	Fructose-1,6-bisphosphatase
TCA cycle	Isocitrate dehydrogenase
Glycogen synthesis	Glycogen synthase
Glycogenolysis	Glycogen phosphorylase
HMP shunt	Glucose-6-phosphate dehydrogenase (G6PD)
De novo pyrimidine synthesis	Carbamoyl phosphate synthetase II
De novo purine synthesis	Glutamine-PRPP amidotransferase
Urea cycle	Carbamoyl phosphate synthetase I
Fatty acid synthesis	Acetyl-CoA carboxylase (ACC)
Fatty acid oxidation	Carnitine acyltransferase I
Ketogenesis	HMG-CoA synthase
Cholesterol synthesis	HMG-CoA reductase

Summary of pathways

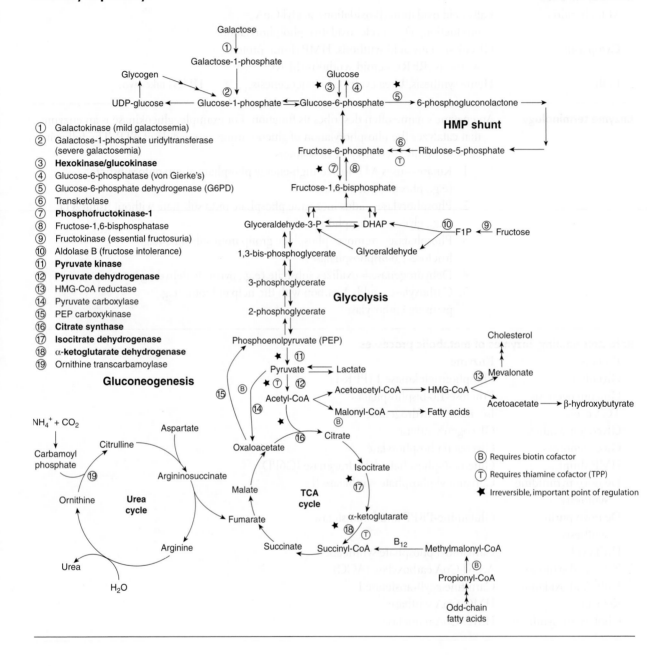

① Galactokinase (mild galactosemia)
② Galactose-1-phosphate uridyltransferase (severe galactosemia)
③ **Hexokinase/glucokinase**
④ Glucose-6-phosphatase (von Gierke's)
⑤ Glucose-6-phosphate dehydrogenase (G6PD)
⑥ Transketolase
⑦ **Phosphofructokinase-1**
⑧ Fructose-1,6-bisphosphatase
⑨ Fructokinase (essential fructosuria)
⑩ Aldolase B (fructose intolerance)
⑪ **Pyruvate kinase**
⑫ **Pyruvate dehydrogenase**
⑬ HMG-CoA reductase
⑭ Pyruvate carboxylase
⑮ PEP carboxykinase
⑯ **Citrate synthase**
⑰ **Isocitrate dehydrogenase**
⑱ **α-ketoglutarate dehydrogenase**
⑲ Ornithine transcarbamoylase

Ⓑ Requires biotin cofactor
Ⓣ Requires thiamine cofactor (TPP)
★ Irreversible, important point of regulation

Glycolysis/ATP production	Aerobic metabolism of glucose produces 32 ATP via malate-aspartate shuttle (heart and liver), 30 ATP via glycerol-3-phosphate shuttle (muscle). Anaerobic glycolysis produces only 2 net ATP per glucose molecule. ATP hydrolysis can be coupled to energetically unfavorable reactions.	

Triphosphate moiety — Base (adenine) — Ribose

Activated carriers	Phosphoryl (ATP). Electrons (NADH, NADPH, $FADH_2$). Acyl (coenzyme A, lipoamide). CO_2 (biotin). 1-carbon units (tetrahydrofolates). CH_3 groups (SAM). Aldehydes (TPP).	
Universal electron acceptors	Nicotinamides (NAD^+, $NADP^+$) and flavin nucleotides (FAD^+). NAD^+ is generally used in **catabolic** processes to carry reducing equivalents away as NADH. **NADPH** is used in **anabolic** processes (steroid and fatty acid synthesis) as a supply of reducing equivalents.	NADPH is a product of the HMP shunt. NADPH is used in: 1. Anabolic processes 2. Respiratory burst 3. P-450 4. Glutathione reductase
Hexokinase vs. glucokinase	Phosphorylation of glucose to yield glucose-6-phosphate serves as the 1st step of glycolysis (also serves as the first step of glycogen synthesis in the liver). Reaction is catalyzed by either hexokinase or glucokinase, depending on the location.	
Hexokinase	Ubiquitous. High affinity (low K_m), low capacity (low V_{max}), uninduced by insulin.	Feedback inhibited by glucose-6-phosphate.
Glucokinase	Liver and β cells of pancreas. Low affinity (high K_m), high capacity (high V_{max}), induced by insulin. (**GLU**cokinase is a **GLU**tton. It has a high V_{max} because it cannot be satisfied.)	No direct feedback inhibition. Phosphorylates excess glucose (e.g., after a meal) to sequester it in the liver. Allows liver to serve as a blood glucose "buffer."

Glycolysis regulation, key enzymes

Net glycolysis (cytoplasm):

$$\text{Glucose} + 2\ P_i + 2\ ADP + 2\ NAD^+ \rightarrow 2\ \text{pyruvate} + 2\ ATP + 2\ NADH + 2H^+ + 2H_2O.$$

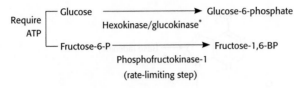

Glucose-6-P $\ominus$.

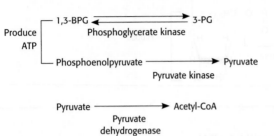

ATP $\ominus$, AMP $\oplus$, **citrate** $\ominus$, fructose-2,6-BP $\oplus$.

ATP $\ominus$, alanine $\ominus$, fructose-1,6-BP $\oplus$.

ATP $\ominus$, NADH $\ominus$, **acetyl-CoA** $\ominus$.

* Glucokinase in liver; hexokinase in all other tissues.

Regulation by F2,6BP

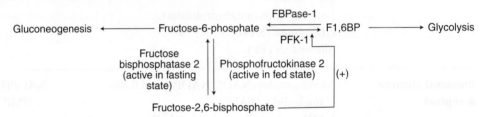

FBPase-2 and PFK-2 are part of the same complex but respond in opposite manners to phosphorylation by protein kinase A.

Fasting state: ↑ glucagon → ↑ cAMP → ↑ protein kinase A → ↑ FBPase-2, ↓ PFK-2.

Fed state: ↑ insulin → ↓ cAMP → ↓ protein kinase A → ↓ FBPase-2, ↑ PFK-2.

Pyruvate dehydrogenase complex	Reaction: pyruvate + NAD^+ + CoA $\rightarrow$ acetyl-CoA + CO_2 + NADH. The complex contains 3 enzymes that require 5 cofactors: 1. Pyrophosphate (B_1, thiamine; TPP) 2. FAD (B_2, riboflavin) 3. NAD (B_3, niacin) 4. CoA (B_5, pantothenate) 5. Lipoic acid Activated by exercise: $\uparrow$ NAD^+/NADH ratio $\uparrow$ ADP $\uparrow$ Ca^{2+}	The complex is similar to the α-ketoglutarate dehydrogenase complex (same cofactors, similar substrate and action), which converts α-ketoglutarate $\rightarrow$ succinyl-CoA (TCA cycle). **Arsenic** inhibits lipoic acid. Findings: vomiting, rice water stools, garlic breath.
Pyruvate dehydrogenase deficiency	Causes backup of substrate (pyruvate and alanine), resulting in lactic acidosis. Can be congenital or acquired (as in alcoholics due to B_1 deficiency). Findings: neurologic defects. Treatment: $\uparrow$ intake of ketogenic nutrients (e.g., high fat content or $\uparrow$ lysine and leucine).	**L**ysine and **L**eucine—the only purely ketogenic amino acids.

Pyruvate metabolism

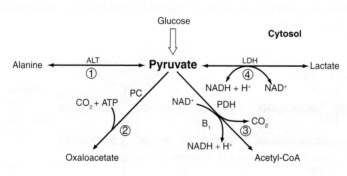

Functions of different pyruvate metabolic pathways:
1. Alanine carries amino groups to the liver from muscle
2. Oxaloacetate can replenish TCA cycle or be used in gluconeogenesis
3. Transition from glycolysis to the TCA cycle
4. End of anaerobic glycolysis (major pathway in RBCs, leukocytes, kidney medulla, lens, testes, and cornea)

**TCA cycle
(Krebs cycle)**

Pyruvate → acetyl-CoA produces 1 NADH, 1 CO_2.

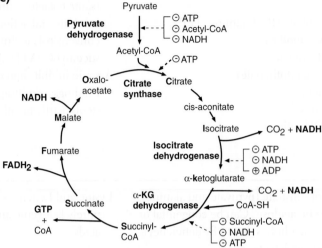

* Enzymes in boldface are irreversible.

The TCA cycle produces
3 NADH, 1 $FADH_2$,
2 CO_2, 1 GTP per acetyl-
CoA = 12 ATP/acetyl-CoA
(2× everything per glucose).
TCA cycle reactions occur in
the mitochondria.

α-ketoglutarate dehydrogenase
complex requires the same
cofactors as the pyruvate
dehydrogenase complex (B_1,
B_2, B_3, B_5, lipoic acid).

Citrate **I**s **K**rebs' **S**tarting
Substrate **F**or **M**aking
Oxaloacetate.

**Electron transport
chain and oxidative
phosphorylation**

NADH electrons from glycolysis and the TCA cycle enter mitochondria via the
malate-aspartate or glycerol-3-phosphate shuttle. $FADH_2$ electrons are transferred to
complex II (at a lower energy level than NADH). The passage of electrons results in
the formation of a proton gradient that, coupled to oxidative phosphorylation, drives
the production of ATP.

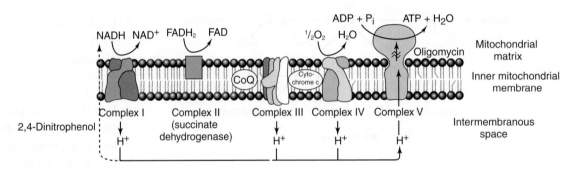

**ATP produced via
ATP synthase:**   1 NADH → 3 ATP; 1 $FADH_2$ → 2 ATP.

Oxidative phosphorylation poisons

Electron transport inhibitors	Directly inhibit electron transport, causing a ↓ proton gradient and block of ATP synthesis.	Rotenone, CN^-, antimycin A, CO.
ATPase inhibitors	Directly inhibit mitochondrial ATPase, causing an ↑ proton gradient. No ATP is produced because electron transport stops.	Oligomycin.
Uncoupling agents	↑ permeability of membrane, causing a ↓ proton gradient and ↑ O_2 consumption. ATP synthesis stops, but electron transport continues. Produces heat.	2,4-DNP, aspirin (fevers often occur after aspirin overdose), thermogenin in brown fat.

Gluconeogenesis, irreversible enzymes

Pyruvate carboxylase	In mitochondria. Pyruvate → oxaloacetate.	Requires biotin, ATP. Activated by acetyl-CoA.
PEP carboxykinase	In cytosol. Oxaloacetate → phosphoenolpyruvate.	Requires GTP.
Fructose-1,6-bisphosphatase	In cytosol. Fructose-1,6-bisphosphate → fructose-6-P.	
Glucose-6-phosphatase	In ER. Glucose-6-P → glucose.	**P**athway **P**roduces **F**resh **G**lucose.

Occurs primarily in liver. Enzymes also found in kidney, intestinal epithelium. Deficiency of the key gluconeogenic enzymes causes hypoglycemia. (Muscle cannot participate in gluconeogenesis because it lacks glucose-6-phosphatase.)

Odd-chain fatty acids yield 1 propionyl-CoA during metabolism, which can enter the TCA cycle (as succinyl-CoA), undergo gluconeogenesis, and serve as a glucose source. Even-chain fatty acids cannot produce new glucose, since they yield only acetyl-CoA equivalents.

HMP shunt (pentose phosphate pathway)

Purpose is to provide a source of NADPH from an abundantly available glucose-6-phosphate (NADPH is required for reductive reactions, e.g., glutathione reduction inside RBCs). Additionally, this pathway yields ribose for nucleotide synthesis and glycolytic intermediates. 2 distinct phases (oxidative and nonoxidative), both of which occur in the cytoplasm. No ATP is used or produced.

Sites: lactating mammary glands, liver, adrenal cortex (sites of fatty acid or steroid synthesis), RBCs.

Reactions	Key enzymes	Products
Oxidative (irreversible)	Glucose-6-P → **Glucose-6-P dehydrogenase** → / Rate-limiting step	CO_2 / 2 NADPH / Ribulose-5-P
Nonoxidative (reversible)	Ribulose-5-P → **Transketolases** → / Requires B_1	Ribose-5-P / G3P / F6P

Respiratory burst (oxidative burst)

Involves the activation of membrane-bound NADPH oxidase (e.g., in neutrophils, macrophages). Plays an important role in the immune response → results in the rapid release of reactive oxygen intermediates (ROIs).

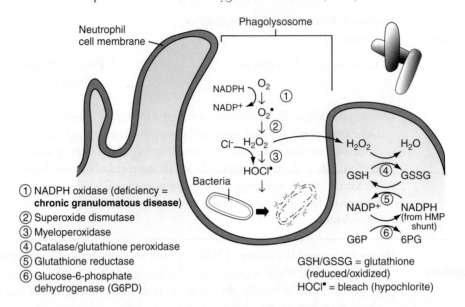

① NADPH oxidase (deficiency = **chronic granulomatous disease**)
② Superoxide dismutase
③ Myeloperoxidase
④ Catalase/glutathione peroxidase
⑤ Glutathione reductase
⑥ Glucose-6-phosphate dehydrogenase (G6PD)

GSH/GSSG = glutathione (reduced/oxidized)
HOClˑ = bleach (hypochlorite)

WBCs of patients with CGD can utilize H_2O_2 generated by invading organisms and convert it to ROIs. Patients are at ↑ risk for infection by catalase-positive species (e.g., *S. aureus*, *Aspergillus*) because they neutralize their own H_2O_2, leaving WBCs without ROIs for fighting infections.

Glucose-6-phosphate dehydrogenase deficiency

NADPH is necessary to keep glutathione reduced, which in turn detoxifies free radicals and peroxides. ↓ NADPH in RBCs leads to **hemolytic anemia** due to poor RBC defense against oxidizing agents (e.g., fava beans, sulfonamides, primaquine, antituberculosis drugs). Infection can also precipitate hemolysis (free radicals generated via inflammatory response can diffuse into RBCs and cause oxidative damage).

X-linked recessive disorder; most common human enzyme deficiency; more prevalent among blacks. ↑ malarial resistance.

Heinz bodies—oxidized Hemoglobin precipitated within RBCs.

Bite cells—result from the phagocytic removal of Heinz bodies by macrophages.

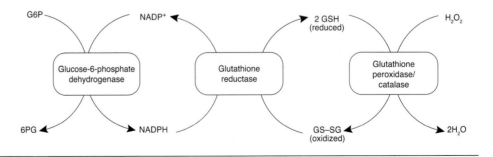

Disorders of fructose metabolism

Essential fructosuria — Involves a defect in **fructokinase.** Autosomal recessive. A benign, asymptomatic condition, since fructose does not enter cells.

Symptoms: fructose appears in blood and urine.

Disorders of fructose metabolism cause milder symptoms than analogous disorders of galactose metabolism.

Fructose intolerance — Hereditary deficiency of **aldolase B.** Autosomal recessive. Fructose-1-phosphate accumulates, causing a ↓ in available phosphate, which results in inhibition of glycogenolysis and gluconeogenesis.

Symptoms: hypoglycemia, jaundice, cirrhosis, vomiting.

Treatment: ↓ intake of both fructose and sucrose (glucose + fructose).

FRUCTOSE METABOLISM (LIVER)

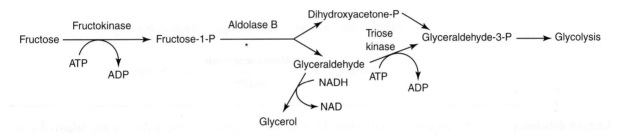

*Fructose bypasses rate-limiting step of glycolysis (PFK) via this pathway.

Disorders of galactose metabolism

Galactokinase deficiency — Hereditary deficiency of **galactokinase.** Galactitol accumulates if galactose is present in diet. Relatively mild condition. Autosomal recessive.

Symptoms: galactose appears in blood and urine, infantile cataracts. May initially present as failure to track objects or to develop a social smile.

Classic galactosemia — Absence of **galactose-1-phosphate uridyltransferase.** Autosomal recessive. Damage is caused by accumulation of toxic substances (including galactitol, which accumulates in the lens of the eye).

Symptoms: failure to thrive, jaundice, hepatomegaly, infantile cataracts, mental retardation.

Treatment: exclude galactose and lactose (galactose + glucose) from diet.

GALACTOSE METABOLISM

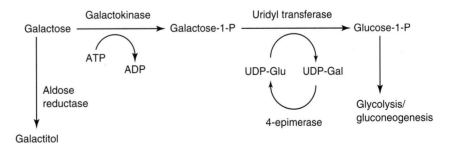

Sorbitol

An alternative method of trapping glucose in the cell is to convert it to its alcohol counterpart, called sorbitol, via **aldose reductase.** Some tissues then convert sorbitol to fructose using **sorbitol dehydrogenase;** tissues lacking this enzyme are at risk for intracellular sorbitol accumulation, causing osmotic damage (e.g., cataracts, retinopathy, and peripheral neuropathy seen with chronic hyperglycemia in diabetes). High blood levels of fructose and galactose also result in conversion to osmotically active alcohol forms via aldose reductase.

Liver, ovaries, and seminal vesicles have both enzymes.

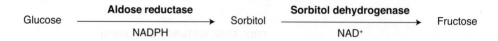

Schwann cells, lens, retina, and kidneys have only aldose reductase.

Glucose $\xrightarrow[\text{NADPH}]{\textbf{Aldose reductase}}$ Sorbitol

---

Lactase deficiency

Age-dependent and/or hereditary lactose intolerance (African Americans, Asians) due to loss of brush-border enzyme. May also follow gastroenteritis.
Symptoms: bloating, cramps, osmotic diarrhea.
Treatment: avoid dairy products or add lactase pills to diet.

Amino acids

Only L-form amino acids are found in proteins.

Essential
Glucogenic: Met, Val, Arg, His.
Glucogenic/ketogenic: Ile, Phe, Thr, Trp.
Ketogenic: Leu, Lys.

All essential AA need to be supplied in the diet.

Acidic
Asp and Glu (negatively charged at body pH).

Basic
Arg, Lys, and His.
Arg is most basic.
His has no charge at body pH.

Arg and His are required during periods of growth. Arg and Lys are ↑ in histones, which bind negatively charged DNA.

| Urea cycle | Amino acid catabolism results in the formation of common metabolites (e.g., pyruvate, acetyl-CoA), which serve as metabolic fuels. Excess nitrogen (NH_4^+) generated by this process is converted to urea and excreted by the kidneys. | Ordinarily, Careless Crappers Are Also Frivolous About Urination. |

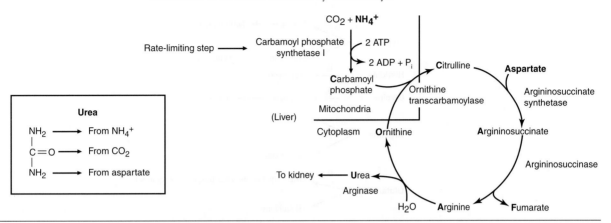

Urea

$$NH_2 \longrightarrow \text{From } NH_4^+$$
$$C=O \longrightarrow \text{From } CO_2$$
$$NH_2 \longrightarrow \text{From aspartate}$$

Transport of ammonium by alanine and glutamate

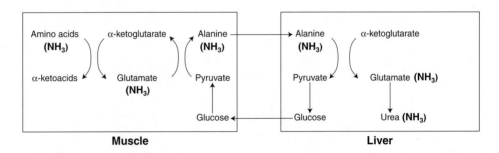

| Muscle | Liver |

| Hyperammonemia | Can be acquired (e.g., liver disease) or hereditary (e.g., urea cycle enzyme deficiencies). Results in excess NH_4^+, which depletes α-ketoglutarate, leading to inhibition of TCA cycle. Treatment: limit protein in diet. Benzoate or phenylbutyrate (both of which bind amino acid and lead to excretion) may be given to ↓ ammonia levels. | **Ammonia intoxication**—tremor, slurring of speech, somnolence, vomiting, cerebral edema, blurring of vision. |

| Ornithine transcarbamoylase (OTC) deficiency | Most common urea cycle disorder. X-linked recessive (vs. other urea cycle enzyme deficiencies, which are autosomal recessive). Interferes with the body's ability to eliminate ammonia. Often evident in the first few days of life, but may present with late onset. Excess carbamoyl phosphate is converted to orotic acid (part of the pyrimidine synthesis pathway).
Findings: orotic acid in blood and urine, ↓ BUN, symptoms of hyperammonemia. |

Amino acid derivatives

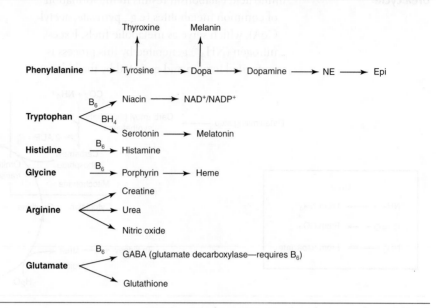

Catecholamine synthesis

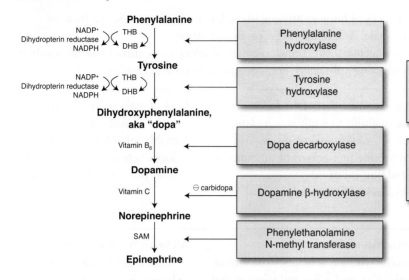

Enzyme legend:
- Hydroxylase adds OH
- Decarboxylase removes COOH
- SAM adds CH$_3$

Breakdown products via MAO and COMT:
Dopamine → HVA
Norepinephrine → VMA
Epinephrine → Metanephrine

Phenylketonuria	Due to ↓ phenylalanine hydroxylase or ↓ tetrahydrobiopterin cofactor. Tyrosine becomes essential. ↑ phenylalanine leads to excess phenylketones in urine.	Screened for 2–3 days after birth (normal at birth because of maternal enzyme during fetal life).
	Findings: mental retardation, growth retardation, seizures, fair skin, eczema, musty body odor.	Phenylketones—phenylacetate, phenyllactate, and phenylpyruvate.
	Treatment: ↓ **phenylalanine** (contained in aspartame, e.g., NutraSweet) and ↑ **tyrosine** in diet.	Autosomal recessive. Incidence ≈ 1:10,000.
	Maternal PKU—lack of proper dietary therapy during pregnancy. Findings in infant: microcephaly, mental retardation, growth retardation, congenital heart defects.	Disorder of **aromatic** amino acid metabolism → musty body **odor**.

Alkaptonuria (ochronosis)

Congenital deficiency of **homogentisic acid oxidase** in the degradative pathway of tyrosine to fumarate. Autosomal recessive. Benign disease.

Findings: dark connective tissue, brown pigmented sclera, urine turns black on standing. May have debilitating arthralgias (homogentisic acid toxic to cartilage).

Albinism

Congenital deficiency of either of the following:
1. Tyrosinase (inability to synthesize melanin from tyrosine)—autosomal recessive
2. Defective tyrosine transporters (↓ amounts of tyrosine and thus melanin)

Can result from a lack of migration of neural crest cells.

Lack of melanin results in an ↑ risk of skin cancer.

Variable inheritance due to locus heterogeneity (vs. ocular albinism—X-linked recessive).

Homocystinuria

3 forms (all autosomal recessive):
1. Cystathionine synthase deficiency (treatment: ↓ Met and ↑ Cys, and ↑ B_{12} and folate in diet)
2. ↓ affinity of cystathionine synthase for pyridoxal phosphate (treatment: ↑↑ vitamin B_6 in diet)
3. Homocysteine methyltransferase deficiency

All forms result in excess homocysteine. Cysteine becomes essential.

Findings: ↑↑ homocysteine in urine, mental retardation, osteoporosis, tall stature, kyphosis, lens subluxation (downward and inward), and atherosclerosis (stroke and MI).

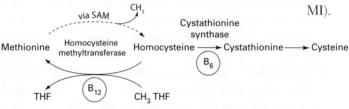

Cystinuria

Hereditary defect of renal tubular amino acid transporter for cysteine, ornithine, lysine, and arginine in the PCT of the kidneys.

Excess cystine in urine can lead to the precipitation of **cystine kidney stones** (cystine staghorn calculi).

Autosomal recessive. Common (1:7000). Treatment: acetazolamide to alkalinize the urine.

Cystine is made of 2 cysteines connected by a disulfide bond.

Maple syrup urine disease

Blocked degradation of **branched** amino acids (Ile, Leu, Val) due to ↓ α-ketoacid dehydrogenase. Causes ↑ α-ketoacids in the blood, especially Leu.

Causes severe CNS defects, mental retardation, and death.

Urine smells like maple syrup.

I Love **V**ermont maple syrup from maple trees (with **branches**).

Hartnup disease

An autosomal-recessive disorder characterized by defective neutral amino acid transporter on renal and intestinal epithelial cells.

Causes tryptophan excretion in urine and ↓ absorption from the gut. **Leads to pellagra.**

Glycogen regulation by insulin and glucagon/epinephrine

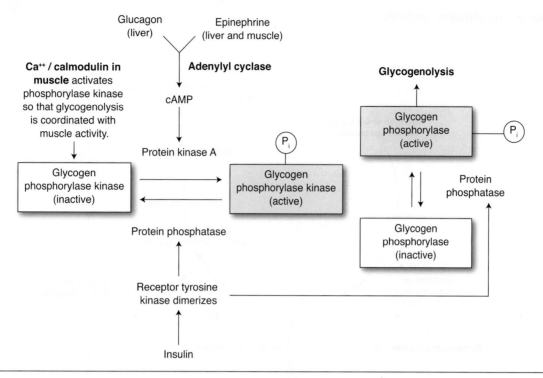

Glycogen	Branches have α (1,6) bonds; linkages have α (1,4) bonds.
Skeletal muscle	Glycogen undergoes glycogenolysis to form glucose, which is rapidly metabolized during exercise.
Hepatocytes	Glycogen is stored and undergoes glycogenolysis to maintain blood sugar at appropriate levels.

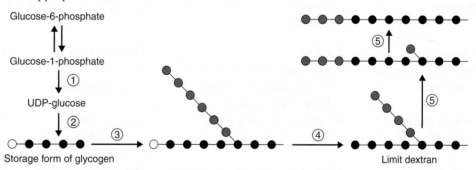

① UDP-glucose pyrophosphorylase
② Glycogen synthase
③ Branching enzyme
④ Glycogen phosphorylase
⑤ Debranching enzyme

Note: A small amount of glycogen is degraded in lysosomes by α-1,4-glucosidase.

Glycogenolysis/glycogen synthesis

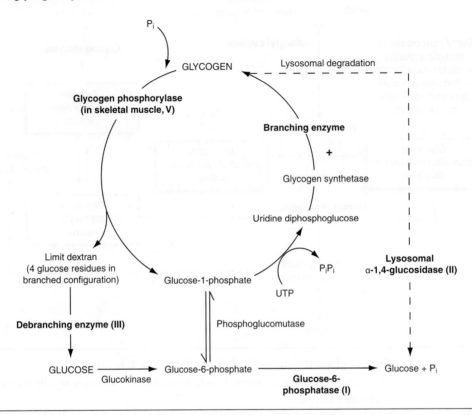

Glycogen storage diseases	12 types, all resulting in abnormal glycogen metabolism and an accumulation of glycogen within cells.		**V**ery **P**oor **C**arbohydrate **M**etabolism.

Disease	Findings	Deficient enzyme	Comments
Von Gierke's disease (type I)	Severe fasting hypoglycemia, ↑↑ glycogen in liver, ↑ blood lactate, hepatomegaly	Glucose-6-phosphatase	
Pompe's disease (type II)	Cardiomegaly and systemic findings leading to early death	Lysosomal α-1,4-glucosidase (acid maltase)	**P**ompe's trashes the **P**ump (heart, liver, and muscle). Gluconeogenesis is intact.
Cori's disease (type III)	Milder form of type I with normal blood lactate levels	Debranching enzyme (α-1,6-glucosidase)	
McArdle's disease (type V)	↑ glycogen in muscle, but cannot break it down, leading to painful muscle cramps, myoglobinuria with strenuous exercise	Skeletal muscle glycogen phosphorylase	**M**cArdle's = **M**uscle.

Lysosomal storage diseases

Each is caused by a deficiency in one of the many lysosomal enzymes. Results in an accumulation of abnormal metabolic products.

Disease	Findings	Deficient enzyme	Accumulated substrate	Inheritance
Sphingolipidoses				
Fabry's disease	Peripheral neuropathy of hands/feet, angiokeratomas, cardiovascular/renal disease	α-galactosidase A	Ceramide trihexoside	**XR**
Gaucher's disease (most common)	Hepatosplenomegaly, aseptic necrosis of femur, bone crises, Gaucher's cells (macrophages that look like crumpled tissue paper)	β-glucocerebrosidase	Glucocerebroside	AR
Niemann-Pick disease	Progressive neurodegeneration, hepatosplenomegaly, cherry-red spot on macula, foam cells	Sphingomyelinase	Sphingomyelin	AR
Tay-Sachs disease	Progressive neurodegeneration, developmental delay, cherry-red spot on macula, lysosomes with onion skin, no hepatosplenomegaly (vs. Niemann-Pick)	Hexosaminidase A	GM_2 ganglioside	AR
Krabbe's disease	Peripheral neuropathy, developmental delay, optic atrophy, globoid cells	Galactocerebrosidase	Galactocerebroside	AR
Metachromatic leukodystrophy	Central and peripheral demyelination with ataxia, dementia	Arylsulfatase A	Cerebroside sulfate	AR
Mucopolysaccharidoses				
Hurler's syndrome	Developmental delay, gargoylism, airway obstruction, corneal clouding, hepatosplenomegaly	α-L-iduronidase	Heparan sulfate, dermatan sulfate	AR
Hunter's syndrome	Mild Hurler's + aggressive behavior, no corneal clouding	Iduronate sulfatase	Heparan sulfate, dermatan sulfate	**XR**

No man picks (**Niemann-Pick**) his nose with his **sphinger** (**sphing**omyelinase).

Tay-Sa**X** (**Tay-Sachs**) lacks he**X**osaminidase.

Hunters see clearly (no corneal clouding) and aim for the **X** (**X**-linked recessive).

↑ incidence of Tay-Sachs, Niemann-Pick, and some forms of Gaucher's disease in Ashkenazi Jews.

Fatty acid metabolism

SYtrate = SYnthesis.
CARnitine = CARnage of fatty acids.

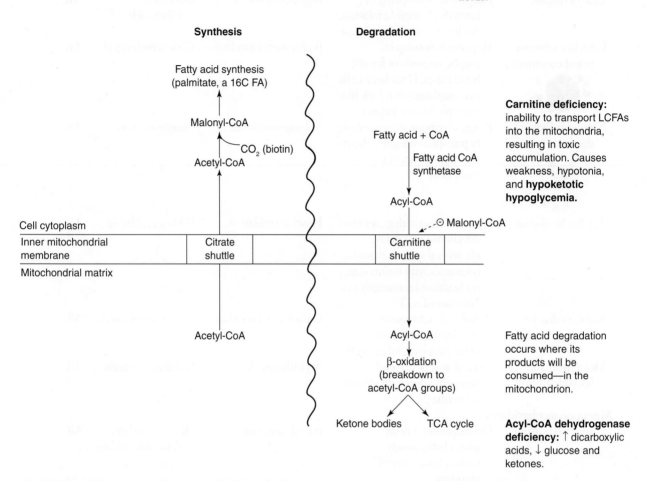

Carnitine deficiency: inability to transport LCFAs into the mitochondria, resulting in toxic accumulation. Causes weakness, hypotonia, and **hypoketotic hypoglycemia.**

Fatty acid degradation occurs where its products will be consumed—in the mitochondrion.

Acyl-CoA dehydrogenase deficiency: ↑ dicarboxylic acids, ↓ glucose and ketones.

Ketone bodies	In the liver, fatty acids and amino acids are metabolized to **acetoacetate** and **β-hydroxybutyrate** (to be used in muscle and brain). In prolonged starvation and diabetic ketoacidosis, oxaloacetate is depleted for gluconeogenesis. In alcoholism, excess NADH shunts oxaloacetate to malate. Both processes stall the TCA cycle, which shunts glucose and FFA toward the production of ketone bodies. Made from HMG-CoA. Metabolized by the brain to 2 molecules of acetyl-CoA. Excreted in urine.	Breath smells like acetone (fruity odor). Urine test for ketones does not detect β-hydroxybutyrate (favored by high redox state).

Metabolic fuel use

Exercise	As distances ↑, ATP is obtained from additional sources.	1 g protein or carbohydrate = 4 kcal.
100-meter sprint (seconds)	Stored ATP, creatine phosphate, anaerobic glycolysis.	1 g fat = 9 kcal.
1000-meter run (minutes)	Above + oxidative phosphorylation.	
Marathon (hours)	Glycogen and FFA oxidation; glucose conserved for final sprinting.	
Fasting and starvation	Priorities are to supply sufficient glucose to the brain and RBCs and to preserve protein.	
Fed state (after a meal)	Glycolysis and aerobic respiration.	Insulin stimulates storage of lipids, proteins, glycogen.
Fasting (between meals)	Hepatic glycogenolysis (major); hepatic gluconeogenesis, adipose release of FFA (minor).	Glucagon, adrenaline stimulate use of fuel reserves.
Starvation days 1–3	Blood glucose level maintained by: 1. Hepatic glycogenolysis 2. Adipose release of FFA 3. Muscle and liver, which shift fuel use from glucose to FFA 4. Hepatic gluconeogenesis from peripheral tissue lactate and alanine, and from adipose tissue glycerol and propionyl-CoA (from odd-chain FFA —the only triacylglycerol components that contribute to gluconeogenesis)	Glycogen reserves depleted after day 1.
Starvation after day 3	Adipose stores (ketone bodies become the main source of energy for the brain and heart). After these are depleted, vital protein degradation accelerates, leading to organ failure and death.	Amount of adipose stores determines survival time.

Cholesterol synthesis	Rate-limiting step is catalyzed by **HMG-CoA reductase,** which converts HMG-CoA to mevalonate. ⅔ of plasma cholesterol is esterified by lecithin-cholesterol acyltransferase (LCAT).	Statins (e.g., lovastatin) inhibit HMG-CoA reductase.

Lipid transport, key enzymes

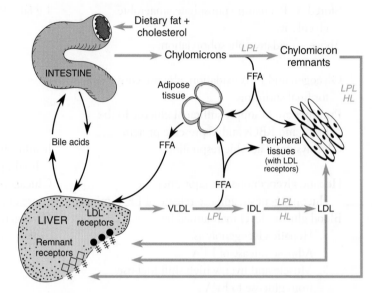

(Reproduced, with permission, from Brunton LL et al. *Goodman & Gilman's The Pharmacological Basis of Therapeutics,* 11th ed. New York: McGraw-Hill, 2005: Fig. 35-1.)

Pancreatic lipase—degradation of dietary TG in small intestine.
Lipoprotein lipase (LPL)—degradation of TG circulating in chylomicrons and VLDLs.
Hepatic TG lipase (HL)—degradation of TG remaining in IDL.
Hormone-sensitive lipase—degradation of TG stored in adipocytes.

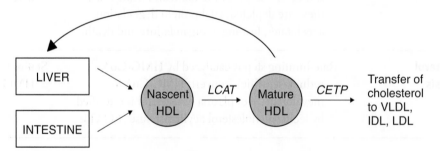

Lecithin-cholesterol acyltransferase (LCAT)—catalyzes esterification of cholesterol.
Cholesterol ester transfer protein (CETP)—mediates transfer of cholesterol esters to other lipoprotein particles.

Major apolipoproteins	A-I—Activates LCAT.
	B-100—**B**inds to LDL receptor, mediates VLDL secretion.
	C-II—**C**ofactor for lipoprotein lipase.
	B-48—Mediates chylomicron secretion.
	E—Mediates **E**xtra (remnant) uptake.

Lipoprotein functions   Lipoproteins are composed of varying proportions of cholesterol, triglycerides (TGs), and phospholipids. LDL and HDL carry most cholesterol.

LDL transports cholesterol from liver to tissues.   LDL is Lousy.
HDL transports it from periphery to liver.   HDL is Healthy.

	Function and route	Apolipoproteins
Chylomicron	Delivers dietary TGs to peripheral tissue. Delivers cholesterol to liver in the form of chylomicron remnants, which are mostly depleted of their triacylglycerols. Secreted by intestinal epithelial cells.	B-48, A-IV, C-II, and E
VLDL	Delivers hepatic TGs to peripheral tissue. Secreted by liver.	B-100, C-II, and E
IDL	Formed in the degradation of VLDL. Delivers triglycerides and cholesterol to liver, where they are degraded to LDL.	B-100 and E
LDL	Delivers hepatic cholesterol to peripheral tissues. Formed by lipoprotein lipase modification of VLDL in the peripheral tissue. Taken up by target cells via receptor-mediated endocytosis.	B-100
HDL	Mediates reverse cholesterol transport from periphery to liver. Acts as a repository for apoC and apoE (which are needed for chylomicron and VLDL metabolism). Secreted from both liver and intestine.	

Familial dyslipidemias

Type	Increased	Elevated blood levels	Pathophysiology
I—hyperchylomicronemia	Chylomicrons	TG, cholesterol	Lipoprotein lipase deficiency or altered apolipoprotein C-II. Causes pancreatitis, hepatosplenomegaly, and eruptive/pruritic xanthomas (no ↑ risk for atherosclerosis).
IIa—familial hypercholesterolemia	LDL	Cholesterol	Autosomal dominant; absent or ↓ LDL receptors. Causes accelerated atherosclerosis, tendon (Achilles) xanthomas, and corneal arcus.
IV—hypertriglyceridemia	VLDL	TG	Hepatic overproduction of VLDL. Causes pancreatitis.

Abeta-lipoproteinemia   Hereditary inability to synthesize lipoproteins due to deficiencies in apoB-100 and apoB-48. Autosomal recessive. Symptoms appear in the first few months of life. Intestinal biopsy shows accumulation within enterocytes due to inability to export absorbed lipid as chylomicrons.
Findings: failure to thrive, steatorrhea, acanthocytosis, ataxia, night blindness.

Embryology

"Zygote. This cell, formed by the union of an ovum and a sperm, represents the beginning of a human being."

—Keith Moore and Vid Persaud,
Before We Are Born

"The humour and illnesses are already on the sperm and are transmitted to the embryo."

—Asaph ben Berechiah

"Is life worth living? This is a question for an embryo, not for a man."
—Samuel Butler

Embryology is traditionally one of the higher-yield areas within anatomy. This topic can be crammed closer to the exam date. Many questions focus on underlying mechanisms of congenital malformations (e.g., failure of fusion of the maxillary and medial nasal processes leading to cleft lip).

Important genes of embryogenesis

Sonic hedgehog gene	Produced at base of limbs in zone of polarizing activity. Involved in patterning along anterior-posterior axis.
Wnt-7 gene	Produced at apical ectodermal ridge (thickened ectoderm at distal end of each developing limb). Necessary for proper organization along dorsal-ventral axis.
FGF gene	Produced at apical ectodermal ridge. Stimulates mitosis of underlying mesoderm, providing for lengthening of limbs.
Homeobox gene	Involved in segmental organization of embryo in a craniocaudal direction.

Fetal landmarks

Day 0	Fertilization by sperm forming zygote, initiating embryogenesis.
Within week 1	hCG secretion begins after implantation of blastocyst.
Within week 2	Bilaminar disk (epiblast, hypoblast).
Within week 3	Gastrulation. Primitive streak, notochord, and neural plate begin to form.
Weeks 3–8 (embryonic period)	Neural tube formed by neuroectoderm and closes by week 4. Organogenesis. Extremely susceptible to teratogens.
Week 4	Heart begins to beat. Upper and lower limb buds begin to form.
Week 8 (fetal period)	Fetal movement, fetus looks like a baby.
Week 10	Genitalia have male/female characteristics.

Alar plate (dorsal)	Sensory	Same orientation as spinal cord.
Basal plate (ventral)	Motor	

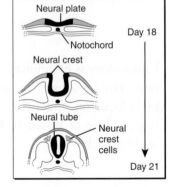

Neural development

Notochord induces overlying ectoderm to differentiate into neuroectoderm and form the neural plate.

Neural plate gives rise to the neural tube and neural crest cells.

Notochord becomes nucleus pulposus of the intervertebral disk in adults.

Rules of early development

Rule of 2's for 2nd week	2 germ layers (bilaminar disk): epiblast, hypoblast. 2 cavities: amniotic cavity, yolk sac. 2 components to placenta: cytotrophoblast, syncytiotrophoblast.	The epiblast (precursor to ectoderm) invaginates to form primitive streak. Cells from the primitive streak give rise to both intraembryonic mesoderm and part of the endoderm.
Rule of 3's for 3rd week	3 germ layers (gastrula): ectoderm, mesoderm, endoderm.	
Rule of 4's for 4th week	4 heart chambers. 4 limb buds grow.	

Embryologic derivatives

Ectoderm

Surface ectoderm — Adenohypophysis (from Rathke's pouch); lens of eye; epithelial linings of oral cavity, sensory organs of ear, and olfactory epithelium; epidermis; salivary, sweat, and mammary glands.

Craniopharyngioma—benign Rathke's pouch tumor with cholesterol crystals, calcifications.

Neuroectoderm — Brain (neurohypophysis, CNS neurons, oligodendrocytes, astrocytes, ependymal cells, pineal gland), retina, spinal cord.

Neuroectoderm—think CNS and brain.

Neural crest — ANS, dorsal root ganglia, cranial nerves, celiac ganglion, melanocytes, chromaffin cells of adrenal medulla, parafollicular (C) cells of thyroid, Schwann cells, pia and arachnoid, bones of the skull, odontoblasts, aorticopulmonary septum.

Neural crest—think PNS and non-neural structures nearby.
Odonto = teeth. Think **Crest** toothpaste.

Endoderm

Gut tube epithelium and derivatives (e.g., lungs, liver, pancreas, thymus, parathyroid, thyroid follicular cells).

Mesoderm

Muscle, bone, connective tissue, serous linings of body cavities (e.g., peritoneum), spleen (derived from foregut mesentery), cardiovascular structures, lymphatics, blood, bladder, urethra, vagina, eustachian tube, kidneys, adrenal cortex, skin dermis, testes, ovaries.

Notochord induces ectoderm to form neuroectoderm (neural plate). Its postnatal derivative is the nucleus pulposus of the intervertebral disk.

Mesodermal defects = **VACTERL**: **V**ertebral defects, **A**nal atresia, **C**ardiac defects, **T**racheo-**E**sophageal fistula, **R**enal defects, **L**imb defects (bone and muscle).

Types of errors in organ morphogenesis

Malformation—intrinsic disruption; occurs during the embryonic period (weeks 3–8).
Deformation—extrinsic disruption; occurs after the embryonic period.
Agenesis—absent organ due to absent primordial tissue.
Hypoplasia—incomplete organ development; primordial tissue present.
Aplasia—absent organ despite present primordial tissue.

Teratogens	Most susceptible in 3rd–8th weeks (embryonic period—organogenesis) of pregnancy. Before week 3: all-or-none effects. After week 8: growth and function affected.

Examples	Effects on fetus
ACE inhibitors	Renal damage
Alcohol	Leading cause of birth defects and mental retardation; fetal alcohol syndrome
Alkylating agents	Absence of digits, multiple anomalies
Aminoglycosides	CN VIII toxicity
Cocaine	Abnormal fetal development and fetal addiction; placental abruption
Diethylstilbestrol (DES)	Vaginal clear cell adenocarcinoma
Folate antagonists	Neural tube defects
Iodide (lack or excess)	Congenital goiter or hypothyroidism
Lithium	Ebstein's anomaly (atrialized right ventricle)
Maternal diabetes	Caudal regression syndrome (anal atresia to sirenomelia)
Smoking (nicotine, CO)	Preterm labor, placental problems, IUGR, ADHD
Tetracyclines	Discolored teeth
Thalidomide	Limb defects ("flipper" limbs)
Valproate	Inhibition of intestinal folate absorption
Vitamin A (excess)	Extremely high risk for spontaneous abortions and birth defects (cleft palate, cardiac abnormalities)
Warfarin	Bone deformities, fetal hemorrhage, abortion
X-rays, anticonvulsants	Multiple anomalies

Fetal infections and certain antibiotics can also cause congenital malformations (see the Microbiology chapter).

Fetal alcohol syndrome	Leading cause of congenital malformations in the United States. Newborns of mothers who consumed significant amounts of alcohol during pregnancy have an ↑ incidence of congenital abnormalities, including pre- and postnatal developmental retardation, microcephaly, holoprosencephaly, facial abnormalities, limb dislocation, and heart and lung fistulas. Mechanism may include inhibition of cell migration.

Twinning

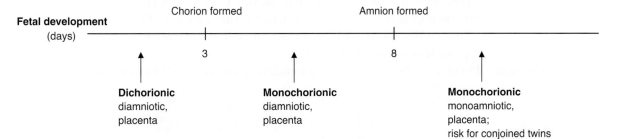

Fetal development
(days)

Chorion formed | Amnion formed

3 | 8

Dichorionic
diamniotic,
placenta

Monochorionic
diamniotic,
placenta

Monochorionic
monoamniotic,
placenta;
risk for conjoined twins

Dizygotic (fraternal) or monozygotic

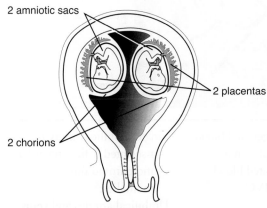

2 amniotic sacs

2 placentas

2 chorions

Monozygotes that split early to develop 2 placentas (separate/fused), chorions, and amniotic sacs.

Dizygotes develop individual placentas, chorions, and amniotic sacs.

Monozygotic

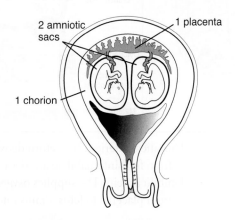

2 amniotic sacs

1 placenta

1 chorion

1 zygote splits evenly to develop 2 amniotic sacs with a single common chorion and placenta.

Conjoined twins have 1 chorion, 1 amniotic sac.

Placental development   1° site of nutrient and gas exchange between mother and fetus.

Fetal component   Cytotrophoblast—inner layer of chorionic villi. **C**yto makes **C**ells.

Syncytiotrophoblast—outer layer of chorionic villi; secretes hCG (structurally similar to LH; stimulates corpus luteum to secrete progesterone during first trimester).

Maternal component   Decidua basalis—derived from the endometrium. Maternal blood in lacunae.

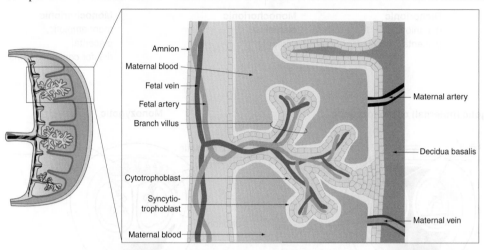

Umbilical cord   Umbilical arteries (2)—return deoxygenated blood from fetal internal iliac arteries to placenta.

Umbilical vein (1)—supplies oxygenated blood from placenta to fetus; drains into IVC.

Single umbilical artery is associated with congenital and chromosomal anomalies.

Umbilical arteries and veins are derived from allantois.

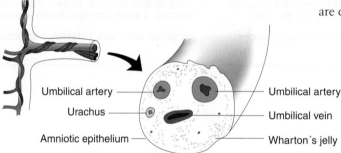

Urachal duct abnormalities:

3rd week—yolk sac forms allantois, which extends into urogenital sinus. Allantois becomes urachus, a duct between bladder and yolk sac.

Failure of urachus to obliterate:

1. Patent urachus—urine discharge from umbilicus
2. Vesicourachal diverticulum—outpouching of bladder

Vitelline duct abnormalities:

7th week—obliteration of vitelline duct (omphalo-mesenteric duct), which connects yolk sac to midgut lumen.

Vitelline fistula—failure of duct to close → meconium discharge from umbilicus. Meckel's diverticulum—partial closure, with patent portion attached to ileum. May have ectopic gastric mucosa → melena and periumbilical pain.

Heart embryology	Embryonic structure	Gives rise to
	Truncus arteriosus (TA)	Ascending aorta and pulmonary trunk
	Bulbus cordis	Right ventricle and smooth parts (outflow tract) of left and right ventricle
	Primitive ventricle	Portion of the left ventricle
	Primitive atria	Trabeculated left and right atrium
	Left horn of sinus venosus (SV)	Coronary sinus
	Right horn of SV	Smooth part of right atrium
	Right common cardinal vein and right anterior cardinal vein	SVC

Truncus arteriosus	Neural crest migration → truncal and bulbar ridges that spiral and fuse to form the aorticopulmonary septum → **ascending aorta and pulmonary trunk.**
	*Pathology—transposition of great vessels (failure to spiral), tetralogy of Fallot (skewed AP septum development), persistent TA (partial AP septum development).

Interventricular septum development

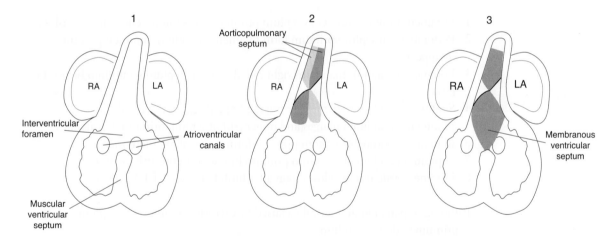

1. Muscular ventricular septum forms. Opening is called interventricular foramen.
2. AP septum meets and fuses with muscular ventricular septum to form membranous interventricular septum, closing interventricular foramen.
3. Growth of endocardial cushions separates atria from ventricles and contributes to both atrial separation and membranous portion of the interventricular septum.

Pathology—membranous septal defect causes initial left-to-right shunting, which then becomes right-to-left shunting (Eisenmenger complex).
Note: Eisenmenger complex is described in detail in the Cardiovascular chapter.

Interatrial septum development

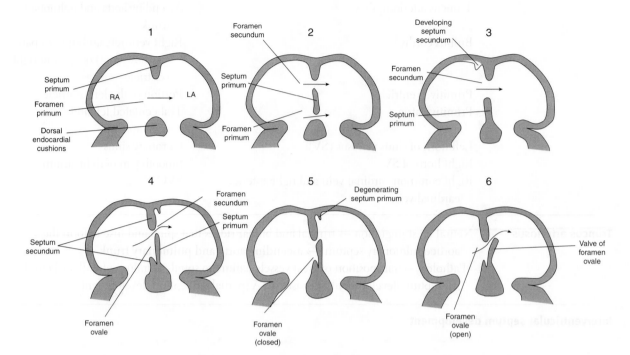

1. Foramen primum narrows as septum primum grows toward endocardial cushions.
2. Perforations in septum primum form foramen secundum (foramen primum disappears).
3. Foramen secundum maintains right-to-left shunt as septum secundum begins to grow.
4. Septum secundum contains a permanent opening (foramen ovale).
5. Foramen secundum enlarges and upper part of septum primum degenerates.
6. Remaining portion of septum primum forms valve of foramen ovale.
7. Septum secundum and septum primum fuse to form the atrial septum.
8. Foramen ovale usually closes soon after birth because of ↑ LA pressure.

Pathology—patent foramen ovale, caused by excessive resorption of septum primum and/or secundum.

Fetal erythropoiesis	Fetal erythropoiesis occurs in: 1. **Y**olk sac (3–8 wk) 2. **L**iver (6–30 wk) 3. **S**pleen (9–28 wk) 4. **B**one marrow (28 wk onward)	**Y**oung **L**iver **S**ynthesizes **B**lood. Fetal hemoglobin = $\alpha_2\gamma_2$. Adult hemoglobin = $\alpha_2\beta_2$.

Fetal circulation

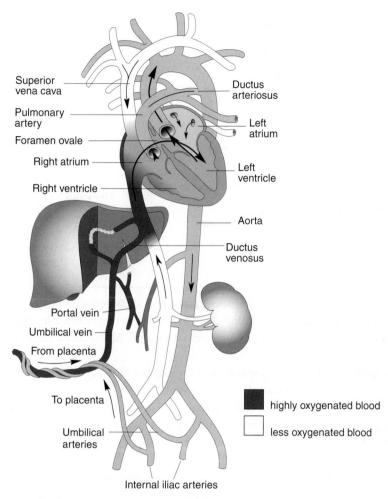

Superior vena cava

Pulmonary artery

Foramen ovale

Right atrium

Right ventricle

Ductus arteriosus

Left atrium

Left ventricle

Aorta

Ductus venosus

Portal vein

Umbilical vein

From placenta

To placenta

Umbilical arteries

Internal iliac arteries

■ highly oxygenated blood

□ less oxygenated blood

(Adapted, with permission, from Ganong WF. *Review of Medical Physiology,* 19th ed. Stamford, CT: Appleton & Lange, 1999: 600.)

Blood in umbilical vein is ≈ 80% saturated with O_2. Umbilical arteries have low O_2 saturation.

3 important shunts:

1. Blood entering the fetus through the umbilical vein is conducted via the **ductus venosus** into the IVC to bypass the hepatic circulation

2. Most oxygenated blood reaching the heart via the IVC is diverted through the **foramen ovale** and pumped out the aorta to the head and body

3. Deoxygenated blood from the SVC is expelled into the pulmonary artery and **ductus arteriosus** to the lower body of the fetus

At birth, infant takes a breath; ↓ resistance in pulmonary vasculature causes ↑ left atrial pressure vs. right atrial pressure; foramen ovale closes (now called fossa ovalis); ↑ in O_2 leads to ↓ in prostaglandins, causing closure of ductus arteriosus.

Indomethacin helps close PDA. Prostaglandins keep PDA open.

Regional specification of developing brain

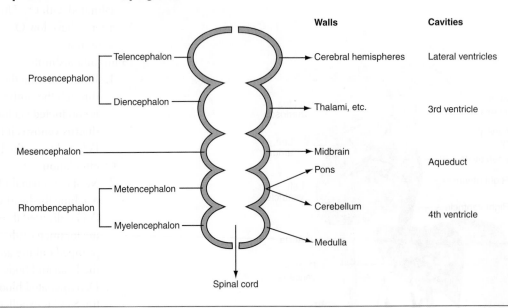

	Walls	Cavities
Prosencephalon — Telencephalon	Cerebral hemispheres	Lateral ventricles
Prosencephalon — Diencephalon	Thalami, etc.	3rd ventricle
Mesencephalon	Midbrain	Aqueduct
Rhombencephalon — Metencephalon	Pons / Cerebellum	4th ventricle
Rhombencephalon — Myelencephalon	Medulla	

Spinal cord

Neural tube defects

Neuropores fail to fuse (4th week) → persistent connection between amniotic cavity and spinal canal. Associated with low folic acid intake during pregnancy. Elevated α-fetoprotein (AFP) in amniotic fluid and maternal serum. ↑ AFP + acetylcholinesterase in CSF.

Spina bifida occulta—failure of bony spinal canal to close, but no structural herniation. Usually seen at lower vertebral levels. Dura is intact.

Meningocele—meninges herniate through spinal canal defect.

Myelomeningocele—meninges and spinal cord herniate through spinal canal defect (see Image 93).

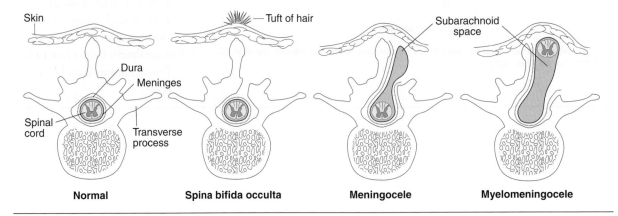

Normal   Spina bifida occulta   Meningocele   Myelomeningocele

Forebrain anomalies

Anencephaly   Malformation of anterior end of neural tube; no brain/calvarium, elevated AFP, polyhydramnios (no swallowing center in brain).

Holoprosencephaly   ↓ separation of hemispheres across midline; results in cyclopia; associated with Patau's syndrome, severe fetal alcohol syndrome, and cleft lip/palate.

Posterior fossa malformations   Chiari II—cerebellar tonsillar herniation through foramen magnum with aqueductal stenosis and hydrocephaly. Often presents with syringomyelia, thoraco-lumbar myelomeningocele.

Dandy-Walker—large posterior fossa; absent cerebellar vermis with cystic enlargement of 4th ventricle. Can lead to hydrocephalus and spina bifida.

Syringomyelia

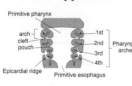

Enlargement of the central canal of spinal cord. Crossing fibers of spinothalamic tract are typically damaged first. "Cape-like," bilateral loss of pain and temperature sensation in upper extremities with preservation of touch sensation.

Syrinx (Greek) = tube, as in syringe.
Associated with Chiari II malformation.
Most common at C8–T1.

Aortic arch derivatives

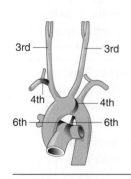

Develop into the arterial system:
1st—part of **MAX**illary artery (branch of external carotid).
2nd—**S**tapedial artery and hyoid artery.
3rd—common **C**arotid artery and proximal part of internal carotid artery.
4th—on left, aortic arch; on right, proximal part of right subclavian artery.
6th—proximal part of pulmonary arteries and (on left only) ductus arteriosus.

1st arch is **MAX**imal.

Second = **S**tapedial.
C is 3rd letter of alphabet.

4th arch (4 limbs) = systemic.

6th arch = pulmonary and the pulmonary-to-systemic shunt (ductus arteriosus).

Branchial apparatus

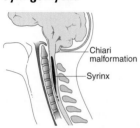

Also called pharyngeal apparatus. Composed of branchial clefts, arches, and pouches.
Branchial clefts—derived from ectoderm. Also called branchial grooves.
Branchial arches—derived from mesoderm (muscles, arteries) and neural crests (bones, cartilage).
Branchial pouches—derived from endoderm.

CAP covers outside from inside:
Clefts = ectoderm
Arches = mesoderm
Pouches = endoderm

Branchial cleft derivatives

1st cleft develops into external auditory meatus.
2nd through 4th clefts form temporary cervical sinuses, which are obliterated by proliferation of 2nd arch mesenchyme.
Persistent cervical sinus → branchial cleft cyst within lateral neck.

Branchial arch derivatives

Derivative	Cartilage	Muscles	Nerves[a]	Abnormalities/ Comments
1	Meckel's cartilage: Mandible, Malleus, incus, spheno-Mandibular ligament	Muscles of Mastication (temporalis, Masseter, lateral and Medial pterygoids), Mylohyoid, anterior belly of digastric, tensor tympani, tensor veli palatini, anterior ⅔ of tongue	CN V_2 and V_3 (chewing)	Treacher Collins syndrome: 1st-arch neural crest fails to migrate → mandibular hypoplasia, facial abnormalities
2	Reichert's cartilage: Stapes, Styloid process, lesser horn of hyoid, Stylohyoid ligament	Muscles of facial expression, Stapedius, Stylohyoid, posterior belly of digastric	CN VII (facial expression)	
3	Cartilage: greater horn of hyoid	Stylopharyngeus (think of stylo-**pharyngeus** innervated by glosso**pharyngeal** nerve)	CN IX (stylo-pharyngeous)	Congenital pharyngo-cutaneous fistula: persistence of cleft and pouch → fistula between tonsillar area, cleft in lateral neck
4–6	Cartilages: thyroid, cricoid, arytenoids, corniculate, cuneiform	4th arch: most pharyngeal constrictors; **cricothyroid**, levator veli palatini 6th arch: all intrinsic muscles of larynx **except cricothyroid**	4th arch: CN X (superior laryngeal branch— **swallowing**) 6th arch: CN X (recurrent laryngeal branch— **speaking**)	Arches 3 and 4 form posterior ⅓ of tongue; arch 5 makes no major developmental contributions

[a]These are the only CNs with both motor and sensory components (except V_2, which is sensory only).

Branchial pouch derivatives	1st pouch develops into middle ear cavity, eustachian tube, mastoid air cells.	1st pouch contributes to endoderm-lined structures of ear.
	2nd pouch develops into epithelial lining of palatine tonsil.	3rd pouch contributes to 3 structures (thymus, left and right inferior parathyroids).
	3rd pouch (dorsal wings) develops into **inferior** parathyroids.	3rd-pouch structures end up **below** 4th-pouch structures.
	3rd pouch (ventral wings) develops into thymus.	Aberrant development of 3rd and 4th pouches →
	4th pouch (dorsal wings) develops into **superior** parathyroids.	**DiGeorge syndrome** → leads to T-cell deficiency (thymic aplasia) and hypocalcemia (failure of parathyroid development).

MEN 2A: mutation of germline *RET* (neural crest cells).
—Adrenal medulla (pheochromocytoma).
—Parathyroid (tumor): 3rd/4th pharyngeal pouch.
—Parafollicular cells (medullary thyroid cancer): derived from neural crest cells; associated with the 4th/5th pharyngeal pouches.

Tongue development	1st branchial arch forms anterior 2/3 (thus sensation via CN V$_3$, taste via CN VII).	Taste—CN VII, IX, X (solitary nucleus).
	3rd and 4th arches form posterior 1/3 (thus sensation and taste mainly via CN IX, extreme posterior via CN X).	Pain—CN V$_3$, IX, X. Motor—CN XII.
	Motor innervation is via CN XII.	
	Muscles of the tongue are derived from occipital myotomes.	

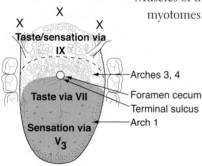

Thyroid development

Thyroid diverticulum arises from floor of primitive pharynx, descends into neck. Connected to tongue by thyroglossal duct, which normally disappears but may persist as pyramidal lobe of thyroid. Foramen cecum is normal remnant of thyroglossal duct. Most common ectopic thyroid tissue site is the tongue.

Thyroglossal duct cyst in midline neck and will move with swallowing (vs. persistent cervical sinus leading to branchial cleft cyst in lateral neck).

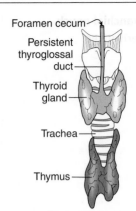

Cleft lip and cleft palate

Cleft lip—failure of fusion of the maxillary and medial nasal processes (formation of 1° palate).

Cleft palate—failure of fusion of the lateral palatine processes, the nasal septum, and/or the median palatine process (formation of 2° palate).

Cleft lip and cleft palate have two distinct etiologies, but often occur together.

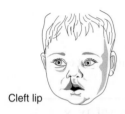

Cleft lip

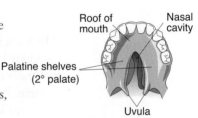

GI embryology

1. Foregut—pharynx to duodenum
2. Midgut—duodenum to transverse colon
3. Hindgut—distal transverse colon to rectum

Developmental defects of anterior abdominal wall due to failure of:
  —Rostral fold closure: sternal defects
  —Lateral fold closure: omphalocele, gastroschisis
  —Caudal fold closure: bladder exstrophy

Duodenal atresia—failure to recanalize (trisomy 21).

Jejunal, ileal, colonic atresia—due to vascular accident (apple peel atresia).

Midgut development:
  6th week—midgut herniates through umbilical ring.
  10th week—returns to abdominal cavity + rotates around SMA.

Pathology—malrotation of midgut, omphalocele, intestinal atresia or stenosis, volvulus.

Gastroschisis—extrusion of abdominal contents through abdominal folds; not covered by peritoneum.

Omphalocele—persistence of herniation of abdominal contents into umbilical cord, covered by peritoneum (see Image 94).

Tracheoesophageal fistula

Abnormal connection between esophagus and trachea.

Most common subtype is blind upper esophagus with lower esophagus connected to trachea. Results in cyanosis, choking and vomiting with feeding, air bubble in stomach on CXR, polyhydramnios, failure to pass NG tube into stomach, and pneumonitis.

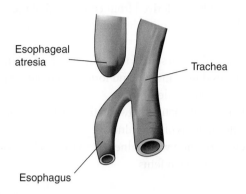

Esophageal atresia

Trachea

Esophagus

Congenital pyloric stenosis

Hypertrophy of the pylorus causes obstruction. Palpable "olive" mass in epigastric region and nonbilious projectile vomiting at ≈ 2 weeks of age. Treatment is surgical incision. Occurs in 1/600 live births, often in 1st-born males.

Pancreas and spleen embryology

Pancreas—derived from foregut. Dorsal and ventral pancreatic buds contribute to the pancreatic head, uncinate process (lower half of head), and main pancreatic duct. Dorsal pancreatic bud becomes everything else (body, tail, isthmus, and accessory pancreatic duct).

Annular pancreas—ventral pancreatic bud abnormally encircles 2nd part of duodenum; forms a ring of pancreatic tissue that may cause duodenal narrowing.

Pancreas divisum—ventral and dorsal parts fail to fuse at 8 weeks.

Spleen—arises from dorsal mesentery (hence is mesodermal) but is supplied by artery of foregut (celiac artery).

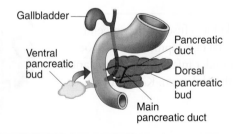

Gallbladder

Ventral pancreatic bud

Pancreatic duct

Dorsal pancreatic bud

Main pancreatic duct

Kidney embryology	1. Pronephros—week 4; then degenerates
	2. Mesonephros—functions as interim kidney for 1st trimester; later contributes to male genital system
	3. Metanephros—permanent; beginnings first appear during 5th week of gestation; nephrogenesis continues through 32–36 weeks of gestation

—Ureteric bud—derived from caudal end of mesonephros; gives rise to ureter, pelvises, and, through branching, calyces and collecting ducts; fully canalized by 10th week

—Metanephric mesenchyme—ureteric bud interacts with this tissue; interaction induces differentiation and formation of glomerulus and renal tubules to distal convoluted tubule

—Aberrant interaction between these 2 tissues may result in several congenital malformations of the kidney

Uteropelvic junction with kidney—last to canalize → most common site of obstruction (hydronephrosis) in fetus.

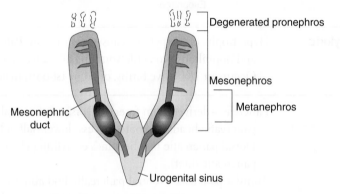

| **Potter's syndrome** | Bilateral renal agenesis → oligohydramnios → limb deformities, facial deformities, pulmonary hypoplasia. Caused by malformation of ureteric bud. | Babies who can't "Pee" in utero develop Potter's. |

| **Horseshoe kidney** | Inferior poles of both kidneys fuse. As they ascend from pelvis during fetal development, horseshoe kidneys get trapped under inferior mesenteric artery and remain low in the abdomen. Kidney functions normally. | 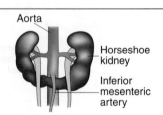 |

Genital embryology

Female	Default development. Mesonephric duct degenerates and paramesonephric duct develops.	Mesonephric duct must be induced to remain; default program for embryo development is for paramesonephric duct to develop into female.
Male	*SRY* gene on Y chromosome—produces testis-determining factor (testes development).	
	Müllerian inhibitory factor from Sertoli cells— suppresses development of paramesonephric ducts.	
	↑ androgens from Leydig cells—stimulates development of mesonephric ducts.	
Mesonephric (wolffian) duct	Develops into male internal structures (except prostate)—**S**eminal vesicles, **E**pididymis, **E**jaculatory duct, and **D**uctus deferens.	**SEED.**
Paramesonephric (müllerian) duct	Develops into female internal structures— fallopian tube, uterus, and upper ⅓ of vagina (lower ⅔ from urogenital sinus).	

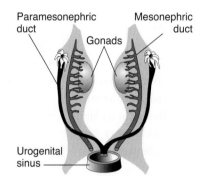

Bicornuate uterus

Results from incomplete fusion of the paramesonephric ducts. Associated with urinary tract abnormalities and infertility.

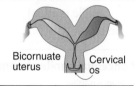

Male/female genital homologues

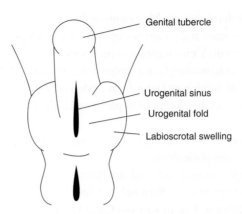

Genital tubercle

Urogenital sinus

Urogenital fold

Labioscrotal swelling

Male	Dihydrotestosterone		Estrogen	Female
Glans penis	←	Genital tubercle	→	Glans clitoris
Corpus cavernosum and spongiosum	←	Genital tubercle	→	Vestibular bulbs
Bulbourethral glands (of Cowper)	←	Urogenital sinus	→	Greater vestibular glands (of Bartholin)
Prostate gland	←	Urogenital sinus	→	Urethral and paraurethral glands (of Skene)
Ventral shaft of penis (penile urethra)	←	Urogenital folds	→	Labia minora
Scrotum	←	Labioscrotal swelling	→	Labia majora

Congenital penile abnormalities

Hypospadias

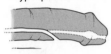

Epispadias

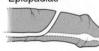

Hypospadias—abnormal opening of penile urethra on inferior (ventral) side of penis due to failure of urethral folds to close.

Epispadias—abnormal opening of penile urethra on superior (dorsal) side of penis due to faulty positioning of genital tubercle.

Hypospadias is more common than epispadias. Fix hypospadias to prevent UTIs.

Hypo is **below.**

Exstrophy of the bladder is associated with Epispadias.

When you have Epispadias, you hit your Eye when you pEE.

Descent of testes and ovaries	Female remnant	Male remnant
Gubernaculum (band of fibrous tissue)	Ovarian ligament + round ligament of uterus.	Anchors testes within scrotum.
Processus vaginalis (evagination of peritoneum)	Obliterated.	Forms tunica vaginalis.

Microbiology

"Support bacteria. They're the only culture some people have."

—Anonymous

"What lies behind us and what lies ahead of us are tiny matters compared to what lies within us."

—Oliver Wendell Holmes

This high-yield material covers the basic concepts of microbiology. The emphasis in previous examinations has been approximately 40% bacteriology (20% basic, 20% quasi-clinical), 25% immunology, 25% virology (10% basic, 15% quasi-clinical), 5% parasitology, and 5% mycology.

Microbiology questions on the Step 1 exam often require two steps: Given a certain clinical presentation, you will first need to identify the most likely causative organism, and you will then need to provide an answer regarding some feature of that organism. For example, a description of a child with fever and a petechial rash will be followed by a question that reads, "From what site does the responsible organism usually enter the blood?"

This section therefore presents organisms in two major ways: in individual microbial "profiles" and in the context of the systems they infect and the clinical presentations they produce. You should become familiar with both formats. When reviewing the systems approach, remind yourself of the features of each microbe by returning to the individual profiles. Also be sure to memorize the laboratory characteristics that allow you to identify microbes.

Additional tables that organize infectious diseases and syndromes according to the most commonly affected hosts and the most likely microbes are available on the First Aid team blog at www.firstaidteam.com.

Bacterial structures

Structure	Function	Chemical composition
Peptidoglycan	Gives rigid support, protects against osmotic pressure.	Sugar backbone with cross-linked peptide side chains.
Cell wall/cell membrane (gram positives)	Major surface antigen.	Peptidoglycan for support. Teichoic acid induces TNF and IL-1.
Outer membrane (gram negatives)	Site of endotoxin (lipopolysaccharide); major surface antigen.	Lipid A induces TNF and IL-1; polysaccharide is the antigen.
Plasma membrane	Site of oxidative and transport enzymes.	Lipoprotein bilayer.
Ribosome	Protein synthesis.	50S and 30S subunits.
Periplasm	Space between the cytoplasmic membrane and peptidoglycan wall in gram-negative bacteria.	Contains many hydrolytic enzymes, including β-lactamases.
Capsule	Protects against phagocytosis.	Polysaccharide (except *Bacillus anthracis*, which contains D-glutamate).
Pilus/fimbria	Mediate adherence of bacteria to cell surface; sex pilus forms attachment between 2 bacteria during conjugation.	Glycoprotein.
Flagellum	Motility.	Protein.
Spore	Provides resistance to dehydration, heat, and chemicals.	Keratin-like coat; dipicolinic acid.
Plasmid	Contains a variety of genes for antibiotic resistance, enzymes, and toxins.	DNA.
Glycocalyx	Mediates adherence to surfaces, especially foreign surfaces (e.g., indwelling catheters).	Polysaccharide.

Cell walls

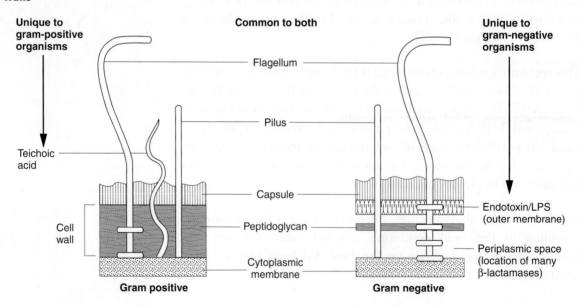

(Adapted, with permission, from Levinson W, Jawetz E. *Medical Microbiology and Immunology: Examination and Board Review,* 9th ed. New York: McGraw-Hill, 2006: 7.)

Bacterial taxonomy

Morphology	Gram Positive	Gram Negative
Circular (coccus)	*Staphylococcus* *Streptococcus*	*Neisseria*
Rod (bacillus)	*Clostridium* *Corynebacterium* *Bacillus* *Listeria* *Mycobacterium* (acid fast)	Enterics: ■ *E. coli* ■ *Shigella* ■ *Salmonella* ■ *Yersinia* ■ *Klebsiella* ■ *Proteus* ■ *Enterobacter* ■ *Serratia* ■ *Vibrio* ■ *Campylobacter* ■ *Helicobacter* ■ *Pseudomonas* ■ *Bacteroides* *Haemophilus* *Legionella* (silver) *Bordetella* *Francisella* *Brucella* *Pasteurella* *Bartonella* *Gardnerella* (gram variable)
Branching filamentous	*Actinomyces* *Nocardia* (weakly acid fast)	
Pleomorphic		Rickettsiae Chlamydiae (Giemsa)
Spiral		Spirochetes: ■ *Leptospira* ■ *Borrelia* (Giemsa) ■ *Treponema*
No cell wall	*Mycoplasma*	

Bacteria with unusual cell membranes/walls

Mycoplasma	Contain sterols and have no cell wall.
Mycobacteria	Contain mycolic acid. High lipid content.

Gram stain limitations	These bugs do not Gram stain well:	These Rascals May Microscopically Lack Color.
	Treponema (too thin to be visualized).	Treponemes—darkfield microscopy and fluorescent antibody staining.
	Rickettsia (intracellular parasite).	
	Mycobacteria (high-lipid-content cell wall requires acid-fast stain).	
	Mycoplasma (no cell wall).	
	Legionella pneumophila (primarily intracellular).	*Legionella*—silver stain.
	Chlamydia (intracellular parasite; lacks muramic acid in cell wall).	

Stains

Giemsa	*Borrelia, Plasmodium,* trypanosomes, *Chlamydia.*	
PAS (periodic acid-Schiff)	Stains glycogen, mucopolysaccharides; used to diagnose Whipple's disease (*Tropheryma whippelii*).	PASs the sugar.
Ziehl-Neelsen	Acid-fast organisms.	
India ink	*Cryptococcus neoformans* (mucicarmine can also be used to stain thick polysaccharide capsule red).	
Silver stain	Fungi (e.g., *Pneumocystis*), *Legionella.*	

Special culture requirements

Bug	Media used for isolation
H. influenzae	Chocolate agar with factors V (NAD$^+$) and X (hematin)
N. gonorrhoeae	Thayer-Martin (or **VPN**) media—**V**ancomycin (inhibits gram-positive organisms), **P**olymyxin (inhibits gram-negative organisms), and **N**ystatin (inhibits fungi); "to connect to *Neisseria*, please use your **VPN** client"
B. pertussis	Bordet-Gengou (potato) agar (**Bordet** for *Bordetella*)
C. diphtheriae	Tellurite plate, Löffler's media
M. tuberculosis	Löwenstein-Jensen agar
M. pneumoniae	Eaton's agar
Lactose-fermenting enterics	Pink colonies on MacConkey's agar (fermentation produces acid, turning plate pink); *E. coli* is also grown on eosin–methylene blue (EMB) agar as blue-black colonies with metallic sheen
Legionella	Charcoal yeast extract agar buffered with cysteine
Fungi	Sabouraud's agar

Obligate aerobes	Use an O$_2$-dependent system to generate ATP.	**N**agging **P**ests **M**ust **B**reathe.
	Examples include **N**ocardia, **P**seudomonas aeruginosa, **M**ycobacterium tuberculosis, and **B**acillus.	P. **AER**uginosa is an **AER**obe seen in burn wounds, nosocomial pneumonia, and pneumonias in cystic fibrosis patients.
	Reactivation of *M. tuberculosis* (e.g., after immune compromise or anti-TNF-α use) has a predilection for the apices of the lung, which have the highest PO$_2$.	

Obligate anaerobes	Examples include *Clostridium*, *Bacteroides*, and *Actinomyces*. They lack catalase and/or superoxide dismutase and are thus susceptible to oxidative damage. Generally foul smelling (short-chain fatty acids), are difficult to culture, and produce gas in tissue (CO_2 and H_2).	Anaerobes Can't Breathe Air. Anaerobes are normal flora in GI tract, pathogenic elsewhere. AminO$_2$glycosides are ineffective against anaerobes because these antibiotics require O_2 to enter into bacterial cell.
Intracellular bugs		
Obligate intracellular	*Rickettsia*, *Chlamydia*. Can't make own ATP.	Stay inside (cells) when it is Really Cold.
Facultative intracellular	*Salmonella*, *Neisseria*, *Brucella*, *Mycobacterium*, *Listeria*, *Francisella*, *Legionella*.	Some Nasty Bugs May Live FacultativeLy.
Encapsulated bacteria	Positive **quellung** reaction—if encapsulated bug is present, capsule **swells** when specific anticapsular antisera are added. Examples are *Streptococcus pneumoniae*, *Klebsiella pneumoniae*, *Haemophilus influenzae* type B, *Neisseria meningitidis*, *Salmonella*, group **B** strep. Their capsules serve as an antiphagocytic virulence factor.	**Q**uellung = capsular "swellung." Some Killers Have Nice Shiny Bodies. Capsule, conjugated with a protein, serves as antigen in vaccines.
Vaccines	For vaccines containing polysaccharide capsule antigens, a protein is conjugated to the polysaccharide antigen to promote T-cell activation and subsequent class switching. A polysaccharide antigen alone would not be recognized and presented by T cells; therefore, only IgM antibodies would be produced.	Pneumovax *H. influenzae* type B Meningococcal vaccines
Urease-positive bugs	*Proteus*, *Klebsiella*, *H. pylori*, *Ureaplasma*.	Particular Kinds Have Urease.
Pigment-producing bacteria	*Actinomyces israelii*—yellow "sulfur" **granules**, which are composed of a mass of filaments and formed in pus. *S. aureus*—yellow pigment. *Pseudomonas aeruginosa*—blue-**green** pigment. *Serratia marcescens*—red pigment.	Israel has **yellow** sand. *Aureus* (Latin) = gold. **AERUG**ula is **green**. *Serratia marcescens*—think red maraschino cherries!

Bacterial virulence factors

These promote evasion of host immune response.

Protein A (*S. aureus*)	Binds Fc region of Ig. Prevents opsonization and phagocytosis.
IgA protease	Enzyme that cleaves IgA. Secreted by **S.** *pneumoniae*, **H.** *influenzae* type B, and *Neisseria* (**SHiN**) in order to colonize respiratory mucosa.
M protein (group A streptococcus)	Helps prevent phagocytosis.

Main features of exotoxins and endotoxins

Property	Exotoxin	Endotoxin
Source	Certain species of some gram-positive and gram-negative bacteria	Outer cell membrane of most gram-negative bacteria
Secreted from cell	Yes	No
Chemistry	Polypeptide	Lipopolysaccharide (structural part of bacteria; released when lysed)
Location of genes	Plasmid or bacteriophage	Bacterial chromosome
Toxicity	High (fatal dose on the order of 1 µg)	Low (fatal dose on the order of hundreds of micrograms)
Clinical effects	Various effects (see text)	Fever, shock
Mode of action	Various modes (see text)	Includes TNF and IL-1
Antigenicity	Induces high-titer antibodies called antitoxins	Poorly antigenic
Vaccines	Toxoids used as vaccines	No toxoids formed and no vaccine available
Heat stability	Destroyed rapidly at 60°C (except staphylococcal enterotoxin)	Stable at 100°C for 1 hour
Typical diseases	Tetanus, botulism, diphtheria	Meningococcemia, sepsis by gram-negative rods

Bugs with exotoxins

Superantigens
Bind directly to MHC II and T-cell receptor simultaneously, activating large numbers of T cells to stimulate release of IFN-γ and IL-2.

S. aureus
TSST-1 superantigen causes toxic shock syndrome (fever, rash, shock). Other *S. aureus* toxins include enterotoxins that cause food poisoning as well as exfoliatin, which causes staphylococcal scalded skin syndrome.

S. pyogenes
Scarlet fever–erythrogenic toxin causes toxic shock–like syndrome.

ADP ribosylating A-B toxins
Interfere with host cell function. B (binding) component binds to a receptor on surface of host cell, enabling endocytosis. A (active) component then attaches an ADP-ribosyl to a host cell protein (ADP ribosylation), altering protein function.

Corynebacterium diphtheriae
Inactivates elongation factor (EF-2) (similar to *Pseudomonas* exotoxin A); causes pharyngitis and "pseudomembrane" in throat.

Vibrio cholerae
ADP ribosylation of G protein stimulates adenylyl cyclase; ↑ pumping of Cl^- into gut and ↓ Na^+ absorption. H_2O moves into gut lumen; causes voluminous rice-water diarrhea.

E. coli
Heat-labile toxin stimulates **A**denylate cyclase. Heat-stable toxin stimulates **G**uanylate cyclase. Both cause watery diarrhea. "Labile like the **A**ir, stable like the **G**round."

Bordetella pertussis
Increases cAMP by inhibiting $G\alpha_i$; causes whooping cough; inhibits chemokine receptor, causing lymphocytosis.

Other toxins
Clostridium perfringens
α toxin, a lecithinase that acts as a phospholipase to cleave cell membranes and causes gas gangrene; get double zone of hemolysis on blood agar.

C. tetani
Blocks the release of inhibitory neurotransmitters GABA and glycine; causes "lockjaw."

C. botulinum
Blocks the release of acetylcholine; causes anticholinergic symptoms, CNS paralysis, especially cranial nerves; spores found in canned food, honey (causes floppy baby).

Bacillus anthracis
Edema factor, part of the toxin complex, is an adenylate cyclase.

Shigella
Shiga toxin (also produced by *E. coli* O157:H7) cleaves host cell rRNA (inactivates 60S ribosome); also enhances cytokine release, causing HUS.

S. pyogenes
Streptolysin O is a hemolysin; antigen for ASO antibody, which is used in the diagnosis of rheumatic fever.

---

cAMP inducers
1. *Vibrio cholerae* toxin permanently activates G_s, causing rice-water diarrhea.
2. Pertussis toxin permanently disables G_i, causing whooping cough.
3. *E. coli* (ETEC)—heat-labile toxin.
4. *Bacillus anthracis* toxin includes edema factor, a bacterial adenylate cyclase (↑ cAMP).

Cholera, pertussis, and *E. coli* toxins act via ADP ribosylation to permanently activate endogenous adenylate cyclase (↑ cAMP), while the anthrax edema factor is itself an adenylate cyclase.

Cholera turns the "on" on.
Pertussis turns the "off" off.
Pertussis toxin also promotes lymphocytosis by inhibiting chemokine receptors.

Endotoxin

A lipopolysaccharide found in outer membrane of gram-negative bacteria.

N-dotoxin is an integral part of gram-**N**egative outer membrane. Endotoxin is heat stable.

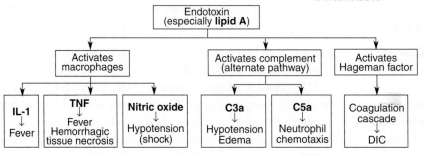

(Adapted, with permission, from Levinson W, Jawetz E. *Medical Microbiology and Immunology: Examination and Board Review,* 6th ed. New York: McGraw-Hill, 2000: 39.)

Bacterial growth curve

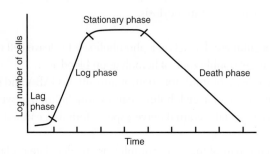

Lag—metabolic activity without division.
Log—rapid cell division.
Stationary—nutrient depletion slows growth. Spore formation in some bacteria.
Death—prolonged nutrient depletion and buildup of waste products lead to death.

Bacterial genetics

Transformation

Ability to take up DNA from environment (also known as "competence"). A feature of many bacteria, especially **S**. *pneumoniae*, **H**. *influenzae* type B, and **N**eisseria (**SHiN**). Any DNA can be used.

Conjugation

F⁺ × F⁻

F⁺ plasmid contains genes required for conjugation process. Bacteria without this plasmid are termed F⁻. Plasmid is replicated and transferred through pilus from F⁺ cell. Plasmid DNA only; no transfer of chromosomal genes.

Hfr × F⁻

F⁺ plasmid can become incorporated into bacterial chromosomal DNA, termed Hfr cell. Replication of incorporated plasmid DNA may include some flanking chromosomal DNA. Transfer of plasmid and chromosomal genes.

Transposition

Segment of DNA that can "jump" (excision and reincorporation) from one location to another, can transfer genes from plasmid to chromosome and vice versa. When excision occurs, may include some flanking chromosomal DNA, which can be incorporated into a plasmid and transferred to another bacterium.

Transduction

Generalized

A "packaging" event. Lytic phage infects bacterium, leading to cleavage of bacterial DNA and synthesis of viral proteins. Parts of bacterial chromosomal DNA may become packaged in viral capsid. Phage infects another bacterium, transferring these genes.

Specialized

An "excision" event. Lysogenic phage infects bacterium; viral DNA incorporated into bacterial chromosome. When phage DNA is excised, flanking bacterial genes may be excised with it. DNA is packaged into phage viral capsid and can infect another bacterium.

Lysogeny, specialized transduction

Genes for the following 5 bacterial toxins encoded in a lysogenic phage:

ShigA-like toxin   ABCDE.
Botulinum toxin (certain strains)
Cholera toxin
Diphtheria toxin
Erythrogenic toxin of *Streptococcus pyogenes*

Gram-positive lab algorithm

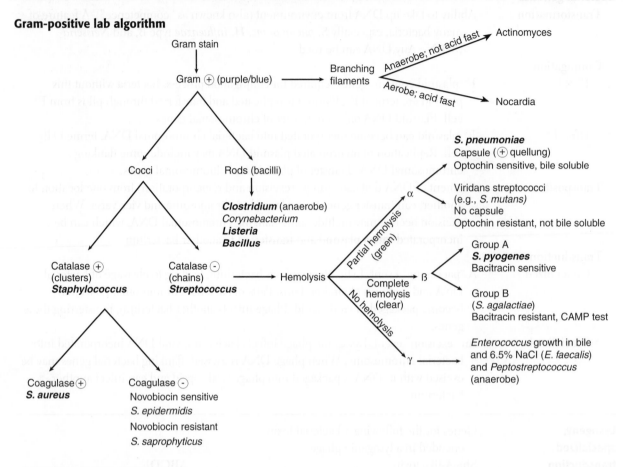

Important pathogens are in **bold type.**

Note: *Enterococcus* is either α- or γ-hemolytic.

Identification of gram-positive cocci

Staphylococci	NOvobiocin—*Saprophyticus* is Resistant; *Epidermidis* is Sensitive.	On the office's **staph** retreat, there was **NO StRES.**
Streptococci	Optochin—*Viridans* is Resistant; *Pneumoniae* is Sensitive.	OVRPS (overpass).
	Bacitracin—group **B** strep are Resistant; group **A** strep are Sensitive.	**B-BRAS.**

α-hemolytic bacteria

Form green ring around colonies on blood agar. Include the following organisms:
1. *Streptococcus pneumoniae* (catalase negative and optochin sensitive) (see Image 1)
2. Viridans streptococci (catalase negative and optochin resistant)

β-hemolytic bacteria

Form clear area of hemolysis on blood agar. Include the following organisms:
1. *Staphylococcus aureus* (catalase and coagulase positive)
2. *Streptococcus pyogenes*—group A strep (catalase negative and bacitracin sensitive)
3. *Streptococcus agalactiae*—group B strep (catalase negative and bacitracin resistant)
4. *Listeria monocytogenes* (tumbling motility, meningitis in newborns, unpasteurized milk)

Catalase/coagulase (gram-positive cocci)	Catalase degrades H_2O_2 before it can be converted to microbicidal products by the enzyme myeloperoxidase. Staphylococci make catalase, whereas streptococci do not. *S. aureus* makes coagulase, whereas *S. epidermidis* and *S. saprophyticus* do not.	**Staph** make catalase because they have more "**staff**." Bad staph (*aureus*, because *epidermidis* is skin flora) make coagulase and toxins. Catalase-producing microbes easily degrade what little H_2O_2 is present in people with chronic granulomatous disease (NADPH oxidase deficiency), thereby causing recurrent infections.
Staphylococcus aureus	Protein A (virulence factor) binds Fc-IgG, inhibiting complement fixation and phagocytosis. Causes: 1. Inflammatory disease—skin infections, organ abscesses, pneumonia 2. Toxin-mediated disease—toxic shock syndrome (TSST-1 toxin), scalded skin syndrome (exfoliative toxin), rapid-onset food poisoning (enterotoxins) (see Image 3) 3. MRSA (methicillin-resistant *S. aureus*) infection—important cause of serious nosocomial and community-acquired infections. Resistant to β-lactams due to altered penicillin-binding protein.	TSST is a superantigen that binds to MHC II and T-cell receptor, resulting in polyclonal T-cell activation. *S. aureus* food poisoning is due to ingestion of preformed toxin. Causes acute bacterial endocarditis, osteomyelitis.
Staphylococcus epidermidis	Infects prosthetic devices and intravenous catheters by producing adherent biofilms. Component of normal skin flora; contaminates blood cultures.	
Streptococcus pneumoniae	Most common cause of: Meningitis Otitis media (in children) Pneumonia Sinusitis Lancet shaped. Encapsulated. IgA protease.	*S. pneumoniae* **MOPS** are Most **OP**tochin Sensitive. Pneumococcus is associated with "rusty" sputum, sepsis in sickle cell anemia and splenectomy.
Viridans group streptococci	Viridans streptococci are α-hemolytic. They are normal flora of the oropharynx and cause dental caries (*Streptococcus mutans*) and subacute bacterial endocarditis (*S. sanguis*). Resistant to optochin, differentiating them from *S. pneumoniae*, which is α-hemolytic but is optochin sensitive.	*Sanguis* (Latin) = blood. There is lots of blood in the heart (endocarditis). Viridans group strep live in the mouth because they are not afraid **of-the-chin** (**op-to-chin** resistant).

HIGH-YIELD PRINCIPLES

MICROBIOLOGY

145

***Streptococcus pyogenes* (group A streptococci)**	Causes: 1. Pyogenic—pharyngitis, cellulitis, impetigo 2. Toxigenic—scarlet fever, toxic shock–like syndrome 3. Immunologic—rheumatic fever, acute glomerulonephritis Bacitracin sensitive. Antibodies to **M protein** enhance host defenses against *S. pyogenes* but can give rise to rheumatic fever. ASO titer detects recent *S. pyogenes* infection.	**PH**aryngitis can result in rheumatic "**PH**ever" and glomerulone**PH**ritis. No "**rheum**" for SPEC**C**ulation: **S**ubcutaneous plaques, **P**olyarthritis, **E**rythema marginatum, **C**horea, **C**arditis.
***Streptococcus agalactiae* (group B streptococci)**	Bacitracin resistant, β-hemolytic, colonizes vagina; causes pneumonia, meningitis, and sepsis, mainly in babies. Produces CAMP factor, which enlarges the area of hemolysis formed by *S. aureus*. (Note: CAMP stands for the authors of the test, not cyclic AMP.) Screen pregnant women at 35–37 weeks. Patients with positive culture receive intrapartum penicillin prophylaxis.	**B** for **B**abies!
Enterococci (group D streptococci) 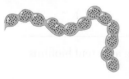	Enterococci (*Enterococcus faecalis* and *E. faecium*) are normal colonic flora that are penicillin G resistant and cause UTI and subacute endocarditis. Lancefield group D includes the enterococci and the nonenterococcal group D streptococci. Lancefield grouping is based on differences in the C carbohydrate on the bacterial cell wall. Variable hemolysis. VRE (vancomycin-resistant enterococci) are an important cause of nosocomial infection.	Enterococci, hardier than nonenterococcal group D, can thus grow in 6.5% NaCl and bile (lab test). *Entero* = intestine, *faecalis* = feces, *strepto* = twisted (chains), *coccus* = berry.
***Streptococcus bovis* (group D streptococci)**	Colonizes the gut. Can cause bacteremia and subacute endocarditis in colon cancer patients.	
Corynebacterium diphtheria	Causes diphtheria via exotoxin encoded by β-prophage. Potent exotoxin inhibits protein synthesis via ADP ribosylation of EF-2. Symptoms include pseudomembranous pharyngitis (grayish-white membrane) with lymphadenopathy. Lab diagnosis based on gram-positive rods with metachromatic (blue and red) granules. Toxoid vaccine prevents diphtheria.	*Coryne* = club shaped. Grows on tellurite agar. **ABCDEFG:** **A**DP ribosylation **B**eta-prophage ***C**orynebacterium* ***D**iphtheria* **E**longation **F**actor 2 **G**ranules

Spores: bacterial	Only certain gram-positive rods form spores when nutrients are limited (at end of stationary phase). Spores are highly resistant to destruction by heat and chemicals. Have dipicolinic acid in their core. Have no metabolic activity. Must autoclave to kill spores (as is done to surgical equipment) by steaming at 121°C for 15 minutes.	Spore-forming gram-positive bacteria found in soil: *Bacillus anthracis, Clostridium perfringens, C. tetani*. Other spore formers include *B. cereus, C. botulinum*.
Clostridia (with exotoxins)	Gram-positive, spore-forming, obligate anaerobic bacilli. *Clostridium tetani* produces tetanospasmin, an exotoxin causing tetanus.	**TET**anus is **TET**anic paralysis (blocks glycine and GABA release [inhibitory neurotransmitters]) from Renshaw cells in spinal cord. Causes spastic paralysis, trismus (lockjaw, and risus sardonicus).
	C. botulinum produces a preformed, heat-labile toxin that inhibits ACh release at the neuromuscular junction, causing botulism. In adults, disease is caused by ingestion of preformed toxin. In babies, ingestion of bacterial spores in honey causes disease (floppy baby syndrome).	***BOT**ulinum* is from bad **BOT**tles of food and honey (causes a flaccid paralysis).
	C. perfringens produces α toxin ("lecithinase," a phospholipase) that can cause myonecrosis (gas gangrene) and hemolysis.	***PERF**ringens* **PERF**orates a gangrenous leg.
	C. difficile produces 2 toxins. Toxin A, enterotoxin, binds to the brush border of the gut. Toxin B, cytotoxin, destroys the cytoskeletal structure of enterocytes, causing pseudomembranous colitis. Often 2° to antibiotic use, especially clindamycin or ampicillin. Diagnosed by detection of one or both toxins in stool.	**DI**ficile causes **DI**arrhea. Treatment: metronidazole.
Anthrax	Caused by *Bacillus anthracis*, a gram-positive, spore-forming rod that produces anthrax toxin. The only bacterium with a polypeptide capsule (contains D-glutamate). Cutaneous anthrax—contact → black eschar (painless ulcer); can progress to bacteremia and death.	Black skin lesions—black eschar (necrosis) surrounded by edematous ring. Caused by lethal factor and edema factor.
	Pulmonary anthrax—inhalation of spores → flulike symptoms that rapidly progress to fever, pulmonary hemorrhage, mediastinitis, and shock.	Woolsorters' disease—inhalation of spores from contaminated wool.

Listeria
monocytogenes

Facultative intracellular microbe; acquired by ingestion of unpasteurized milk/cheese and deli meats or by vaginal transmission during birth. Form "actin rockets" by which they move from cell to cell. Characteristic tumbling motility.

Can cause amnionitis, septicemia, and spontaneous abortion in pregnant women; granulomatosis infantiseptica; neonatal meningitis; meningitis in immunocompromised patients; mild gastroenteritis in healthy individuals.

Actinomyces vs.
Nocardia

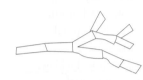

Both are gram-positive rods forming long branching filaments resembling fungi.

Actinomyces israelii, a gram-positive anaerobe, causes oral/facial abscesses that may drain through sinus tracts in skin. Normal oral flora.

Nocardia asteroides, a gram-positive and also a weakly acid-fast aerobe in soil, causes pulmonary infection in immunocompromised patients.

A. israelii forms yellow "sulfur granules" in sinus tracts.

SNAP:

Sulfa for

Nocardia;

Actinomyces use

Penicillin

1° and 2° tuberculosis

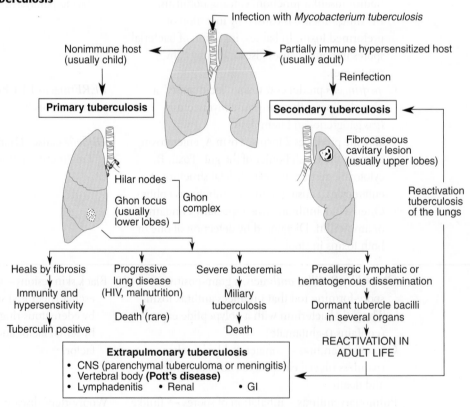

(Adapted, with permission, from Chandrasoma P, Taylor CR. *Concise Pathology*, 3rd ed. Stamford, CT: Appleton & Lange, 1998: 523.)

PPD+ if current infection, past exposure, or BCG vaccinated.

PPD– if no infection or anergic (steroids, malnutrition, immunocompromise, sarcoidosis).

Ghon complex

TB granulomas (Ghon focus + lobar and perihilar lymph node involvement). Reflects 1° infection or exposure.

Mycobacteria	*Mycobacterium tuberculosis* (TB, often resistant to multiple drugs). *M. kansasii* (pulmonary TB-like symptoms). *M. avium–intracellulare* (often resistant to multiple drugs; causes disseminated disease in AIDS). Prophylactic treatment with azithromycin. All mycobacteria are acid-fast organisms.	TB symptoms i night sweats, and hemopt
Leprosy (Hansen's disease) 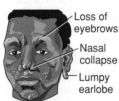 "Leonine facies" of lepromatous leprosy	Caused by *Mycobacterium leprae*, an acid-fast bacillus that likes cool temperatures (infects skin and superficial nerves) and cannot be grown in vitro. Reservoir in United States: armadillos. Treatment: long-term oral dapsone; toxicity is hemolysis and methemoglobinemia. Alternate treatments include rifampin and combination of clofazimine and dapsone.	Hansen's disease has 2 forms: lepromatous (see Image 14) and tuberculoid; lepromatous presents diffusely over skin and is communicable (patients with weak T-cell–mediated immunity); tuberculoid is limited to a few hypoesthetic skin nodules (patients with intact T-cell response). **LE**promatous can be **LE**thal.

Loss of eyebrows
Nasal collapse
Lumpy earlobe

Gram-negative lab algorithm

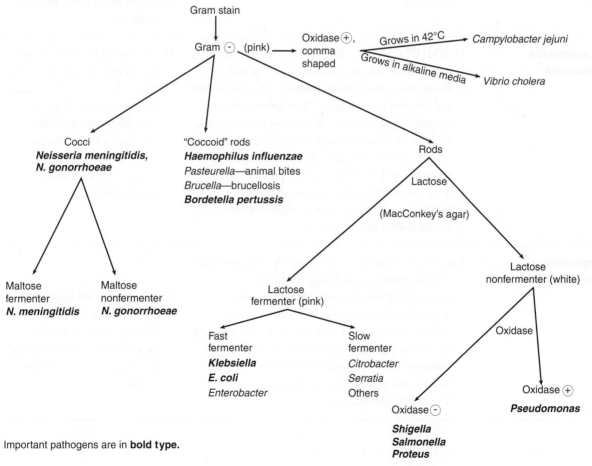

Important pathogens are in **bold type.**

Lactose-fermenting enteric bacteria

Grow pink colonies on MacConkey's agar. Examples include *Citrobacter*, *Klebsiella*, *E. coli*, *Enterobacter*, and *Serratia*. *E. coli* produces β-galactosidase, which breaks down lactose into glucose and galactose.

Lactose is **KEE**.
Test with MacCon**KEE'S** agar.

Penicillin and gram-negative bugs

Gram-negative bacilli are resistant to penicillin G but may be susceptible to penicillin derivatives such as ampicillin. The gram-negative outer membrane layer inhibits entry of penicillin G and vancomycin.

Neisseria

Gram-negative cocci (see Image 4). Both ferment glucose and produce IgA proteases. Menin**G**ococci ferment **M**altose and **G**lucose. **G**onococci ferment **G**lucose.

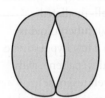

Gonococci	Meningococci
No polysaccharide capsule	Polysaccharide capsule
No maltose fermentation	Maltose fermentation
No vaccine (due to rapid antigenic variation of pilus proteins)	Vaccine (none for type B)
Sexually transmitted	Respiratory and oral secretions
Causes gonorrhea, septic arthritis, neonatal conjunctivitis, PID, and Fitz-Hugh–Curtis syndrome	Causes meningococcemia and meningitis, Waterhouse-Friderichsen syndrome
	Rifampin prophylaxis in close contacts

Haemophilus influenzae

*Ha**EMOP**hilus* causes **E**piglottitis ("cherry red" in children), **M**eningitis, **O**titis media, and **P**neumonia. Small gram-negative (coccobacillary) rod. Aerosol transmission. Most invasive disease caused by capsular type B. Produces IgA protease. Culture on **chocolate agar** requires factors **V** (NAD⁺) and **X** (hematin) for growth; can also be grown with *S. aureus*, which provides factor V. Treat meningitis with ceftriaxone. Rifampin prophylaxis in close contacts. Does not cause the flu (influenza virus does).

When a child has "flu," mom goes to five (**V**) and dime (**X**) store to buy some **chocolate**. Vaccine contains type B capsular polysaccharide conjugated to diphtheria toxoid or other protein. Given between 2 and 18 months of age.

Legionella pneumophila

Legionnaires' disease = severe pneumonia and fever. Pontiac fever = mild flulike syndrome.
Gram-negative rod. Gram stains poorly—use silver stain. Grow on charcoal yeast extract culture with iron and cysteine. Detected clinically by presence of antigen in urine. Aerosol transmission from environmental water source habitat. No person-to-person transmission. Treatment: erythromycin.

Think of a French legionnaire (soldier) with his silver helmet, sitting around a campfire (charcoal) with his iron dagger—he is no **sissy** (**cysteine**).

Pseudomonas aeruginosa	*PSEUDOmonas* is associated with wound and burn infections, Pneumonia (especially in cystic fibrosis), Sepsis (black lesions on skin), External otitis (swimmer's ear), UTI, Drug use and Diabetic Osteomyelitis, and hot tub folliculitis. Malignant otitis externa in diabetics. Aerobic gram-negative rod. Non–lactose fermenting, oxidase positive. Produces pyocyanin (blue-green) pigment; has a grapelike odor. Water source. Produces endotoxin (fever, shock) and exotoxin A (inactivates EF-2). Treatment: aminoglycoside plus extended-spectrum penicillin (e.g., piperacillin, ticarcillin).	AERuginosa—AERobic. Think water connection and blue-green pigment. Think *Pseudomonas* in burn victims.
E. coli	*E. coli* virulence factors: fimbriae—cystitis and pyelonephritis; K capsule—pneumonia, neonatal meningitis; LPS endotoxin—septic shock.	

Strain	Toxin and Mechanism	Presentation
EIEC	Produces Shiga-like toxin. Microbe invades intestinal mucosa **and** toxin causes necrosis and inflammation.	Invasive; dysentery.
ETEC	Labile toxin/stable toxin. No inflammation or invasion.	Traveler's diarrhea (watery).
EPEC	No toxin produced. Adheres to apical surface, flattens villi, prevents absorption.	Diarrhea usually in children (Pediatrics).
EHEC	O157:H7 is the most common serotype. Produces Shiga-like toxin and Hemolytic-uremic syndrome (triad of anemia, thrombocytopenia, and acute renal failure). Endothelium swells and narrows lumen, leading to mechanical hemolysis and reduced renal blood flow; damaged endothelium consumes platelets.	Dysentery (toxin alone causes necrosis and inflammation). Does not ferment sorbitol (distinguishes it from other *E. coli*).

Klebsiella	An intestinal flora that causes lobar pneumonia in alcoholics and diabetics when aspirated. Red currant jelly sputum. Also cause of nosocomial UTIs.	4 A's: Aspiration pneumonia Abscess in lungs Alcoholics di-A-betics

Salmonella* vs. *Shigella	Both are non–lactose fermenters; both invade intestinal mucosa and can cause bloody diarrhea. *Salmonella* have flagella and can disseminate hematogenously. Only *Salmonella* produce H_2S. Symptoms of salmonellosis may be prolonged with antibiotic treatments, and there is typically a monocytic response. *Shigella* is more virulent (10^1 organisms) than *Salmonella* (10^5 organisms). *Salmonella typhi* causes typhoid fever—fever, diarrhea, headache, rose spots on abdomen. Can remain in gallbladder chronically.	**Salmon swim** (motile and disseminate). *Salmonella* have an animal reservoir (except *S. typhi*, which is found only in humans); *Shigella* do not have flagella but can propel themselves while within a cell by actin polymerization. Transmission is via "**F**ood, **F**ingers, **F**eces, and **F**lies."

Campylobacter jejuni	Major cause of bloody diarrhea, especially in children. Fecal-oral transmission through foods such as poultry, meat, unpasteurized milk. Comma or S-shaped, oxidase positive, grows at 42°C ("*Campylobacter* likes the hot **camp**fire."). Common antecedent to Guillain-Barré syndrome.

Vibrio cholerae	Produces profuse rice-water diarrhea via toxin that permanently activates G_s, ↑ cAMP. Prompt oral rehydration is necessary. Comma shaped, oxidase positive, grows in alkaline media. Endemic to developing countries.

Yersinia enterocolitica	Usually transmitted from pet feces (e.g., puppies), contaminated milk, or pork. Outbreaks of **diarrhea** are common in day care centers. **Causes mesenteric adenitis that can mimic Crohn's or appendicitis.**

Helicobacter pylori 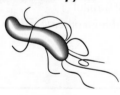	Causes gastritis and up to 90% of duodenal ulcers. Risk factor for peptic ulcer, gastric adenocarcinoma, and lymphoma. Gram-negative rod. Urease positive (e.g., urease breath test). Creates alkaline environment. Treat with triple therapy: (1) metronidazole, bismuth (Pepto-Bismol), and either tetracycline or amoxicillin; or (2) (more costly) metronidazole, omeprazole, and clarithromycin.

Spirochetes 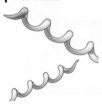	The spirochetes are spiral-shaped bacteria with axial filaments and include *Borrelia* (big size), *Leptospira*, and *Treponema*. Only *Borrelia* can be visualized using aniline dyes (Wright's or Giemsa stain) in light microscopy. *Treponema* is visualized by dark-field microscopy.	**BLT. B** is **B**ig.

Leptospira interrogans 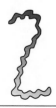	Question mark–shaped bacteria found in water contaminated with animal urine. Leptospirosis includes flulike symptoms, fever, headache, abdominal pain, jaundice, and photophobia with conjunctivitis. Most prevalent among surfers and in the tropics. Weil's disease (icterohemorrhagic leptospirosis)—severe form with jaundice and azotemia from liver and kidney dysfunction; fever, hemorrhage, and anemia.

Lyme disease	Caused by *Borrelia burgdorferi*, which is transmitted by the tick *Ixodes* (also vector for *Babesia*). Presents with erythema chronicum migrans, an expanding "bull's eye" red rash with central clearing. Also affects joints, CNS, and heart. Mice are important reservoirs. Deer required for tick life cycle. Treatment: doxycycline, ceftriaxone. Named after Lyme, Connecticut; disease is common in northeastern United States.	3 stages of Lyme disease: Stage 1—erythema chronicum migrans, flulike symptoms. Stage 2—neurologic (Bell's palsy) and cardiac (AV nodal block) manifestations. Stage 3—chronic monoarthritis, and migratory polyarthritis. **BAKE** a Key **Lyme** pie: **B**ell's palsy (bilateral), **A**rthritis, **K**ardiac block, **E**rythema migrans.
Syphilis	Caused by spirochete *Treponema pallidum*.	Treatment: penicillin G.
1° syphilis	Presents with painless chancre (localized disease).	
2° syphilis	Disseminated disease with constitutional symptoms, maculopapular rash (palms and soles), condylomata lata. Many treponemes are present in chancres of 1° and condylomata lata of 2° syphilis.	Secondary syphilis = Systemic.
3° syphilis	Gummas (chronic granulomas), aortitis (vasa vasorum destruction), neurosyphilis (tabes dorsalis), Argyll Robertson pupil.	Signs: broad-based ataxia, positive Romberg, Charcot joint, stroke without hypertension. Screen with: VDRL. Confirm with: FTA-ABS.
Congenital syphilis	Saber shins, saddle nose, CN VIII deafness, Hutchinson's teeth, mulberry molars.	
Argyll Robertson pupil	Argyll Robertson pupil constricts with accommodation but is not reactive to light. Associated with 3° syphilis.	"Prostitute's pupil"— accommodates but does not react.
VDRL false positives	VDRL detects nonspecific antibody that reacts with beef cardiolipin. Used for diagnosis of syphilis, but many biologic false positives, including viral infection (mononucleosis, hepatitis), some drugs, rheumatic fever, SLE, and leprosy.	**VDRL:** **V**iruses (mono, hepatitis) **D**rugs **R**heumatic fever **L**upus and leprosy

Zoonotic bacteria

Species	Disease	Transmission and source	
Bartonella spp.	Cat scratch fever	Cat scratch; can cause bacillary angiomatosis in immunocompromised patients (often confused with Kaposi's sarcoma)	**B**ig **B**ad **B**ed **B**ugs **F**rom **Y**our **P**et named **Ella**.
Borrelia burgdorferi	Lyme disease	Tick bite; *Ixodes* ticks that live on deer and mice	
Borrelia recurrentis	Recurrent fever from variable surface antigens	Louse	
Brucella spp.	Brucellosis/ undulant fever	Dairy products, contact with animals	**U**npasteurized dairy products give you **U**ndulant fever.
Francisella tularensis	Tularemia	Tick bite; rabbits, deer	
Yersinia pestis	Plague	Flea bite; rodents, especially prairie dogs	
Pasteurella multocida	Cellulitis, osteomyelitis	Animal bite; cats, dogs	

Gardnerella vaginalis	A pleomorphic, gram-variable rod that causes vaginosis presenting as a gray vaginal discharge with a **fishy** smell; nonpainful. *Mobiluncus*, an anaerobe, is also involved. Associated with sexual activity, but not an STD. Bacterial vaginosis is characterized by overgrowth of certain bacteria in vagina. Treatment: metronidazole. **Clue** cells, or vaginal epithelial cells covered with bacteria, are visible under the microscope (see Image 13).	I don't have a **clue** why I smell **fish** in the **vagina garden!**
Rickettsiae	Rickettsiae are obligate intracellular organisms that need CoA and NAD$^+$. All except *Coxiella* are transmitted by an arthropod vector and cause headache, fever, and rash; *Coxiella* is an atypical rickettsia because it is transmitted by aerosol and causes pneumonia. Treatment: doxycycline.	Classic triad—headache, fever, rash (vasculitis).

Rickettsial diseases and vectors	Rocky Mountain spotted fever (tick)—*Rickettsia rickettsii.* Endemic typhus (fleas)—*R. typhi.* Epidemic typhus (human body louse)—*R. prowazekii.* Ehrlichiosis (tick)—*Ehrlichia.* No rash. Granulocytes with berry cluster organisms. Q fever (tick feces and cattle placenta release spores that are inhaled as aerosols)—*Coxiella burnetii.* Treatment for all: doxycycline.	Rickettsial rash starts on hands and feet; typhus rash starts centrally and spreads outward without involving palms or soles: "**R**ickettsia on the w**R**ists, **T**yphus on the **T**runk." **Q** fever is **Q**ueer because it has no rash, has no vector, and has negative Weil-Felix, and its causative organism can survive outside for a long time and does not have *Rickettsia* as its genus name.
Weil-Felix reaction	Patients with rickettsial infection have antibodies against *Rickettsia.* When patient serum is mixed with *Proteus* antigens, antirickettsial antibodies cross-react to *Proteus* O antigens and agglutinate (Weil-Felix is negative in *Coxiella* infection).	
Rocky Mountain spotted fever	Caused by *Rickettsia rickettsii.* Symptoms: rash on palms and soles (migrating to wrists, ankles, then trunk), headache, fever. Endemic to East Coast (in spite of name).	**Palm** and **sole** rash is seen in Coxsackievirus **A** infection (hand, foot, and mouth disease), **R**ocky Mountain spotted fever, and **S**yphilis (you drive **CARS** using your **palms** and **soles**).

Chlamydiae

Chlamydiae cannot make their own ATP. They are obligate intracellular organisms that cause mucosal infections. 2 forms:
1. Elementary body (small, dense) is **E**nfectious and **E**nters cell via endocytosis
2. **R**eticulate body **R**eplicates in cell by fission; form seen on tissue culture.

Chlamydia trachomatis causes reactive arthritis, conjunctivitis, nongonococcal urethritis, and pelvic inflammatory disease (PID).

C. pneumoniae and *C. psittaci* cause atypical pneumonia; transmitted by aerosol.

Treatment: azithromycin or doxycycline.

Chlamys = cloak (intracellular).
Chlamydia psittaci—notable for an avian reservoir.

The chlamydial cell wall is unusual in that it lacks muramic acid.

Lab diagnosis: cytoplasmic inclusions seen on Giemsa or fluorescent antibody–stained smear.

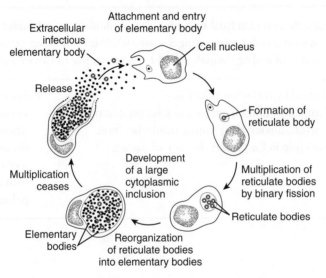

Chlamydia trachomatis serotypes

Types A, B, and C—chronic infection, cause blindness due to follicular conjunctivitis in Africa.

Types D–K—urethritis/PID, ectopic pregnancy, neonatal pneumonia (staccato cough), or neonatal conjunctivitis.

Types L1, L2, and L3—lymphogranuloma venereum. Do not confuse with granuloma inguinale (donovanosis), which is caused by *Klebsiella granulomatis*.

ABC = **A**frica/**B**lindness/ **C**hronic infection.

L1–3 = **L**ymphogranuloma venereum.

D–K = everything else.
Neonatal disease can be acquired during passage through infected birth canal.
Treatment: azithromycin.

Mycoplasma pneumoniae

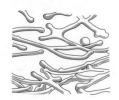

Classic cause of atypical "walking" pneumonia (insidious onset, headache, nonproductive cough, diffuse interstitial infiltrate). X-ray looks worse than patient. High titer of cold agglutinins (IgM), which can agglutinate or lyse RBCs. Grown on Eaton's agar.

Treatment: tetracycline or erythromycin (bugs are penicillin resistant because they have no cell wall).

No cell wall. Not seen on gram stain.

Only bacterial membrane containing cholesterol.

Mycoplasmal pneumonia is more common in patients < 30 years of age.

Frequent outbreaks in military recruits and prisons.

Systemic mycoses

All of the following can cause **pneumonia** and can disseminate. All are caused by dimorphic fungi: cold (20°C) = mold; heat (37°C) = yeast. The only exception is coccidioidomycosis, which is a spherule (not yeast) in tissue. Treatment: fluconazole or ketoconazole for **local** infection; amphotericin B for **systemic** infection. Systemic mycoses can mimic TB (granuloma formation), except, unlike TB, have no person-person transmission.

Disease	Endemic location and pathologic features	Notes
Histoplasmosis  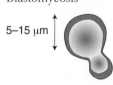 3–5 μm	Mississippi and Ohio river valleys. Causes pneumonia. Macrophage filled with *Histoplasma* (smaller than RBC)	Histo Hides (within macrophages). Bird or bat droppings.
Blastomycosis 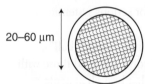 5–15 μm	States east of Mississippi River and Central America. Causes inflammatory lung disease and can disseminate to skin and bone. Forms granulomatous nodules. Broad-base budding (same size as RBC)	Blasto Buds (Broadly).
Coccidioidomycosis 20–60 μm	Southwestern United States, California. Causes pneumonia and meningitis; can disseminate to bone and skin. Case rate ↑ after earthquakes (spherules in dust are thrown up in the air). Spherule filled with endospores (much larger than RBC)	Coccidio Crowds. San Joaquin Valley or desert (desert bumps) "valley fever" (see Image 7).
Paracoccidioidomy-cosis 40–50 μm	Latin America. Budding yeast with "captain's wheel" formation (much larger than RBC)	"Captain's wheel" appearance. Paracoccidio Parasails with the **captain's wheel** all the way to **Latin America**.

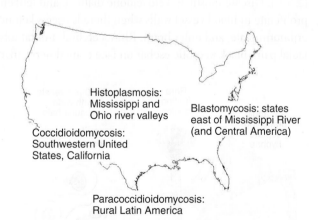

Histoplasmosis: Mississippi and Ohio river valleys

Blastomycosis: states east of Mississippi River (and Central America)

Coccidioidomycosis: Southwestern United States, California

Paracoccidioidomycosis: Rural Latin America

Cutaneous mycoses

Tinea versicolor

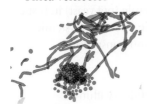

Caused by *Malassezia furfur*. Degradation of lipids produces acids that damage melanocytes and cause hypopigmented and/or hyperpigmented patches. Occurs in hot, humid weather. Treatment: topical miconazole, selenium sulfide (Selsun). "Spaghetti and meatball" appearance on KOH prep.

Tinea pedis (foot), Tinea cruris (groin), Tinea corporis (ringworm, on body), Tinea capitis (head, scalp)

Pruritic lesions with central clearing resembling a ring, caused by dermatophytes (*Microsporum*, *Trichophyton*, and *Epidermophyton*). See mold hyphae in KOH prep, not dimorphic. Pets are a reservoir for *Microsporum* and can be treated with topical azoles.

Opportunistic fungal infections

Candida albicans (*alba* = white)

Systemic or superficial fungal infection. **Dimorphic:** yeast with pseudohyphae in culture at 20°C; germ tube formation at 37°C (diagnostic). Oral and esophageal thrush in immunocompromised (neonates, steroids, diabetes, AIDS), vulvovaginitis (diabetes, use of antibiotics), diaper rash, endocarditis in IV drug users, disseminated candidiasis (to any organ), chronic mucocutaneous candidiasis (see Image 9).
Treatment: nystatin for superficial infection; amphotericin B for serious systemic infection.

Aspergillus fumigatus

Allergic bronchopulmonary aspergillosis, lung cavity aspergilloma ("fungus ball"), invasive aspergillosis, especially in immunocompromised individuals and those with chronic granulomatous disease. **Mold** with septate hyphae that branch at acute angles (≤ 45°). Think "A" for Acute Angles in Aspergillus. Not dimorphic.

Cryptococcus neoformans

Cryptococcal meningitis, cryptococcosis. Heavily encapsulated **yeast.** Not dimorphic. Found in soil, pigeon droppings. Culture on Sabouraud's agar. Stains with India ink. Latex agglutination test detects polysaccharide capsular antigen and is more specific (see Image 8). "Soap bubble" lesions in brain.

Mucor and *Rhizopus* spp.

Mucormycosis. **Mold** with irregular nonseptate hyphae branching at wide angles (≥ 90°). Disease mostly in ketoacidotic diabetic and leukemic patients. Fungi proliferate in blood vessel walls when there is excess ketone and glucose, penetrate cribiform plate, and enter brain. Rhinocerebral, frontal lobe abscesses. Headache, facial pain, black necrotic eschar on face cranial nerve involvement.

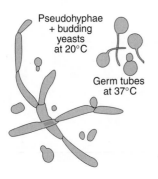

Pseudohyphae + budding yeasts at 20°C

Germ tubes at 37°C

Candida

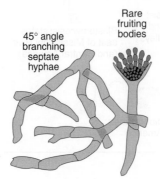

45° angle branching septate hyphae

Rare fruiting bodies

Aspergillus

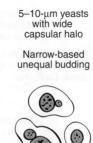

5–10-μm yeasts with wide capsular halo

Narrow-based unequal budding

Cryptococcus

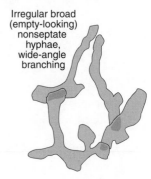

Irregular broad (empty-looking) nonseptate hyphae, wide-angle branching

Mucor

Pneumocystis jiroveci (formerly carinii) Saucer-shaped yeast forms	Causes diffuse interstitial pneumonia. Yeast (originally classified as protozoan). Inhaled. Most infections are asymptomatic. Immunosuppression (e.g., AIDS) predisposes to disease. Diffuse, bilateral CXR appearance. Diagnosed by lung biopsy or lavage. Identified by methenamine silver stain of lung tissue. Treatment: TMP-SMX, pentamidine, dapsone. Start prophylaxis when CD4 drops < 200 cells/mL in HIV patients (see Image 19).	
Sporothrix schenckii Cigar-shaped yeast forms, unequal budding	Sporotrichosis. **Dimorphic fungus** that lives on vegetation. When traumatically introduced into the skin, typically by a thorn (**"rose gardener's"** disease), causes local pustule or ulcer with nodules along draining lymphatics (ascending lymphangitis). Little systemic illness. Treatment: itraconazole or **pot**assium iodide. ("Plant a **rose** in the **pot**.")	

HIGH-YIELD PRINCIPLES

MICROBIOLOGY

Medically important protozoa—single-celled organisms

Organism	Disease	Transmission	Diagnosis	Treatment
GI infections				
Giardia lamblia (see Image 5) Trophozoite Cyst	Giardiasis: bloating, flatulence, foul-smelling, fatty diarrhea (often seen in campers/hikers)—think fat-rich **Ghirardelli** chocolates for fatty stools of *Giardia*	Cysts in water	Trophozoites or cysts in stool	Metronidazole
Entamoeba histolytica RBCs Trophozoite Cyst with 4 nuclei	Amebiasis: bloody diarrhea (dysentery), liver abscess (reddish brown), RUQ pain (histology shows flask-shaped ulcer if submucosal abscess of colon ruptures)	Cysts in water	Serology and/or trophozoites or cysts in stool; RBCs in cytoplasm of entamoeba	Metronidazole and iodoquinol
Cryptosporidium Acid-fast cysts	Severe diarrhea in AIDS Mild disease (watery diarrhea) in non-immunocompromised	Cysts in water	Cysts on acid-fast stain	Prevention (by filtering city water supplies); no treatment
CNS infections				
Toxoplasma gondii	Brain abscess in HIV (seen as ring-enhancing brain lesions on CT/MRI); congenital toxoplasmosis = "classic triad" of chorioretinitis, hydrocephalus, and intracranial calcifications	Cysts in meat or cat feces; crosses placenta (pregnant women should avoid cats)	Serology, biopsy	Sulfadiazine + pyrimethamine
Naegleria fowleri	Rapidly fatal meningoencephalitis	Swimming in freshwater lakes (think **Nalgene** bottle filled with **freshwater** containing *Naegleria*); enter via cribriform plate	Amoebas in spinal fluid	Amphotericin has been effective for a few survivors

Medically important protozoa—single-celled organisms *(continued)*

Organism	Disease	Transmission	Diagnosis	Treatment
CNS infections *(continued)*				
Trypanosoma brucei *T. gambiense* *T. rhodesiense*	African sleeping sickness: enlarged lymph nodes, recurring fever (due to antigenic variation), somnolence, coma	Tsetse fly, a painful bite	Blood smear	**SUR**amin for blood-borne disease or **MELA**rsoprol for CNS penetration (it **SUR**e is nice to go to sleep; **ME-LA**tonin helps with sleep)
Visceral infections				
Trypanosoma cruzi RBC Blood smear	Chagas' disease (dilated cardiomyopathy, megacolon, megaesophagus); predominantly in South America	Reduviid bug ("kissing bug"), a painless bite (much like a kiss)	Blood smear	Nifurtimox
Leishmania donovani	Visceral leishmaniasis (kala-azar): spiking fevers, hepatosplenomegaly, pancytopenia	Sandfly	Macrophages containing "amastigotes" (form that lacks flagella)	Sodium stibogluconate
Hematologic infections				
Plasmodium *P. vivax/ovale* *P. falciparum* *P. malariae* Trophozoite ring form in RBC RBC schizont with merozoites	Malaria: 48-hr (tertian) cyclic fever, headache, anemia, splenomegaly *P. vivax/ovale*— cycles occur every other day; dormant form in liver is treated with primaquine *P. falciparum*— severe; daily cycles; parasitized RBCs occlude capillaries in brain (cerebral malaria), kidneys, lungs	Mosquito (*Anopheles*)	Blood smear	Begin with chloroquine; if resistant, use mefloquine *Vivax/ovale*—add primaquine for dormant forms in liver (hypnozoite)
Babesia RBC Maltese cross and ring forms	Babesiosis: fever and hemolytic anemia; predominantly in northeastern United States	*Ixodes* tick (same as *Borrelia burgdorferi* of Lyme disease; may often coinfect humans)	Blood smear, no RBC pigment, appears as "Maltese cross"	Quinine, clindamycin
STDs				
Trichomonas vaginalis (see Image 10)	Vaginitis: foul-smelling, greenish discharge; itching and burning; do not confuse with *Gardnerella vaginalis*, a gram-negative bacterium that causes vaginosis	Sexual (cannot exist outside human because it cannot form cysts)	Trophozoites (motile) on wet mount	Metronidazole

Medically important helminths/worms

Multicellular organisms. Life cycle involves stages in other organisms.

Organism	Transmission/Disease	Treatment
Nematodes (roundworms)		
Intestinal		
Enterobius vermicularis (pinworm)	Food contaminated with eggs; intestinal infection; causes anal pruritus (the Scotch tape test).	-bendazoles or pyrantel pamoate (worms are **BEND**y; treat with me**BEND**azole)
Ascaris lumbricoides (giant roundworm)	Eggs are visible in feces; intestinal infection.	-bendazoles or pyrantel pamoate
Trichinella spiralis	Undercooked meat, usually pork; inflammation of muscle (larvae encyst in muscle), periorbital edema.	-bendazoles
Strongyloides stercoralis	Larvae in soil penetrate the skin; intestinal infection; causes vomiting, diarrhea, and anemia.	-bendazoles or ivermectin
Ancylostoma duodenale, Necator americanus (hookworms)	Larvae penetrate skin of feet; intestinal infection can cause anemia (sucks blood from intestinal walls).	-bendazoles or pyrantel pamoate
Tissue		
Dracunculus medinensis	In drinking water; skin inflammation and ulceration.	Niridazole
Onchocerca volvulus	Transmitted by female blackflies; causes hyperpigmented skin and **river** blindness (remember **black**flies, **black** skin nodules, "**black** sight"). Can have allergic reaction to microfilaria.	**Ivermectin (IVER**mectin for r**IVER** blindness)
Loa loa	Transmitted by deer fly, horse fly, and mango fly; causes swelling in skin (can see worm crawling in conjunctiva).	Diethylcarbamazine
Wuchereria bancrofti	Female mosquito; causes blockage of lymphatic vessels (elephantiasis). Takes 9 months to 1 year after bite to get elephantiasis symptoms.	Diethylcarbamazine
Toxocara canis	Food contaminated with eggs; causes granulomas (if in retina → blindness) and visceral larva migrans.	Diethylcarbamazine
Cestodes (tapeworms)		
Taenia solium	Ingestion of larvae encysted in undercooked pork leads to intestinal tapeworms. Ingestion of eggs causes cysticercosis and neurocysticercosis, mass lesions in brain ("swiss cheese" appearance).	Praziquantel (use -bendazoles for neurocysticercosis)
Diphyllobothrium latum	Ingestion of larvae in raw freshwater fish. Causes vitamin B_{12} deficiency, resulting in anemia.	Praziquantel
Echinococcus granulosus	Eggs in dog feces when ingested can cause cysts in liver; causes anaphylaxis if echinococcal antigens are released from cysts (surgeons inject ethanol before removal to kill daughter cysts).	-bendazoles

Medically important helminths/worms *(continued)*

Organism	Transmission/Disease	Treatment
Trematodes (flukes)		
Schistosoma	Snails are host; cercariae penetrate skin of humans; causes granulomas, fibrosis, and inflammation of the spleen and liver. Chronic infection with *S. haematobium* can lead to squamous cell carcinoma of the bladder.	Praziquantel
Clonorchis sinensis	Undercooked fish; causes inflammation of the biliary tract → pigmented gallstones. Also associated with cholangiocarcinoma.	Praziquantel
Paragonimus westermani	Undercooked crab meat; causes inflammation and 2° bacterial infection of the lung, causing hemoptysis.	Praziquantel

---

Nematode routes of infection	Ingested—*Enterobius, Ascaris, Trichinella.* Cutaneous—*Strongyloides, Ancylostoma, Necator.*	You'll get sick if you **EAT** these! These get into your feet from the **SAN**d.

Parasite hints

Findings	Organism
Brain cysts, seizures	*Taenia solium* (cysticercosis)
Liver cysts	*Echinococcus granulosus*
B_{12} deficiency	*Diphyllobothrium latum*
Biliary tract disease, cholangiocarcinoma	*Clonorchis sinensis*
Hemoptysis	*Paragonimus westermani*
Portal hypertension	*Schistosoma mansoni*
Hematuria, bladder cancer	*Schistosoma haematobium*
Microcytic anemia	*Ancylostoma, Necator*
Perianal pruritus	*Enterobius*

"Tricky T's"

Typhoid fever	Caused by bacterium *Salmonella typhi*.
Typhus	Caused by bacteria *Rickettsia prowazekii* (epidemic), *Rickettsia typhi* (endemic), and *Rickettsia tsutsugamushi* (scrub typhus).
Chlamydia **trach**omatis	Bacteria, STD.
Treponema	Spirochete; causes syphilis (*T. pallidum*) or yaws (*T. pertenue*).
Trichomonas vaginalis	Protozoan, STD.
Trypanosoma	Protozoan, causes Chagas' disease (*T. cruzi*) or African sleeping sickness.
Toxoplasma	Protozoan, a TORCH infection.
Trichinella spiralis	Nematode in undercooked meat.
Taenia solium	Tapeworm larvae (intestinal infection) in pork or eggs (neurocysticercosis) in food/water contaminated with human feces.

Viral structure—general features

Naked icosahedral

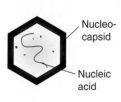

Nucleo-
capsid

Nucleic
acid

Enveloped icosahedral

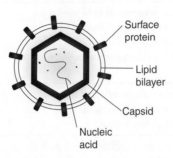

Surface
protein

Lipid
bilayer

Capsid

Nucleic
acid

Enveloped helical

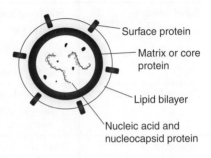

Surface protein

Matrix or core
protein

Lipid bilayer

Nucleic acid and
nucleocapsid protein

Viral genetics

Recombination	Exchange of genes between 2 chromosomes by crossing over within regions of significant base sequence homology.
Reassortment	When viruses with segmented genomes (e.g., influenza virus) exchange segments. High-frequency recombination. Cause of worldwide influenza pandemics.
Complementation	When 1 of 2 viruses that infect the cell has a mutation that results in a nonfunctional protein. The nonmutated virus "complements" the mutated one by making a functional protein that serves both viruses.
Phenotypic mixing	Occurs with simultaneous infection of a cell with 2 viruses. Genome of virus A can be partially or completely coated (forming pseudovirion) with the surface proteins of virus B. Type B protein coat determines the infectivity of the phenotypically mixed virus. However, the progeny from this infection have a type A coat that is encoded by its type A genetic material.

Viral vaccines

Live attenuated vaccines induce humoral and cell-mediated immunity but have reverted to virulence on rare occasions. Killed/inactivated vaccines induce only humoral immunity but are stable.

No booster needed for live attenuated vaccines.
Dangerous to give live vaccines to immunocompromised patients or their close contacts.

Live attenuated—**small**pox, **yellow** fever, **chicken**pox (VZV), **Sabin's** polio virus, **MMR**.

"**Live!** One night only! See **small yellow chickens** get vaccinated with **Sabin's** and **MMR!**"
MMR = measles, mumps, rubella (the only live attenuated vaccine that can be given to HIV-positive patients).

Killed—**R**abies, **I**nfluenza, Salk **P**olio, and HAV vaccines.
Recombinant—HBV (antigen = recombinant HBsAg), HPV (types 6, 11, 16, and 18).

Sal**K** = **K**illed.
RIP Always.

DNA viral genomes	All DNA viruses except the Parvoviridae are dsDNA. All are linear except papilloma, polyoma, and hepadnaviruses (circular).	All are dsDNA (like our cells), except **"part-of-a-virus"** (**parvovirus**) is ssDNA. *Parvus* = small.
RNA viral genomes	All RNA viruses except Reoviridae and Rotavirus are ssRNA. Positive-stranded RNA viruses: I went to a **RETRO** (**RETRO**virus) **TOGA** (**TOGA**virus) party, where I drank **FLAV**ored (**FLAVI**virus) **CORONA** (**CORONA**virus) and ate **HIPPY** (**HEPE**virus) **CALI**FORNIA (**CALI**civirus) **PICKLES** (**PICO**rnavirus).	All are ssRNA (like our mRNA), except "repeato-virus" (**reo**virus) is dsRNA.
Naked viral genome infectivity	Purified nucleic acids of most dsDNA (except poxviruses and HBV) and (+) strand ssRNA (≈ mRNA) viruses are infectious. Naked nucleic acids of (−) strand ssRNA and dsRNA viruses are not infectious. They require enzymes contained in the complete virion.	
Virus ploidy	All viruses are haploid (with 1 copy of DNA or RNA) except retroviruses, which have 2 identical ssRNA molecules (≈ diploid).	
Viral replication		
DNA viruses	All replicate in the nucleus (except poxvirus).	
RNA viruses	All replicate in the cytoplasm (except influenza virus and retroviruses).	
Viral envelopes	**Naked** (nonenveloped) viruses include **C**alicivirus, **P**icornavirus, **R**eovirus, **P**arvovirus, **A**denovirus, **P**apilloma, and **P**olyoma. Generally, enveloped viruses acquire their envelopes from plasma membrane when they exit from cell. Exceptions are herpesviruses, which acquire envelopes from nuclear membrane.	**Naked CPR** and **PAPP** smear.

Viral pathogens

Structure	Viruses
DNA enveloped viruses	Herpesviruses (HSV types 1 and 2, VZV, CMV, EBV), HBV, smallpox virus
DNA nucleocapsid viruses	Adenovirus, papillomaviruses, parvovirus
RNA enveloped viruses	Influenza virus, parainfluenza virus, RSV, measles virus, mumps virus, rubella virus, rabies virus, HTLV, HIV
RNA nucleocapsid viruses	Enteroviruses (poliovirus, coxsackievirus, echovirus, HAV), rhinovirus, reovirus (rotavirus)

DNA virus characteristics

Some general rules—all DNA viruses:

1. Are **HHAPPPP**y viruses   **H**epadna, **H**erpes, **A**deno, **P**ox, **P**arvo, **P**apilloma, **P**olyoma.
2. Are double stranded   EXCEPT parvo (single stranded).
3. Are linear   EXCEPT papilloma and polyoma (circular, supercoiled) and hepadna (circular, incomplete).
4. Are icosahedral   EXCEPT pox (complex).
5. Replicate in the nucleus   EXCEPT pox (carries own DNA-dependent RNA polymerase).

DNA viruses

Viral Family	Envelope	DNA Structure	Medical Importance
Herpesviruses	Yes	DS – linear	HSV-1—oral (and some genital) lesions, spontaneous temporal lobe encephalitis, keratoconjunctivitis HSV-2—genital (and some oral) lesions VZV (HHV-3)—chickenpox, zoster (shingles) EBV (HHV-4)—mononucleosis, Burkitt's lymphoma CMV (HHV-5)—infection in immunosuppressed patients (AIDS retinitis), especially transplant recipients; congenital defects HHV-6—roseola (exanthem subitum) HHV-7–clinically insignificant (included only to complete family) HHV-8—Kaposi's sarcoma–associated herpesvirus (KSHV)
Hepadnavirus	Yes	DS – partial circular	HBV Acute or chronic hepatitis Vaccine available—contains HBV surface antigen Not a retrovirus but has reverse transcriptase
Adenovirus	No	DS – linear	Febrile pharyngitis—sore throat; acute hemorrhagic cystitis° Pneumonia Conjunctivitis—"pink eye" (watery)
Parvovirus	No	SS – linear (−) (smallest DNA virus)	B19 virus—aplastic crises in sickle cell disease, "slapped cheeks" rash in children—erythema infectiosum (fifth disease), RBC destruction in fetus leads to hydrops fetalis and death, pure RBC aplasia and rheumatoid arthritis–like symptoms in adults
Papillomavirus*	No	DS – circular	HPV—warts (1, 2, 6, 11), CIN, cervical cancer (16, 18) vaccine available
Polyomavirus*	No	DS – circular	JC—progressive multifocal leukoencephalopathy (PML) in HIV
Poxvirus	Yes	DS – linear (largest DNA virus)	Smallpox, although eradicated, could be used in germ warfare Vaccinia—cowpox ("milkmaid's blisters") Molluscum contagiosum—flesh-colored dome lesions with central dimple

*Papillomavirus and polyomavirus are two new classifications originally grouped as "papovavirus."

Herpesviruses

Virus	Diseases	Route of transmission	
HSV-1	Gingivostomatitis, keratoconjunctivitis, temporal lobe encephalitis (most common cause of sporadic encephalitis in the United States), herpes labialis	Respiratory secretions, saliva	Get herpes in a **CHEV**rolet: CMV HSV
HSV-2	Herpes genitalis (see Image 11), neonatal herpes	Sexual contact, perinatal	EBV VZV
VZV	Varicella-zoster (shingles), encephalitis, pneumonia (see Image 15)	Respiratory secretions	Herpesviruses can remain
EBV	Infectious mononucleosis, Burkitt's lymphoma, nasopharyngeal carcinoma	Respiratory secretions, saliva	latent in ganglia or cells:
CMV	Congenital infection, mononucleosis (negative Monospot), pneumonia. Infected cells have characteristic "owl's eye" inclusions (see Image 6)	Congenital, transfusion, sexual contact, saliva, urine, transplant	HSV-1 (trigeminal ganglia), HSV-2 (sacral
HHV-6	Roseola: high fevers for several days that can cause seizures, followed by a diffuse macular rash	Not determined	ganglia), VZV (trigeminal and dorsal
HHV-8	Kaposi's sarcoma (HIV patients)	Sexual contact	root ganglia), EBV (B cells), CMV (mononuclear cells).

HSV identification	Tzanck test—a smear of an opened skin vesicle to detect multinucleated giant cells. Used to assay for HSV-1, HSV-2, and VZV. Infected cells also have intranuclear Cowdry A inclusions.	**Tzanck** heavens I do not have herpes.

EBV	A herpesvirus. Can cause mononucleosis. Infects B cells. Characterized by fever, hepatospleno-megaly, pharyngitis, and lymphadenopathy (especially posterior cervical nodes). Peak incidence 15–20 years of age. Reactive circulating cytotoxic T cells (termed "atypical lymphocytes" but are actually normal T cells simply reacting to EBV-infected cells). Also associated with development of Hodgkin's and endemic Burkitt's lymphomas as well as nasopharyngeal carcinoma.	Most common during peak kissing years ("kissing disease"). Positive Monospot test—heterophil antibodies detected by agglutination of sheep RBCs.

RNA viruses

Viral Family	Envelope	RNA Structure	Capsid Symmetry	Medical Importance
Reoviruses	No	**DS** linear 10–12 segments	Icosahedral (double)	Reovirus—Colorado tick fever Rotavirus—#1 cause of fatal diarrhea in children

Picornaviruses	No	SS + linear	Icosahedral	Poliovirus—polio-Salk/Sabin vaccines—IPV/OPV
				Echovirus—aseptic meningitis
				Rhinovirus—"common cold"
				Coxsackievirus—aseptic meningitis
				    herpangina—febrile pharyngitis
				    hand, foot, and mouth disease
				    myocarditis
				HAV—acute viral hepatitis

Hepevirus	No	SS + linear	Icosahedral	HEV
Caliciviruses	No	SS + linear	Icosahedral	Norwalk virus—viral gastroenteritis
Flaviviruses	Yes	SS + linear	Icosahedral	HCV Yellow fever* Dengue* St. Louis encephalitis* West Nile virus*
Togaviruses	Yes	SS + linear	Icosahedral	Rubella (German measles) Eastern equine encephalitis* Western equine encephalitis*
Retroviruses	Yes	SS + linear	Icosahedral	Have reverse transcriptase HIV—AIDS HTLV—T-cell leukemia
Coronaviruses	Yes	SS + linear	Helical	Coronavirus—"common cold" and SARS
Orthomyxoviruses	Yes	SS – linear 8 segments	Helical	Influenza virus

Paramyxoviruses	Yes	SS – linear Nonsegmented	Helical	**PaRaM**yxovirus:
				    Parainfluenza—croup
				    RSV—bronchiolitis in babies; Rx—ribavirin
				    Rubeola (**M**easles)
				    Mumps

Rhabdoviruses	Yes	SS – linear	Helical	Rabies
Filoviruses	Yes	SS – linear	Helical	Ebola/Marburg hemorrhagic fever—often fatal!
Arenaviruses	Yes	SS – circular 2 segments	Helical	LCMV—lymphocytic choriomeningitis virus Lassa fever encephalitis—spread by mice
Bunyaviruses	Yes	SS – circular 3 segments	Helical	California encephalitis* Sandfly/Rift Valley fevers* Crimean-Congo hemorrhagic fever* Hantavirus—hemorrhagic fever, pneumonia
Deltavirus	Yes	SS – circular	Helical	HDV

SS, single-stranded; DS, double-stranded; +, + sense; –, – sense; *= arbovirus, transmitted by arthropods (mosquitoes, ticks)

(Adapted, with permission, from Levinson W, Jawetz E. *Medical Microbiology and Immunology: Examination and Board Review,* 6th ed. New York: McGraw-Hill, 2000: 182.)

Negative-stranded viruses	Must transcribe negative strand to positive. Virion brings its own RNA-dependent RNA polymerase. They include **A**renaviruses, **B**unyaviruses, **P**aramyxoviruses, **O**rthomyxoviruses, **F**iloviruses, and **R**habdoviruses.	Always **B**ring **P**olymerase **O**r **F**ail **R**eplication.
Segmented viruses	All are RNA viruses. They include **B**unyaviruses, **O**rthomyxoviruses (influenza viruses), **A**renaviruses, and **R**eoviruses. Influenza virus consists of 8 segments of negative-stranded RNA. These segments can undergo high-frequency recombination via reassortment, causing antigenic shifts that lead to worldwide pandemics of the flu.	**BOAR.**
Picornavirus	Includes **P**oliovirus, **E**chovirus, **R**hinovirus, **C**oxsackievirus, **H**AV. RNA is translated into 1 large polypeptide that is cleaved by proteases into functional viral proteins. Can cause aseptic (viral) meningitis (except rhinovirus and HAV). All are **enteroviruses** (fecal-oral spread) except rhinovirus.	Pico**RNA**virus = small **RNA** virus. **PERCH** on a "peak" (pico).
Rhinovirus	A picornavirus. Nonenveloped RNA virus. Cause of common cold; > 100 serologic types. Acid labile—destroyed by stomach acid; therefore, does not infect the GI tract (unlike the other picornaviruses).	**Rhino** has a runny nose.
Yellow fever virus	A flavivirus (also an arbovirus) transmitted by *Aedes* mosquitos. Virus has a monkey or human reservoir. Symptoms: high fever, black vomitus, and jaundice.	*Flavi* = yellow, jaundice.
Rotavirus	Rotavirus, the most important global cause of infantile gastroenteritis, is a segmented dsRNA virus (a reovirus). Major cause of acute diarrhea in the United States during winter, especially in day-care centers, kindergartens. Villous destruction with atrophy leads to ↓ absorption of Na^+ and water.	**ROTA** = **R**ight **O**ut **T**he **A**nus.

Influenza viruses	Orthomyxoviruses. Enveloped, single-stranded RNA viruses with segmented genome. Contain hemagglutinin (promotes viral entry) and neuraminidase (promotes progeny virion release) antigens. Responsible for worldwide influenza epidemics; patients at risk for fatal bacterial superinfection. Rapid genetic changes.	Killed viral vaccine is major mode of protection; reformulated vaccine offered each fall to elderly, health-care workers, etc.
Genetic shift (pandemic)	Reassortment of viral genome (such as when human flu A virus recombines with swine flu A virus).	Sudden **Shift** is more deadly than gra**Dual Drift**.
Genetic drift (epidemic)	Minor (antigenic drift) changes based on random mutation.	
Rubella virus	A togavirus. Causes German (3-day) measles. Fever, postauricular tenderness, lymphadenopathy, arthralgias, fine truncal rash. Causes mild disease in children but serious congenital disease (a TORCH infection).	
Paramyxoviruses	Paramyxoviruses cause disease in children. They include those that cause parainfluenza (croup: seal-like barking cough), mumps, and measles as well as RSV, which causes respiratory tract infection (bronchiolitis, pneumonia) in infants. All contain surface F (fusion) protein, which causes respiratory epithelial cells to fuse and form multinucleated cells. Palivizumab is used in RSV to neutralize F protein.	
Rubeola (measles) virus	A paramyxovirus that causes measles. Koplik spots (red spots with blue-white center on buccal mucosa; see Image 17) are diagnostic. SSPE (years later), encephalitis (1:2000), and giant cell pneumonia (rarely, in immunosuppressed) are possible sequelae. Rash presents last and spreads from head to toe (see Image 18). Includes hands and feet (vs. truncal rash in rubella). Do not confuse with roseola (caused by HHV-6).	3 C's of measles: Cough Coryza Conjunctivitis Also look for **K**oplik spots.
Mumps virus	A paramyxovirus. Symptoms: **P**arotitis, **O**rchitis (inflammation of testes), and aseptic **M**eningitis. Can cause sterility (especially after puberty).	Mumps makes your parotid glands and testes as big as **POM**-poms.
Rabies virus	Negri bodies are characteristic cytoplasmic inclusions in neurons infected by rabies virus; commonly found in Purkinje cells of cerebellum. Has bullet-shaped capsid. Rabies has long incubation period (weeks to months) before symptom onset. However, prophylactic vaccination should occur immediately upon exposure. Progression of disease: fever, malaise → agitation, photophobia, hydrophobia → paralysis, coma → death. More commonly from bat, raccoon, and skunk bites than from dog bites in the United States.	Travels to the CNS by migrating in a retrograde fashion up nerve axons. Negri bodies

"Lots of spots"

Rubella	Togavirus; German 3-day measles.
Rubeola	Paramyxovirus; measles.
Roseola	Herpesvirus (HHV-6). High fevers followed by diffuse maculopapular rash.
Varicella	Herpesvirus; chickenpox and zoster.
Variola	Poxvirus; smallpox (no longer present outside of labs).

Hepatitis viruses

The hepatitis viruses belong to 5 different viral families. Signs and symptoms: episodes of fever, jaundice, elevated ALT and AST.

HAV (RNA picornavirus) is transmitted primarily by fecal-oral route. Short incubation (3 weeks). No carriers.

> Hep A: Asymptomatic (usually), Acute, Alone (no carriers).

HBV (DNA hepadnavirus) is transmitted primarily by parenteral, sexual, and maternal-fetal routes. Long incubation (3 months). Carriers. Cellular RNA polymerase transcribes RNA from DNA template. Reverse transcriptase transcribes DNA genome from RNA intermediate. However, the virion enzyme is a DNA-dependent DNA polymerase.

> Hep B: Blood borne.

HCV (RNA flavivirus) is transmitted primarily via blood and resembles HBV in its course and severity. Carriers. Common cause of post-transfusion hepatitis and of hepatitis among IV drug users in the United States.

> Hep C: Chronic, Cirrhosis, Carcinoma, Carriers.

HDV (delta agent) is a defective virus that requires HBsAg as its envelope. HDV can coinfect with HBV or superinfect; the latter has a worse prognosis. Carriers.

> Hep D: Defective, Dependent on HBV.

HEV (RNA hepevirus) is transmitted enterically and causes water-borne epidemics. Resembles HAV in course, severity, incubation. High mortality rate in pregnant women.

> Hep E: Enteric, Expectant mothers, Epidemics.

Both HBV and HCV predispose a patient to chronic active hepatitis, cirrhosis, and hepatocellular carcinoma.

> A and E by fecal-oral route: "The **vowels** hit your **bowels.**" (Because naked viruses do not rely on an envelope, they are not destroyed in the gut.)

Hepatitis serologic markers

Anti-HAVAb (IgM)	IgM antibody to HAV; best test to detect active hepatitis A.
Anti-HAVAb (IgG)	IgG antibody indicates prior HAV infection; protects against reinfection.
HBsAg	Antigen found on surface of HBV; indicates **hepatitis B infection**.
Anti-HBsAg	Antibody to HBsAg; indicates **immunity to hepatitis B**.
HBcAg	Antigen associated with core of HBV.
Anti-HBcAg	Antibody to HBcAg; IgM = acute/recent infection; IgG = chronic disease. Positive during **window period**.
HBeAg	A second, different antigenic determinant in the HBV core. HBeAg indicates active viral replication and therefore **high transmissibility**.
Anti-HBeAg	Antibody to e antigen; indicates **low transmissibility**.

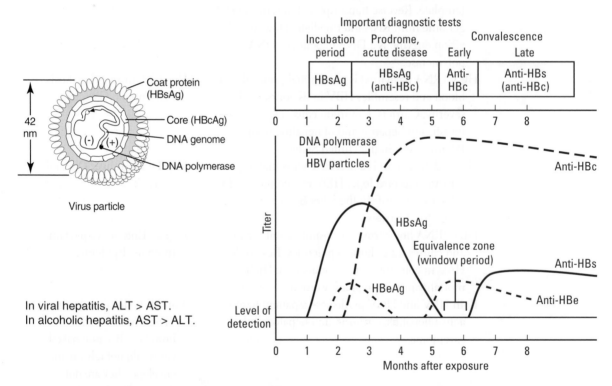

In viral hepatitis, ALT > AST.
In alcoholic hepatitis, AST > ALT.

	HBsAg	Anti-HBsAb	HBeAg	Anti-HBeAb	Anti-HBcAb
Acute HBV	+		+		IgM
Window					+
Chronic HBV (high infectivity)	+		+		IgG
Chronic HBV (low infectivity)	+			+	IgG
Recovery		+		+	IgG
Immunized		+			

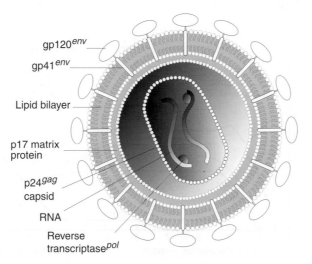

gp120*env*
gp41*env*
Lipid bilayer
p17 matrix protein
p24*gag* capsid
RNA
Reverse transcriptase*pol*

(Adapted, with permission, from Levinson W. *Medical Microbiology and Immunology: Examination and Board Review,* 8th ed. New York: McGraw-Hill, 2004: 314.)

Diploid genome (2 molecules of RNA).

p24 = capsid protein.

gp41 (fusion and entry) and gp120 (attachment to host T cell) = envelope proteins.

Reverse transcriptase synthesizes dsDNA from RNA; dsDNA integrates into host genome.

The 3 structural genes (protein coded for):
env (gp120 and gp41)
gag (p24)
pol (reverse transcriptase)

Virus binds CXCR4 and CD4 on T cells; binds CCR5 and CD4 on macrophages. Homozygous CCR5 mutation = immunity. Heterozygous CCR5 mutation = slower course.

| **HIV diagnosis** | Presumptive diagnosis made with ELISA (sensitive, high false-positive rate and low threshold, RULE OUT test); positive results are then confirmed with Western blot assay (specific, high false-negative rate and high threshold, RULE IN test).
 HIV PCR/viral load tests are increasing in popularity: they allow physician to monitor the effect of drug therapy on viral load.
 AIDS diagnosis ≤ 200 CD4+ (normal: 500–1500). HIV positive with AIDS indicator condition (e.g., *Pneumocystis jiroveci* pneumonia, formerly known as PCP) or CD4/CD8 ratio < 1.5. | ELISA/Western blot tests look for antibodies to viral proteins; these tests are often falsely negative in the first 1–2 months of HIV infection and falsely positive initially in babies born to infected mothers (anti-gp120 crosses placenta). |

Time course of HIV infection

4 stages of infection:
1. Flulike (acute)
2. Feeling fine (latent)
3. Falling count
4. Final crisis

During latent phase, virus replicates in lymph nodes.

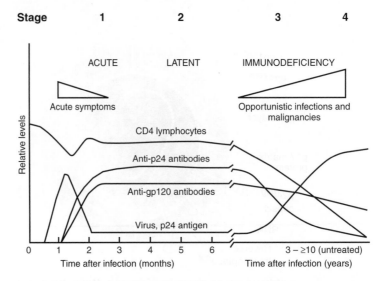

(Adapted, with permission, from Levinson W. *Medical Microbiology and Immunology: Examination and Board Review,* 8th ed. New York: McGraw-Hill, 2004: 318.)

Opportunistic infections and disease in AIDS

Organ system	Infection/disease
Brain	Cryptococcal meningitis, toxoplasmosis, CMV encephalopathy, AIDS dementia, PML (JC virus)
Eyes	CMV retinitis
Mouth and throat	Thrush (*Candida albicans*), HSV, CMV, oral hairy leukoplakia (EBV)
Lungs	*Pneumocystis jiroveci* pneumonia (formerly known as PCP), TB, histoplasmosis
GI	Cryptosporidiosis, *Mycobacterium avium–intracellulare* complex, CMV colitis, non-Hodgkin's lymphoma (EBV), *Isospora belli*
Skin	Shingles (VZV), Kaposi's sarcoma (HHV-8)
Genitals	Genital herpes, warts, and cervical cancer (HPV)

HIV-associated infections and CD4 count

CD4 level	Increased risk of infection
< 400	Oral thrush, tinea pedis, reactivation VZV, reactivation TB, other bacterial infections (e.g., *H. influenzae, S. pneumoniae, Salmonella*)
< 200	Reactivation HSV, cryptosporidiosis, *Isospora*, disseminated coccidioidomycosis, *Pneumocystis* pneumonia
< 100	Candidal esophagitis, toxoplasmosis, histoplasmosis
< 50	CMV retinitis and esophagitis, disseminated *M. avium–intracellulare*, cryptococcal meningoencephalitis

Neoplasms associated with HIV

Kaposi's sarcoma (HHV-8), invasive cervical carcinoma (HPV), 1° CNS lymphoma, non-Hodgkin's lymphoma.

| **Prions** | Prion diseases are caused by the conversion of a normal cellular protein termed *prion protein* (PrP^c) to a β-pleated form (PrP^{sc}), which is transmissible. PrP^{sc} resists degradation and facilitates the conversion of still more PrP^c to PrP^{sc}. Accumulation of PrP^{sc} results in spongiform encephalopathy and dementia, ataxia, and death. It can be **sporadic** (Creutzfeldt-Jakob disease—rapidly progressive dementia), **inherited** (Gerstmann-Sträussler-Scheinker syndrome), or **acquired** (kuru). | |

| **Normal flora: dominant** | Skin—*Staphylococcus epidermidis*.
 Nose—*S. epidermidis*; colonized by *S. aureus*.
 Oropharynx—viridans group streptococci.
 Dental plaque—*Streptococcus mutans*.
 Colon—*Bacteroides fragilis* > *E. coli*.
 Vagina—*Lactobacillus*, colonized by *E. coli* and group B strep. | Neonates delivered by cesarean section have no flora but are rapidly colonized after birth. |
| **Bugs causing food poisoning** | *Vibrio parahaemolyticus* and *V. vulnificus* in contaminated seafood. *V. vulnificus* can also cause wound infections from contact with contaminated water or shellfish.
 Bacillus cereus in reheated rice.
 S. aureus in meats, mayonnaise, custard. Preformed toxin.
 Clostridium perfringens in reheated meat dishes.
 C. botulinum in improperly canned foods (bulging cans).
 E. coli O157:H7 in undercooked meat.
 Salmonella in poultry, meat, and eggs. | *S. aureus* and *B. cereus* food poisoning starts quickly and ends quickly.
 "Food poisoning from reheated rice? **Be serious!**"
 (**B. cereus**). |

Bugs causing diarrhea

Type	Species	Findings
Bloody diarrhea	*Campylobacter*	Comma- or S-shaped organisms; growth at 42°C
	Salmonella	Lactose negative; flagellar motility
	Shigella	Lactose negative; very low ID_{50}; produces Shiga toxin
	Enterohemorrhagic *E. coli*	O157:H7; can cause HUS; makes Shiga-like toxin
	Enteroinvasive *E. coli*	Invades colonic mucosa
	Yersinia enterocolitica	Day-care outbreaks, pseudoappendicitis
	C. difficile (can cause both watery and bloody diarrhea)	Pseudomembranous colitis
	Entamoeba histolytica	Protozoan
Watery diarrhea	Enterotoxigenic *E. coli*	Traveler's diarrhea; produces ST and LT toxins
	Vibrio cholerae	Comma-shaped organisms; rice-water diarrhea
	C. perfringens	Also causes gas gangrene
	Protozoa	*Giardia, Cryptosporidium* (in immunocompromised)
	Viruses	Rotavirus, adenovirus, Norwalk virus (norovirus)

Common causes of pneumonia

Neonates (< 4 wk)	Children (4 wk–18 yr)	Adults (18–40 yr)	Adults (40–65 yr)	Elderly
Group B streptococci	Viruses (**R**SV)	*Mycoplasma*	*S. pneumoniae*	*S. pneumoniae*
E. coli	**M**ycoplasma	*C. pneumoniae*	*H. influenzae*	Influenza virus
	Chlamydia pneumoniae	*S. pneumoniae*	Anaerobes	Anaerobes
	Streptococcus *pneumoniae*		Viruses	*H. influenzae*
	Runts **M**ay **C**ough **S**putum		*Mycoplasma*	Gram-negative rods

Special groups:

Nosocomial (hospital acquired)	*Staphylococcus*, enteric gram-negative rods
Immunocompromised	*Staphylococcus*, enteric gram-negative rods, fungi, viruses, *Pneumocystis jiroveci* — with HIV
Aspiration	Anaerobes
Alcoholic/IV drug user	*S. pneumoniae, Klebsiella, Staphylococcus*
Cystic fibrosis	*Pseudomonas*
Postviral	*Staphylococcus, H. influenzae*
Atypical	*Mycoplasma, Legionella, Chlamydia*

**Common causes
of meningitis**

Newborn (0–6 mos)	Children (6 mos–6 yrs)	6–60 yrs	60 yrs +
Group B streptococci	Streptococcus pneumoniae	N. meningitidis	S. pneumoniae
E. coli	Neisseria meningitidis	Enteroviruses	Gram- negative rods
Listeria	Haemophilus influenzae type B	S. pneumoniae	Listeria
	Enteroviruses	HSV	

⊕ Kernig's and/or Brudzinski's sign.

Viral causes of meningitis—enteroviruses (esp. coxsackievirus), HSV, HIV, West Nile virus, VZV.

In HIV—*Cryptococcus*, CMV, toxoplasmosis (brain abscess), JC virus (PML).

Note: Incidence of *H. influenzae* meningitis has ↓ greatly with introduction of *H. influenzae* vaccine in last 10–15 years. Today, cases are usually seen in unimmunized children.

CSF findings in meningitis

	Pressure	Cell type	Protein	Sugar
Bacterial	↑	↑ PMNs	↑	↓
Fungal/TB	↑	↑ lymphocytes	↑	↓
Viral	Normal/↑	↑ lymphocytes	Normal/↑	Normal

Osteomyelitis

Most people—*S. aureus*.

Sexually active—*Neisseria gonorrhoeae* (rare), septic arthritis more common.

Diabetics and drug addicts—*Pseudomonas aeruginosa*.

Sickle cell—*Salmonella*.

Prosthetic replacement—*S. aureus* and *S. epidermidis*.

Vertebral—*Mycobacterium tuberculosis* (Pott's disease).

Cat and dog bites or scratches—*Pasteurella multocida*.

Assume *S. aureus* if no other information.

Most osteomyelitis occurs in children.

Elevated CRP and ESR classic but nonspecific.

Urinary tract infections

Presents with dysuria, frequency, urgency, suprapubic pain, and WBCs (but not WBC casts) in urine. Primarily caused by ascension of microbes from urethra to bladder. Males—infants with congenital defects, vesicoureteral reflux. Elderly—enlarged prostate. Ascension to kidney results in pyelonephritis, which presents with fever, chills, flank pain, CVA tenderness, hematuria, and WBC casts.

Ten times more common in women (shorter urethras colonized by fecal flora). Other predisposing factors include obstruction, kidney surgery, catheterization, GU malformation, diabetes, and pregnancy.

Diagnostic markers:

Positive leukocyte esterase test = bacterial UTI.

Positive nitrite test = gram-negative bacterial UTI.

UTI bugs

Species	Features of the organism	
Escherichia coli	Leading cause of UTI. Colonies show metallic sheen on EMB agar.	Diagnostic markers:
Staphylococcus saprophyticus	2nd leading cause of community-acquired UTI in sexually active women.	Leukocyte esterase— positive = bacterial.
Klebsiella pneumoniae	3rd leading cause of UTI. Large mucoid capsule and viscous colonies.	Nitrite test—positive = gram negative (except *S. saprophyticus*).
Serratia marcescens	Some strains produce a red pigment; often nosocomial and drug resistant.	
Enterobacter cloacae	Often nosocomial and drug resistant.	
Proteus mirabilis	Motility causes "swarming" on agar; produces urease; associated with struvite stones.	
Pseudomonas aeruginosa	Blue-green pigment and fruity odor; usually nosocomial and drug resistant.	

ToRCHeS infections   Microbes that may pass from mother to fetus. Nonspecific signs common to many ToRCHeS infections include hepatosplenomegaly, jaundice, thrombocytopenia, and growth retardation.

Other important infectious agents include *Streptococcus agalactiae* (group B streptococci), *E. coli*, and *Listeria monocytogenes*—all causes of meningitis in neonates.

Agent	Mode of Transmission	Maternal Manifestations	Neonatal Manifestions
Toxoplasma gondii	Aerosolized cat feces or ingestion of undercooked meat	Usually asymptomatic; lymphadenopathy (rarely)	Classic triad: chorioretinitis, hydrocephalus, and intracranial calcifications
Rubella	Respiratory droplets	Rash, lymphadenopathy, arthritis	Classic triad: PDA (or pulmonary artery hypoplasia), cataracts, and deafness ± "blueberry muffin" rash
CMV	Sexual contact, organ transplants	Usually asymptomatic; mononucleosis-like illness	Hearing loss, seizures, petechial rash
HIV	Sexual contact	Variable presentation depending on CD4+ count	Recurrent infections, chronic diarrhea
Herpes simplex virus	Skin or mucous membrane contact	Usually asymptomatic; herpetic (vesicular) lesions	Temporal encephalitis, herpetic (vesicular) lesions
Syphilis	Sexual contact	Chancre (1°), disseminated rash (2°), or cardiac/neurologic disease (3°)	Often results in stillbirth, hydrops fetalis; if child survives, presents with facial abnormalities (notched teeth, saddle nose, short maxilla), saber shins

Red rashes of childhood

Agent	Associated Syndrome/Disease	Clinical Presentation
Rubella virus	German measles	Rash begins at head and moves down; postauricular lymphadenopathy.
Measles virus	Rubeola, measles	A paramyxovirus; beginning at head and moving down; rash is preceded by cough, coryza, conjunctivitis, and blue-white (Koplik) spots on buccal mucosa.
Mumps virus	Mumps	A paramyxovirus; no rash, but can present with parotitis, meningitis (orchitis or oophoritis in young adults).
VZV	Chickenpox	Rash begins on trunk; spreads to face and extremities with lesions of different age.
HHV-6	Roseola	A macular rash over body appears after several days of high fever; usually affects infants.
Parvovirus B19	Erythema infectiosum	"Slapped cheek" rash on face later appears over body in reticular, "lace-like" pattern. (Can cause hydrops fetalis in pregnant women.)
Streptococcus pyogenes	Scarlet fever	Erythematous, sandpaper-like rash with fever and sore throat.
Coxsackievirus type A	Hand-foot-mouth disease	Vesicular rash on palms and soles; ulcers in oral mucosa.

Sexually transmitted diseases

Disease	Clinical features	Organism
Gonorrhea	Urethritis, cervicitis, PID, prostatitis, epididymitis, arthritis, creamy purulent discharge	*Neisseria gonorrhoeae*
1° syphilis	Painless chancre	*Treponema pallidum*
2° syphilis	Fever, lymphadenopathy, skin rashes, condylomata lata	
3° syphilis	Gummas, tabes dorsalis, general paresis, aortitis, Argyll Robertson pupil	
Chancroid	Painful genital ulcer, inguinal adenopathy	*Haemophilus **ducreyi*** (it's so painful, you "**do cry**")
Genital herpes	Painful penile, vulvar, or cervical vesicles and ulcers; can cause systemic symptoms such as fever, headache, myalgia.	HSV-2
Chlamydia	Urethritis, cervicitis, conjunctivitis, Reiter's syndrome, PID	*Chlamydia trachomatis* (D–K)
Lymphogranuloma venereum	Ulcers, lymphadenopathy, rectal strictures	*C. trachomatis* (L1–L3)
Trichomoniasis	Vaginitis, strawberry-colored mucosa, corkscrew motility on wet prep	*Trichomonas vaginalis*
AIDS	Opportunistic infections, Kaposi's sarcoma, lymphoma	HIV
Condylomata acuminata	Genital warts, koilocytes	HPV 6 and 11
Hepatitis B	Jaundice	HBV
Bacterial vaginosis	Noninflammatory, malodorous discharge (fishy smell); positive whiff test, clue cells	*Gardnerella vaginalis*

Pelvic inflammatory disease	Top bugs—*Chlamydia trachomatis* (subacute, often undiagnosed), *Neisseria gonorrhoeae* (acute, high fever). *C. trachomatis*—the most common STD in the United States. Cervical motion tenderness (chandelier sign), purulent cervical discharge. PID may include salpingitis, endometritis, hydrosalpinx, and tubo-ovarian abscess. Can lead to Fitz-Hugh–Curtis syndrome—infection of the liver capsule and "violin string" adhesions of parietal peritoneum to liver.	Salpingitis is a risk factor for ectopic pregnancy, infertility, chronic pelvic pain, and adhesions.

Nosocomial infections

Pathogen	Risk factor	Notes
CMV, RSV	Newborn nursery	The 2 most common causes of nosocomial infections are *E. coli* (UTI) and *S. aureus* (wound infection).
E. coli, Proteus mirabilis	Urinary catheterization	
Pseudomonas aeruginosa	Respiratory therapy equipment	Presume *Pseudomonas **AIR**uginosa* when **AIR** or burns are involved.
HBV	Work in renal dialysis unit	
Candida albicans	Hyperalimentation	
Legionella	Water aerosols	*Legionella* when water source is involved.

Bugs affecting HIV-positive adults

Clinical Presentation	Findings/Labs	Pathogen
Systemic		
Low-grade fevers, cough, hepato-splenomegaly	Oval yeast cells within macrophages	*Histoplasma capsulatum* (causes only pulmonary symptoms in immunocompetent hosts)
Dermatologic		
Fluffy white cottage-cheese lesions, often in mouth	Pseudohyphae	*C. albicans* (causes thrush)
Superficial vascular proliferation	Biopsy reveals neutrophilic inflammation	*Bartonella henselae* (causes bacillary angiomatosis)
Superficial neoplastic proliferation of vasculature	Biopsy reveals lymphocytic inflammation	HHV-8 (causes Kaposi's sarcoma)
Gastrointestinal		
Chronic, watery diarrhea	Acid-fast cysts seen in stool	*Cryptosporidium* spp.
Neurologic		
Meningitis	India ink stain reveals yeast with narrow-based budding and large capsule	*Cryptococcus neoformans* (may also cause encephalitis)
Encephalopathy	Due to reactivation of a latent virus; results in demyelination	JC virus (cause of PML)
Abscesses	Many ring-enhancing lesions on imaging	*Toxoplasma gondii*
Retinitis	Cotton-wool spots on funduscopic exam	CMV
Oncologic		
Hairy leukoplakia	Often on lateral tongue	EBV
Non-Hodgkin's lymphoma (large cell type)	Often on oropharynx (Waldeyer's ring)	EBV
Squamous cell carcinoma	Often in anus (MSM) or cervix (females)	HPV
Respiratory		
Interstitial pneumonia	Biopsy reveals cells with intranuclear (Owl's eye) inclusion bodies	CMV
Invasive aspergillosis	Pleuritic pain, hemoptysis, infiltrates on imaging	*Aspergillus fumigatus*
Pneumonia	Especially with CD4 < 200 cells/mm^3	*Pneumocystis jiroveci* (formerly *carinii*)
Tuberculosis-like disease	Especially with CD4 < 50 cells/mm^3	*Mycobacterium avium–intracellulare*

HIGH-YIELD PRINCIPLES

MICROBIOLOGY

Bugs affecting unimmunized children

Clinical Presentation	Findings/Labs	Pathogen
Dermatologic		
Rash	Beginning at head and moving down with postauricular lymphadenopathy	Rubella virus
	Beginning at head and moving down; rash preceded by cough, coryza, conjunctivitis, and blue-white (Koplik) spots on buccal mucosa	Measles virus (paramyxovirus; "rubeola")
Neurologic		
Meningitis	Microbe colonizes nasopharynx Can also lead to myalgia and paralysis	*H. influenzae* type B Poliovirus
Respiratory		
Pharyngitis	Grayish oropharyngeal exudate ("pseudomembranes" may obstruct airway); painful throat	*Corynebacterium diphtheriae* (elaborates toxin that causes necrosis in pharynx, cardiac, and CNS tissue)
Epiglottitis	Fever with dysphagia, drooling, and difficulty breathing due to edematous "cherry red" epiglottis	*H. influenzae* type B (also capable of causing epiglottitis in fully immunized children)

Bug hints (if all else fails)

Pus, empyema, abscess	*S. aureus.*
Pediatric infection	*Haemophilus influenzae* (including epiglottitis).
Pneumonia in cystic fibrosis, burn infection	*Pseudomonas aeruginosa.*
Branching rods in oral infection, sulfur granules	*Actinomyces israelii.*
Traumatic open wound	*Clostridium perfringens.*
Surgical wound	*S. aureus.*
Dog or cat bite	*Pasteurella multocida.*
Currant jelly sputum	*Klebsiella.*
Positive PAS stain	*Tropheryma whippelii* (Whipple's disease).
Sepsis/meningitis in newborn	Group B strep.
Health care provider	HBV (from needle stick).
Fungal infection in diabetic	*Mucor* or *Rhizopus* spp.
Asplenic patient	Encapsulated microbes, especially **SHiN** (**S.** *pneumoniae*, **H.** *influenzae* type B, **N.** *meningitidis*).
Chronic granulomatous disease	Catalase-positive microbes—*S. aureus*, *Nocardia* spp., *Aspergillus* spp.
Neutropenic patients	*Candida albicans* (systemic), *Aspergillus.*
Bilateral Bell's palsy	*Borrelia burgdorferi* (Lyme disease).

Antimicrobial therapy

Mechanism of action	Drugs
1. Block cell wall synthesis by inhibition of peptidoglycan cross-linking	Penicillin, ampicillin, ticarcillin, piperacillin, imipenem, aztreonam, cephalosporins
2. Block peptidoglycan synthesis	Bacitracin, vancomycin
3. Disrupt bacterial cell membranes	Polymyxins
4. Block nucleotide synthesis	Sulfonamides, trimethoprim
5. Block DNA topoisomerases	Fluoroquinolones
6. Block mRNA synthesis	Rifampin
7. Block protein synthesis at 50S ribosomal subunit	Chloramphenicol, macrolides, clindamycin, streptogramins (quinupristin, dalfopristin), linezolid
8. Block protein synthesis at 30S ribosomal subunit	Aminoglycosides, tetracyclines

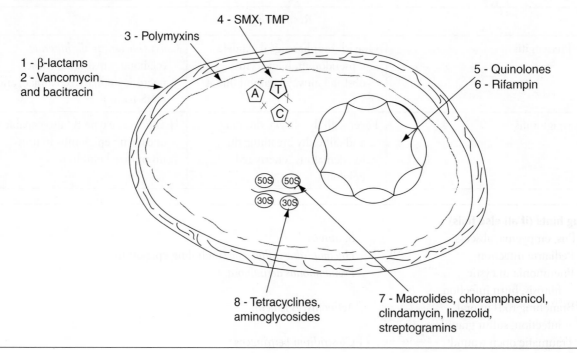

Bacteriostatic vs. bactericidal antibiotics

Bacteriostatic	Erythromycin, Clindamycin, Sulfamethoxazole, Trimethoprim, Tetracyclines, Chloramphenicol.	"We're **ECSTaTiC** about bacteriostatics."
Bactericidal	Vancomycin, Fluoroquinolones, Penicillin, Aminoglycosides, Cephalosporins, Metronidazole.	"**V**ery **F**inely **P**roficient **A**t **C**ell **M**urder."

Penicillin

Penicillin G (IV form), penicillin V (oral). Prototype β-lactam antibiotics.

Mechanism	1. Bind penicillin-binding proteins 2. Block transpeptidase cross-linking of cell wall 3. Activate autolytic enzymes	
Clinical use	Mostly used for **gram-positive organisms** (*S. pneumoniae*, *S.pyogenes*, *Actinomyces*) and **syphilis**. Bactericidal for gram-positive cocci, gram-positive rods, gram-negative cocci, and spirochetes. Not penicillinase resistant.	
Toxicity	Hypersensitivity reactions, hemolytic anemia.	

Methicillin, nafcillin, dicloxacillin (penicillinase-resistant penicillins)

Mechanism	Same as penicillin. Narrow spectrum; penicillinase resistant because of bulkier R group.	"Use **naf** (nafcillin) for **staph**."
Clinical use	*S. aureus* (except MRSA; resistant because of altered penicillin-binding protein target site).	
Toxicity	Hypersensitivity reactions; methicillin—interstitial nephritis.	

Ampicillin, amoxicillin (aminopenicillins)

Mechanism	Same as penicillin. Wider spectrum; penicillinase sensitive. Also combine with clavulanic acid to enhance spectrum. Am**O**xicillin has greater **O**ral bioavailability than ampicillin.	**AMP**ed up penicillin.
Clinical use	Extended-spectrum penicillin—certain gram-positive bacteria and gram-negative rods (*Haemophilus influenzae*, *E. coli*, *Listeria monocytogenes*, *Proteus mirabilis*, *Salmonella*, enterococci).	Coverage: ampicillin/ amoxicillin **HELPS** kill enterococci.
Toxicity	Hypersensitivity reactions; ampicillin rash; pseudomembranous colitis.	

Ticarcillin, carbenicillin, piperacillin (antipseudomonals)

Mechanism	Same as penicillin. Extended spectrum.	**TCP**: **T**akes **C**are of ***P**seudomonas*.
Clinical use	*Pseudomonas* spp. and gram-negative rods; susceptible to penicillinase; use with clavulanic acid.	
Toxicity	Hypersensitivity reactions.	

β-lactamase inhibitors

	Include **c**lavulanic acid, **s**ulbactam, **t**azobactam. Often added to penicillin antibiotics to protect the antibiotic from destruction by β-lactamase (penicillinase).	**CAST**.

Cephalosporins

Mechanism	β-lactam drugs that inhibit cell wall synthesis but are less susceptible to penicillinases. Bactericidal.	
Clinical use	1st generation (cefazolin, cephalexin)—gram-positive cocci, *Proteus mirabilis, E. coli, Klebsiella pneumoniae.*	1st generation—**PEcK.**
	2nd generation (cefoxitin, cefaclor, cefuroxime)—gram-positive cocci, *Haemophilus influenzae, Enterobacter aerogenes, Neisseria* spp., *Proteus mirabilis, E. coli, Klebsiella pneumoniae, Serratia marcescens.*	2nd generation—**HEN PEcKS.**
	3rd generation (ceftriaxone, cefotaxime, ceftazidime)—serious gram-negative infections resistant to other β-lactams.	**Ceftriaxone**—meningitis and gonorrhea. **Ceftazidime**—*Pseudomonas.*
	4th generation (cefepime)—↑ activity against *Pseudomonas* and gram-positive organisms.	
Toxicity	Hypersensitivity reactions, vitamin K deficiency. Cross-hypersensitivity with penicillins occurs in 5–10% of patients. ↑ nephrotoxicity of aminoglycosides; disulfiram-like reaction with ethanol (in cephalosporins with a methylthiotetrazole group, e.g., cefamandole).	

Aztreonam

Mechanism	A monobactam resistant to β-lactamases. Inhibits cell wall synthesis (binds to PBP3). Synergistic with aminoglycosides. No cross-allergenicity with penicillins.
Clinical use	**Gram-negative rods only**—No activity against gram-positives or anaerobes. For penicillin-allergic patients and those with renal insufficiency who cannot tolerate aminoglycosides.
Toxicity	Usually nontoxic; occasional GI upset. No cross-sensitivity with penicillins or cephalosporins.

Imipenem/cilastatin, meropenem

Mechanism	Imipenem is a broad-spectrum, β-lactamase-resistant carbapenem. Always administered with cilastatin (inhibitor of renal dihydropeptidase I) to ↓ inactivation of drug in renal tubules.	With imipenem, "the kill is **LASTIN'** with ci**LASTATIN**."
Clinical use	Gram-positive cocci, gram-negative rods, and anaerobes. Wide spectrum, but the significant side effects limit use to life-threatening infections, or after other drugs have failed. Meropenem, however, has a reduced risk of seizures and is stable to dihydropeptidase I.	
Toxicity	GI distress, skin rash, and CNS toxicity (seizures) at high plasma levels.	

Vancomycin

Mechanism	Inhibits cell wall mucopeptide formation by binding D-ala D-ala portion of cell wall precursors. Bactericidal.
Clinical use	**Gram positive only**—serious, multidrug-resistant organisms, including S. *aureus*, enterococci and *Clostridium difficile* (pseudomembranous colitis).
Toxicity	**N**ephrotoxicity, **O**totoxicity, **T**hrombophlebitis, diffuse flushing—"red man syndrome" (can largely prevent by pretreatment with antihistamines and slow infusion rate). Well tolerated in general—does **NOT** have many problems.
Resistance	Occurs with amino acid change of D-ala D-ala to D-ala D-lac.

Protein synthesis inhibitors

Specifically target smaller bacterial ribosome (70S, made of 30S and 50S subunits), leaving human ribosome (80S) unaffected.

"Buy **AT 30, CCELL** (sell) at **50**."

30S inhibitors:

A = **A**minoglycosides [bacteri**cidal**]

T = **T**etracyclines [bacteriostatic]

50S inhibitors:

C = **C**hloramphenicol, **C**lindamycin [bacteriostatic]

E = **E**rythromycin [bacteriostatic]

L = **L**incomycin [bacteriostatic]

L = **L**inezolid [variable]

Aminoglycosides

Gentamicin, **N**eomycin, **A**mikacin, **T**obramycin, **S**treptomycin.

"**Mean**" GNATS can**NOT** kill anaerobes.

Mechanism	Bactericidal; inhibit formation of initiation complex and cause misreading of mRNA. Require O_2 for uptake; therefore ineffective against anaerobes.
Clinical use	Severe **gram-negative rod** infections. Synergistic with β-lactam antibiotics. Neomycin for bowel surgery.
Toxicity	**N**ephrotoxicity (especially when used with cephalosporins), **O**totoxicity (especially when used with loop diuretics). **T**eratogen.
Resistance	Transferase enzymes that inactivate the drug by acetylation, phosphorylation, or adenylation.

Tetracyclines	Tetracycline, doxycycline, demeclocycline, minocycline.	Demeclocycline—ADH antagonist; acts as a **Diuretic in SIADH.**
Mechanism	Bacteriostatic; bind to 30S and prevent attachment of aminoacyl-tRNA; limited CNS penetration. Doxycycline is fecally eliminated and can be used in patients with renal failure. Must NOT take with milk, antacids, or iron-containing preparations because divalent cations inhibit its absorption in the gut.	
Clinical use	*Borrelia burgdorferi, H. pylori, M. pneumoniae.* Drug's ability to accumulate intracellularly makes it very effective against *Rickettsia* and *Chlamydia.*	
Toxicity	GI distress, discoloration of teeth and inhibition of bone growth in children, photosensitivity. Contraindicated in pregnancy.	
Resistance	↓ uptake into cells or ↑ efflux out of cell by plasmid-encoded transport pumps.	

Macrolides	Erythromycin, azithromycin, clarithromycin.
Mechanism	Inhibit protein synthesis by blocking translocation; bind to the 23S rRNA of the 50S ribosomal subunit. Bacteriostatic.
Clinical use	**Atypical pneumonias (*Mycoplasma, Chlamydia, Legionella*),** URIs, STDs, gram-positive cocci (streptococcal infections in patients allergic to penicillin), and *Neisseria.*
Toxicity	Prolonged QT interval (especially erythromycin), GI discomfort (most common cause of noncompliance), acute cholestatic hepatitis, eosinophilia, skin rashes. Increases serum concentration of theophyllines, oral anticoagulants.
Resistance	Methylation of 23S rRNA binding site.

Chloramphenicol	
Mechanism	Inhibits 50S peptidyltransferase activity. Bacteriostatic.
Clinical use	**Meningitis** (*Haemophilus influenzae, Neisseria meningitidis, Streptococcus pneumoniae*). Conservative use owing to toxicities but often still used in developing countries due to low cost.
Toxicity	Anemia (dose dependent), aplastic anemia (dose independent), gray baby syndrome (in premature infants because they lack liver UDP-glucuronyl transferase).
Resistance	Plasmid-encoded acetyltransferase that inactivates drug.

Clindamycin		
Mechanism	Blocks peptide bond formation at 50S ribosomal subunit. Bacteriostatic.	Treats anaerobes **above** the diaphragm vs. metronidazole (anaerobic infections **below** diaphragm).
Clinical use	**Anaerobic infections** (e.g., *Bacteroides fragilis, Clostridium perfringens*) in aspiration pneumonia or lung abscesses.	
Toxicity	Pseudomembranous colitis (*C. difficile* overgrowth), fever, diarrhea.	

HIGH-YIELD PRINCIPLES

MICROBIOLOGY

Sulfonamides   Sulfamethoxazole (SMX), sulfisoxazole, sulfadiazine.
   Mechanism   PABA antimetabolites inhibit dihydropteroate synthetase. Bacteriostatic.
   Clinical use   Gram-positive, gram-negative, *Nocardia*, *Chlamydia*. Triple sulfas or SMX for simple UTI.
   Toxicity   Hypersensitivity reactions, hemolysis if G6PD deficient, nephrotoxicity (tubulointerstitial nephritis), photosensitivity, kernicterus in infants, displace other drugs from albumin (e.g., warfarin).
   Resistance   Altered enzyme (bacterial dihydropteroate synthetase), ↓ uptake, or ↑ PABA synthesis.

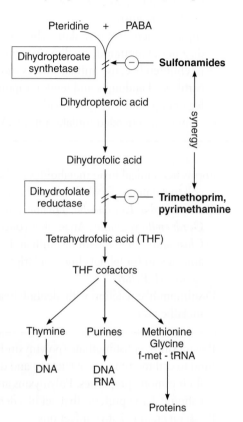

(Adapted, with permission, from Katzung BG. *Basic and Clinical Pharmacology*, 7th ed. Stamford, CT: Appleton & Lange, 1997: 762.)

Trimethoprim
   Mechanism   Inhibits bacterial dihydrofolate reductase. Bacteriostatic.   Trimethoprim = **TMP:**
   Clinical use   Used in combination with sulfonamides   "Treats **M**arrow **P**oorly."
                (trimethoprim-sulfamethoxazole [TMP-SMX]), causing sequential block of folate synthesis. Combination used for recurrent UTIs, *Shigella*, *Salmonella*, *Pneumocystis jiroveci* pneumonia.
   Toxicity   Megaloblastic anemia, leukopenia, granulocytopenia. (May alleviate with supplemental folinic acid [leucovorin rescue].)

Sulfa drug allergies   Patients who do not tolerate sulfa drugs should not be given sulfonamides or other sulfa drugs, such as sulfasalazine, sulfonylureas, thiazide diuretics, acetazolamide, furosemide, celecoxib, or probenecid.

Fluoroquinolones | Ciprofloxacin, norfloxacin, ofloxacin, sparfloxacin, moxifloxacin, gatifloxacin, enoxacin (fluoroquinolones), nalidixic acid (a quinolone).

Mechanism — Inhibit DNA gyrase (topoisomerase II). Bactericidal. Must not be taken with antacids.

FluoroquinoLONES hurt attachments to your BONES.

Clinical use — Gram-negative rods of urinary and GI tracts (including *Pseudomonas*), *Neisseria*, some gram-positive organisms.

Toxicity — GI upset, superinfections, skin rashes, headache, dizziness. Contraindicated in pregnant women and in children because animal studies show damage to cartilage. Tendonitis and tendon rupture in adults; leg cramps and myalgias in kids.

Resistance — Chromosome-encoded mutation in DNA gyrase.

Metronidazole

Mechanism — Forms free radical toxic metabolites in the bacterial cell that damage DNA. Bactericidal, antiprotozoal.

Clinical use — Treats *Giardia*, *Entamoeba*, *Trichomonas*, *Gardnerella vaginalis*, **A**naerobes (*Bacteroides*, *Clostridium*). Used with bismuth and amoxicillin (or tetracycline) for "triple therapy" against *H. Pylori*.

GET GAP on the **Metro!** Anaerobic infection below the diaphragm.

Toxicity — Disulfiram-like reaction with alcohol; headache, metallic taste.

Polymyxins | Polymyxin B, colistimethate (polymyxin E).

'MYXins MIX up membranes.

Mechanism — Bind to cell membranes of bacteria and disrupt their osmotic properties. Polymyxins are cationic, basic proteins that act like detergents.

Clinical use — Resistant gram-negative infections.

Toxicity — Neurotoxicity, acute renal tubular necrosis.

Antimycobacterial drugs

Bacterium	Prophylaxis	Treatment
M. tuberculosis	Isoniazid	Rifampin, Isoniazid, Pyrazinamide, Ethambutol (**RIPE** for **treatment**)
M. avium–intracellulare	Azithromycin	Azithromycin, rifampin, ethambutol, streptomycin
M. leprae	N/A	Dapsone, rifampin, clofazimine

Anti-TB drugs	Streptomycin, Pyrazinamide, Isoniazid (INH), Rifampin, Ethambutol. Cycloserine (2nd-line therapy). Important side effect of ethambutol is optic neuropathy (red-green color blindness). For other drugs, hepatotoxicity.	**INH-SPIRE** (inspire). Pyrazinamide—effective in acidic pH of phagolysosomes, where TB engulfed by macrophages is found. Ethambutol—↓ carbohydrate polymerization of mycobacterium cell wall by blocking arabinosyltransferase.

Isoniazid (INH)

Mechanism	↓ synthesis of mycolic acids. Bacteria catalase-peroxidase needed to convert INH to active metabolite.	**INH I**njures **N**eurons and **H**epatocytes.
Clinical use	*Mycobacterium tuberculosis.* The only agent used as solo prophylaxis against TB.	Different INH half-lives in fast vs. slow acetylators.
Toxicity	Neurotoxicity, hepatotoxicity, lupus. Pyridoxine (vitamin B_6) can prevent neurotoxicity, lupus.	

Rifampin

Mechanism	Inhibits DNA-dependent RNA polymerase.	Rifampin's **4 R's**:
Clinical use	*Mycobacterium tuberculosis*; delays resistance to dapsone when used for leprosy. Used for meningococcal prophylaxis and chemoprophylaxis in contacts of children with *Haemophilus influenzae* type B.	**R**NA polymerase inhibitor **R**evs up microsomal P-450 **R**ed/orange body fluids **R**apid resistance if used alone
Toxicity	Minor hepatotoxicity and drug interactions (↑ P-450); orange body fluids (nonhazardous side effect).	

Nonsurgical antimicrobial prophylaxis	Meningococcal infection	Rifampin (drug of choice), minocycline.
	Gonorrhea	Ceftriaxone.
	Syphilis	Benzathine penicillin G.
	History of recurrent UTIs	TMP-SMX.
	Pneumocystis jiroveci pneumonia	TMP-SMX (drug of choice), aerosolized pentamidine.
	Endocarditis with surgical or dental procedures	Penicillins.
	Mycobacterium avium-intracellulare	Azithromycin.

Treatment of highly resistant bacteria	MRSA—vancomycin. VRE—linezolid and streptogramins (quinupristin/dalfopristin).

Antifungal therapy

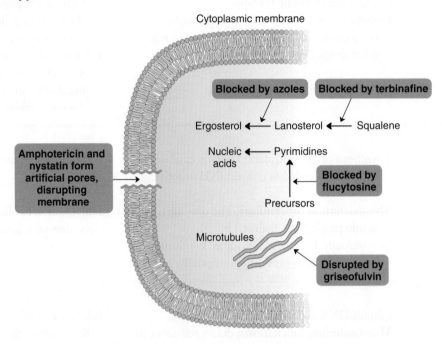

(Adapted, with permission, from Katzung BG, Trevor AJ. *USMLE Road Map: Pharmacology*, 1st ed. New York: McGraw-Hill, 2003: 120.)

Amphotericin B

Mechanism	Binds ergosterol (unique to fungi); forms membrane pores that allow leakage of electrolytes.	Amphotericin "tears" holes in the fungal membrane by forming pores.
Clinical use	**Serious, systemic** mycoses. *Cryptococcus, Blastomyces, Coccidioides, Aspergillus, Histoplasma, Candida, Mucor* (systemic mycoses). Intrathecally for fungal meningitis; does not cross blood-brain barrier.	
Toxicity	Fever/chills ("shake and bake"), hypotension, nephrotoxicity, arrhythmias, anemia, IV phlebitis ("amphoterrible"). Hydration reduces nephrotoxicity. Liposomal amphotericin reduces toxicity.	

Nystatin

Mechanism	Same as amphotericin B. **Topical** form because too toxic for systemic use.
Clinical use	"Swish and swallow" for oral candidiasis (thrush); topical for diaper rash or vaginal candidiasis.

Azoles   Fluconazole, ketoconazole, clotrimazole, miconazole, itraconazole, voriconazole.

  Mechanism   Inhibit fungal sterol (ergosterol) synthesis, by inhibiting the P-450 enzyme that converts lanosterol to ergosterol.

  Clinical use   Systemic mycoses. Fluconazole for **cryptococcal meningitis in AIDS** patients (because it can cross blood-brain barrier) and **candidal infections** of all types.
                 Ketoconazole for *Blastomyces, Coccidioides, Histoplasma, Candida albicans*; hypercortisolism. Clotrimazole and miconazole for topical fungal infections.

  Toxicity   Hormone synthesis inhibition (gynecomastia), liver dysfunction (inhibits cytochrome P-450), fever, chills.

Flucytosine

  Mechanism   Inhibits DNA synthesis by conversion to 5-fluorouracil.

  Clinical use   Used in systemic fungal infections (e.g., ***Candida, Cryptococcus***) in combination with amphotericin B.

  Toxicity   Nausea, vomiting, diarrhea, bone marrow suppression.

Caspofungin

  Mechanism   Inhibits cell wall synthesis by inhibiting synthesis of β-glucan.

  Clinical use   **Invasive aspergillosis.**

  Toxicity   GI upset, flushing.

Terbinafine

  Mechanism   Inhibits the fungal enzyme squalene epoxidase.

  Clinical use   Used to treat dermatophytoses (especially **onychomycosis**—fungal infection of finger or toe nails).

Griseofulvin

  Mechanism   Interferes with microtubule function; disrupts mitosis. Deposits in keratin-containing tissues (e.g., nails).

  Clinical use   Oral treatment of superficial infections; inhibits growth of **dermatophytes** (tinea, ringworm).

  Toxicity   Teratogenic, carcinogenic, confusion, headaches, ↑ P-450 and warfarin metabolism.

Antiprotozoan therapy

Drug	Mechanism
Pyrimethamine	Selectively inhibits plasmodial dihydrofolate reductase (best for *P. falciparum*). Drug of choice for toxoplasmosis when combined with sulfadiazine.
Suramin	Inhibits enzymes involved in energy metabolism. No CNS involvement.
Melarsoprol	Inhibits sulfhydryl groups in parasite enzymes. CNS involvement.
Nifurtimox	Forms intracellular oxygen radicals, which are toxic to the organism.
Sodium stibogluconate	Inhibits glycolysis at PFK reaction.
Chloroquine	Blocks plasmodium heme polymerase, leading to accumulation of toxic hemoglobin breakdown products that destroy the organism.
Mefloquine	Unknown.
Quinine	For chloroquine-resistant species when used in combination with pyrimethamine/sulfonamide.

Antihelminthic therapy

Mebendazole	Inhibits glucose uptake and microtubule synthesis.
Pyrantel pamoate	Stimulates nicotinic receptors at neuromuscular junctions. Contraction occurs, followed by depolarization-induced paralysis. No effect on tapeworms or flukes.
Ivermectin	Intensifies GABA-mediated neurotransmission and causes immobilization. Does not cross the blood-brain barrier; therefore, no effect on humans.
Diethylcarbamazine	Unknown.
Praziquantel	Increases membrane permeability to calcium, causing contraction and paralysis of tapeworms and flukes.

Antiviral chemotherapy

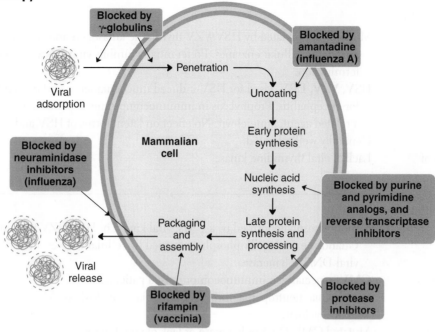

(Adapted, with permission, from Katzung BG, Trevor AJ. *USMLE Road Map: Pharmacology*, 1st ed. New York: McGraw-Hill, 2003: 120.)

Amantadine

Mechanism	Blocks viral penetration/un**coat**ing (M2 protein). Also causes the release of dopamine from intact nerve terminals.	"**A man to dine**" takes off his **coat**.
Clinical use	Prophylaxis and treatment for influenza A only; **Parkinson's disease**.	**A**mantadine blocks influenza **A** and causes problems with the cerebell**A**.
Toxicity	Ataxia, dizziness, slurred speech.	Rimantidine is a derivative
Mechanism of resistance	Mutated M2 protein. 90% of all influenza A strains are resistant to amantadine, so not used.	with fewer CNS side effects. Does not cross the blood-brain barrier.

Zanamivir, oseltamivir

Mechanism	Inhibit influenza neuraminidase, decreasing the release of progeny virus.
Clinical use	Both **influenza A and B**.

Ribavirin

Mechanism	Inhibits synthesis of guanine nucleotides by competitively inhibiting IMP dehydrogenase.
Clinical use	**RSV, chronic hepatitis C**.
Toxicity	Hemolytic anemia. Severe teratogen.

Acyclovir

Mechanism	Monophosphorylated by HSV/VZV thymidine kinase. Guanosine analog. Triphosphate formed by cellular enzymes. Preferentially inhibits viral DNA polymerase by chain termination.
Clinical use	**HSV, VZV, EBV**. Used for HSV-induced mucocutaneous and genital lesions as well as for encephalitis. Prophylaxis in immunocompromised patients. For herpes zoster, use a related agent, famciclovir. No effect on latent forms of HSV and VZV.
Toxicity	Generally well tolerated.
Mechanism of resistance	Lack of viral thymidine kinase.

Ganciclovir

Mechanism	5'-monophosphate formed by a CMV viral kinase or HSV/VZV thymidine kinase. Guanosine analog. Triphosphate formed by cellular kinases. Preferentially inhibits viral DNA polymerase.
Clinical use	**CMV**, especially in immunocompromised patients.
Toxicity	Leukopenia, neutropenia, thrombocytopenia, renal toxicity. More toxic to host enzymes than acyclovir.
Mechanism of resistance	Mutated CMV DNA polymerase or lack of viral kinase.

Foscarnet

Mechanism	Viral DNA polymerase inhibitor that binds to the pyrophosphate-binding site of the enzyme. Does not require activation by viral kinase.	**FOS**carnet = pyro**FOS**phate analog.
Clinical use	**CMV retinitis** in immunocompromised patients **when ganciclovir fails**; acyclovir-resistant HSV.	
Toxicity	Nephrotoxicity.	
Mechanism of resistance	Mutated DNA polymerase.	

HIV therapy

Highly active antiretroviral therapy (HAART): Initiated when patients present with AIDS-defining illness, low CD4 cell counts (< 350 cells/mm³), or high viral load. Regimen consists of 3 drugs to prevent resistance:

[2 nucleoside reverse transcriptase inhibitors (NRTIs) + 1 protease inhibitor] OR

[2 NRTIs + 1 non-nucleoside reverse transcriptase inhibitor (NNRTI)]

Drug	Mechanism	Toxicity
Protease inhibitors		
Saqui**navir** Rito**navir** Indi**navir** Nelfi**navir** Ampre**navir**	Assembly of virions depends on HIV-1 protease (*pol* gene), which cleaves the polypeptide products of HIV mRNA into their functional parts. Thus, protease inhibitors prevent maturation of new viruses. All protease inhibitors end in *-navir*. **NAVIR** (never) **TEASE** a pro**TEASE**.	Hyperglycemia, GI intolerance (nausea, diarrhea), lipodystrophy, thrombocytopenia (indinavir). *metabolic Sx*
NRTIs		
Zidovudine (ZDV, formerly AZT) Didanosine (ddI) Zalcitabine (ddC) Stavudine (d4T)	Competitively inhibit nucleotide binding to reverse transcriptase and terminate the DNA chain (lack a 3'-OH group). Must be phosphorylated by thymidine kinase to be active. ZDV is used for general prophylaxis and during pregnancy to reduce risk of fetal transmission. Have **you dined (vudine)** with my **nuclear (nucleosides)** family?	Bone marrow suppression (can be reversed with G-CSF and erythropoietin), peripheral neuropathy, lactic acidosis (nucleosides), rash (non-nucleosides), megaloblastic anemia (ZDV).
NNRTIs		
Nevirapine Efavirenz Declaviridine	Bind to reverse transcriptase at site different from NRTIs. Do not require phosphorylation to be active or compete with nucleotides. **N**ever **E**ver **D**eliver nucleosides.	Same as NRTIs.
Fusion inhibitors		
Enfuvirtide	Bind viral gp41 subunit; inhibit conformational change required for fusion with CD4 cells, blocking entry and replication. Used in patients with persistent viral replication despite antiretroviral therapy.	Hypersensitivity reactions, reactions at subcutaneous injection site, ↑ risk of bacterial pneumonia.

Interferons

Mechanism	Glycoproteins synthesized by virus-infected cells block replication of both RNA and DNA viruses.
Clinical use	IFN-α—chronic hepatitis B and C, Kaposi's sarcoma. IFN-β—MS. IFN-γ—NADPH oxidase deficiency.
Toxicity	Neutropenia.

Antibiotics to avoid in pregnancy	Sulfonamides—kernicterus.	**SAFE** Moms Take Really Good Care.
	Aminoglycosides—ototoxicity.	
	Fluoroquinolones—cartilage damage.	
	Erythromycin—acute cholestatic heptatitis in mom (and clarithromycin—embryotoxic).	
	Metronidazole—mutagenesis.	
	Tetracyclines—discolored teeth, inhibition of bone growth.	
	Ribavirin (antiviral)—teratogenic.	
	Griseofulvin (antifungal)—teratogenic.	
	Chloramphenicol—"gray baby."	

Immunology

"I hate to disappoint you, but my rubber lips are immune to your charms."
—*Batman & Robin*

"No State shall abridge the privileges or immunities of its citizens."
—The United States Constitution

▶ **Lymphoid Structures**

▶ **Lymphocytes**

▶ **Immune Responses**

▶ **Immunosuppressants**

Immunology can be confusing and complicated, but luckily the USMLE tests only basic principles and facts in this area. Cell surface markers are important to know because they are clinically useful (i.e., in identifying specific types of immune deficiency or cancer) and are functionally critical to the jobs immune cells carry out. By spending a little extra effort here, it is possible to turn a traditionally difficult subject into one that is high yield.

Lymph node   A 2° lymphoid organ that has many afferents, 1 or more efferents. Encapsulated, with trabeculae. Functions are nonspecific filtration by macrophages, storage and activation of B and T cells, antibody production.

Follicle   Site of B-cell localization and proliferation. In outer cortex. 1° follicles are dense and dormant. 2° follicles have pale central germinal centers and are active.

Medulla   Consists of medullary cords (closely packed lymphocytes and plasma cells) and medullary sinuses. Medullary sinuses communicate with efferent lymphatics and contain reticular cells and macrophages.

Paracortex   Houses T cells. Region of cortex between follicles and medulla. Contains high endothelial venules through which T and B cells enter from blood. In an extreme cellular immune response, paracortex becomes greatly enlarged. Not well developed in patients with DiGeorge syndrome.

Paracortex enlarges in an extreme cellular immune response (i.e., viral).

Lymph drainage

Area of body	**1° lymph node drainage site**
1. Upper limb, lateral breast	1. Axillary
2. Stomach	2. Celiac
3. Duodenum jejunum,	3. Superior mesenteric
4. Sigmoid colon	4. Colic → inferior mesenteric
5. Rectum (lower above pectinate line	5. Internal iliac part), anal canal
6. Anal canal below	6. Superficial inguinal pectinate line
7. Testes	7. Superficial and deep plexuses → para-aortic
8. Scrotum	8. Superficial inguinal
9. Thigh (superficial)	9. Superficial inguinal
10. Lateral side of dorsum of foot	10. Popliteal

Right lymphatic duct—drains right arm and right half of head.
Thoracic duct—drains everything else.

| **Sinusoids of spleen** | Long, vascular channels in red pulp with fenestrated "barrel hoop" basement membrane. Macrophages found nearby. | T cells are found in the periarterial lymphatic sheath (PALS) and in the white pulp of the spleen. B cells are found in follicles within the white pulp of the spleen. |

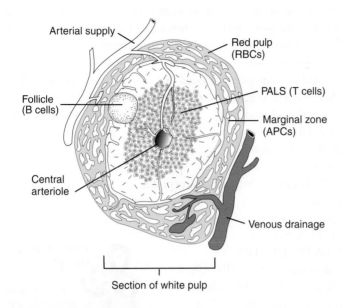

Section of white pulp

Macrophages in the spleen remove encapsulated bacteria.

Splenic dysfunction: ↓ IgM → ↓ complement activation → ↓ C3b opsonization → ↑ susceptibility to encapsulated organisms "S SHiN":
Salmonella,
S. pneumoniae,
H. influenzae,
N. meningitidis.

Postsplenectomy:
—Howell-Jolly bodies (nuclear remnants)
—Target cells
—Thrombocytosis

| **Thymus** | Site of T-cell differentiation and maturation. Encapsulated. From epithelium of 3rd branchial pouches. Lymphocytes of mesenchymal origin. Cortex is dense with immature T cells; medulla is pale with mature T cells and epithelial reticular cells and contains Hassall's corpuscles. Positive (MHC restriction) and negative selection (nonreactive to self) occur at the corticomedullary junction. | **T** cells = **T**hymus. **B** cells = **B**one marrow. |

HIGH-YIELD PRINCIPLES

IMMUNOLOGY

Innate vs. adaptive immunity

Innate—receptors that recognize pathogens are germline encoded. Response to pathogens is fast and nonspecific. No memory. Consists of neutrophils, macrophages, dendritic cells, natural killer cells (lymphoid origin), and complement.

Adaptive—receptors that recognize pathogens undergo V(D)J recombination during lymphocyte development. Response is slow on first exposure, but memory response is faster and more robust. Consists of T cells, B cells, and circulating antibody.

MHC I and II

MHC = major histocompatibility complex, encoded by Human Leukocyte Antigen (HLA) genes; present antigen fragments to T cells and bind TCR.

MHC I = HLA-A, HLA-B, HLA-C.
  Expressed on almost all nucleated cells.
    Not expressed on RBC.
  Antigen is loaded in RER of mostly intracellular peptides.
  Mediates viral immunity.
  Pairs with β_2-microglobulin (aids in transport to cell surface). Binds TCR and CD8.

MHC II = HLA-DR, HLA-DP, HLA-DQ.
  Expressed only on antigen-presenting cells (APCs).
  Antigen is loaded following release of invariant chain in an acidified endosome. Binds TCR and CD4.

MHC I—binds TCR and CD8.
MHC II—binds TCR and CD4.

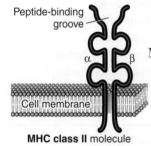

MHC class II molecule

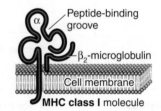

MHC class I molecule

HLA subtypes associated with diseases

A3	Hemochromatosis	
B27	Psoriasis, Ankylosing spondylitis, Inflammatory bowel disease, Reiter's syndrome.	**PAIR.**
B8	Graves' disease.	
DR2	Multiple sclerosis, hay fever, SLE, Goodpasture's.	
DR3	Diabetes mellitus type 1.	
DR4	Rheumatoid arthritis, diabetes mellitus type 1.	
DR5	Pernicious anemia → B_{12} deficiency, Hashimoto's thyroiditis.	
DR7	Steroid-responsive nephrotic syndrome.	

Natural killer cells

Use perforin and granzymes to induce apoptosis of virally infected cells and tumor cells.
Only lymphocyte member of innate immune system.
Activity enhanced by IL-12, IFN-β, and IFN-α.
Induced to kill when exposed to a nonspecific activation signal on target cell and/or to an absence of class I MHC on target cell surface.

Major functions of B and T cells

B-cell functions

Make antibody—opsonize bacteria, neutralize viruses (IgG); activate complement (IgM, IgG); sensitize mast cells (IgE).

Allergy (type I hypersensitivity): IgE.

Cytotoxic (type II) and immune complex (type III) hypersensitivity: IgG.

Hyperacute organ rejection (antibody mediated).

T-cell functions

CD4+ T cells help B cells make antibody and produce γ-interferon, which activates macrophages.

CD8+ T cells kill virus-infected cells directly.

Delayed cell-mediated hypersensitivity (type IV).

Acute and chronic organ rejection.

Differentiation of T cells

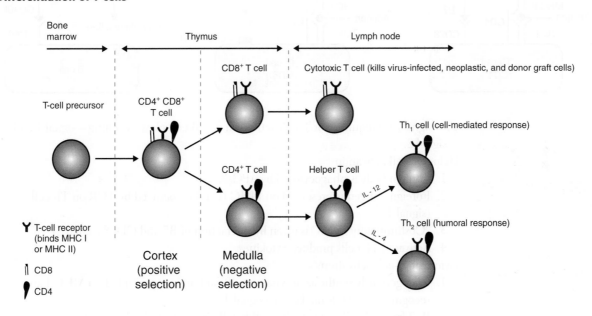

T- and B-cell activation

Antigen-presenting cells (APCs):
1. Macrophage
2. Dendritic cell
3. B cell

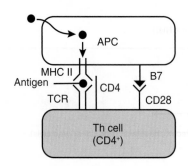
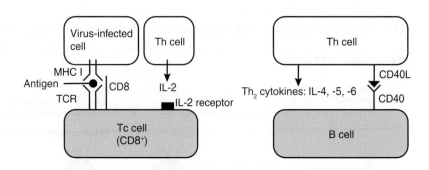

Two signals are required for T-cell activation and B-cell class switching—signal 1 and signal 2.

Helper T-cell activation:
1. Foreign body is phagocytosed by APC
2. Foreign antigen is presented on MHC II and recognized by TCR on Th cell (signal 1)
3. "Costimulatory signal" is given by interaction of B7 and CD28 (signal 2)
4. Activated Th cells produce cytokines

Cytotoxic T-cell activation:
1. Endogenously synthesized (viral or self) proteins are presented on MHC I and recognized by TCR on Tc cell (signal 1)
2. IL-2 from Th cell activates Tc cell to kill virus-infected cell (signal 2)

B-cell class switching:
1. IL-4, IL-5, IL-6 from Th_2 cell (signal 1)
2. CD40 receptor on B cell binds CD40 ligand on Th cell (signal 2)

Helper T cells

Th_1 cell	Th_2 cell
Regulates cell-mediated response	Regulates humoral response
Secretes Th_1 cytokines: IL-2, IFN-γ	Secretes Th_2 cytokines: IL-4, IL-5, IL-10
Activates macrophage and $CD8^+$ T cell	Helps B cells make antibody (IgE > IgG)
Inhibited by IL-10 (from Th_2 cell)	Inhibited by IFN-γ (from Th_1 cell)

Macrophage-lymphocyte interaction—activated lymphocytes (release IFN-γ) and macrophages (release IL-1, TNF-α) stimulate one another.

Helper T cells have CD4, which binds to MHC II on APCs.

Cytotoxic T cells

Kill virus-infected, neoplastic, and donor graft cells by inducing apoptosis.

Release cytotoxic granules containing preformed proteins (perforin—helps to deliver the content of granules into target cell; granzyme—a serine protease, activates apoptosis inside target cell; granulysin—antimicrobial, induces apoptosis).

Cytotoxic T cells have CD8, which binds to MHC I on virus-infected cells.

Antibody structure and function

Variable part of L and H chains recognizes antigens. Fc portion of IgM and IgG fixes complement. Heavy chain contributes to Fc and Fab fractions. Light chain contributes only to Fab fraction.

Fab:

  Antigen-binding fragment

  Determines idiotype: unique antigen-binding pocket; only 1 antigenic specificity expressed per B cell

Fc:

  Constant

  Carboxy terminal

  Complement binding at C_H2 (IgG + IgM only)

  Carbohydrate side chains

  Determines isotype (IgM, IgD, etc.)

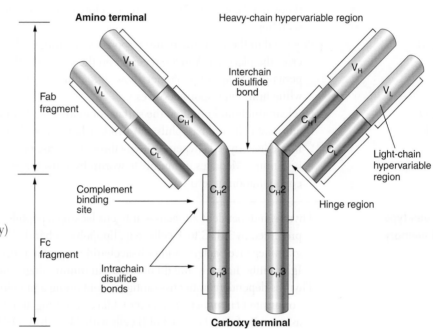

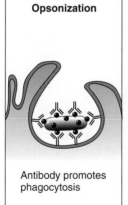 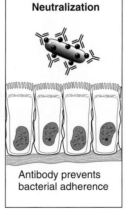 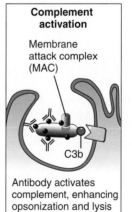

Opsonization	Neutralization	Complement activation
Antibody promotes phagocytosis	Antibody prevents bacterial adherence	Antibody activates complement, enhancing opsonization and lysis

Antibody diversity is generated by:

1. Random "recombination" of VJ (light-chain) or V(D)J (heavy-chain) genes
2. Random combination of heavy chains with light chains
3. Somatic hypermutation (following antigen stimulation)
4. Addition of nucleotides to DNA during "recombination" (see #1) by terminal deoxynucleotidyl transferase

Immunoglobulin isotypes	Mature B lymphocytes express IgM and IgD on their surfaces. They may differentiate by isotype switching (alternative splicing of mRNA; mediated by cytokines and CD40 ligand) into plasma cells that secrete IgA, IgE, or IgG.
IgG	Main antibody in 2° (**delayed**) response to an antigen. Most abundant in blood. Fixes complement, crosses the placenta (provides infants with passive immunity), opsonizes bacteria, neutralizes bacterial toxins and viruses.
IgA	Prevents attachment of bacteria and viruses to mucous membranes; does not fix complement. Monomer (in circulation) or dimer (when secreted). Crosses epithelial cells by transcytosis. Found in secretions (tears, saliva, mucus) and breast milk (known as "colostrum"). Picks up secretory component from epithelial cells before secretion.
IgM	Produced in the 1° (**immediate**) response to an antigen. Fixes complement but does not cross the placenta. Antigen receptor on the surface of B cells. Monomer on B cell or pentamer. Shape of pentamer allows it to efficiently trap free antigens out of tissue while humoral response evolves.
IgD	Unclear function. Found on the surface of many B cells and in serum.
IgE	Binds mast cells and basophils; cross-links when exposed to allergen, mediating immediate (type I) hypersensitivity through release of inflammatory mediators such as histamine. Mediates immunity to worms by activating eosinophils. Lowest concentration in serum.
Antigen type and memory	Thymus-independent antigens—antigens lacking a peptide component; cannot be presented by MHC to T cells (e.g., lipopolysaccharide from cell envelope of gram-negative bacteria and polysaccharide capsular antigen). Stimulate release of IgM antibodies only and do not result in immunologic memory.
	Thymus-dependent antigens—antigens containing a protein component (e.g., conjugated *H. influenzae* vaccine). Class switching and immunologic memory occur as a result of direct contact of B cells with Th cells (CD40–CD40 ligand interaction) and release of IL-4, IL-5, and IL-6.

Complement

System of proteins that interact to play a role in humoral immunity and inflammation.

Membrane attack complex of complement defends against gram-negative bacteria. Activated by IgG or IgM in the **classic** pathway, and activated by molecules on the surface of microbes (especially endotoxin) in the **alternative** pathway.

C3b and IgG are the two 1° opsonins in bacterial defense. C3b aids in clearance of immune complexes.

Decay-accelerating factor (DAF) and C1 esterase inhibitor help prevent complement activation on self-cells (e.g., RBC).

GM makes **classic** cars.

C1, C2, C3, C4—viral neutralization.

C3b—opsonization. **B**inds **B**acteria.

C3a, C5a—**A**naphylaxis.

C5a—neutrophil chemotaxis.

C5b-9—cytolysis by membrane attack complex (MAC).

Deficiency of C1 esterase inhibitor leads to hereditary angioedema.

Deficiency of C3 leads to severe, recurrent pyogenic sinus and respiratory tract infections; ↑ susceptibility to type III hypersensitivity reactions.

Deficiency of C5–C8 leads to *Neisseria* bacteremia.

Deficiency of DAF (GPI-anchored enzyme) leads to complement-mediated lysis of RBCs and paroxysmal nocturnal hemoglobinuria (PNH).

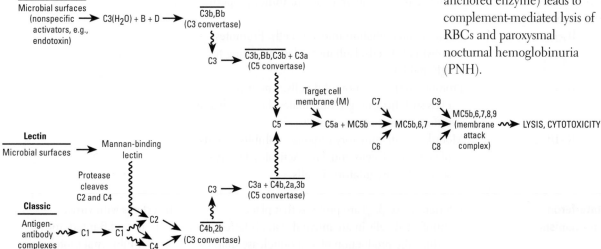

(Adapted, with permission, from Levinson W. *Medical Microbiology and Immunology: Examination and Board Review,* 8th ed. New York: McGraw-Hill, 2004: 432.)

Important cytokines

Secreted by macrophages

IL-1	An endogenous pyrogen. Causes fever, acute inflammation. Activates endothelium to express adhesion molecules; induces chemokine secretion to recruit leukocytes.	"Hot T-Bone stEAk": IL-1: fever (hot). IL-2: stimulates T cells. IL-3: stimulates Bone marrow.
IL-6	An endogenous pyrogen. Also secreted by Th cells. Causes fever and stimulates production of acute-phase proteins.	IL-4: stimulates IgE production. IL-5: stimulates IgA production.
IL-8	Major chemotactic factor for neutrophils.	"Clean up on aisle 8."
IL-12	Induces differentiation of T cells into Th_1 cells. Activates NK cells. Also secreted by B cells.	Neutrophils are recruited by IL-8 to clear infections.
TNF-α	Mediates septic shock. Activates endothelium. Causes leukocyte recruitment, vascular leak.	

Secreted by T cells

IL-3	Supports the growth and differentiation of bone marrow stem cells. Functions like GM-CSF.

From Th_1 cells

IL-2	Stimulates growth of helper and cytotoxic T cells.
Interferon-γ	Activates macrophages and Th_1 cells. Suppresses Th_2 cells. Has antiviral and antitumor properties.

From Th_2 cells

IL-4	Induces differentiation into Th_2 cells. Promotes growth of B cells. Enhances class switching to IgE and IgG.
IL-5	Promotes differentiation of B cells. Enhances class switching to IgA. Stimulates the growth and differentiation of eosinophils.
IL-10	Modulates inflammatory response. Inhibits actions of activated T cells and Th_1. Activates Th_2. Also secreted by **Regulatory T cells.**

Interferon mechanism	Interferons (α, β, γ) are proteins that place uninfected cells in an antiviral state. Interferons induce the production of a ribonuclease that inhibits viral protein synthesis by degrading viral mRNA (but not host mRNA).	Interferes with viruses: 1. α- and β-interferons inhibit viral protein synthesis 2. γ-interferons ↑ MHC I and II expression and antigen presentation in all cells 3. Activates NK cells to kill virus-infected cells

Cell surface proteins

T cells	TCR (binds antigen-MHC complex), CD3 (associated with TCR, for signal transduction), CD28 (binds B7 on APC). Helper T cells: CD4, CD40L (binds CD40 on B cells). Cytotoxic T cells: CD8.
B cells	Ig (binds antigen), CD19, CD20, CD21 (receptor for EBV), CD40, MHC II, B7.
Macrophages	MHC II, B7, CD40, CD14, receptors for Fc and C3b.
NK cells	Receptors for MHC I, CD16 (binds Fc of IgG), CD56 (unique marker for NK).
All cells except mature red cells	MHC I.

"You can drink **B**eer at the **B**ar when you're 21": **B** cells; Epstein-**B**arr virus; CD-**21**.

Anergy

Self-reactive T cells become nonreactive without costimulatory molecule. B cells also become anergic, but tolerance is less complete than in T cells.

Effects of bacterial toxins

Superantigens (*S. pyogenes* and *S. aureus*)—cross-link the β-region of the T-cell receptor to the MHC class II on APCs. Results in the uncoordinated release of IFN-γ from Th$_1$ cells and subsequent release of IL-1, IL-6, and TNF-α from macrophages.
Endotoxins/lipopolysaccharide (gram-negative bacteria)—directly stimulate macrophages by binding to endotoxin receptor CD14; Th cells are not involved.

Antigen variation

Classic examples:
Bacteria—*Salmonella* (2 flagellar variants), *Borrelia* (relapsing fever), *Neisseria gonorrhoeae* (pilus protein).
Virus—influenza (major = shift, minor = drift).
Parasites—trypanosomes (programmed rearrangement).

Some mechanisms for variation include DNA rearrangement and RNA segment reassortment (e.g., influenza major shift).

Passive vs. active immunity

Active	Induced after exposure to foreign antigens. Slow onset. Long-lasting protection (memory).
Passive	Based on receiving preformed antibodies from another host. Rapid onset. Short life span of antibodies (half-life = 3 weeks). Example: IgA in breast milk.

After exposure to **T**etanus toxin, **B**otulinum toxin, **H**BV, or **R**abies virus, patients are given preformed antibodies (passive)—**To Be H**ealed **R**apidly.

HIGH-YIELD PRINCIPLES

IMMUNOLOGY

Hypersensitivity

Type I

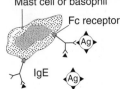

Mast cell or basophil

Fc receptor

Ag

IgE

Ag

Anaphylactic and atopic—free antigen cross-links IgE on presensitized mast cells and basophils, triggering release of vasoactive amines that act at postcapillary venules (i.e., histamine). Reaction develops rapidly after antigen exposure due to preformed antibody.

First and Fast (anaphylaxis). Types I, II, and III are all antibody mediated.
Test: scratch test and radioimmunosorbent assay.

Type II

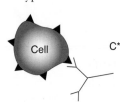

Cell

C*

Antibody mediated—IgM, IgG bind to fixed antigen on "enemy" cell, leading to lysis (by complement) or phagocytosis.

3 mechanisms:
1. Opsonize cells or activate complement
2. Antibodies recruit neutrophils and macrophages that incite tissue damage
3. Bind to normal cellular receptors and interfere with functioning

Cy-2-toxic.
Antibody and complement lead to membrane attack complex (MAC).
Test: direct and indirect Coombs.

Type III

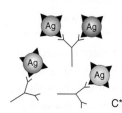

Ag   Ag

Ag

Ag

C*

Immune complex—antigen-antibody (IgG) complexes activate complement, which attracts neutrophils; neutrophils release lysosomal enzymes.

Serum sickness—an immune complex disease (type III) in which antibodies to the foreign proteins are produced (takes 5 days). Immune complexes form and are deposited in membranes, where they fix complement (leads to tissue damage). More common than Arthus reaction.

Arthus reaction—a local subacute antibody-mediated hypersensitivity (type III) reaction. Intradermal injection of antigen induces antibodies, which form antigen-antibody complexes in the skin. Characterized by edema, necrosis, and activation of complement.

Imagine an immune complex as **3** things stuck together: antigen-antibody-complement.
Most serum sickness is now caused by drugs (not serum). Fever, urticaria, arthralgias, proteinuria, lymphadenopathy 5–10 days after antigen exposure.
Antigen-antibody complexes cause the Arthus reaction.
Test: immunofluorescent staining.

Type IV

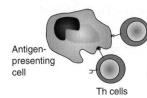

Antigen-presenting cell

Th cells

C* = complement

Delayed (T-cell-mediated) type—sensitized T lymphocytes encounter antigen and then release lymphokines (leads to macrophage activation; no antibody involved).

ACID:
Anaphylactic and Atopic (type I)
Cytotoxic (antibody mediated) (type II)
Immune complex (type III)
Delayed (cell mediated) (type IV)

4th and last—delayed. Cell mediated; therefore, it is not transferable by serum.
4 T's = T lymphocytes, Transplant rejections, TB skin tests, Touching (contact dermatitis).
Test: patch test (e.g., PPD).

Hypersensitivity disorders

Reaction	Disorder	Presentation
Type I	Anaphylaxis (e.g., bee sting, some food/drug allergies) Allergic and atopic disorders (e.g., rhinitis, hay fever, eczema, hives, asthma)	Immediate, anaphylactic, atopic
Type II	Hemolytic anemia Pernicious anemia Idiopathic thrombocytopenic purpura Erythroblastosis fetalis Acute hemolytic transfusion reactions Rheumatic fever Goodpasture's syndrome Bullous pemphigoid Pemphigus vulgaris Graves' disease Myasthenia gravis	Disease tends to be specific to tissue or site where antigen is found
Type III	SLE Rheumatoid arthritis Polyarteritis nodosum Poststreptococcal glomerulonephritis Serum sickness Arthus reaction (e.g., swelling and inflammation following tetanus vaccine) Hypersensitivity pneumonitis (e.g., farmer's lung)	Can be associated with vasculitis and systemic manifestations
Type IV	Type 1 DM Multiple sclerosis Guillain-Barré syndrome Hashimoto's thyroiditis Graft-versus-host disease PPD (test for *M. tuberculosis*) Contact dermatitis (e.g., poison ivy, nickel allergy)	Response is delayed and does **not** involve antibodies (vs. types I, II, and III)

HIGH-YIELD PRINCIPLES

IMMUNOLOGY

Autoantibodies	Autoantibody	Associated disorder
	Antinuclear antibodies (ANA)	SLE, nonspecific
	Anti-dsDNA, anti-Smith	SLE
	Antihistone	Drug-induced lupus
	Anti-IgG (rheumatoid factor)	Rheumatoid arthritis
	Anticentromere	Scleroderma (CREST)
	Anti-Scl-70 (anti-DNA topoisomerase I)	Scleroderma (diffuse)
	Antimitochondrial	1° biliary cirrhosis
	Antigliadin, antiendomysial	Celiac disease
	Anti–basement membrane	Goodpasture's syndrome
	Anti-desmoglein	Pemphigus vulgaris
	Antimicrosomal, antithyroglobulin	Hashimoto's thyroiditis
	Anti-Jo-1	Polymyositis, dermatomyositis
	Anti-SS-A (anti-Ro)	Sjögren's syndrome
	Anti-SS-B (anti-La)	Sjögren's syndrome
	Anti-U1 RNP (ribonucleoprotein)	Mixed connective tissue disease
	Anti–smooth muscle	Autoimmune hepatitis
	Anti–glutamate decarboxylase	Type 1 diabetes mellitus
	c-ANCA	Wegener's granulomatosis
	p-ANCA	Other vasculitides

Immune deficiencies

Disease	Defect	Presentation	Labs
B-cell disorders			
Bruton's agammaglobulinemia	X-linked recessive (↑ in **B**oys). Defect in *BTK*, a **tyrosine kinase** gene → blocks B-cell differentiation/ maturation.	Recurrent bacterial infections after 6 months (↓ maternal IgG) due to opsonization defect.	Normal pro-B, ↓ maturation, ↓ number of B cells, ↓ immunoglobulins of all classes.
Hyper-IgM syndrome	Defective CD40L on helper T cells = inability to class switch.	Severe pyogenic infections early in life.	↑ IgM; ↓↓ IgG, IgA, IgE.
Selective Ig deficiency	Defect in isotype switching → deficiency in specific class of immunoglobulins.	Sinus and lung infections, milk allergies and diarrhea, Anaphylaxis on exposure to blood products with Ig**A**.	IgA deficiency most common. Failure to mature into plasma cells. ↓ secretory IgA.
Common variable immunodeficiency (CVID)	Defect in B-cell maturation; many causes.	Can be acquired in 20s–30s; ↑ risk of autoimmune disease, lymphoma, sinopulmonary infections.	Normal number of B cells; ↓ plasma cells, immunoglobulin.
T-cell disorders			
Thymic aplasia (DiGeorge syndrome)	22q11 deletion; failure to develop 3rd and 4th pharyngeal pouches.	Tetany (hypocalcemia), recurrent viral/fungal infections (T-cell deficiency), congenital heart and great vessel defects.	Thymus and parathyroids fail to develop → ↓ T cells, ↓ PTH, ↓ Ca^{2+}. Absent thymic shadow on CXR.
IL-12 receptor deficiency	↓ Th$_1$ response.	Disseminated mycobacterial infections.	↓ IFN-γ.
Hyper-IgE syndrome (Job's syndrome)	Th cells fail to produce IFN-γ → inability of neutrophils to respond to chemotactic stimuli.	**FATED:** coarse **F**acies, cold (noninflamed) staphylococcal **A**bscesses, retained primary **T**eeth, ↑ Ig**E**, **D**ermatologic problems (eczema).	↑ IgE.
Chronic mucocutaneous candidiasis	T-cell dysfunction.	*Candida albicans* infections of skin and mucous membranes.	

HIGH-YIELD PRINCIPLES

IMMUNOLOGY

Immune deficiencies (continued)

Disease	Defect	Presentation	Labs
B- and T-cell disorders			
Severe combined immunodeficiency (SCID)	Several types: defective IL-2 receptor (most common, X-linked), adenosine deaminase deficiency, failure to synthesize MHC II antigens.	Recurrent viral, bacterial, fungal, and protozoal infections due to both B- and T-cell deficiency. Treatment: bone marrow transplant (no allograft rejection).	↓ IL-2R = ↓ T-cell activation. ↑ adenine = toxic to B and T cells. (↓ dNTPs, ↓ DNA synthesis.)
Ataxia-telangiectasia	Defect in DNA repair enzymes.	Triad: cerebellar defects (ataxia), spider angiomas (telangiectasia), IgA deficiency.	IgA deficiency.
Wiskott-Aldrich syndrome	X-linked recessive defect. Progressive deletion of B and T cells.	Triad (TIE): Thrombocytopenic purpura, Infections, Eczema.	↑ IgE, IgA; ↓ IgM.
Phagocyte dysfunction			
Leukocyte adhesion deficiency (type 1)	Defect in LFA-1 integrin (CD18) protein on phagocytes.	Recurrent bacterial infections, absent pus formation, delayed separation of umbilicus.	Neutrophilia.
Chédiak-Higashi syndrome	Autosomal recessive; defect in microtubular function with ↓ phagocytosis.	Recurrent pyogenic infections by staphylococci and streptococci; partial albinism, peripheral neuropathy.	
Chronic granulomatous disease	Lack of NADPH oxidase → ↓ reactive oxygen species (e.g., superoxide) and absent respiratory burst in neutrophils.	↑ susceptibility to catalase-positive organisms (e.g., S. aureus, E. coli, Aspergillus).	Negative Nitroblue tetrazolium dye reduction test.

Grafts

Autograft	From self.
Syngeneic graft	From identical twin or clone.
Allograft	From nonidentical individual of same species.
Xenograft	From different species.

Transplant rejection

Hyperacute rejection	Antibody mediated (type II) due to the presence of preformed antidonor antibodies in the transplant recipient. Occurs within minutes after transplantation. Occludes graft vessels, causing ischemia and necrosis.
Acute rejection	Cell mediated due to cytotoxic T lymphocytes reacting against foreign MHCs. Occurs weeks after transplantation. Reversible with immunosuppressants such as cyclosporine and OKT3. Vasculitis of graft vessels with dense interstitial lymphocytic infiltrate.
Chronic rejection	T-cell- and antibody-mediated vascular damage (obliterative vascular fibrosis); occurs months to years after transplantation. Irreversible. Class I-MHC$_{non-self}$ is perceived by CTLs as class I-MHC$_{self}$ presenting a non-self antigen. Fibrosis of graft tissue and blood vessels.
Graft-versus-host disease	Grafted immunocompetent T cells proliferate in the irradiated immunocompromised host and reject cells with "foreign" proteins, resulting in severe organ dysfunction. Major symptoms include a maculopapular rash, jaundice, hepatosplenomegaly, and diarrhea. Usually in bone marrow and liver transplant (organs rich in lymphocytes). Potentially beneficial in bone marrow transplant.

▶ IMMUNOLOGY—IMMUNOSUPPRESSANTS

Cyclosporine

Mechanism	Binds to cyclophilins. Complex blocks the differentiation and activation of T cells by inhibiting calcineurin, thus preventing the production of IL-2 and its receptor.
Clinical use	Suppresses organ rejection after transplantation; selected autoimmune disorders.
Toxicity	Predisposes patients to viral infections and lymphoma; nephrotoxic (preventable with mannitol diuresis).

Tacrolimus (FK506)

Mechanism	Similar to cyclosporine; binds to FK-binding protein, inhibiting secretion of IL-2 and other cytokines.
Clinical use	Potent immunosuppressive used in organ transplant recipients.
Toxicity	Significant—nephrotoxicity, peripheral neuropathy, hypertension, pleural effusion, hyperglycemia.

HIGH-YIELD PRINCIPLES

IMMUNOLOGY

Sirolimus (rapamycin)

Mechanism	Binds to mTOR. Inhibits T-cell proliferation in response to IL-2.
Clinical use	Immunosuppression after kidney transplantation in combination with cyclosporine and corticosteroids.
Toxicity	Hyperlipidemia, thrombocytopenia, leukopenia.

Daclizumab

Mechanism	Monoclonal antibody with high affinity for the IL-2 receptor on activated T cells.

Azathioprine

Mechanism	Antimetabolite precursor of 6-mercaptopurine that interferes with the metabolism and synthesis of nucleic acids. Toxic to proliferating lymphocytes.
Clinical use	Kidney transplantation, autoimmune disorders (including glomerulonephritis and hemolytic anemia).
Toxicity	Bone marrow suppression. Active metabolite mercaptopurine is metabolized by xanthine oxidase; thus, toxic effects may be ↑ by allopurinol.

Muromonab-CD3 (OKT3)

Mechanism	Monoclonal antibody that binds to CD3 (epsilon chain) on the surface of T cells. Blocks cellular interaction with CD3 protein responsible for T-cell signal transduction.
Clinical use	Immunosuppression after kidney transplantation.
Toxicity	Cytokine release syndrome, hypersensitivity reaction.

Recombinant cytokines and clinical uses

Agent	Clinical uses
Aldesleukin (interleukin-2)	Renal cell carcinoma, metastatic melanoma
Erythropoietin (epoetin)	Anemias (especially in renal failure)
Filgrastim (granulocyte colony-stimulating factor)	Recovery of bone marrow
Sargramostim (granulocyte-macrophage colony-stimulating factor)	Recovery of bone marrow
α-interferon	Hepatitis B and C, Kaposi's sarcoma, leukemias, malignant melanoma
β-interferon	Multiple sclerosis
γ-interferon	Chronic granulomatous disease
Oprelvekin (interleukin-11)	Thrombocytopenia
Thrombopoietin	Thrombocytopenia

Therapeutic antibodies

Agent	Target	Clinical use
Muromonab-CD3 (OKT3)	CD3	Prevent acute transplant rejection
Daclizumab	IL-2 receptor	Prevent acute rejection of renal transplant
Digoxin Immune Fab	Digoxin	Antidote for digoxin intoxication
Infliximab	TNF-α	Crohn's disease, rheumatoid arthritis, psoriatic arthritis, ankylosing spondylitis
Adalimumab	TNF-α	Crohn's disease, rheumatoid arthritis, psoriatic arthritis
Abciximab	Glycoprotein IIb/IIIa	Prevent cardiac ischemia in unstable angina and in patients treated with percutaneous coronary intervention
Trastuzumab (Herceptin)	*erb*-B2	HER-2–overexpressing breast cancer
Rituximab	CD20	B-cell non-Hodgkin's lymphoma

Pathology

"Digressions, objections, delight in mockery, carefree mistrust are signs of health; everything unconditional belongs in pathology."

—Friedrich Nietzsche

▶ Inflammation

▶ Neoplasia

The fundamental principles of pathology are key to understanding diseases in all organ systems. Major topics such as inflammation and neoplasia appear frequently in questions aimed at many different organ systems, and such topics are definitely high yield. For example, the concepts of cell injury and inflammation are key to understanding the inflammatory response that follows myocardial infarction, a very common subject of boards questions. Similarly, a familiarity with the early cellular changes that culminate in the development of neoplasias—for example, esophageal or colon cancer—is critical. Finally, make sure you recognize the major tumor-associated genes and are comfortable with key cancer concepts such as tumor staging and metastasis.

Apoptosis	Programmed cell death; ATP required. Intrinsic or extrinsic pathway.
	Intrinsic pathway—occurs during embryogenesis, hormone induction (e.g., menstruation), and atrophy (e.g., endometrial lining during menopause) and as a result of injurious stimuli (e.g., radiation, toxins, hypoxia). Changes in the levels of anti- and pro-apoptotic factors lead to ↑ mitochondrial permeability and release of cytochrome c.
	Extrinsic pathway—occurs with ligand-receptor interactions (e.g., Fas ligand binding to Fas [CD95]) or immune cell (T_{killer}) release of perforin and granzyme B.
	Both pathways lead to activation of cytosolic caspases that mediate cellular breakdown.
	Characterized by cell shrinkage, nuclear shrinkage and basophilia (pyknosis), membrane blebbing, pyknotic nuclear fragmentation (karyorrhexis), nuclear fading (karyolysis), and formation of apoptotic bodies, which are then phagocytosed. No significant inflammation.

Necrosis	Enzymatic degradation and protein denaturation of a cell resulting from exogenous injury. Intracellular components extravasate. Inflammatory process (unlike apoptosis).
	Types of necrosis
	1. Coagulative—heart, liver, kidney
	2. Liquefactive—brain, bacterial abscess, pleural effusion
	3. Caseous—TB, systemic fungi
	4. Fatty—pancreas (saponification)
	5. Fibroid—blood vessels
	6. Gangrenous—dry (ischemic coagulative) OR wet (with bacteria); common in limbs and in GI tract

Apoptosis vs. necrosis

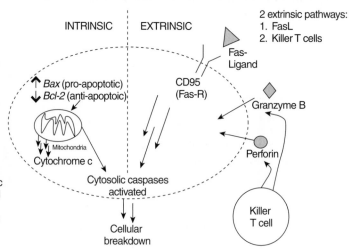

The intrinsic pathway occurs during embryogenesis, hormone induction (e.g., menstruation), and atrophy (e.g., endometrial lining during menstruation) and as a result of injurious stimuli (e.g, radiation, toxins, hypoxia).

Changes in proportions of anti- and pro-apoptotic factors lead to increased mitochondria permeability and cytochrome c release.

Cell injury	**Reversible with O₂**	**Irreversible**

Cell injury

Reversible with O_2
↓ ATP synthesis
Cellular swelling (no ATP →
 impaired Na⁺/K⁺ pump)
Nuclear chromatin clumping
↓ glycogen
Fatty change
Ribosomal detachment
 (↓ protein synthesis)

Irreversible
Nuclear pyknosis, karyolysis,
 karyorrhexis
Ca^{2+} influx → caspase activation
Plasma membrane damage
Lysosomal rupture
Mitochondrial permeability

Infarcts: red vs. pale

Red (hemorrhagic) infarcts occur in loose tissues
 with collaterals, such as liver, lungs, or intestine,
 or following reperfusion.
Pale infarcts occur in solid tissues with single blood
 supply, such as heart, kidney, and spleen.

REd = **RE**perfusion.
Reperfusion injury is due to
 damage by free radicals.

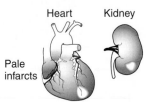

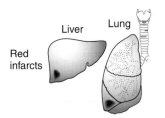

Atrophy

Reduction in the size or number of cells. Causes include:
1. ↓ hormones (uterus/vagina)
2. ↓ innervation (motor neuron damage)
3. ↓ blood flow
4. ↓ nutrients
5. ↑ pressure (nephrolithiasis)
6. Occlusion of secretory ducts (cystic fibrosis)

Inflammation

Characterized by *rubor* (redness), *dolor* (pain), *calor* (heat), *tumor* (swelling), and
 functio laesa (loss of function).

Fluid exudation

↑ vascular permeability,
 vasodilation, endothelial injury.

Fibrosis

Fibroblast emigration and proliferation;
 deposition of extracellular matrix.

Resolution

Restoration of normal structure.
Granulation tissue—highly vascularized, fibrotic.
Abscess—fibrosis surrounding pus.
Fistula—abnormal communication.
Scarring—collagen deposition resulting in altered
 structure and function.

Acute—Neutrophil, eosinophil, and antibody mediated. Acute inflammation is rapid onset (seconds to minutes),
 lasts minutes to days.
Chronic—Mononuclear cell mediated: Characterized by persistent destruction and repair. Associated with
 blood vessel proliferation, fibrosis. Granuloma: nodular collections of epithelioid macrophages and giant
 cells.

Leukocyte extravasation

Neutrophils exit from blood vessels at sites of tissue injury and inflammation in 4 steps:

Step	Vasculature/Stroma	Leukocyte
1. Rolling	E-selectin P-selectin	Sialyl Lewis^X
2. Tight binding	ICAM-1	LFA-1 ("integrin")
3. Diapedesis—leukocyte travels between endothelial cells and exits blood vessel	PECAM-1	PECAM-1

4. Migration—leukocyte travels through interstitium to site of injury or infection guided by chemotactic signals	Bacterial products
	CILK:
	  C5a
	  IL-8
	  LTB4
	  Kallikrein
		Various

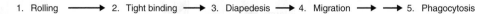

1. Rolling ⟶ 2. Tight binding ⟶ 3. Diapedesis ⟶ 4. Migration ⟶ ⟶ 5. Phagocytosis

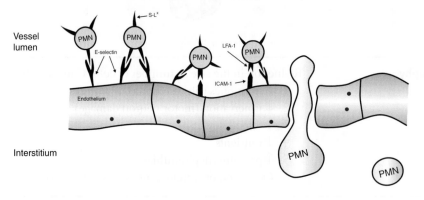

Free radical injury

Free radicals damage cells via membrane lipid peroxidation, protein modification, and DNA breakage.

Initiated via radiation exposure, metabolism of drugs (phase I), redox reaction, nitric oxide, transition metals, leukocyte oxidative burst.

Free radicals can be eliminated by enzymes (catalase, superoxide dismutase, glutathione peroxidase), spontaneous decay, antioxidants (vitamins A, C, E).

Pathologies include:
1. Retinopathy of prematurity
2. Bronchopulmonary dysplasia
3. CCi$_4$ leading to liver necrosis (fatty change)
4. Acetaminophen
5. Iron overload
6. Reperfusion after anoxia, (e.g., superoxide) especially after thrombolytic therapy

Granulomatous diseases	1. Tuberculosis 2. Fungal infections (e.g., histoplasmosis) 3. Syphilis 4. Leprosy 5. Cat scratch fever 6. Sarcoidosis 7. Crohn's disease 8. Berylliosis	Th_1 cells secrete γ-interferon, activating macrophages. TNF-α from macrophages induce and maintain granuloma formation. Anti-TNF drugs can break down granulomas, leading to disseminated disease. T cells secrete IFN-γ, macrophages secrete TNF-α, contributing to granuloma formation.

Transudate vs. exudate	**Transudate**
	 Hypocellular
	 Protein poor
	 Specific gravity < 1.012
	 Due to:
	   $\uparrow$ hydrostatic pressure
	   $\downarrow$ oncotic pressure
	   Na^+ retention
		Exudate
		 Cellular
		 Protein rich
		 Specific gravity > 1.020
		 Due to:
		   Lymphatic obstruction
		   Inflammation

Erythrocyte sedimentation rate (ESR)

Products of inflammation (e.g., fibrinogen) coat RBCs and cause aggregation. When aggregated, RBCs fall at a faster rate within the test tube.

$\uparrow$ **ESR**	$\downarrow$ **ESR**
Infections Inflammation (e.g., temporal arteritis) Cancer Pregnancy SLE	Sickle cell (altered shape) Polycythemia (too many) CHF (unknown)

Iron poisoning   One of the leading causes of fatality from toxicologic agents in children.
  Mechanism   Cell death due to peroxidation of membrane lipids.
  Symptoms   Acute—gastric bleeding.
    Chronic—metabolic acidosis, scarring leading to GI obstruction.

Amyloidosis   β-pleated sheet demonstrable by apple-green birefringence of Congo red stain under polarized light; affected tissue has waxy appearance.

Types	Protein	Derived from	
Primary	AL	Ig light chains (multiple myeloma)	**AL** = **L**ight chain.
Secondary	AA	Serum amyloid-associated (SAA) protein (chronic inflammatory disease)	**AA** = **A**cute-phase reactant.
Senile cardiac	Transthyretin	AF	**AF** = old **F**ogies.
Diabetes mellitus type 2	Amylin	AE	**AE** = **E**ndocrine.
Medullary carcinoma of the thyroid	A-CAL	Calcitonin	**A-CAL** = **CAL**citonin.
Alzheimer's disease	β-amyloid	Amyloid precursor protein (APP)	
Dialysis-associated	β₂-microglobulin	MHC class I proteins	

Shock

Hypovolemic/cardiogenic	Septic
Low-output failure	**High**-output failure
↑ TPR	↓ TPR
Low cardiac output	Dilated arterioles, high venous return
Cold, clammy patient	Hot patient

Neoplastic progression Hallmarks of cancer—evading apoptosis, self-sufficiency in growth signals, insensitivity to anti-growth signals, sustained angiogenesis, limitless replicative potential, tissue invasion, and metastasis.

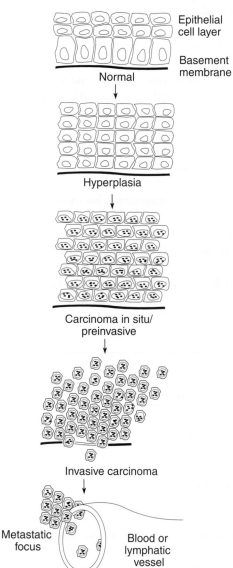

Normal
Epithelial cell layer
Basement membrane

- Normal cells with basal → apical differentiation

Hyperplasia

- Cells have increased in number—**hyperplasia**
- Abnormal proliferation of cells with loss of size, shape, and orientation—**dysplasia**

Carcinoma in situ/preinvasive

- **In situ carcinoma**
- Neoplastic cells have not invaded basement membrane
- High nuclear/cytoplasmic ratio and clumped chromatin
- Neoplastic cells encompass entire thickness
- Tumor cells are monoclonal

Invasive carcinoma

- Cells have invaded basement membrane using **collagenases** and **hydrolases**
- Can metastasize if they reach a blood or lymphatic vessel

Metastatic focus
Blood or lymphatic vessel

Metastasis—spread to distant organ
- Must survive immune attack
- "Seed and soil" theory of metastasis
  - Seed = tumor embolus
  - Soil = target organ—liver, lungs, bone, brain, etc.
  - Angiogenesis allows for tumor survival
  - ↓ cadherin, ↑ laminin, integrin receptors

(Adapted, with permission, from McPhee SJ et al. *Pathophysiology of Disease: An Introduction to Clinical Medicine,* 3rd ed. New York: McGraw-Hill, 2000: 84.)

-plasia definitions

Reversible	**Hyperplasia**— ↑ in number of cells.
	Metaplasia—one adult cell type is replaced by another. Often 2° to irritation and/or environmental exposure (e.g., squamous metaplasia in trachea and bronchi of smokers).
	Dysplasia—abnormal growth with loss of cellular orientation, shape, and size in comparison to normal tissue maturation; commonly preneoplastic.
Irreversible	**Anaplasia**—abnormal cells lacking differentiation; like primitive cells of same tissue, often equated with undifferentiated malignant neoplasms. Little or no resemblance to tissue of origin.
	Neoplasia—a clonal proliferation of cells that is uncontrolled and excessive.
	Desmoplasia—fibrous tissue formation in response to neoplasm.

Tumor grade vs. stage

Grade	Degree of cellular differentiation based on histologic appearance of tumor. Usually graded I–IV based on degree of differentiation and number of mitoses per high-power field; character of tumor itself.	Stage usually has more prognostic value than grade. Stage = Spread. TNM staging system: **T** = size of **T**umor
Stage	Degree of localization/spread based on site and size of 1° lesion, spread to regional lymph nodes, presence of metastases; spread of tumor in a specific patient.	**N** = **N**ode involvement **M** = **M**etastases

Tumor nomenclature

Cell type	Benign	Malignant[a]
Epithelium	Adenoma, papilloma	Adenocarcinoma, papillary carcinoma
Mesenchyme		
Blood cells		Leukemia, lymphoma
Blood vessels	Hemangioma	Angiosarcoma
Smooth muscle	Leiomyoma	Leiomyosarcoma
Skeletal muscle	Rhabdomyoma	Rhabdomyosarcoma
Bone	Osteoma	Osteosarcoma
Fat	Lipoma	Liposarcoma
> 1 cell type	Mature teratoma (women)	Immature teratoma and mature teratoma (men)

[a]The term **carcinoma** implies epithelial origin, whereas **sarcoma** denotes mesenchymal origin. Both terms imply malignancy.

Tumor differences

Benign	Usually well differentiated, slow growing, well demarcated, no metastasis.
Malignant	May be poorly differentiated, erratic growth, locally invasive/diffuse, may metastasize.

Disease conditions associated with neoplasms	Condition	Neoplasm
	1. **Down** syndrome	1. **ALL** (we **ALL** fall **Down**), AML
	2. Xeroderma pigmentosum, albinism	2. Melanoma, basal cell carcinoma, and especially squamous cell carcinomas of skin
	3. Chronic atrophic gastritis, pernicious anemia, postsurgical gastric remnants	3. Gastric adenocarcinoma
	4. Tuberous sclerosis (facial angiofibroma, seizures, mental retardation)	4. Astrocytoma, angiomyolipoma, and cardiac rhabdomyoma
	5. Actinic keratosis	5. Squamous cell carcinoma of skin
	6. Barrett's esophagus (chronic GI reflux)	6. Esophageal adenocarcinoma
	7. Plummer-Vinson syndrome (atrophic glossitis, esophageal webs, anemia; all due to iron deficiency)	7. Squamous cell carcinoma of esophagus
	8. Cirrhosis (alcoholic, hepatitis B or C)	8. Hepatocellular carcinoma
	9. Ulcerative colitis	9. Colonic adenocarcinoma
	10. Paget's disease of bone	10. 2° osteosarcoma and fibrosarcoma
	11. Immunodeficiency states	11. Malignant lymphomas
	12. AIDS	12. Aggressive malignant lymphomas (non-Hodgkin's) and Kaposi's sarcoma
	13. Autoimmune diseases (e.g., Hashimoto's thyroiditis, myasthenia gravis)	13. Lymphoma
	14. Acanthosis nigricans (hyperpigmentation and epidermal thickening)	14. Visceral malignancy (stomach, lung, breast, uterus)
	15. Dysplastic nevus	15. Malignant melanoma
	16. Radiation exposure	16. Sarcoma, papillary thyroid cancer

Oncogenes	Gain of function → cancer. Need damage to only 1 allele.	
Gene	**Associated tumor**	**Gene product**
abl	CML	Tyrosine kinase
c-*myc*	Burkitt's lymphoma	Transcription factor
bcl-2	Follicular and undifferentiated lymphomas (inhibits apoptosis)	Anti-apoptotic molecule
erb-B2	Breast, ovarian, and gastric carcinomas	Tyrosine kinase
ras	Colon carcinoma	GTPase
L-*myc*	Lung tumor	Transcription factor
N-*myc*	Neuroblastoma	Transcription factor
ret	Multiple endocrine neoplasia (MEN) types II and III	Tyrosine kinase
c-*kit*	Gastrointestinal stromal tumor (GIST)	Cytokine receptor

HIGH-YIELD PRINCIPLES

PATHOLOGY

Tumor suppressor genes

Loss of function → cancer; both alleles must be lost for expression of disease.

Gene	Associated tumor	Gene products
Rb (13q)	Retinoblastoma, osteosarcoma	*Rb* gene product blocks G1 → S phase of the cell cycle
p53 (17p)	Most human cancers, Li-Fraumeni syndrome	p53 gene product blocks G1 → S phase of the cell cycle
BRCA1 (17q)	Breast and ovarian cancer	DNA repair protein
BRCA2 (13q)	Breast cancer	DNA repair protein
p16 (9p)	Melanoma	
APC (5q)	Colorectal cancer (associated with FAP)	
WT1 (11p)	Wilms' tumor	
NF1 (17q)	Neurofibromatosis type 1	
NF2 (22q)	Neurofibromatosis type 2	Type 2 = 22.
DPC (18q)	Pancreatic cancer	**DPC**—**D**eleted in **P**ancreatic **C**ancer.
DCC (18q)	Colon cancer	**DCC**—**D**eleted in **C**olon **C**ancer.

Tumor markers

PSA	Prostate-specific antigen. Used to screen for prostate carcinoma. Can also be elevated in BPH and prostatitis.	Tumor markers should not be used as the 1° tool for cancer diagnosis. They may be used to confirm diagnosis, to monitor for tumor recurrence, and to monitor response to therapy.
Prostatic acid phosphatase	Prostate carcinoma.	
CEA	Carcinoembryonic antigen. Very nonspecific but produced by ∼ 70% of colorectal and pancreatic cancers; also produced by gastric, breast, and thyroid medullary carcinomas.	
α-fetoprotein	Normally made by fetus. Hepatocellular carcinomas. Nonseminomatous germ cell tumors of the testis (e.g., yolk sac tumor).	
β-hCG	Hydatidiform moles, Choriocarcinomas, and Gestational trophoblastic tumors.	
CA-125	Ovarian, malignant epithelial tumors.	
S-100	Melanoma, neural tumors, astrocytomas.	
Alkaline phosphatase	Metastases to bone, obstructive biliary disease, Paget's disease of bone.	
Bombesin	Neuroblastoma, lung and gastric cancer.	
TRAP	Tartrate-resistant acid phosphatase. **Hairy** cell leukemia—a B-cell neoplasm.	**TRAP** the **hairy** animal.
CA-19-9	Pancreatic adenocarcinoma.	
Calcitonin	Thyroid medullary carcinoma.	

Oncogenic microbes	Virus	Associated cancer
	HTLV-1	Adult T-cell leukemia/lymphoma
	HBV, HCV	Hepatocellular carcinoma
	EBV	Burkitt's lymphoma, nasopharyngeal carcinoma
	HPV	Cervical carcinoma (16, 18), penile/anal carcinoma
	HHV-8 (Kaposi's sarcoma–associated herpesvirus)	Kaposi's sarcoma, body cavity fluid B-cell lymphoma
	HIV	Primary CNS lymphoma
	H. pylori	Gastric adenocarcinoma and lymphoma
	Schistosoma	Squamous cell carcinoma of transitional epithelium, e.g., bladder

Chemical carcinogens	Toxin	Affected organ
	Aflatoxins (produced by *Aspergillus*)	Liver (hepatocellular carcinoma)
	Vinyl chloride	Liver (angiosarcoma)
	CCl_4	Liver (centrilobular necrosis, fatty change)
	Nitrosamines (e.g., in smoked foods)	Esophagus, stomach
	Cigarette smoke	Larynx (squamous cell carcinoma), lung (squamous cell and small cell carcinomas), kidney (renal cell carcinoma), bladder (transitional cell carcinoma)
	Asbestos	Lung (mesothelioma and bronchogenic carcinoma)
	Arsenic	Skin (squamous cell carcinoma), liver (angiosarcoma)
	Naphthalene (aniline) dyes	Bladder (transitional cell carcinoma)
	Alkylating agents	Blood (leukemia)

Paraneoplastic effects of tumors

Neoplasm	Causes	Effect
Small cell lung carcinoma	ACTH or ACTH-like peptide	Cushing's syndrome
Small cell lung carcinoma and intracranial neoplasms	ADH	SIADH
Squamous cell lung carcinoma, renal cell carcinoma, and breast carcinoma	PTH-related peptide, TGF-β, TNF, IL-1	Hypercalcemia
Renal cell carcinoma, hemangioblastoma	Erythropoietin	Polycythemia
Thymoma, small cell lung carcinoma	Antibodies against presynaptic Ca^{2+} channels at neuromuscular junction	Lambert-Eaton syndrome (muscle weakness)
Leukemias and lymphomas	Hyperuricemia due to excess nucleic acid turnover (i.e., cytotoxic therapy)	Gout, urate nephropathy

Psammoma bodies	Laminated, concentric, calcific spherules seen in:
	  1. Papillary adenocarcinoma of thyroid
	  2. Serous papillary cystadenocarcinoma of ovary
	  3. Meningioma
	  4. Malignant mesothelioma
			PSaMMoma:
			  Papillary (thyroid)
			  Serous (ovary)
			  Meningioma
			  Mesothelioma

Cancer epidemiology

	Male	Female	
Incidence	Prostate (32%) Lung (16%) Colon and rectum (12%)	Breast (32%) Lung (13%) Colon and rectum (13%)	Deaths from lung cancer have plateaued in males but continue to ↑ in females.
Mortality	Lung (33%) Prostate (13%)	Lung (23%) Breast (18%)	Cancer is the 2nd leading cause of death in the United States (heart disease is 1st).

Metastasis to brain	1° tumors that metastasize to brain—Lung, Breast, Skin (melanoma), Kidney (renal cell carcinoma), GI. Overall, approximately 50% of brain tumors are from metastases.	Lots of Bad Stuff Kills Glia. Typically multiple well-circumscribed tumors at gray/white matter junction.
Metastasis to liver	The liver and lung are the most common sites of metastasis after the regional lymph nodes. 1° tumors that metastasize to the liver—Colon > Stomach > Pancreas > Breast > Lung.	Metastases >> 1° liver tumors. Cancer Sometimes Penetrates Benign Liver.
Metastasis to bone	These 1° tumors metastasize to bone—Prostate, Thyroid, Testes, Breast, Lung, Kidney. Metastases from breast and prostate are most common. Metastatic bone tumors are far more common than 1° bone tumors.	P. T. Barnum Loves Kids. Lung = Lytic. Prostate = blastic. Breast = Both lytic and blastic.

Pharmacology

"Take me, I am the drug; take me, I am hallucinogenic."

—Salvador Dali

"I was under medication when I made the decision not to burn the tapes."
—Richard Nixon

"I wondher why ye can always read a doctor's bill an' ye niver can read his purscription."

—Finley Peter Dunne

"Once you get locked into a serious drug collection, the tendency is to push it as far as you can."

—Hunter S. Thompson

▶ **Pharmacodynamics**

▶ **Autonomic Drugs**

▶ **Toxicities and Side Effects**

▶ **Miscellaneous**

Preparation for questions on pharmacology is straightforward. Memorizing all the key drugs and their characteristics (e.g., mechanisms, clinical use, and important side effects) is high yield. Focus on understanding the prototype drugs in each class. Avoid memorizing obscure derivatives. Learn the "classic" and distinguishing toxicities of the major drugs. Do not bother with drug dosages or trade names. Reviewing associated biochemistry, physiology, and microbiology can be useful while studying pharmacology. There is a strong emphasis on ANS, CNS, antimicrobial, and cardiovascular agents as well as on NSAIDs. Much of the material is clinically relevant. Newer drugs on the market are also fair game.

Enzyme kinetics

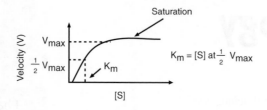

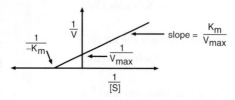

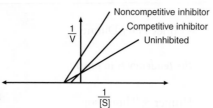

K_m reflects the affinity of the enzyme for its substrate.

V_{max} is directly proportional to the enzyme concentration.

$\downarrow K_m$, $\uparrow$ affinity.

$\uparrow$ y-intercept, $\downarrow V_{max}$. The further to the right the x-intercept, the greater the K_m.

HINT: Competitive inhibitors cross each other competitively, while noncompetitive inhibitors do not.

	Competitive inhibitors	Noncompetitive inhibitors
Resemble substrate	Yes	No
Overcome by $\uparrow$ [S]	Yes	No
Bind active site	Yes	No
Effect on V_{max}	Unchanged	$\downarrow$
Effect on K_m	$\uparrow$	Unchanged
Pharmacodynamics	$\downarrow$ potency	$\downarrow$ efficacy

Pharmacokinetics

Volume of distribution (V_d)	Relates the amount of drug in the body to the plasma concentration. V_d of plasma protein–bound drugs can be altered by liver and kidney disease.

$$V_d = \frac{\text{amount of drug in the body}}{\text{plasma drug concentration}}$$

Drugs with:

Low V_d (4–8 L) distribute in blood.

Medium V_d distribute in extracellular space or body water.

High V_d (> body weight) distribute into all tissues.

Clearance (CL)	Relates the rate of elimination to the plasma concentration.

$$CL = \frac{\text{rate of elimination of drug}}{\text{plasma drug concentration}} = V_d \times K_e \text{ (elimination constant)}$$

Half-life ($t_{1/2}$)	The time required to change the amount of drug in the body by ½ during elimination (or constant infusion). Property of first-order elimination. A drug infused at a constant rate takes 4–5 half-lives to reach steady state.

$$t_{1/2} = \frac{0.7 \times V_d}{CL}$$

# of half-lives	1	2	3	4
Concentration	50%	75%	87.5%	93.75%

| **Dosage calculations** | Loading dose = $C_p \times V_d/F$.
Maintenance dose = $C_p \times CL/F$.
C_p = target plasma concentration and
F = bioavailability = 1 when drug is given IV. | In renal or liver disease, maintenance dose ↓ and loading dose is unchanged. |

Elimination of drugs

| Zero-order elimination | Rate of elimination is constant regardless of C_p (i.e., constant **amount** of drug eliminated per unit time).
C_p ↓ linearly with time. Examples of drugs—**P**henytoin, **E**thanol, and **A**spirin (at high or toxic concentrations). | **PEA.** (A pea is round, shaped like the "0" in "zero-order.") |
| First-order elimination | Rate of elimination is proportional to the drug concentration (i.e., constant **fraction** of drug eliminated per unit time).
C_p ↓ exponentially with time. | |

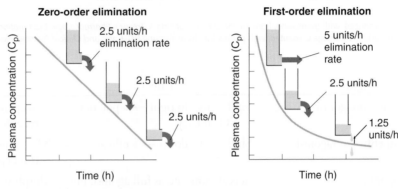

(Adapted, with permission, from Katzung BG, Trevor AJ. *Pharmacology: Examination & Board Review,* 5th ed. Stamford, CT: Appleton & Lange, 1998: 5.)

Urine pH and drug elimination	Ionized species are trapped in urine and cleared quickly. Neutral forms can be reabsorbed.
Weak acids	Examples: phenobarbital, methotrexate, aspirin. Trapped in basic environments. Treat overdose with bicarbonate. $$RCOOH \rightleftharpoons RCOO^- + H^+$$ (lipid soluble) (trapped)
Weak bases	Example: amphetamines. Trapped in acidic environments. Treat overdose with ammonium chloride. $$RNH_3^+ \rightleftharpoons RNH_2 + H^+$$ (trapped) (lipid soluble)

| **Phase I vs. phase II metabolism** | Phase I (reduction, oxidation, hydrolysis) usually yields slightly polar, water-soluble metabolites (often still active).
Phase II (acetylation, glucuronidation, sulfation) usually yields very polar, inactive metabolites (renally excreted). | Phase I—cytochrome P-450.
Phase II—conjugation.
Geriatric patients lose phase I first. |

| **Efficacy vs. potency** | Efficacy—maximal effect a drug can produce.
Potency—amount of drug needed for a given effect. |

Pharmacodynamics

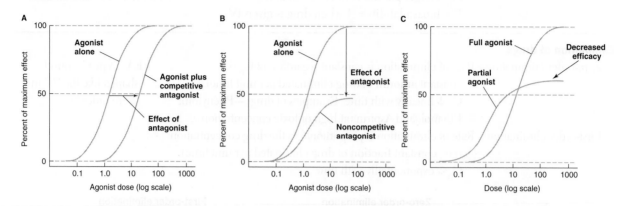

(Image A and B reproduced, with permission, from Trevor AJ et al. *Katzung & Trevor's Pharmacology: Examination & Board Review,* 8th ed. New York: McGraw-Hill, 2008: 14. Image C adapted, with permission, from Katzung BG. *Basic and Clinical Pharmacology,* 7th ed. Stamford, CT: Appleton & Lange, 1997: 13.)

Figure	Effect	Example
A. Competitive antagonist	Shifts curve to right → ↓ potency, NC efficacy.	Diazepam + flumazenil on GABA receptor.
B. Noncompetitive antagonist	Shifts curve down → ↓ efficacy.	NE + phenoxybenzamine on α-receptors.
C. Partial agonist	Acts at same site as full agonist, but with reduced maximal effect → ↓ efficacy. Potency is a different variable and can be ↑ or ↓.	Morphine + buprenorphine at opioid μ-receptor.

Physiologic antagonism	Substance that produces the opposite physiologic effect of an agonist but does not act at the same receptor.	Example: In a patient with asthma due to muscarinic overactivity, epinephrine can act as a bronchodilator by stimulating β_2 receptors.

Therapeutic index	Measurement of drug safety. $$\frac{LD_{50}}{ED_{50}} = \frac{\text{median lethal dose}}{\text{median effective dose}}$$	TILE: $TI = LD_{50} / ED_{50}$. Safer drugs have higher TI values.

Central and peripheral nervous system

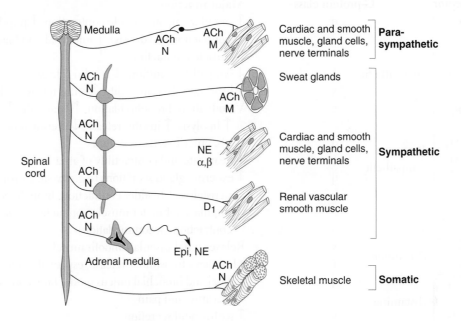

(Adapted, with permission, from Katzung BG. *Basic and Clinical Pharmacology,* 7th ed. Stamford, CT: Appleton & Lange, 1997: 74.)

Note that the adrenal medulla and sweat glands are part of the sympathetic NS but are innervated by cholinergic fibers. Botulinum toxin prevents release of neurotransmitter at all cholinergic terminals.

ACh receptors	Nicotinic ACh receptors are ligand-gated Na^+/K^+ channels; N_N (found in autonomic ganglia) and N_M (found in neuromuscular junction) subtypes.
	Muscarinic ACh receptors are G-protein-coupled receptors that act through 2nd messengers; 5 subtypes: M_1, M_2, M_3, M_4, and M_5.

G-protein–linked 2nd messengers

Receptor	G-protein class	Major functions
α_1	q	↑ vascular smooth muscle contraction, ↑ pupillary dilator muscle contraction (mydriasis), ↑ intestinal and bladder sphincter muscle contraction
α_2 Sympathetic	i	↓ sympathetic outflow, ↓ insulin release
β_1	s	↑ heart rate, ↑ contractility, ↑ renin release, ↑ lipolysis
β_2	s	Vasodilation, bronchodilation, ↑ heart rate, ↑ contractility, ↑ lipolysis, ↑ insulin release, ↓ uterine tone
M_1 Para-	q	CNS, enteric nervous system
M_2 sympathetic	i	↓ heart rate and contractility of atria
M_3	q	↑ exocrine gland secretions (e.g., sweat, gastric acid), ↑ gut peristalsis, ↑ bladder contraction, bronchoconstriction, ↑ pupillary sphincter muscle contraction (miosis), ciliary muscle contraction (accommodation)
D_1 Dopamine	s	Relaxes renal vascular smooth muscle
D_2	i	Modulates transmitter release, especially in brain
H_1 Histamine	q	↑ nasal and bronchial mucus production, contraction of bronchioles, pruritus, and pain
H_2	s	↑ gastric acid secretion
V_1 Vasopressin	q	↑ vascular smooth muscle contraction
V_2	s	↑ H_2O permeability and reabsorption in the collecting tubules of the kidney (V2 is found in the 2 kidneys)

"**Q**iss (kiss) and **qiq** (kick) till you're **siq** (sick) of **sqs** (sex)."

H₁, α₁, V₁,
M₁, M₃ Receptor $\xrightarrow{G_q}$ Phospholipase **C** ⟶

Lipids
↓
PIP_2 ⟶ IP_3 ⟶ ↑ $[Ca^{2+}]_{in}$
⟶ DAG ⟶ Protein kinase **C**

HAVe 1 M&M.

β₁, β₂, D₁,
H₂, V₂ Receptor $\xrightarrow{G_s}$ **A**denylyl cyclase ⟶

ATP
↓
cAMP ⟶ Protein kinase **A**

M₂, α₂, D₂ Receptor $\xrightarrow{G_i}$ **A**denylyl cyclase ⟶ cAMP ↓ ⟶ Protein kinase **A** ↓

MAD 2's.

Autonomic drugs

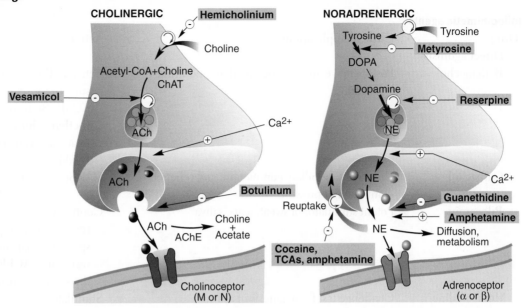

(Adapted, with permission, from Katzung BG, Trevor AJ. *Pharmacology: Examination & Board Review,* 5th ed. Stamford, CT: Appleton & Lange, 1998: 42.)

Circles with rotating arrows represent transporters; ChAT, choline acetyltransferase; ACh, acetylcholine; AChE, acetylcholinesterase; NE, norepinephrine.

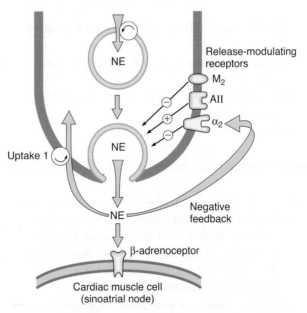

(Adapted, with permission, from Katzung BG, Trevor AJ. *Pharmacology: Examination & Board Review,* 5th ed. Stamford, CT: Appleton & Lange, 1998: 42.)

Release of NE from a sympathetic nerve ending is modulated by NE itself, acting on presynaptic α_2 autoreceptors, and by ACh, angiotensin II, and other substances.

Cholinomimetic agents

Drug	Clinical applications	Action
1. Direct agonists		
Bethanechol	Postoperative and neurogenic ileus and urinary retention	Activates **B**owel and **B**ladder smooth muscle; resistant to AChE. **Beth Anne, call (bethanechol)** me if you want to activate your **B**owels and **B**ladder.
Carbachol	Glaucoma, pupillary contraction, and relief of intraocular pressure	**CARB**on copy of acetylcholine.
Pilocarpine	Potent stimulator of sweat, tears, saliva	Contracts ciliary muscle of eye (open angle), pupillary sphincter (narrow angle); resistant to AChE. **PILE** on the sweat and tears.
Methacholine	Challenge test for diagnosis of asthma	Stimulates muscarinic receptors in airway when inhaled.
2. Indirect agonists (anticholinesterases)		
Neostigmine	Postoperative and neurogenic ileus and urinary retention, myasthenia gravis, reversal of neuromuscular junction blockade (postoperative)	↑ endogenous ACh; no CNS penetration. **NEO** CNS = **NO** CNS penetration.
Pyridostigmine	Myasthenia gravis (long acting); does not penetrate CNS	↑ endogenous ACh; ↑ strength.
Edrophonium	Diagnosis of myasthenia gravis (extremely short acting)	↑ endogenous ACh.
Physostigmine	Glaucoma (crosses blood-brain barrier → CNS) and atropine overdose	↑ endogenous ACh. **PHYS** is for **EYES**.
Echothiophate	Glaucoma	↑ endogenous ACh.

Note: With all cholinomimetic agents, watch for exacerbation of COPD, asthma, and peptic ulcers when giving to susceptible patients.

Cholinesterase inhibitor poisoning	Often due to organophosphates, such as parathion, that irreversibly inhibit AchE. Causes **D**iarrhea, **U**rination, **M**iosis, **B**ronchospasm, **B**radycardia, **E**xcitation of skeletal muscle and CNS, **L**acrimation, **S**weating, and **S**alivation. Antidote—atropine + pralidoxime (regenerates active AchE).	**DUMBBELSS.** Organophosphates are components of insecticides; poisoning usually seen in farmers.

Muscarinic antagonists

Drug	Organ system	Application
Atropine, homatropine, tropicamide	Eye	Produce mydriasis and cycloplegia
Benztropine	CNS	**PARK**inson's disease—**PARK** my **BENZ**
Scopolamine	CNS	Motion sickness
Ipratropium	Respiratory	Asthma, COPD (**I pray** I can breathe soon!)
Oxybutynin, glycopyrrolate	Genitourinary	Reduce urgency in mild cystitis and reduce bladder spasms
Methscopolamine, pirenzepine, propantheline	Gastrointestinal	Peptic ulcer treatment

Atropine

Muscarinic antagonist.

Organ system

Eye	↑ pupil dilation, cycloplegia.	Blocks **DUMBBELSS** (see previous page).
Airway	↓ secretions.	
Stomach	↓ acid secretion.	
Gut	↓ motility.	
Bladder	↓ urgency in cystitis.	

Toxicity

↑ body temperature (due to ↓ sweating); rapid pulse; dry mouth; dry, flushed skin; cycloplegia; constipation; disorientation.

Can cause acute angle-closure glaucoma in elderly, urinary retention in men with prostatic hyperplasia, and hyperthermia in infants.

Side effects:
Hot as a hare
Dry as a bone
Red as a beet
Blind as a bat
Mad as a hatter

Hexamethonium

Nicotinic antagonist.

Put a **hex** on smokers (**nicotine**) to help them quit.

Clinical use

Ganglionic blocker. Used in experimental models to prevent vagal reflex responses to changes in blood pressure—e.g., prevents reflex bradycardia caused by NE.

Toxicity

Severe orthostatic hypotension, blurred vision, constipation, sexual dysfunction.

Sympathomimetics

Drug	Mechanism/selectivity	Applications
1. Direct sympatho-mimetics		
Epinephrine	$\alpha_1, \alpha_2, \beta_1, \beta_2$, **low** doses selective for β_1 (**Blow**)	Anaphylaxis, glaucoma (open angle), asthma, hypotension
NE	$\alpha_1, \alpha_2 > \beta_1$	Hypotension (but ↓ renal perfusion)
Isoproterenol	$\beta_1 = \beta_2$ (isolated to β)	AV block (rare)
Dopamine	$D_1 = D_2 > \beta > \alpha$, inotropic and chronotropic	Shock (↑ renal perfusion), heart failure
Dobutamine	$\beta_1 > \beta_2$, inotropic but not chronotropic	Heart failure, cardiac stress testing
Phenylephrine	$\alpha_1 > \alpha_2$	Pupillary dilation, vasoconstriction, nasal decongestion
Metaproterenol, albuterol, salmeterol, terbutaline	Selective β_2-agonists ($\beta_2 > \beta_1$)	**MAST: M**etaproterenol and **A**lbuterol for acute asthma; **S**almeterol for long-term treatment; **T**erbutaline to reduce premature uterine contractions
Ritodrine	β_2	Reduces premature uterine contractions
2. Indirect sympatho-mimetics		
Amphetamine	Indirect general agonist, releases stored catecholamines	Narcolepsy, obesity, attention deficit disorder
Ephedrine	Indirect general agonist, releases stored catecholamines	Nasal decongestion, urinary incontinence, hypotension
Cocaine	Indirect general agonist, uptake inhibitor	Causes vasoconstriction and local anesthesia

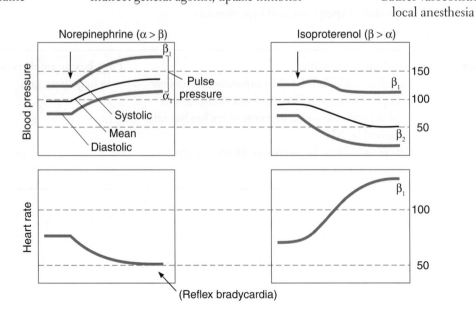

(Adapted, with permission, from Katzung BG, Trevor AJ. *Pharmacology: Examination & Board Review,* 5th ed. Stamford, CT: Appleton & Lange, 1998: 72.)

Sympatholplegics

Clonidine, α-methyldopa	Centrally acting $α_2$-agonists, ↓ central adrenergic outflow	Hypertension, especially with renal disease (no ↓ in blood flow to kidney)

α-blockers

Drug	Application	Toxicity
Nonselective		
Phenoxybenzamine (irreversible) and phentolamine (reversible)	Pheochromocytoma (use phenoxybenzamine before removing tumor, since high levels of released catecholamines will not be able to overcome blockage)	Orthostatic hypotension, reflex tachycardia
$α_1$ selective (-zosin ending)		
Prazosin, terazosin, doxazosin	Hypertension, urinary retention in BPH	1st-dose orthostatic hypotension, dizziness, headache
$α_2$ selective		
Mirtazapine	Depression	Sedation, ↑ serum cholesterol, ↑ appetite

α-blockade of epinephrine vs. phenylephrine

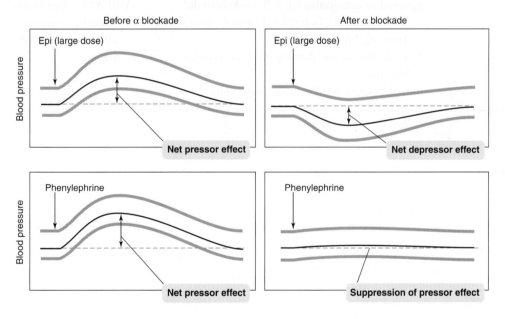

(Adapted, with permission, from Katzung BG, Trevor AJ. *Pharmacology: Examination & Board Review,* 5th ed. Stamford, CT: Appleton & Lange, 1998: 80.)

Shown above are the effects of an α-blocker (e.g., phentolamine) on blood pressure responses to epinephrine and phenylephrine. The epinephrine response exhibits reversal of the mean blood pressure change, from a net increase (the α response) to a net decrease (the $β_2$ response). The response to phenylephrine is suppressed but not reversed because phenylephrine is a "pure" α-agonist without β action.

β-blockers
Acebutolol, betaxolol, esmolol, atenolol, metoprolol, propranolol, timolol, pindolol, labetalol.

Application	Effect
Hypertension	↓ cardiac output, ↓ renin secretion (due to β-receptor blockade on JGA cells)
Angina pectoris	↓ heart rate and contractility, resulting in ↓ O_2 consumption
MI	β-blockers ↓ mortality
SVT (propranolol, esmolol)	↓ AV conduction velocity (class II antiarrhythmic)
CHF	Slows progression of chronic failure
Glaucoma (timolol)	↓ secretion of aqueous humor

Toxicity
Impotence, exacerbation of asthma, cardiovascular adverse effects (bradycardia, AV block, CHF), CNS adverse effects (sedation, sleep alterations); use with caution in diabetics

Selectivity
Nonselective antagonists ($\beta_1 = \beta_2$)—propranolol, timolol, nadolol, and pindolol

β_1-selective antagonists ($\beta_1 > \beta_2$)—**A**cebutolol (partial agonist), **B**etaxolol, **E**smolol (short acting), **A**tenolol, **M**etoprolol

Nonselective α- and β-antagonists—carvedilol, labetalol

Partial β-Agonists—Pindolol, Acebutolol

A BEAM of β_1-blockers. Advantageous in patients with comorbid pulmonary disease.

Specific antidotes

Toxin	Antidote/treatment
1. Acetaminophen	1. N-acetylcysteine
2. Salicylates	2. NaHCO$_3$ (alkalinize urine), dialysis
3. Amphetamines (basic)	3. NH$_4$Cl (acidify urine)
4. Acetylcholinesterase inhibitors, organophosphates	4. Atropine, pralidoxime
5. Antimuscarinic, anticholinergic agents	5. Physostigmine salicylate
6. β-blockers	6. Glucagon
7. Digitalis	7. Stop dig, normalize K$^+$, lidocaine, anti-dig Fab fragments, Mg^{2+}
8. Iron	8. Deferoxamine
9. Lead	9. CaEDTA, dimercaprol, succimer, penicillamine
10. Mercury, arsenic, gold	10. Dimercaprol (BAL), succimer
11. Copper, arsenic, gold	11. Penicillamine
12. Cyanide	12. Nitrite, hydroxocobalamin, thiosulfate
13. **Meth**emoglobin	13. **Meth**ylene blue, vitamin C
14. Carbon monoxide	14. 100% O$_2$, hyperbaric O$_2$
15. Methanol, ethylene glycol (antifreeze)	15. Ethanol, dialysis, fomepizole
16. Opioids	16. Naloxone/naltrexone
17. Benzodiazepines	17. Flumazenil
18. TCAs	18. NaHCO$_3$ (plasma alkalinization)
19. Heparin	19. Protamine
20. Warfarin	20. Vitamin K, fresh frozen plasma
21. tPA, streptokinase	21. Aminocaproic acid
22. Theophylline	22. β-blocker

Drug reactions

Drug reaction by system	Causal agent
1. Cardiovascular	
Atropine-like side effects	TCAs
Coronary vasospasm	Cocaine, sumatriptan
Cutaneous flushing	**VANC: V**ancomycin, **A**denosine, **N**iacin, **C**a^{2+} channel blockers
Dilated cardiomyopathy	Doxorubicin (Adriamycin), daunorubicin
Torsades de pointes	Class III (sotalol), class IA (quinidine) antiarrhythmics
2. Hematologic	
Agranulocytosis	Clozapine, carbamazepine, colchicine, propylthiouracil, methimazole, dapsone
Aplastic anemia	Chloramphenicol, benzene, NSAIDs, propylthiouracil, methimazole
Direct Coombs-positive hemolytic anemia	Methyldopa
Gray baby syndrome	Chloramphenicol
Hemolysis in G6PD-deficient patients	**I**soniazid (INH), **S**ulfonamides, **P**rimaquine, **A**spirin, **I**buprofen, **N**itrofurantoin (hemolysis **IS PAIN**)
Megaloblastic anemia	**P**henytoin, **M**ethotrexate, **S**ulfa drugs (having a **blast** with **PMS**)
Thrombotic complications	OCPs (e.g., estrogens and progestins)
3. Respiratory	
Cough	ACE inhibitors (note: ARBs like losartan—no cough)
Pulmonary fibrosis	**BL**eomycin, **A**miodarone, **B**usulfan (it's hard to **BLAB** when you have pulmonary fibrosis)
4. GI	
Acute cholestatic hepatitis	Macrolides
Focal to massive hepatic necrosis	Halothane, valproic acid, acetaminophen, *Amanita phalloides*
Hepatitis	INH
Pseudomembranous colitis	Clindamycin, ampicillin
5. Reproductive/endocrine	
Adrenocortical insufficiency	Glucocorticoid withdrawal (HPA suppression)
Gynecomastia	**S**pironolactone, **D**igitalis, **C**imetidine, chronic **A**lcohol use, estrogens, **K**etoconazole (**S**ome **D**rugs **C**reate **A**wesome **K**nockers)
Hot flashes	Tamoxifen, clomiphene
Hypothyroidism	Lithium, amiodarone

HIGH-YIELD PRINCIPLES

PHARMACOLOGY

Drug reactions *(continued)*

6. **Musculoskeletal/ connective tissue**

Gingival hyperplasia	Phenytoin
Gout	Furosemide, thiazides
Osteoporosis	Corticosteroids, heparin
Photosensitivity	Sulfonamides, **A**miodarone, **T**etracycline (**SAT** for a **photo**)
Rash (Stevens-Johnson syndrome)	Ethosuximide, lamotrigine, carbamazepine, phenobarbital, phenytoin, sulfa drugs, penicillin, allopurinol
SLE-like syndrome	**H**ydralazine, **INH**, **P**rocainamide, **P**henytoin (it's not **HIPP** to have lupus)
Tendonitis, tendon rupture, and cartilage damage (kids)	Fluoroquinolones

7. **Renal/GU**

Fanconi's syndrome	Expired tetracycline
Interstitial nephritis	Methicillin, NSAIDs, furosemide
Hemorrhagic cystitis	Cyclophosphamide, ifosfamide (prevent by coadministering with mesna)

8. **Neurologic**

Cinchonism	Quinidine, quinine
Diabetes insipidus	Lithium, demeclocycline
Parkinson-like syndrome	Haloperidol, chlorpromazine, reserpine, metoclopramide
Seizures	Bupropion, imipenem/cilastatin, isoniazid
Tardive dyskinesia	Antipsychotics

9. **Multiorgan**

Disulfiram-like reaction	Metronidazole, certain cephalosporins, procarbazine, 1st-generation sulfonylureas
Nephrotoxicity/ neurotoxicity	Polymyxins
Nephrotoxicity/ ototoxicity	Aminoglycosides, vancomycin, loop diuretics, cisplatin

---

P-450 interactions	**Inducers (+)**	**Inhibitors (−)**	**Inducers:**
	Quinidine*	HIV protease inhibitors	**Q**ueen **B**arb **S**teals **Phen**-phen
	Barbiturates	Ketoconazole	and **R**efuses **G**reasy **C**arbs
	St. John's wort	Erythromycin	**Chronic**ally.
	Phenytoin	Grapefruit juice	
	Rifampin	**A**cute alcohol use	**Inhibitors:**
	Griseofulvin	Sulfonamides	**Inhib**it yourself from drinking
	Carbamazepine	Isoniazid	beer from a **KEG** because it
	Chronic alcohol use	Cimetidine	makes you **A**cutely **SICk**.

*Quinidine can both induce and inhibit different isoforms of P-450. Induction is the more important effect.

Alcohol toxicity

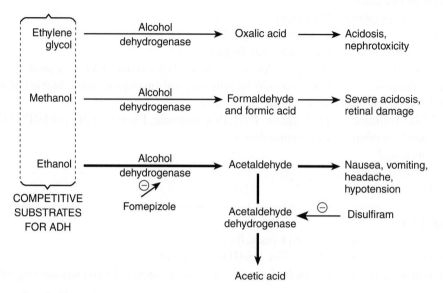

(Adapted, with permission, from Katzung BG, Trevor AJ. *Pharmacology: Examination & Board Review*, 5th ed. Appleton & Lange, 1998: 181.)

Alcohol metabolism depletes NAD^+, which is needed for fatty acid oxidation in the liver and conversion of pyruvate to lactate → fatty liver and lactic acidosis.

Polymorphism in the gene that codes for acetaldehyde dehydrogenase leads to facial flushing and a build-up of acetaldehyde. Responsible for the "glow" seen in some individuals after drinking.

Sulfa drugs	Celecoxib, furosemide, probenecid, thiazides, TMP-SMX, sulfasalazine, sulfonylureas, acetazolamide, sulfonamide antibiotics.
	Patients with sulfa allergies may develop fever, pruritic rash, Stevens-Johnson syndrome, hemolytic anemia, thrombocytopenia, agranulocytosis, and urticaria (hives). Symptoms range from mild to life-threatening.

Drug name

Ending	Category	Example
-afil	Erectile dysfunction	Sildenafil
-ane	Inhalational general anesthetic	Halothane
-azepam	Benzodiazepine	Diazepam
-azine	Phenothiazine (neuroleptic, antiemetic)	Chlorpromazine
-azole	Antifungal	Ketoconazole
-barbital	Barbiturate	Phenobarbital
-caine	Local anesthetic	Lidocaine
-cillin	Penicillin	Methicillin
-cycline	Antibiotic, protein synthesis inhibitor	Tetracycline
-etine	SSRI	Fluoxetine
-ipramine	TCA	Imipramine
-navir	Protease inhibitor	Saquinavir
-olol	β antagonist	Propranolol
-operidol	Butyrophenone (neuroleptic)	Haloperidol
-oxin	Cardiac glycoside (inotropic agent)	Digoxin
-phylline	Methylxanthine	Theophylline
-pril	ACE inhibitor	Captopril
-terol	β_2 agonist	Albuterol
-tidine	H_2 antagonist	Cimetidine
-triptan	$5\text{-HT}_{1B/1D}$ agonists (migraine)	Sumatriptan
-triptyline	TCA	Amitriptyline
-tropin	Pituitary hormone	Somatotropin
-zolam	Benzodiazepine	Alprazolam
-zosin	α_1 antagonist	Prazosin

High-Yield Organ Systems

"Symptoms, then, are in reality nothing but the cry from suffering organs."
—Jean Martin Charcot

In this section, we have divided the High-Yield Facts into the major **Organ Systems.** Within each Organ System are several subsections, including **Anatomy, Physiology, Pathology,** and **Pharmacology.** As you progress through each Organ System, refer back to information in the previous subsections to organize these basic science subsections into a "vertical" framework for learning. Below is some general advice for studying the organ systems by these subsections.

Anatomy

Several topics fall under this heading, including embryology, gross anatomy, histology, and neuroanatomy. Do not memorize all the small details; however, do not ignore anatomy altogether. Review what you have already learned and what you wish you had learned. Many questions require two steps. The first step is to identify a structure on anatomic cross section, electron micrograph, or photomicrograph. The second step may require an understanding of the clinical significance of the structure.

When studying, stress clinically important material. For example, be familiar with gross anatomy related to specific diseases (e.g., Pancoast's tumor, Horner's syndrome), traumatic injuries (e.g., fractures, sensory and motor nerve deficits), procedures (e.g., lumbar puncture), and common surgeries (e.g., cholecystectomy). There are also many questions on the exam involving x-rays, CT scans, and neuro MRI scans. Many students suggest browsing through a general radiology atlas, pathology atlas, and histology atlas. Focus on learning basic anatomy at key levels in the body (e.g., sagittal brain MRI; axial CT of the midthorax, abdomen, and pelvis). Basic neuroanatomy (especially pathways, blood supply, and functional anatomy) also has good yield. Use this as an opportunity to learn associated neuropathology and neurophysiology. Basic embryology (especially congenital malformations) is worth reviewing as well.

Physiology

The portion of the examination dealing with physiology is broad and concept oriented and thus does not lend itself as well to fact-based review. Diagrams are often the best study aids, especially given the increasing number of questions requiring the interpretation of diagrams. Learn to apply basic physiologic relationships in a variety of ways (e.g., the Fick equation, clearance equations). You are seldom asked to perform complex calculations. Hormones are the focus of many questions, so learn their sites of production and action as well as their regulatory mechanisms.

A large portion of the physiology tested on the USMLE Step 1 is now clinically relevant and involves understanding physiologic changes associated with pathologic processes (e.g., changes in pulmonary function with COPD). Thus, it is worthwhile to review the physiologic changes that are found with common pathologies of the major organ systems (e.g., heart, lungs, kidneys, GI tract) and endocrine glands.

Pathology

Questions dealing with this discipline are difficult to prepare for because of the sheer volume of material involved. Review the basic principles and hallmark characteristics of the key diseases. Given the increasingly clinical orientation of Step 1, it is no longer sufficient to know only the "trigger word" associations of certain diseases (e.g., café-au-lait macules and neurofibromatosis); you must also know the clinical descriptions of these findings.

Given the clinical slant of the USMLE Step 1, it is also important to review the classic presenting signs and symptoms of diseases as well as their associated laboratory findings. Delve into the signs, symptoms, and pathophysiology of major diseases that have a high prevalence in the United States (e.g., alcoholism, diabetes, hypertension, heart failure, ischemic heart disease, infectious disease). Be prepared to think one step beyond the simple diagnosis to treatment or complications.

The examination includes a number of color photomicrographs and photographs of gross specimens that are presented in the setting of a brief clinical history. However, read the question and the choices carefully before looking at the illustration, because the history will help you identify the pathologic process. Flip through an illustrated pathology textbook, color atlases, and appropriate Web sites in order to look at the pictures in the days before the exam. Pay attention to potential clues such as age, sex, ethnicity, occupation, recent activities and exposures, and specialized lab tests.

Pharmacology

Preparation for questions on pharmacology is straightforward. Memorizing all the key drugs and their characteristics (e.g., mechanisms, clinical use, and important side effects) is high yield. Focus on understanding the prototype drugs in each class. Avoid memorizing obscure derivatives. Learn the "classic" and distinguishing toxicities of the major drugs. Do not bother with drug dosages or trade names. Reviewing associated biochemistry, physiology, and microbiology can be useful while studying pharmacology. There is a strong emphasis on ANS, CNS, antimicrobial, and cardiovascular agents as well as on NSAIDs. Much of the material is clinically relevant. Newer drugs on the market are also fair game.

Cardiovascular

"As for me, except for an occasional heart attack, I feel as young as I ever did."
—Robert Benchley

"Hearts will never be practical until they are made unbreakable."
—The Wizard of Oz

"As the arteries grow hard, the heart grows soft."
—H. L. Mencken

"Nobody has ever measured, not even poets, how much the heart can hold."
—Zelda Fitzgerald

"Only from the heart can you touch the sky."
—Rumi

▶ Anatomy

▶ Physiology

▶ Pathology

▶ Pharmacology

Starting in 2008, the USMLE Step 1 began to include audio questions, which include heart sounds.

Coronary artery anatomy

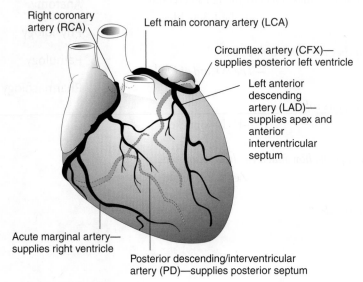

Right coronary artery (RCA)

Left main coronary artery (LCA)

Circumflex artery (CFX)—supplies posterior left ventricle

Left anterior descending artery (LAD)—supplies apex and anterior interventricular septum

Acute marginal artery—supplies right ventricle

Posterior descending/interventricular artery (PD)—supplies posterior septum

(Adapted, with permission, from Ganong WF. *Review of Medical Physiology,* 19th ed. Stamford, CT: Appleton & Lange, 1999: 592.)

In the majority of cases, the SA and AV nodes are supplied by the RCA. 80% of the time, the RCA supplies the inferior portion of the left ventricle via the PD artery (= right dominant). 20% of the time, the PD arises from the CFX.

Coronary artery occlusion most commonly occurs in the LAD, which supplies the anterior interventricular septum.

Coronary arteries fill during diastole.

The most posterior part of the heart is the left atrium; enlargement can cause dysphagia (due to compression of the esophageal nerve) or hoarseness (due to compression of the recurrent laryngeal nerve, a branch of the vagus).

Cardiac output (CO)

Cardiac output (CO) = (stroke volume) × (heart rate). Fick principle:

$$CO = \frac{\text{rate of } O_2 \text{ consumption}}{\text{arterial } O_2 \text{ content} - \text{venous } O_2 \text{ content}}$$

$$\text{Mean arterial pressure} = \left(\begin{array}{c}\text{cardiac}\\\text{output}\end{array}\right) \times \left(\begin{array}{c}\text{total peripheral}\\\text{resistance}\end{array}\right)$$

MAP = ⅔ diastolic pressure + ⅓ systolic pressure.
Pulse pressure = systolic pressure – diastolic pressure.
Pulse pressure ∝ stroke volume.

$$SV = \frac{CO}{HR} = EDV - ESV$$

During exercise, CO ↑ initially as a result of an ↑ in HR.

If HR is too high, diastolic filling is incomplete and CO ↓ (e.g., ventricular tachycardia).

Cardiac output variables	Stroke Volume affected by **C**ontractility, **A**fterload, and **P**reload. ↑ SV when ↑ preload, ↓ afterload, or ↑ contractility.	**SV CAP.**
	Contractility (and SV) ↑ with:	SV ↑ in anxiety, exercise, and pregnancy.
	1. Catecholamines (↑ activity of Ca^{2+} pump in sarcoplasmic reticulum)	A failing heart has ↓ SV.
	2. ↑ intracellular calcium	Myocardial O_2 demand is ↑ by:
	3. ↓ extracellular sodium (↓ activity of Na^+/Ca^{2+} exchanger)	1. ↑ afterload ($\propto$ arterial pressure)
	4. Digitalis (↑ intracellular Na^+, resulting in ↑ Ca^{2+})	2. ↑ contractility
	Contractility (and SV) ↓ with:	3. ↑ heart rate
	1. β_1 blockade (↓ cAMP)	4. ↑ heart size (↑ wall tension)
	2. Heart failure (systolic dysfunction)	
	3. Acidosis	
	4. Hypoxia/hypercapnea (↓ Po_2/↑ Pco_2)	
	5. Non-dihydropyridine Ca^{2+} channel blockers	
Preload and afterload	Preload = ventricular EDV.	Preload ↑ with exercise (slightly), ↑ blood volume (overtransfusion), and excitement (sympathetics).
	Afterload = mean arterial pressure (proportional to peripheral resistance).	
	Venodilators (e.g., nitroglycerin) ↓ preload.	
	Vasodilators (e.g., hydr**AlA**zine) ↓ **A**fterload (**A**rterial).	Preload pumps up the heart.
Starling curve	Force of contraction is proportional to initial length of cardiac muscle fiber (preload).	

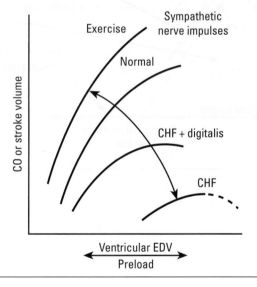

CONTRACTILE STATE OF MYOCARDIUM

⊕	⊖
Circulating catecholamines	Pharmacologic depressants
Digitalis	Loss of myocardium (MI)
Sympathetic stimulation	

Ejection fraction (EF)	$$EF = \frac{SV}{EDV} = \frac{EDV - ESV}{EDV}$$	EF ↓ in heart failure.
	EF is an index of ventricular contractility.	
	EF is normally ≥ 55%.	

HIGH-YIELD SYSTEMS

CARDIOVASCULAR

Resistance, pressure, flow

$\Delta P = Q \times R$

Similar to Ohm's law: $\Delta V = IR$.

$$\text{Resistance} = \frac{\text{driving pressure } (\Delta P)}{\text{flow } (Q)} = \frac{8\eta \text{ (viscosity)} \times \text{length}}{\pi r^4}$$

Total resistance of vessels in series = $R_1 + R_2 + R_3 \ldots$

1/Total resistance of vessels in parallel = $1/R_1 + 1/R_2 + 1/R_3 \ldots$

Viscosity depends mostly on hematocrit.

Viscosity ↑ in:
1. Polycythemia
2. Hyperproteinemic states (e.g., multiple myeloma)
3. Hereditary spherocytosis

Pressure gradient drives flow from high pressure to low.

Resistance is directly proportional to viscosity and inversely proportional to the radius to the 4th power.

Arterioles account for most of total peripheral resistance → regulate capillary flow.

Cardiac and vascular function curves

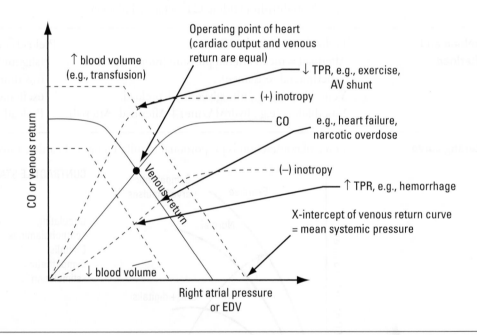

Cardiac cycle

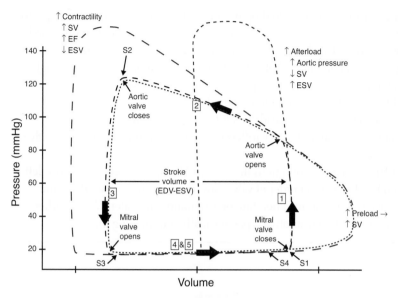

↑ Contractility
↑ SV
↑ EF
↓ ESV

↑ Afterload
↑ Aortic pressure
↓ SV
↑ ESV

S2

Aortic valve closes

Stroke volume (EDV-ESV)

Aortic valve opens

Mitral valve opens

Mitral valve closes

↑ Preload →
↑ SV

S3   S4 S1

Pressure (mmHg) — 140, 120, 100, 80, 60, 40, 20

Volume

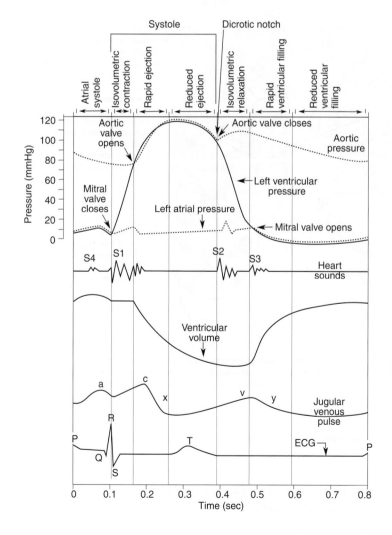

Systole

Dicrotic notch

Atrial systole | Isovolumetric contraction | Rapid ejection | Reduced ejection | Isovolumetric relaxation | Rapid ventricular filling | Reduced ventricular filling

Aortic valve opens

Aortic valve closes

Aortic pressure

Left ventricular pressure

Mitral valve closes

Left atrial pressure

Mitral valve opens

S4 S1   S2 S3   Heart sounds

Ventricular volume

a   c
x   v   y   Jugular venous pulse

P   R   T   ECG   P
Q
S

Pressure (mmHg) — 120, 100, 80, 60, 40, 20, 0

Time (sec) — 0 0.1 0.2 0.3 0.4 0.5 0.6 0.7 0.8

Phases—left ventricle:
1. Isovolumetric contraction—period between mitral valve closure and aortic valve opening; period of highest O_2 consumption
2. Systolic ejection—period between aortic valve opening and closing
3. Isovolumetric relaxation—period between aortic valve closing and mitral valve opening
4. Rapid filling—period just after mitral valve opening
5. Reduced filling—period just before mitral valve closure

Sounds:
S1—mitral and tricuspid valve closure. Loudest at mitral area.
S2—aortic and pulmonary valve closure. Loudest at left sternal border.
S3—in early diastole during rapid ventricular filling phase. Associated with ↑ filling pressures and more common in dilated ventricles (but normal in children and pregnant women).
S4 ("atrial kick")—in late diastole. High atrial pressure. Associated with ventricular hypertrophy. Left atrium must push against stiff LV wall.

Jugular venous pulse (JVP):
a wave—atrial contraction.
c wave—RV contraction (closed tricuspid valve bulging into atrium).
v wave—↑ right atrial pressure due to filling against closed tricuspid valve.

S2 splitting: aortic valve closes before pulmonic; inspiration ↑ this difference.

Normal:
Expiration | | |
                  S_1 A_2 P_2
Inspiration | | |

Wide splitting (associated with pulmonic stenosis or right bundle branch block):
Expiration | | |
                  S_1 A_2 P_2
Inspiration | | |

Fixed splitting (associated with ASD):
Expiration | | |
                  S_1 A_2 P_2
Inspiration | | |

Paradoxical splitting (associated with aortic stenosis or left bundle branch block):
Expiration | | |
                  S_1 P_2 A_2
Inspiration | | |

Splitting

Normal splitting—inspiration leads to drop in intrathoracic pressure, which ↑ capacity of pulmonary circulation. Pulmonic valve closes later to accommodate more blood entering lungs; aortic valve closes earlier because of ↓ return to left heart.

Wide splitting—seen in conditions that delay RV emptying (pulmonic stenosis, right bundle branch block). Delay in RV emptying causes delayed pulmonic sound (regardless of breath). An exaggeration of normal splitting.

Fixed splitting—seen in ASD. ASD leads to left-to-right shunt and therefore ↑ flow through pulmonic valve such that, regardless of breath, pulmonic closure is greatly delayed.

Paradoxical splitting—seen in conditions that delay LV emptying (aortic stenosis, left bundle branch block). Normal order of valve closure is reversed so that P2 sound occurs before delayed A2 sound. Therefore on inspiration, the later P2 and earlier A2 sounds move closer to one another, "paradoxically" eliminating the split.

Auscultation of the heart

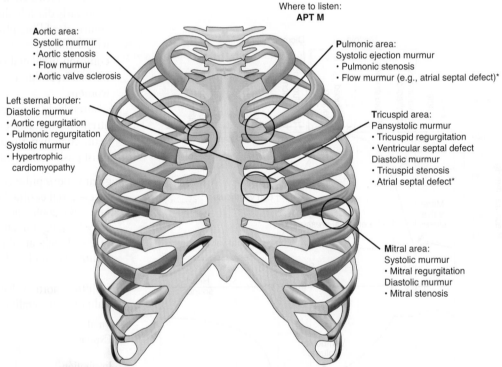

Where to listen:
APT M

Aortic area:
Systolic murmur
• Aortic stenosis
• Flow murmur
• Aortic valve sclerosis

Left sternal border:
Diastolic murmur
• Aortic regurgitation
• Pulmonic regurgitation
Systolic murmur
• Hypertrophic cardiomyopathy

Pulmonic area:
Systolic ejection murmur
• Pulmonic stenosis
• Flow murmur (e.g., atrial septal defect)*

Tricuspid area:
Pansystolic murmur
• Tricuspid regurgitation
• Ventricular septal defect
Diastolic murmur
• Tricuspid stenosis
• Atrial septal defect*

Mitral area:
Systolic murmur
• Mitral regurgitation
Diastolic murmur
• Mitral stenosis

* ASD commonly presents with a pulmonary flow murmur (↑ flow through pulmonary valve) and a diastolic rumble (↑ flow across tricuspid); blood flow across the actual ASD does not cause a murmur because there is no pressure gradient. The murmur later progresses to a louder diastolic murmur of pulmonic regurgitation from dilatation of the pulmonary artery.

Right-sided heart sounds—intensity ↑ with inspiration.
Left-sided heart sounds—intensity ↑ with expiration.

Systolic heart sounds include aortic/pulmonic stenosis, mitral/tricuspid regurgitation.
Diastolic heart sounds include aortic/pulmonic regurgitation, mitral/tricuspid stenosis.

Heart murmurs

S1   S2

Mitral/tricuspid regurgitation (MR/TR)

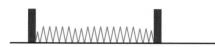

Holosystolic, high-pitched "blowing murmur."
Mitral—loudest at apex and radiates toward axilla. Enhanced by maneuvers that ↑ TPR (e.g., squatting, hand grip) or LA return (e.g., expiration). MR is often due to ischemic heart disease, mitral valve prolapse, or LV dilation.
Tricuspid—loudest at tricuspid area and radiates to right sternal border. Enhanced by maneuvers that ↑ RA return (e.g., inspiration). TR is due to RV dilation or endocarditis. Rheumatic fever can cause both.

Aortic stenosis (AS)

EC

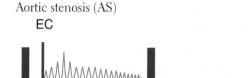

Crescendo-decrescendo systolic ejection murmur following ejection click (EC; due to abrupt halting of valve leaflets). LV >> aortic pressure during systole. Radiates to carotids/apex. "Pulsus parvus et tardus"—pulses weak compared to heart sounds. Can lead to syncope. Often due to age-related calcific aortic stenosis or bicuspid aortic valve (see Image 77).

VSD

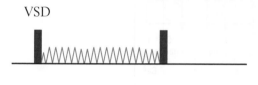

Holosystolic, harsh-sounding murmur. Loudest at tricuspid area.

Mitral prolapse

MC

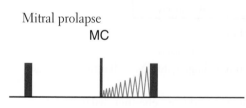

Late systolic crescendo murmur with midsystolic click (MC; due to sudden tensing of chordae tendineae). Most frequent valvular lesion. Loudest at S2. Usually benign. Can predispose to infective endocarditis. Can be caused by myxomatous degeneration, rheumatic fever, or chordae rupture. Enhanced by maneuvers that ↑ TPR (e.g., squatting, hand grip).

Aortic regurgitation (AR)

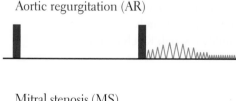

Immediate high-pitched "blowing" diastolic murmur. Wide pulse pressure when chronic; can present with bounding pulses and head bobbing. Often due to aortic root dilation, bicuspid aortic valve, or rheumatic fever. Vasodilators ↓ intensity of murmur.

Mitral stenosis (MS)

OS

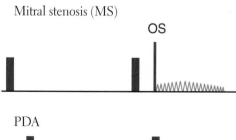

Follows opening snap (OS; due to tensing of chordae tendineae). Delayed rumbling late diastolic murmur. LA >> LV pressure during diastole. Often occurs 2° to rheumatic fever. Chronic MS can result in LA dilation. Enhanced by maneuvers that ↑ LA return (e.g., expiration).

PDA

Continuous machine-like murmur. Loudest at S2. Often due to congenital rubella or prematurity.

Cardiac myocyte physiology

Cardiac muscle contraction depends on extracellular calcium, which enters the cells during plateau of action potential and stimulates calcium release from the cardiac muscle sarcoplasmic reticulum (calcium-induced calcium release).

In contrast to skeletal muscle:

1. Cardiac muscle action potential has a plateau, which is due to Ca^{2+} influx
2. Cardiac nodal cells spontaneously depolarize during diastole (diastolic depolarization), resulting in automaticity due to I_f channels
3. Cardiac myocytes are electrically coupled to each other by gap junctions

Ventricular action potential

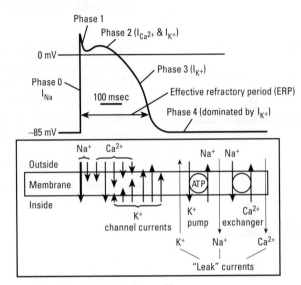

Also occurs in bundle of His and Purkinje fibers.

Phase 0 = rapid upstroke—voltage-gated Na^+ channels open.

Phase 1 = initial repolarization—inactivation of voltage-gated Na^+ channels. Voltage-gated K^+ channels begin to open.

Phase 2 = plateau—Ca^{2+} influx through voltage-gated Ca^{2+} channels balances K^+ efflux. Ca^{2+} influx triggers Ca^{2+} release from sarcoplasmic reticulum and myocyte contraction.

Phase 3 = rapid repolarization—massive K^+ efflux due to opening of voltage-gated slow K^+ channels and closure of voltage-gated Ca^{2+} channels.

Phase 4 = resting potential—high K^+ permeability through K^+ channels.

Pacemaker action potential

Occurs in the SA and AV nodes. Key differences from the ventricular action potential include:

Phase 0 = upstroke—opening of voltage-gated Ca^{2+} channels. These cells lack fast voltage-gated Na^+ channels. Results in a slow conduction velocity that is used by the AV node to prolong transmission from the atria to ventricles.

Phase 2 = plateau is absent.

Phase 3 = inactivation of the Ca^{2+} channels and $\uparrow$ activation of K^+ channels $\rightarrow \uparrow K^+$ efflux.

Phase 4 = slow diastolic depolarization—membrane potential spontaneously depolarizes as Na^+ conductance $\uparrow$ (I_f different from I_{Na} above). Accounts for automaticity of SA and AV nodes. The slope of phase 4 in the SA node determines heart rate. ACh/adenosine $\downarrow$ the rate of diastolic depolarization and $\downarrow$ heart rate, while catecholamines $\uparrow$ depolarization and $\uparrow$ heart rate. Sympathetic stimulation $\uparrow$ the chance that I_f channels are open.

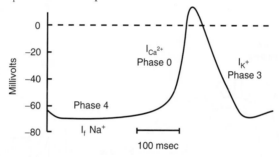

Electrocardiogram

P wave—atrial depolarization.

PR interval—conduction delay through AV node (normally < 200 msec).

QRS complex—ventricular depolarization (normally < 120 msec).

QT interval—mechanical contraction of the ventricles.

T wave—ventricular repolarization. T-wave inversion indicates recent MI.

Atrial repolarization is masked by QRS complex.

ST segment—isoelectric, ventricles depolarized.

U wave—caused by hypokalemia, bradycardia.

Speed of conduction— Purkinje > atria > ventricles > AV node.

Pacemakers—SA > AV > bundle of His/Purkinje/ ventricles.

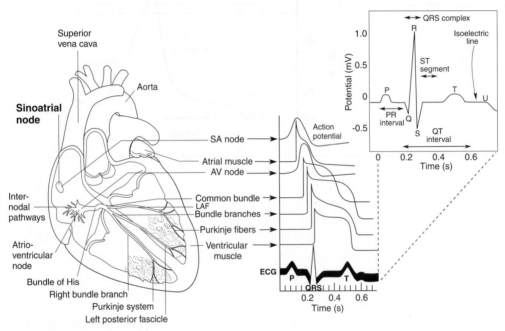

SA node "pacemaker" inherent dominance with slow phase of upstroke
AV node—100-msec delay—atrioventricular delay; allows time for ventricular filling

(Adapted, with permission, from Ganong WF. *Review of Medical Physiology*, 22nd ed. New York: McGraw-Hill, 2005: 548, 550.)

Torsades de pointes

Ventricular tachycardia, characterized by shifting sinusoidal waveforms on ECG. Can progress to V-fib. Anything that prolongs the QT interval can predispose to torsades de pointes.

Congenital long QT syndromes are most often due to defects in cardiac sodium or potassium channels. Can present with severe congenital sensorineural deafness (Jervell and Lange-Nielsen syndrome).

Wolff-Parkinson-White syndrome

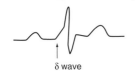

δ wave

Also known as ventricular preexcitation syndrome. Accessory conduction pathway from atria to ventricle (bundle of Kent), bypassing AV node. As a result, ventricles begin to partially depolarize earlier, giving rise to characteristic delta wave on ECG. May result in reentry current leading to supraventricular tachycardia.

ECG tracings

Atrial fibrillation

Chaotic and erratic baseline (**irregularly irregular**) with **no discrete P waves** in between irregularly spaced QRS complexes. Can result in atrial stasis and lead to stroke. Treat with β-blocker or calcium channel blocker; prophylaxis against thromboembolism with warfarin (Coumadin).

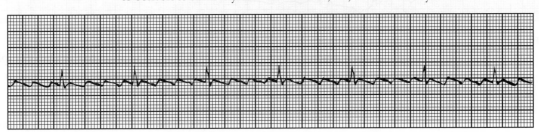

Atrial flutter

A rapid succession of identical, back-to-back atrial depolarization waves. The identical appearance accounts for the **"sawtooth"** appearance of the flutter waves. Attempt to convert to sinus rhythm. Use class IA, IC, or III antiarrhythmics.

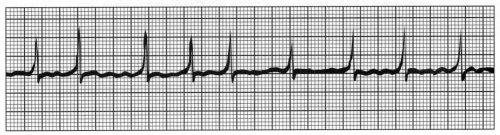

AV block

1st degree

The PR interval is prolonged (> 200 msec). Asymptomatic.

Prolonged PR interval

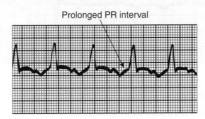

ECG tracings *(continued)*

2nd degree

Mobitz type I
(Wenckebach)

Progressive lengthening of the PR interval until a beat is "dropped" (a P wave not followed by a QRS complex). Usually asymptomatic.

Note progressive increase in PR length before dropped beat

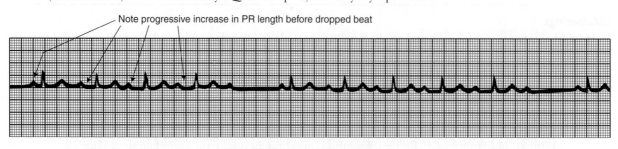

Mobitz type II

Dropped beats that are not preceded by a change in the length of the PR interval (as in type I). These abrupt, nonconducted P waves result in a pathologic condition. It is often found as 2:1 block, where there are 2 P waves to 1 QRS response. May progress to 3rd-degree block.

No QRS following P wave, normal PR intervals

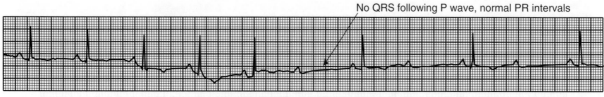

3rd degree
(complete)

The atria and ventricles beat independently of each other. Both P waves and QRS complexes are present, although the **P waves bear no relation to the QRS complexes.** The atrial rate is faster than the ventricular rate. Usually treated with pacemaker. Lyme disease can result in 3rd-degree heart block.

P on T wave   P wave on ST-T complex

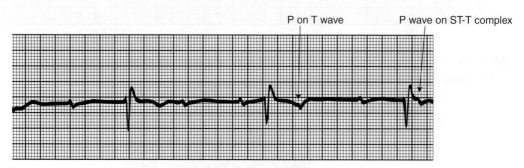

Ventricular fibrillation

A completely erratic rhythm with no identifiable waves. Fatal arrhythmia without immediate CPR and defibrillation.

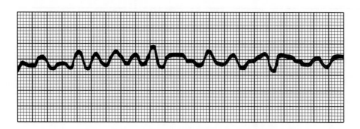

Maintenance of mean arterial pressure

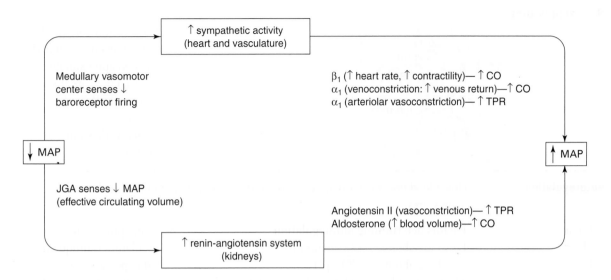

ANP is released from the atria in response to ↑ blood volume and atrial pressure. Causes generalized vascular relaxation. Constricts efferent renal arterioles and dilates afferent arterioles (cGMP mediated), promoting diuresis and contributing to the "escape from aldosterone" mechanism.

Baroreceptors and chemoreceptors

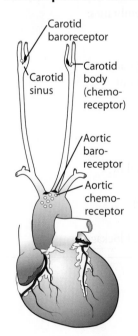

Receptors:
1. Aortic arch transmits via vagus nerve to medulla (responds **only** to ↑ BP)
2. Carotid sinus transmits via glossopharyngeal nerve to solitary nucleus of medulla (responds to ↓ and ↑ in BP).

Baroreceptors:
1. Hypotension—↓ arterial pressure → ↓ stretch → ↓ afferent baroreceptor firing → ↑ efferent sympathetic firing and ↓ efferent parasympathetic stimulation → vasoconstriction, ↑ HR, ↑ contractility, ↑ BP. Important in the response to severe hemorrhage.
2. Carotid massage—↑ pressure on carotid artery → ↑ stretch → ↑ afferent baroreceptor firing → ↓ HR.

Chemoreceptors:
1. Peripheral—carotid and aortic bodies respond to ↓ Po_2 (< 60 mmHg), ↑ Pco_2, and ↓ pH of blood.
2. Central—respond to changes in pH and Pco_2 of brain interstitial fluid, which in turn are influenced by arterial CO_2. Do not directly respond to Po_2. Responsible for Cushing reaction— ↑ intracranial pressure constricts arterioles → cerebral ischemia → hypertension (sympathetic response) → reflex bradycardia. Note: Cushing triad = hypertension, bradycardia, respiratory depression.

Circulation through organs

Liver	Largest share of systemic cardiac output.
Kidney	Highest blood flow per gram of tissue.
Heart	Large arteriovenous O_2 difference because O_2 extraction is always ~ 100%. ↑ O_2 demand is met by ↑ coronary blood flow, not by ↑ extraction of O_2.

Normal pressures

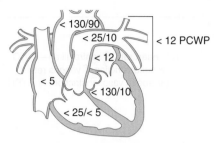

< 130/90
< 25/10
< 12 PCWP
< 12
< 5
< 130/10
< 25/< 5

PCWP—pulmonary capillary wedge pressure (in mmHg) is a good approximation of left atrial pressure. In mitral stenosis, PCWP > LV diastolic pressure.
Measured with Swan-Ganz catheter.

Autoregulation

How blood flow to an organ remains constant over a wide range of perfusion pressures.

Organ	Factors determining autoregulation
Heart	Local metabolites—O_2, adenosine, NO
Brain	Local metabolites—CO_2 (pH)
Kidneys	Myogenic and tubuloglomerular feedback
Lungs	Hypoxia causes vasoconstriction
Skeletal muscle	Local metabolites—lactate, adenosine, K^+
Skin	Sympathetic stimulation most important mechanism—temperature control

Note: the pulmonary vasculature is unique in that hypoxia causes vasoconstriction so that only well-ventilated areas are perfused. In other organs, hypoxia causes vasodilation.

Capillary fluid exchange

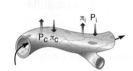

Starling forces determine fluid movement through capillary membranes:
1. P_c = capillary pressure—pushes fluid out of capillary
2. P_i = interstitial fluid pressure—pushes fluid into capillary
3. π_c = plasma colloid osmotic pressure—pulls fluid into capillary
4. π_i = interstitial fluid colloid osmotic pressure—pulls fluid out of capillary

Thus, net filtration pressure = $P_{net} = [(P_c - P_i) - (\pi_c - \pi_i)]$.
K_f = filtration constant (capillary permeability).
Net fluid flow = $(P_{net})(K_f)$.
Edema—excess fluid outflow into interstitium commonly caused by:
1. ↑ capillary pressure (↑ P_c; heart failure)
2. ↓ plasma proteins (↓ π_c; nephrotic syndrome, liver failure)
3. ↑ capillary permeability (↑ K_f; toxins, infections, burns)
4. ↑ interstitial fluid colloid osmotic pressure (↑ π_i; lymphatic blockage)

Congenital heart disease

Right-to-left shunts (early cyanosis)— "blue babies"	1. Tetralogy of Fallot (most common cause of early cyanosis) 2. Transposition of great vessels 3. Truncus arteriosus 4. Tricuspid atresia 5. Total anomalous pulmonary venous return (TAPVR)	The **5 T**'s: Tetralogy Transposition Truncus Tricuspid TAPVR

Persistent truncus arteriosus—failure of truncus arteriosus to divide into pulmonary trunk and aorta.

Tricuspid atresia—characterized by absence of tricuspid valve and hypoplastic right ventricle. Requires both ASD and VSD for viability.

TAPVR—pulmonary veins drain into right heart circulation (SVC, coronary sinus, etc.).

Left-to-right shunts (late cyanosis)— "blue kids"	1. VSD (most common congenital cardiac anomaly) 2. ASD (loud S1; wide, fixed split S2) 3. PDA (close with indomethacin)	Frequency—VSD > ASD > PDA.

Eisenmenger's syndrome

Uncorrected VSD, ASD, or PDA causes compensatory vascular hypertrophy, which results in progressive pulmonary hypertension. As pulmonary resistance ↑, the shunt reverses from L → R to R → L, which causes late cyanosis (clubbing and polycythemia).

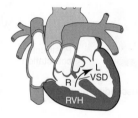

Tetralogy of Fallot

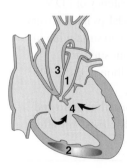

1. Pulmonary stenosis (most important determinant for prognosis)
2. RVH
3. Overriding aorta (overrides the VSD)
4. VSD

Early cyanosis is caused by a right-to-left shunt across the VSD. Right-to-left shunt exists because of the ↑ pressure caused by stenotic pulmonic valve. On x-ray, boot-shaped heart due to RVH. Patients suffer "cyanotic spells."

Tetralogy of Fallot is caused by anterosuperior displacement of the infundibular septum.

PROVe.

Patient learns to squat to improve symptoms: compression of femoral arteries ↑ TPR thereby ↓ the right-to-left shunt and directing more blood from the RV to the lungs. Compression → resistance → pressure.

D-transposition of great vessels

Aorta leaves RV (anterior) and pulmonary trunk leaves LV (posterior) → separation of systemic and pulmonary circulations. Not compatible with life unless a shunt is present to allow adequate mixing of blood (e.g., VSD, PDA, or patent foramen ovale).

Due to failure of the aorticopulmonary septum to spiral.

Without surgical correction, most infants die within the first few months of life.

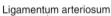

Aorta — Pulmonary artery

Left ventricle

Right ventricle

Ventricular septum

Coarctation of the aorta

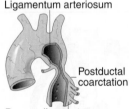

Ligamentum arteriosum

Postductal coarctation

Descending aorta

Infantile type—aortic stenosis proximal to insertion of ductus arteriosus (preductal).
Associated with Turner syndrome.

Adult type—stenosis is distal to ligamentum arteriosum (postductal). Associated with notching of the ribs (due to collateral circulation), hypertension in upper extremities, weak pulses in lower extremities.
Can result in aortic regurgitation.

Check femoral pulses on physical exam.

INfantile: **IN** close to the heart.
ADult: **D**istal to **D**uctus.
Most commonly associated with bicuspid aortic valve.

Patent ductus arteriosus

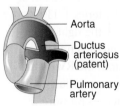

Aorta

Ductus arteriosus (patent)

Pulmonary artery

In fetal period, shunt is right to left (normal). In neonatal period, lung resistance ↓ and shunt becomes left to right with subsequent RVH and failure (abnormal). Associated with a continuous, "machine-like" murmur. Patency is maintained by PGE synthesis and low O_2 tension.
Uncorrected PDA can eventually result in late cyanosis in the lower extremities (differential cyanosis).

ENDomethacin (indomethacin) **END**s patency of PDA; **PGEE** k**EE**ps it open (may be necessary to sustain life in conditions such as transposition of the great vessels).
PDA is normal in utero and normally closes only after birth.

HIGH-YIELD SYSTEMS

CARDIOVASCULAR

Congenital cardiac defect associations	Disorder	Defect
	22q11 syndromes	Truncus arteriosus, tetralogy of Fallot
	Down syndrome	ASD, VSD, AV septal defect (endocardial cushion defect)
	Congenital rubella	Septal defects, PDA, pulmonary artery stenosis
	Turner syndrome	Coarctation of aorta (preductal)
	Marfan's syndrome	Aortic insufficiency (late complication)
	Infant of diabetic mother	Transposition of great vessels

Hypertension

Defined as BP ≥ 140/90.

Risk factors ↑ age, obesity, diabetes, smoking, genetics, black > white > Asian.

Features 90% of hypertension is 1° (essential) and related to ↑ CO or ↑ TPR; remaining 10% mostly 2° to renal disease. Malignant hypertension is severe and rapidly progressing.

Predisposes to Atherosclerosis, left ventricular hypertrophy, stroke, CHF, renal failure, retinopathy, and aortic dissection.

Hyperlipidemia signs

Atheromas Plaques in blood vessel walls.

Xanthomas Plaques or nodules composed of lipid-laden histiocytes in the skin, especially the eyelids (xanthelasma).

Tendinous xanthoma Lipid deposit in tendon, especially Achilles.

Corneal arcus Lipid deposit in cornea, nonspecific (arcus senilis).

Arteriosclerosis

Mönckeberg Calcification in the media of the arteries, especially radial or ulnar. Usually benign; "pipestem" arteries. Does not obstruct blood flow; intima not involved.

Arteriolosclerosis Hyaline thickening of small arteries in essential hypertension or diabetes mellitus. Hyperplastic "onion skinning" in malignant hypertension.

Atherosclerosis Fibrous plaques and atheromas form in intima of arteries.

Atherosclerosis	Disease of elastic arteries and large and medium-sized muscular arteries.
Risk factors	Smoking, hypertension, diabetes mellitus, hyperlipidemia, family history.
Progression	Endothelial cell dysfunction → macrophage and LDL accumulation → foam cell formation → fatty streaks → smooth muscle cell migration (involves PDGF and TGF-β) → fibrous plaque → complex atheromas.
Complications	Aneurysms, ischemia, infarcts, peripheral vascular disease, thrombus, emboli.
Location	Abdominal aorta > coronary artery > popliteal artery > carotid artery.
Symptoms	Angina, claudication, but can be asymptomatic.

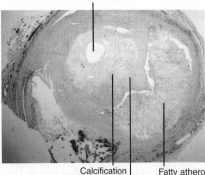

Lumen of vessel
(narrowed to about
5% of original lumen)

Calcification

Fibrous cap

Fatty atherosclerotic
plaque (lipid zone)

Aortic dissection
Longitudinal intraluminal tear forming a false lumen. Associated with hypertension or cystic medial necrosis (component of Marfan's syndrome). Presents with tearing chest pain radiating to the back. CXR shows mediastinal widening. The false lumen occupies most of the descending aorta. Can result in aortic rupture and death.

Ischemic heart disease
Possible manifestations:
1. **Angina** (CAD narrowing > 75%):
    a. Stable—mostly 2° to atherosclerosis; ST depression on ECG (retrosternal chest pain with exertion)
    b. Prinzmetal's variant—occurs at rest 2° to coronary artery spasm; ST elevation on ECG
    c. Unstable/crescendo—thrombosis but no necrosis; ST depression on ECG (worsening chest pain at rest or with minimal exertion)
2. **Myocardial infarction**—most often acute thrombosis due to coronary artery atherosclerosis; results in myocyte necrosis
3. **Sudden cardiac death**—death from cardiac causes within 1 hour of onset of symptoms, most commonly due to a lethal arrhythmia (e.g., V-fib)
4. **Chronic ischemic heart disease**—progressive onset of CHF over many years due to chronic ischemic myocardial damage

Evolution of MI Coronary artery occlusion: LAD > RCA > circumflex.

Symptoms: diaphoresis, nausea, vomiting, severe retrosternal pain, pain in left arm and/or jaw, shortness of breath, fatigue, adrenergic symptoms.

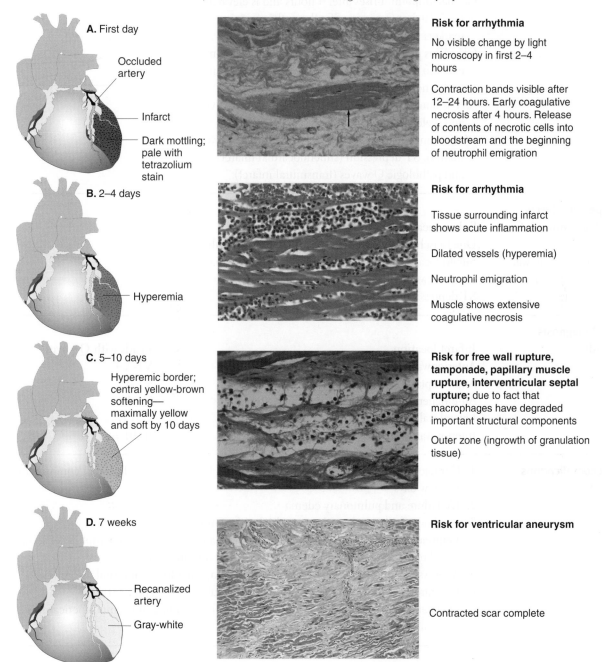

A. First day

Occluded artery

Infarct

Dark mottling; pale with tetrazolium stain

Risk for arrhythmia

No visible change by light microscopy in first 2–4 hours

Contraction bands visible after 12–24 hours. Early coagulative necrosis after 4 hours. Release of contents of necrotic cells into bloodstream and the beginning of neutrophil emigration

B. 2–4 days

Hyperemia

Risk for arrhythmia

Tissue surrounding infarct shows acute inflammation

Dilated vessels (hyperemia)

Neutrophil emigration

Muscle shows extensive coagulative necrosis

C. 5–10 days

Hyperemic border; central yellow-brown softening—maximally yellow and soft by 10 days

Risk for free wall rupture, tamponade, papillary muscle rupture, interventricular septal rupture; due to fact that macrophages have degraded important structural components

Outer zone (ingrowth of granulation tissue)

D. 7 weeks

Recanalized artery

Gray-white

Risk for ventricular aneurysm

Contracted scar complete

Diagnosis of MI

In the first 6 hours, ECG is the gold standard.

Cardiac troponin I rises after 4 hours and is elevated for 7–10 days; more specific than other protein markers.

CK-MB is predominantly found in myocardium but can also be released from skeletal muscle. Useful in diagnosing reinfarction on top of acute MI.

AST is nonspecific and can be found in cardiac, liver, and skeletal muscle cells.

ECG changes can include ST elevation (transmural infarct), ST depression (subendocardial infarct), and pathologic Q waves (transmural infarct).

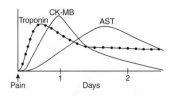

Types of infarcts

Transmural infarcts	Subendocardial infarcts
↑ necrosis	Due to ischemic necrosis of < 50% of ventricle wall
Affects entire wall	Subendocardium especially vulnerable to ischemia
ST elevation on ECG	Due to fewer collaterals, higher pressure
Q waves	ST depression on ECG

ECG diagnosis of MI

Infarct location	Leads with Q waves
Anterior wall (LAD)	V1–V4
Anteroseptal (LAD)	V1–V2
Anterolateral (LCX)	V4–V6
Lateral wall (LCX)	I, aVL
Inferior wall (RCA)	II, III, aVF

MI complications

1. Cardiac arrhythmia—important cause of death before reaching hospital; common in first few days
2. LV failure and pulmonary edema
3. Cardiogenic shock (large infarct—high risk of mortality)
4. Ventricular free wall rupture → cardiac tamponade; papillary muscle rupture → severe mitral regurgitation; and interventricular septal rupture → VSD
5. Aneurysm formation—↓ CO, risk of arrhythmia, embolus from mural thrombus
6. Postinfarction fibrinous pericarditis—friction rub (3–5 days post-MI)
7. Dressler's syndrome—autoimmune phenomenon resulting in fibrinous pericarditis (several weeks post-MI)

HIGH-YIELD SYSTEMS

CARDIOVASCULAR

Cardiomyopathies

Dilated (congestive) cardiomyopathy	Most common cardiomyopathy (90% of cases). Etiologies include chronic **A**lcohol abuse, wet **B**eriberi, **C**oxsackie B virus myocarditis, chronic **C**ocaine use, **C**hagas' disease, **D**oxorubicin toxicity, hemochromatosis, and peripartum cardiomyopathy. Findings: S3, dilated heart on ultrasound, balloon appearance on chest x-ray.	Systolic dysfunction ensues. Eccentric hypertrophy (sarcomeres added in series).
Hypertrophic cardiomyopathy	Hypertrophied IV septum is "too close" to mitral valve leaflet, leading to outflow tract obstruction. 50% of cases are familial, autosomal dominant. Associated with Friedreich's ataxia. Disoriented, tangled, hypertrophied myocardial fibers. Cause of sudden death in young athletes. Findings: normal-sized heart, S4, apical impulses, systolic murmur. Treat with β-blocker or non-dihydropyridine calcium channel blocker (e.g., verapamil).	Diastolic dysfunction ensues. Concentric hypertrophy (sarcomeres added in parallel). Proximity of hypertrophied IV septum to mitral leaflet obstructs outflow tract, resulting in systolic murmur and syncopal episodes.
Restrictive/obliterative cardiomyopathy	Major causes include sarcoidosis, amyloidosis, postradiation fibrosis, endocardial fibroelastosis (thick fibroelastic tissue in endocardium of young children), Löffler's syndrome (endomyocardial fibrosis with a prominent eosinophilic infilitrate), and hemochromatosis (dilated cardiomyopathy can also occur).	Diastolic dysfunction ensues.

CHF

A clinical syndrome that occurs in patients with an inherited or acquired abnormality of cardiac structure or function, who develop a constellation of clinical symptoms (dyspnea, fatigue) and signs (edema, rales).

Abnormality	Cause
Dyspnea on exertion	Failure of LV output to ↑ during exercise.
Cardiac dilation	Greater ventricular end-diastolic volume.
Pulmonary edema, paroxysmal nocturnal dyspnea	LV failure → ↑ pulmonary venous pressure → pulmonary venous distention and transudation of fluid. Presence of hemosiderin-laden macrophages ("heart failure" cells) in the lungs due to microhemorrhages from ↑ pulmonary capillary pressure.
Orthopnea (shortness of breath when supine)	↑ venous return in supine position exacerbates pulmonary vascular congestion.
Hepatomegaly (nutmeg liver)	↑ central venous pressure → ↑ resistance to portal flow. Rarely, leads to "cardiac cirrhosis."
Ankle, sacral edema	RV failure → ↑ venous pressure → fluid transudation.
Jugular venous distention	Right heart failure → ↑ venous pressure.

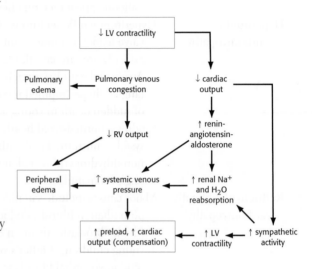

Right heart failure most often results from left heart failure. Isolated right heart failure is usually due to cor pulmonale.

Bacterial endocarditis	Fever (most common symptom), Roth's spots (round white spots on retina surrounded by hemorrhage), Osler's nodes (tender raised lesions on finger or toe pads), new **murmur, Janeway lesions** (small erythematous lesions on palm or sole), anemia, **splinter hemorrhages** on nail bed. Valvular damage may cause new murmur (see damaged aortic valve below). Multiple blood cultures necessary for diagnosis.	Mitral valve is most frequently involved. **Tri**cuspid valve endocarditis is associated with IV **drug** abuse (don't **tri drugs**). Associated with *S. aureus*, *Pseudomonas*, and *Candida*.
	1. Acute—*S. aureus* (high virulence). Large vegetations on previously normal valves. Rapid onset. 2. Subacute—viridans streptococci (low virulence). Smaller vegetations on congenitally abnormal or diseased valves. Sequela of dental procedures. More insidious onset.	Complications: chordae rupture, glomerulonephritis, suppurative pericarditis, emboli. Bacteria **FROM JANE:**
	Endocarditis may also be nonbacterial 2° to malignancy or hypercoagulable state (marantic/thrombotic endocarditis). *S. bovis* is present in colon cancer, *S. epidermidis* on prosthetic valves; HACEK organisms cause culture-negative endocarditis.	**F**ever **R**oth's spots **O**sler's nodes **M**urmur **J**aneway lesions **A**nemia **N**ail-bed hemorrhage **E**mboli

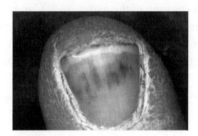

Splinter hemorrhage

(Reproduced, with permission, from USMLERx.)

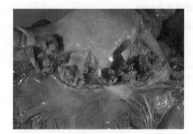

Acute bacterial endocarditis

| **Libman-Sacks endocarditis** | Verrucous (wartlike), sterile vegetations occur on both sides of the valve. Most often benign; can be associated with mitral regurgitation and, less commonly, mitral stenosis. | SLE causes LSE. |

Rheumatic heart disease

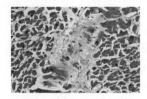

Aschoff body

A consequence of pharyngeal infection with group A β-hemolytic streptococci. Early deaths due to myocarditis. Late sequelae include rheumatic heart disease, which affects heart valves—mitral > aortic >> tricuspid (high-pressure valves affected most). Early lesion is mitral valve prolapse; late lesion is mitral stenosis. Associated with Aschoff bodies (granuloma with giant cells), Anitschkow's cells (activated histiocytes), elevated ASO titers.

Immune mediated (type II hypersensitivity); not direct effect of bacteria. Antibodies to M protein.

FEVERSS:
Fever
Erythema marginatum
Valvular damage (vegetation and fibrosis)
ESR ↑
Red-hot joints (migratory polyarthritis)
Subcutaneous nodules
St. Vitus' dance (chorea)

Cardiac tamponade

Compression of heart by fluid (e.g., blood, effusions) in pericardium, leading to ↓ CO. Equilibration of diastolic pressures in all 4 chambers.

Findings: hypotension, ↑ venous pressure (JVD), distant heart sounds, ↑ HR, pulsus paradoxus.

Pulsus paradoxus (Kussmaul's pulse)—exaggerated ↓ in amplitude of pulse during inspiration. Seen in severe cardiac tamponade, asthma, obstructive sleep apnea, pericarditis, and croup.

Syphilitic heart disease

3° syphilis disrupts the vasa vasorum of the aorta with consequent dilation of the aorta and valve ring. May see calcification of the aortic root and ascending aortic arch. Leads to "tree bark" appearance of the aorta.

Can result in aneurysm of the ascending aorta or aortic arch and aortic valve incompetence.

Cardiac tumors	Myxomas are the most common 1° cardiac tumor in adults (see Image 80). 90% occur in the atria (mostly left atrium). Myxomas are usually described as a "ball-valve" obstruction in the left atrium (associated with multiple syncopal episodes). Rhabdomyomas are the most frequent 1° cardiac tumor in children (associated with tuberous sclerosis). Metastases most common heart tumor (from melanoma, lymphoma). Kussmaul's sign: ↑ in jugular venous pressure on inspiration.	
Varicose veins	Dilated, tortuous superficial veins due to chronically ↑ venous pressure. Predisposes to poor wound healing and varicose ulcers.	Thromboembolism is rare (compare with stasis of deep veins).
Raynaud's disease	↓ blood flow to the skin due to arteriolar vasospasm in response to cold temperature or emotional stress. Most often in the fingers and toes (see Image 97). Called Raynaud's phenomenon when 2° to a mixed connective tissue disease, SLE, or CREST syndrome.	Affects small vessels.
Wegener's granulomatosis	Characterized by triad of focal necrotizing vasculitis, necrotizing granulomas in the **lung and upper airway**, and necrotizing glomerulonephritis.	Affects small vessels.
Symptoms	Hemoptysis, hematuria, perforation of nasal septum, chronic sinusitis, otitis media, mastoiditis, cough, dyspnea.	
Findings	**c-ANCA** is a strong marker of disease; chest x-ray may reveal large nodular densities; hematuria and red cell casts.	
Treatment	Cyclophosphamide and corticosteroids.	

Other ANCA-positive vasculitides

Microscopic polyangiitis	Like Wegener's but lacks granulomas. **p-ANCA.**	All affect small vessels.
1° pauci-immune crescentic glomerulo-nephritis	Vasculitis limited to kidney. **Pauci-**immune = **pauci**ty of antibodies.	
Churg-Strauss syndrome	Granulomatous vasculitis with eosinophilia. Most often presents with asthma, sinusitis, skin lesions, and peripheral neuropathy (e.g., wrist/foot drop); can also involve heart, GI, and kidneys. **p-ANCA.**	

Sturge-Weber disease	Congenital vascular disorder that affects capillary-sized blood vessels. Manifests with port-wine stain (aka nevus flammeus) on face, ipsilateral leptomeningeal angiomatosis (intracerebral AVM), seizures, and early-onset glaucoma.	Affects small vessels.

Henoch-Schönlein purpura	Most common form of childhood systemic vasculitis. Skin rash on buttocks and legs (palpable purpura), arthralgia, intestinal hemorrhage, abdominal pain, and melena. Follows URIs. IgA immune complexes. Association with IgA nephropathy.	Affects small vessels. Common triad: 1. Skin 2. Joints 3. GI Multiple lesions of the same age.
Buerger's disease	Also known as thromboangiitis obliterans; idiopathic, segmental, thrombosing vasculitis of small and medium peripheral arteries and veins. Seen in **heavy smokers.**	Affects small and medium vessels. Note: Medium-vessel diseases cause thrombosis/infarction of arteries.
Symptoms	Intermittent claudication, superficial nodular phlebitis, cold sensitivity (Raynaud's phenomenon), severe pain in affected part. May lead to gangrene and autoamputation of digits.	
Treatment	Smoking cessation.	
Kawasaki disease	Acute, self-limiting necrotizing vasculitis in infants/children. Association with Asian ethnicity.	Affects small and medium vessels.
Symptoms	Fever, conjunctivitis, changes in lips/oral mucosa ("strawberry tongue"), lymphadenitis, desquamative skin rash. May develop coronary aneurysms.	
Treatment	IV immunoglobulin, aspirin.	
Polyarteritis nodosa	Immune complex–mediated transmural vasculitis with fibrinoid necrosis.	Affects small and medium arteries.
Symptoms	Fever, weight loss, malaise, abdominal pain, melena, headache, myalgia, hypertension, neurologic dysfunction, cutaneous eruptions.	Typically involves renal and visceral vessels, **not** pulmonary arteries.
Findings	**Hepatitis B** seropositivity in 30% of patients. Multiple aneurysms and constrictions on arteriogram.	Lesions are of different ages.
Treatment	Corticosteroids, cyclophosphamide.	
Takayasu's arteritis	Known as **"pulseless disease"**—granulomatous thickening of aortic arch and/or proximal great vessels. Associated with an ↑ ESR. Primarily affects Asian females < 40 years of age.	Affects medium and large arteries.
Symptoms	Fever, Arthritis, Night sweats, MYalgia, SKIN nodules, Ocular disturbances, Weak pulses in upper extremities.	FAN MY SKIN On Wednesday.

Temporal arteritis (giant cell arteritis)	Most common vasculitis affecting medium and large arteries, usually branches of carotid artery. Focal, granulomatous inflammation. Affects elderly females.	Affects medium and large arteries. **TEM**poral arteritis has signs near **TEM**ples.
Symptoms	Unilateral headache, jaw claudication, impaired vision (occlusion of ophthalmic artery that may lead to irreversible blindness).	
Findings	Associated with an ↑ ESR. Half of patients have systemic involvement and polymyalgia rheumatica.	
Treatment	High-dose steroids.	

Vascular tumors

Strawberry hemangioma	Benign capillary hemangioma of infancy. Initially grows with child; then spontaneously regresses.
Cherry hemangioma	Benign capillary hemangioma of the elderly. Does not regress. Frequency ↑ with age.
Pyogenic granuloma	Polypoid capillary hemangioma that can ulcerate and bleed. Associated with trauma and pregnancy.
Cystic hygroma	Cavernous lymphangioma of the neck. Associated with Turner syndrome.
Glomus tumor	Benign, painful, red-blue tumor under fingernails. Arises from modified smooth muscle cells of glomus body.
Bacillary angiomatosis	Benign capillary skin papules found in AIDS patients. Caused by *Bartonella henselae* infections. Frequently mistaken for Kaposi's sarcoma.
Angiosarcoma	Highly lethal malignancy of the liver. Associated with vinyl chloride, arsenic, and ThO_2 (Thorotrast) exposure.
Lymphangiosarcoma	Lymphatic malignancy associated with persistent lymphedema (e.g., post–radical mastectomy).
Kaposi's sarcoma	Endothelial malignancy of the skin associated with HHV-8 and HIV. Frequently mistaken for bacillary angiomatosis.

Antihypertensive therapy

Essential hypertension	Diuretics, ACE inhibitors, angiotensin II receptor blockers (ARBs), calcium channel blockers.	See the Renal chapter for more details about diuretics and ACE inhibitors/ARBs.
CHF	Diuretics, ACE inhibitors/ARBs, β-blockers (compensated CHF), K^+-sparing diuretics.	β-blockers are contraindicated in decompensated CHF.
Diabetes mellitus	ACE inhibitors/ARBs, calcium channel blockers, diuretics, β-blockers, α-blockers.	ACE inhibitors are protective against diabetic nephropathy. See the Pharmacology chapter for more details about α-blockers.

Hydralazine

Mechanism	↑ cGMP → smooth muscle relaxation. Vasodilates arterioles > veins; afterload reduction.
Clinical use	Severe hypertension, CHF. First-line therapy for hypertension in pregnancy, with methyldopa. Frequently coadministered with a β-blocker to prevent reflex tachycardia.
Toxicity	Compensatory tachycardia (contraindicated in angina/CAD), fluid retention, nausea, headache, angina. Lupus-like syndrome.

Calcium channel blockers

Nifedipine, verapamil, diltiazem.

Mechanism	Block voltage-dependent L-type calcium channels of cardiac and smooth muscle and thereby reduce muscle contractility. Vascular smooth muscle—nifedipine > diltiazem > verapamil (**V**erapamil = **V**entricle). Heart—verapamil > diltiazem > nifedipine.
Clinical use	Hypertension, angina, arrhythmias (not nifedipine), Prinzmetal's angina, Raynaud's.
Toxicity	Cardiac depression, AV block, peripheral edema, flushing, dizziness, and constipation.

Nitroglycerin, isosorbide dinitrate

Mechanism	Vasodilate by releasing nitric oxide in smooth muscle, causing ↑ in cGMP and smooth muscle relaxation. Dilate veins >> arteries. ↓ preload.
Clinical use	Angina, pulmonary edema. Also used as an aphrodisiac and erection enhancer.
Toxicity	Reflex tachycardia, hypotension, flushing, headache, "Monday disease" in industrial exposure; development of tolerance for the vasodilating action during the work week and loss of tolerance over the weekend, resulting in tachycardia, dizziness, and headache on reexposure.

Malignant hypertension treatment

Nitroprusside	Short acting; ↑ cGMP via direct release of NO. Can cause cyanide toxicity (releases CN).
Fenoldopam	Dopamine D_1 receptor agonist—relaxes renal vascular smooth muscle.
Diazoxide	K^+ channel opener—hyperpolarizes and relaxes vascular smooth muscle. Can cause hyperglycemia (reduces insulin release).

Antianginal therapy

Goal—reduction of myocardial O_2 consumption (MVO_2) by decreasing 1 or more of the determinants of MVO_2: end diastolic volume, blood pressure, heart rate, contractility, ejection time.

Component	Nitrates (affect preload)	β-blockers (affect afterload)	Nitrates + β-blockers
End diastolic volume	↓	↑	No effect or ↓
Blood pressure	↓	↓	↓
Contractility	↑ (reflex response)	↓	Little/no effect
Heart rate	↑ (reflex response)	↓	↓
Ejection time	↓	↑	Little/no effect
MVO_2	↓	↓	↓↓

Calcium channel blockers—**N**ifedipine is similar to **N**itrates in effect; verapamil is similar to β-blockers in effect.

Note: Pindolol and acebutolol are partial β-agonists—contraindicated in angina.

Lipid-lowering agents

Drug	Effect on LDL "Bad Cholesterol"	Effect on HDL "Good Cholesterol"	Effect on Triglycerides	Mechanisms of Action	Side Effects/ Problems
HMG-CoA reductase inhibitors (lovastatin, pravastatin, simvastatin, atorvastatin, rosuvastatin)	↓↓↓	↑	↓	Inhibit cholesterol precursor, mevalonate	Hepatotoxicity (↑ LFTs), rhabdomyolysis
Niacin	↓↓	↑↑	↓	Inhibits lipolysis in adipose tissue; reduces hepatic VLDL secretion into circulation	Red, flushed face, which is ↓ by aspirin or long-term use Hyperglycemia (acanthosis nigricans) Hyperuricemia (exacerbates gout)
Bile acid resins (cholestyramine, colestipol, colesevelam)	↓↓	Slightly ↑	Slightly ↑	Prevent intestinal reabsorption of bile acids; liver must use cholesterol to make more	Patients hate it—tastes bad and causes GI discomfort, ↓ absorption of fat-soluble vitamins Cholesterol gallstones
Cholesterol absorption blockers (ezetimibe)	↓↓	–	–	Prevent cholesterol reabsorption at small intestine brush border	Rare ↑ LFTs
"Fibrates" (gemfibrozil, clofibrate, bezafibrate, fenofibrate)	↓	↑	↓↓↓	Upregulate LPL → ↑ TG clearance	Myositis, hepatotoxicity (↑ LFTs), cholesterol gallstones

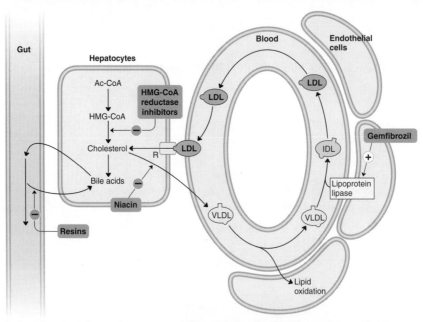

(Adapted, with permission, from Katzung BG, Trevor AJ. *USMLE Road Map: Pharmacology*, 1st ed. New York: McGraw-Hill, 2003: 56.)

Cardiac drugs: sites of action

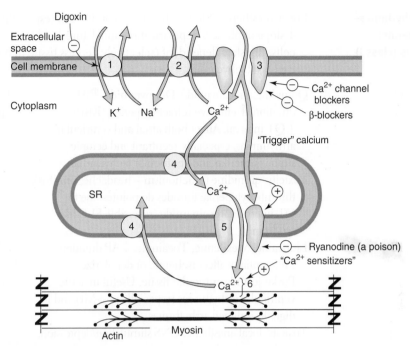

(Adapted, with permission, from Katzung BG. *Basic and Clinical Pharmacology*, 7th ed. Stamford, CT: Appleton & Lange, 1997: 198.)

Cardiac sarcomere is shown above with the cellular components involved in excitation-contraction coupling. Factors involved in excitation-contraction coupling are numbered. (1) Na^+/K^+ ATPase; (2) Na^+-Ca^{2+} exchanger; (3) voltage-gated (L-type) calcium channel; (4) calcium pump in the wall of the sarcoplasmic reticulum (SR); (5) ryanodine receptors and calcium release channels in the SR, which are closely coupled to L-type calcium channels in the cell membrane; (6) site of calcium interaction with troponin-tropomyosin system.

β_1 receptors are G_s and activate protein kinase A, which phosphorylates L-type Ca^{2+} channels and phospholamban, both of which $\uparrow$ intracellular Ca^{2+} during contraction.

Cardiac glycosides	Digoxin—75% bioavailability, 20–40% protein bound, $t_{1/2}$ = 40 hours, urinary excretion.
Mechanism	Direct inhibition of Na^+/K^+ ATPase leads to indirect inhibition of Na^+/Ca^{2+} exchanger/ antiport. $\uparrow$ [Ca^{2+}]$_i$ → positive inotropy. Stimulates vagus nerve.
Clinical use	CHF ($\uparrow$ contractility); atrial fibrillation ($\downarrow$ conduction at AV node and depression of SA node).
Toxicity	Cholinergic—nausea, vomiting, diarrhea, blurry yellow vision (think Van Gogh). ECG—$\uparrow$ PR, $\downarrow$ QT, scooping, T-wave inversion, arrhythmia, hyperkalemia. Worsened by renal failure ($\downarrow$ excretion), hypokalemia (permissive for digoxin binding at K$^+$-binding site on Na^+/K^+ ATPase), quinidine ($\downarrow$ digoxin clearance; displaces digoxin from tissue-binding sites).
Antidote	Slowly normalize K$^+$, lidocaine, cardiac pacer, anti-dig Fab fragments, Mg^{2+}.

Antiarrhythmics—Na⁺ channel blockers (class I)

Local anesthetics. Slow or block (↓) conduction (especially in depolarized cells). ↓ slope of phase 0 depolarization and ↑ threshold for firing in abnormal pacemaker cells. Are state dependent (selectively depress tissue that is frequently depolarized, e.g., fast tachycardia).

Class IA

Quinidine, Procainamide, Disopyramide. ↑ AP duration, ↑ effective refractory period (ERP), ↑ QT interval. Affect both atrial and ventricular arrhythmias, especially reentrant and ectopic supraventricular and ventricular tachycardia.

Toxicity: quinidine (cinchonism—headache, tinnitus); thrombocytopenia; torsades de pointes due to ↑ QT interval; procainamide (reversible SLE-like syndrome).

"The Queen Proclaims Diso's pyramid."

Class IB

Lidocaine, Mexiletine, Tocainide. ↓ AP duration. Preferentially affect ischemic or depolarized Purkinje and ventricular tissue. Useful in acute ventricular arrhythmias (especially post-MI) and in digitalis-induced arrhythmias.

Toxicity: local anesthetic. CNS stimulation/depression, cardiovascular depression.

"I'd Buy Lidy's Mexican Tacos." Phenytoin can also fall into the IB category.

Class IC

Flecainide, Encainide, Propafenone. No effect on AP duration. Useful in V-tachs that progress to VF and in intractable SVT. Usually used only as last resort in refractory tachyarrhythmias. For patients without structural abnormalities.

Toxicity: proarrhythmic, especially post-MI (contraindicated). Significantly prolongs refractory period in AV node.

"Chipotle's Food has Excellent Produce."
IB is Best post-MI.
IC is Contraindicated post-MI.

Hyperkalemia causes ↑ toxicity for all class I drugs.

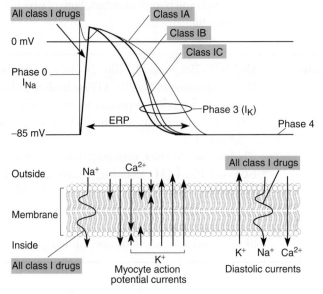

(Adapted, with permission, from Katzung BG, Trevor AJ. *Pharmacology: Examination & Board Review*, 5th ed. Stamford, CT: Appleton & Lange, 1998: 118.)

Antiarrhythmics—β-blockers (class II)	Propranolol, esmolol, metoprolol, atenolol, timolol.
Mechanism	↓ cAMP, ↓ Ca^{2+} currents. Suppress abnormal pacemakers by ↓ slope of phase 4. AV node particularly sensitive—↑ PR interval. Esmolol very short acting.
Clinical use	V-tach, SVT, slowing ventricular rate during atrial fibrillation and atrial flutter.
Toxicity	Impotence, exacerbation of asthma, cardiovascular effects (bradycardia, AV block, CHF), CNS effects (sedation, sleep alterations). May mask the signs of hypoglycemia. Metoprolol can cause dyslipidemia. Treat overdose with glucagon.

Antiarrhythmics—K^+ channel blockers (class III)	Sotalol, ibutilide, bretylium, dofetilide, amiodarone.	
Mechanism	↑ AP duration, ↑ ERP. Used when other antiarrhythmics fail. ↑ QT interval.	
Toxicity	Sotalol—torsades de pointes, excessive β block; ibutilide—torsades; bretylium—new arrhythmias, hypotension; amiodarone—**pulmonary fibrosis, hepatotoxicity, hypothyroidism/hyperthyroidism** (amiodarone is 40% iodine by weight), corneal deposits, skin deposits (blue/gray) resulting in photodermatitis, neurologic effects, constipation, cardiovascular effects (bradycardia, heart block, CHF). Amiodarone has class I, II, III, and IV effects because it alters the lipid membrane.	Remember to check **PFT**s, **LFT**s, and **TFT**s when using amiodarone.

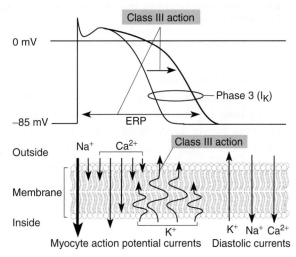

(Adapted, with permission, from Katzung BG, Trevor AJ. *Pharmacology: Examination & Board Review,* 5th ed. Stamford, CT: Appleton & Lange, 1998: 120.)

Antiarrhythmics—
Ca²⁺ channel
blockers (class IV)

Verapamil, diltiazem.

    Mechanism

↓ conduction velocity, ↑ ERP, ↑ PR interval. Used in prevention of nodal arrhythmias (e.g., SVT).

    Toxicity

Constipation, flushing, edema, CV effects (CHF, AV block, sinus node depression).

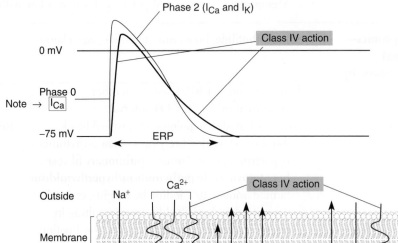

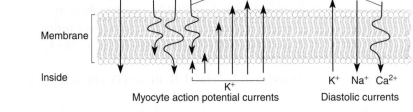

(Adapted, with permission, from Katzung BG, Trevor AJ. *Pharmacology: Examination & Board Review,* 5th ed. Stamford, CT: Appleton & Lange, 1998: 121.)

Other antiarrhythmics

    Adenosine

↑ K⁺ out of cells → hyperpolarizing the cell + ↓ I_{Ca}. Drug of choice in diagnosing/abolishing supraventricular tachycardia. Very short acting (∼ 15 sec). Toxicity includes flushing, hypotension, chest pain. Effects blocked by theophylline.

    K⁺

Depresses ectopic pacemakers in hypokalemia (e.g., digoxin toxicity).

    Mg²⁺

Effective in torsades de pointes and digoxin toxicity.

Endocrine

"Chocolate causes certain endocrine glands to secrete hormones that affect your feelings and behavior by making you happy."

—Elaine Sherman, *Book of Divine Indulgences*

▶ Anatomy

▶ Physiology

▶ Pathology

▶ Pharmacology

Adrenal cortex and medulla

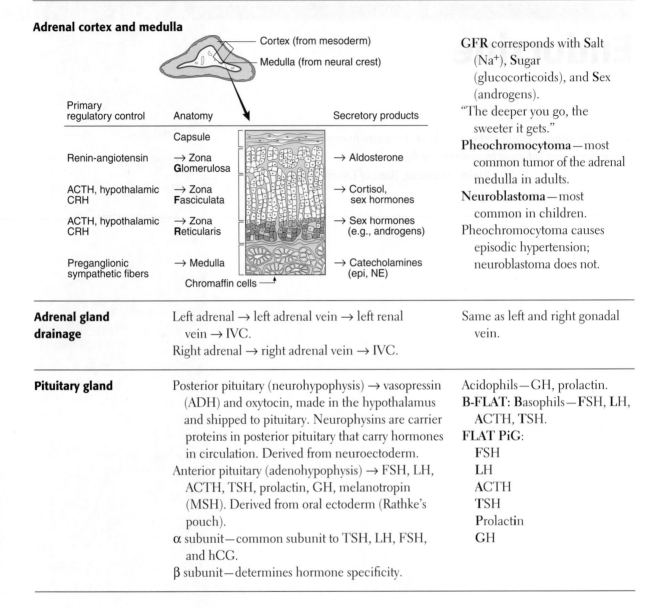

Primary regulatory control	Anatomy	Secretory products
	Capsule	
Renin-angiotensin	→ Zona **G**lomerulosa	→ Aldosterone
ACTH, hypothalamic CRH	→ Zona **F**asciculata	→ Cortisol, sex hormones
ACTH, hypothalamic CRH	→ Zona **R**eticularis	→ Sex hormones (e.g., androgens)
Preganglionic sympathetic fibers	→ Medulla	→ Catecholamines (epi, NE)
	Chromaffin cells —	

Cortex (from mesoderm)
Medulla (from neural crest)

GFR corresponds with **S**alt (Na⁺), **S**ugar (glucocorticoids), and **S**ex (androgens).
"The deeper you go, the sweeter it gets."
Pheochromocytoma—most common tumor of the adrenal medulla in adults.
Neuroblastoma—most common in children.
Pheochromocytoma causes episodic hypertension; neuroblastoma does not.

Adrenal gland drainage

Left adrenal → left adrenal vein → left renal vein → IVC.
Right adrenal → right adrenal vein → IVC.

Same as left and right gonadal vein.

Pituitary gland

Posterior pituitary (neurohypophysis) → vasopressin (ADH) and oxytocin, made in the hypothalamus and shipped to pituitary. Neurophysins are carrier proteins in posterior pituitary that carry hormones in circulation. Derived from neuroectoderm.
Anterior pituitary (adenohypophysis) → FSH, LH, ACTH, TSH, prolactin, GH, melanotropin (MSH). Derived from oral ectoderm (Rathke's pouch).
α subunit—common subunit to TSH, LH, FSH, and hCG.
β subunit—determines hormone specificity.

Acidophils—GH, prolactin.
B-FLAT: Basophils—**F**SH, **L**H, **A**CTH, **T**SH.
FLAT PiG:
FSH
LH
ACTH
TSH
Prolactin
GH

| **Endocrine pancreas cell types** | Islets of Langerhans are collections of α, β, and δ endocrine cells (most numerous in tail of pancreas). Islets arise from pancreatic buds. α = glucagon (peripheral); β = insulin (central); δ = somatostatin (interspersed). | INSulin (β cells) INSide. |

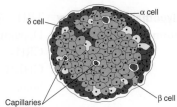

| **Insulin** | Made in β cells of pancreas in response to ATP from glucose metabolism closing K$^+$ channels and depolarizing cells. Required for adipose and skeletal muscle uptake of glucose. | Insulin moves glucose Into cells. |

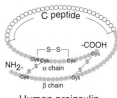

Human proinsulin

Made in β cells of pancreas in response to ATP from glucose metabolism closing K$^+$ channels and depolarizing cells. Required for adipose and skeletal muscle uptake of glucose.

Inhibits glucagon release by α cells of pancreas.

Serum C-peptide is not present with exogenous insulin intake (proinsulin → insulin + C-peptide).

Anabolic effects of insulin:
1. ↑ glucose transport
2. ↑ glycogen synthesis and storage
3. ↑ triglyceride synthesis and storage
4. ↑ Na$^+$ retention (kidneys)
5. ↑ protein synthesis (muscles)
6. ↑ cellular uptake of K$^+$ and amino acids

Insulin moves glucose Into cells.

BRICK L (don't need insulin for glucose uptake):
Brain
RBCs
Intestine
Cornea
Kidney
Liver

GLUT-1: RBCs, brain.

GLUT-2 (bidirectional): β islet cells, liver, kidney, small intestine.

GLUT-4 (insulin responsive): adipose tissue, skeletal muscle.

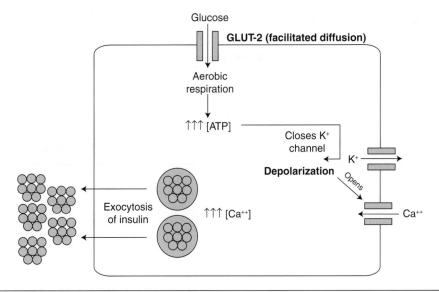

| **Insulin-dependent organs** | Skeletal muscle and adipose tissue depend on insulin for ↑ glucose uptake (GLUT-4). Brain and RBCs take up glucose independent of insulin levels (GLUT-1). Brain depends on glucose for metabolism under normal circumstances and uses ketone bodies in starvation. RBCs always depend on glucose. |

Hypothalamic-pituitary hormone regulation	TRH—⊕→ TSH, prolactin. Dopamine—⊖→ prolactin. CRH—⊕→ ACTH. GHRH—⊕→ GH. Somatostatin—⊖→ GH, TSH. GnRH—⊕→ FSH, LH. Prolactin—⊖→ GnRH.

Prolactin regulation

Regulation—prolactin secretion from anterior pituitary is tonically inhibited by dopamine from hypothalamus. Prolactin in turn inhibits its own secretion by increasing dopamine synthesis and secretion from hypothalamus. TRH ↑ prolactin secretion.

Function—stimulates milk production in breast; inhibits ovulation (in females) and spermatogenesis (in males) by inhibiting GnRH synthesis and release.

Dopamine agonists (bromocriptine) inhibit prolactin secretion and can be used in treatment of prolactinoma.

Dopamine antagonists (most antipsychotics) and estrogens (OCPs, pregnancy) stimulate prolactin secretion.

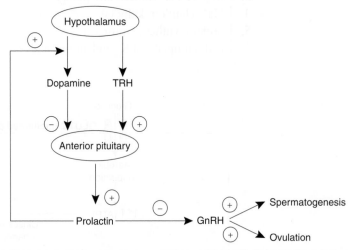

Adrenal steroids

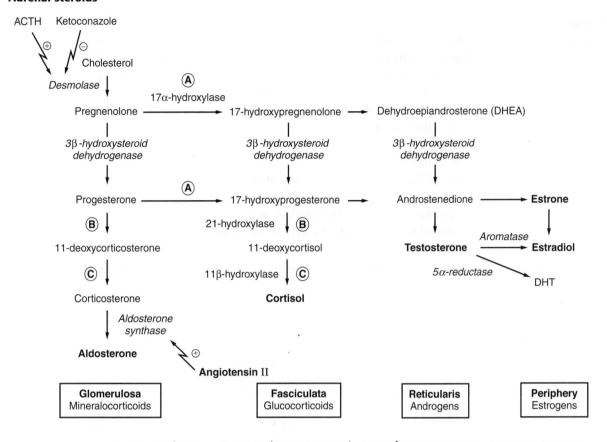

Congenital bilateral adrenal hyperplasias*

A = 17α-hydroxylase deficiency. ↓ sex hormones, ↓ cortisol, ↑ mineralocorticoids. Sx = **HYPER**tension, hypokalemia. XY: ↓ DHT → pseudohermaphroditism (externally phenotypic female, no internal reproductive structures due to MIF). XX: externally phenotypic female with normal internal sex organs, but lacking 2° sexual characteristics ("sexual infantilism").

B = 21-hydroxylase deficiency. Most common form. ↓ cortisol (increased ACTH), ↓ mineralocorticoids, ↑ sex hormones. Sx = masculinization, female pseudohermaphroditism, **HYPO**tension, hyperkalemia, ↑ plasma renin activity, and volume depletion. Salt wasting can lead to hypovolemic shock in the newborn.

C = 11ß-hydroxylase deficiency. ↓ cortisol, ↓ aldosterone and corticosterone, ↑ sex hormones. Sx = masculinization, **HYPER**tension (like aldosterone, 11-deoxycorticosterone is a mineralocorticoid and is secreted in excess).

*All congenital adrenal enzyme deficiencies are characterized by an enlargement of the adrenal glands due to an ↑ in ACTH stimulation because of the ↓ levels of cortisol.

Cortisol

Source	Adrenal zona fasciculata.	Bound to corticosteroid-binding globulin (CBG).
Function	Cortisol is **BBIIG:**	Chronic stress induces prolonged secretion.

Function — Cortisol is **BBIIG:**

1. Maintains **B**lood pressure (permissive effect with epinephrine—upregulates α_1 receptors on arterioles)
2. ↓ **B**one formation
3. Anti-**I**nflammatory
4. ↓ **I**mmune function
5. ↑ **G**luconeogenesis, lipolysis, proteolysis

Regulation — CRH (hypothalamus) stimulates ACTH release (pituitary), causing cortisol production in adrenal zona fasciculata. Excess cortisol ↓ CRH, ACTH, and cortisol secretion.

PTH

Source	Chief cells of parathyroid.
Function	1. ↑ bone resorption of calcium and phosphate
	2. ↑ kidney reabsorption of calcium in distal convoluted tubule
	3. ↓ kidney reabsorption of phosphate
	4. ↑ 1,25-(OH)$_2$ vitamin D (calcitriol) production by stimulating kidney 1α-hydroxylase
Regulation	↓ free serum Ca^{2+} ↑ PTH secretion.
	↓ free serum Mg^{2+} ↓ PTH secretion.
	Common causes of ↓ Mg^{2+} include diarrhea, aminoglycosides, diuretics, and alcohol abuse.

PTH ↑ serum Ca^{2+}, ↓ serum (PO$_4$)$^{3-}$, ↑ urine (PO$_4$)$^{3-}$.
↑ production of M-CSF and RANK-L in osteoBLASTS, stimulating osteoCLASTS.
PTH = **P**hosphate **T**rashing **H**ormone.

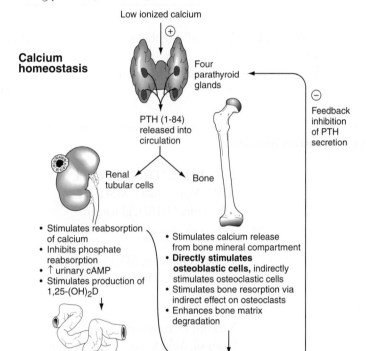

Calcium homeostasis

Low ionized calcium
(+)

Four parathyroid glands

⊖ Feedback inhibition of PTH secretion

PTH (1-84) released into circulation

Renal tubular cells   Bone

• Stimulates reabsorption of calcium
• Inhibits phosphate reabsorption
• ↑ urinary cAMP
• Stimulates production of 1,25-(OH)$_2$D

• Stimulates calcium release from bone mineral compartment
• **Directly stimulates osteoblastic cells,** indirectly stimulates osteoclastic cells
• Stimulates bone resorption via indirect effect on osteoclasts
• Enhances bone matrix degradation

• Increases intestinal calcium absorption → Increases serum calcium

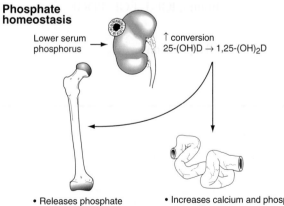

Phosphate homeostasis

Lower serum phosphorus → ↑ conversion 25-(OH)D → 1,25-(OH)$_2$D

• Releases phosphate from matrix

• Increases calcium and phosphate absorption

(Adapted, with permission, from Chandrasoma P et al. *Concise Pathology,* 3rd ed. Stamford, CT: Appleton & Lange, 1998.)

Vitamin D (cholecalciferol)

Source	Vitamin D_3 from sun exposure in skin. D_2 ingested from plants. Both converted to 25-OH vitamin D in liver and to $1,25\text{-}(OH)_2$ vitamin D (active form) in kidney.	Vitamin D deficiency causes rickets in kids and osteomalacia in adults. $24,25\text{-}(OH)_2$ vitamin D is an inactive form of vitamin D. PTH ↑ calcium reabsorption and ↓ phosphate reabsorption, while $1,25\text{-}(OH)_2$ vitamin D ↑ absorption of **both** calcium and phosphate.
Function	1. ↑ absorption of dietary calcium and phosphate 2. ↑ bone resorption of Ca^{2+} and $(PO_4)^{3-}$	
Regulation	↑ PTH, ↓ $[Ca^{2+}]$, ↓ phosphate cause ↑ $1,25\text{-}(OH)_2$ vitamin D production. $1,25\text{-}(OH)_2$ vitamin D feedback inhibits it own production.	

Calcitonin

Source	Parafollicular cells (C cells) of thyroid.	Calcitonin opposes actions of PTH. Not important in normal calcium homeostasis. Calci**TON**in **TON**es down calcium levels.
Function	↓ bone resorption of calcium.	
Regulation	↑ serum Ca^{2+} causes calcitonin secretion.	

Signaling pathways of endocrine hormones

cAMP	FSH, LH, ACTH, TSH, CRH, hCG, ADH (V_2 receptor), MSH, PTH, calcitonin, GHRH, glucagon	**"FLAT CHAMP"**
cGMP	ANP, NO (EDRF)	Think vasodilators
IP_3	GnRH, Oxytocin, ADH (V_1 receptor), TRH	**"GOAT"**
Steroid receptor		
Cytosolic	Vitamin D, Estrogen, Testosterone, Cortisol, Aldosterone, Progesterone	**"VET CAP"**
Nuclear	T_3/T_4	
Intrinsic tyrosine kinase (MAP kinase pathway)	Insulin, IGF-1, FGF, PDGF	Think growth factors
Receptor-associated tyrosine kinase (JAK/STAT pathway)	GH, prolactin	Also cytokine IL-2

Steroid/thyroid hormone mechanism

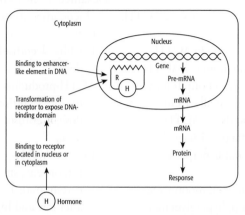

Cytoplasm

Nucleus

Gene
Pre-mRNA
mRNA
mRNA
Protein
Response

Binding to enhancer-like element in DNA

Transformation of receptor to expose DNA-binding domain

Binding to receptor located in nucleus or in cytoplasm

H Hormone

(Adapted, with permission, from Ganong WF. *Review of Medical Physiology,* 22th ed. New York: McGraw-Hill, 2005, Fig. 1-35.)

In men, $\uparrow$ levels of sex hormone–binding globulin (SHBG) lower free testosterone $\rightarrow$ gynecomastia.
In women, $\downarrow$ SHBG raises free testosterone $\rightarrow$ hirsutism.

Steroid hormones are lipophilic and relatively insoluble in plasma; therefore, they must circulate bound to specific binding globulins, which $\uparrow$ solubility and allow for $\uparrow$ delivery of steroid to the target organ. The need for gene transcription and protein synthesis delays the onset of action of these hormones.

Thyroid hormones (T_3/T_4)

Iodine-containing hormones that control the body's metabolic rate.

Source	Follicles of thyroid. Most T_3 formed in blood.
Function	1. Bone growth (synergism with GH)
	2. CNS maturation
	3. $\uparrow$ β_1 receptors in heart = $\uparrow$ CO, HR, SV, contractility
	4. $\uparrow$ basal metabolic rate via $\uparrow$ Na^+/K^+-ATPase activity = $\uparrow$ O_2 consumption, RR, body temperature
	5. $\uparrow$ glycogenolysis, gluconeogenesis, lipolysis
Regulation	TRH (hypothalamus) stimulates TSH (pituitary), which stimulates follicular cells. Negative feedback by free T_3 to anterior pituitary $\downarrow$ sensitivity to TRH. TSI, like TSH, stimulates follicular cells (Graves' disease).

T_3 functions—4 **B**'s:
Brain maturation
Bone growth
Beta-adrenergic effects
BMR $\uparrow$

Thyroxine-binding globulin (TBG) binds most T_3/T_4 in blood; only free hormone is active. $\downarrow$ TBG in hepatic failure; $\uparrow$ TBG in pregnancy or OCP use (estrogen $\uparrow$ TBG).

T_4 is major product; converted to T_3 by peripheral tissue.

T_3 binds receptors with greater affinity than T_4.

Peroxidase is enzyme responsible for oxidation and organification of iodide as well as coupling of MIT and DIT.

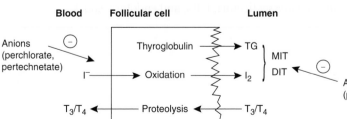

Blood   Follicular cell   Lumen

Anions (perchlorate, pertechnetate)

Thyroglobulin → TG
I^- → Oxidation → I_2

MIT
DIT

Antithyroid drugs (propylthiouracil, methimazole)

T_3/T_4 ← Proteolysis ← T_3/T_4

Cushing's syndrome

↑ cortisol due to a variety of causes.
Exogenous (iatrogenic) steroids—#1 cause; ↓ ACTH.
Endogenous causes:
1. **Cushing's disease** (70%)—due to ACTH secretion from pituitary adenoma; ↑ ACTH
2. **Ectopic ACTH** (15%)—from nonpituitary tissue making ACTH (e.g., small cell lung cancer, bronchial carcinoids); ↑ ACTH
3. **Adrenal** (15%)—adenoma (see Image 68), carcinoma, nodular adrenal hyperplasia; ↓ ACTH

Findings: hypertension, weight gain, moon facies, truncal obesity, buffalo hump, hyperglycemia (insulin resistance), skin changes (thinning, striae), osteoporosis, amenorrhea, and immune suppression (see Image 70).

Dexamethasone (synthetic glucocorticoid) suppression test:
Healthy: ↓ cortisol after low dose.
ACTH-producing pituitary tumor: ↑ cortisol after low dose; ↓ cortisol after high dose.
Ectopic ACTH-producing tumor (e.g., small cell carcinoma): ↑ cortisol after low and high dose.
Cortisol-producing tumor: ↑ cortisol after low and high dose.

Hyperaldosteronism

Primary (Conn's syndrome)

Caused by an aldosterone-secreting tumor, resulting in hypertension, hypokalemia, metabolic alkalosis, and **low** plasma renin. May be bilateral or unilateral.

Treatment: surgery to remove the tumor and/or spironolactone, a K^+-sparing diuretic that works by acting as an aldosterone antagonist.

Secondary

Kidney perception of low intravascular volume results in an overactive renin-angiotensin system. Due to renal artery stenosis, chronic renal failure, CHF, cirrhosis, or nephrotic syndrome. Associated with **high** plasma renin.

Addison's disease

Chronic 1° adrenal insufficiency due to adrenal atrophy or destruction by disease (e.g., autoimmune, TB, metastasis). Deficiency of aldosterone and cortisol, causing hypotension (hyponatremic volume contraction), hyperkalemia, acidosis, and skin hyperpigmentation (due to MSH, a by-product of ↑ ACTH production from POMC). Characterized by **A**drenal **A**trophy and **A**bsence of hormone production; involves **A**ll 3 cortical divisions (spares medulla). Distinguish from 2° adrenal insufficiency (↓ pituitary ACTH production), which has no skin hyperpigmentation and no hyperkalemia.

Waterhouse-Friderichsen syndrome

Acute 1° adrenal insufficiency due to adrenal hemorrhage associated with *Neisseria meningitidis* septicemia, DIC, and endotoxic shock.

Pheochromocytoma	Most common tumor of the adrenal medulla in adults. Derived from chromaffin cells (arise from neural crest; see Image 69).	Rule of 10's:

Pheochromocytoma — Most common tumor of the adrenal medulla in adults. Derived from chromaffin cells (arise from neural crest; see Image 69).

Most tumors secrete epinephrine, NE, and dopamine and can cause episodic hypertension. Urinary VMA (a breakdown product of norepinephrine) and plasma catecholamines are elevated. Associated with neurofibromatosis, MEN types 2A and 2B. Treatment: α-antagonists, especially **phenoxybenzamine**, a nonselective, **irreversible** α-blocker, followed by surgery to remove the tumor.

Episodic hyperadrenergic symptoms (**5 P's**):
Pressure (elevated blood pressure)
Pain (headache)
Perspiration
Palpitations (tachycardia)
Pallor

Rule of 10's:
10% malignant
10% bilateral
10% extra-adrenal
10% calcify
10% kids
10% familial
Symptoms occur in "spells"— relapse and remit.

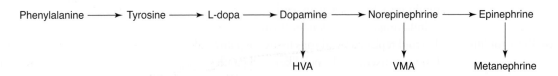

Phenylalanine ⟶ Tyrosine ⟶ L-dopa ⟶ Dopamine ⟶ Norepinephrine ⟶ Epinephrine

Dopamine ↓ HVA   Norepinephrine ↓ VMA   Epinephrine ↓ Metanephrine

Neuroblastoma — The most common tumor of the adrenal medulla in children. Can occur anywhere along the sympathetic chain. Homovanillic acid (HVA), a breakdown product of dopamine, elevated in urine. Less likely to develop hypertension. Overexpression of N-*myc* oncogene associated with rapid tumor progression.

Hypothyroidism vs. hyperthyroidism

	Hypothyroidism	Hyperthyroidism
Signs/symptoms	Cold intolerance (↓ heat production)	Heat intolerance (↑ heat production)
	Weight gain, ↓ appetite	Weight loss, ↑ appetite
	Hypoactivity, lethargy, fatigue, weakness	Hyperactivity
	Constipation	Diarrhea
	↓ reflexes	↑ reflexes
	Myxedema (facial/periorbital)	Pretibial myxedema (Graves' disease)
	Dry, cool skin; coarse, brittle hair	Warm, moist skin; fine hair
	Bradycardia, dyspnea on exertion	Chest pain, palpitations, arrhythmias
Lab findings	↑ TSH (sensitive test for 1° hypothyroidism)	↓ TSH (if 1°)
	↓ total T_4	↑ total T_4
	↓ free T_4	↑ free T_4
	↓ T_3 uptake	↑ T_3 uptake

Hypothyroidism

Hashimoto's thyroiditis	Most common cause of hypothyroidism; an autoimmune disorder (antimicrosomal, antithyroglobulin antibodies). Associated with HLA-DR5. Histology: Hürthle cells, lymphocytic infiltrate with germinal centers. Findings: moderately enlarged, nontender thyroid.	May be hyperthyroid early in course (thyrotoxicosis during follicular rupture).
Cretinism	Due to severe fetal hypothyroidism. Endemic cretinism occurs wherever endemic goiter is prevalent (lack of dietary iodine); sporadic cretinism is caused by defect in T_4 formation or developmental failure in thyroid formation. Findings: pot-bellied, pale, puffy-faced child with protruding umbilicus and protuberant tongue.	Cretin means Christlike (French *chrétien*). Those affected were considered so mentally retarded as to be incapable of sinning. Still common in China.
Subacute thyroiditis (de Quervain's)	Self-limited hypothyroidism often following a flulike illness. Histology: granulomatous inflammation. Findings: ↑ ESR, jaw pain, early inflammation, very tender thyroid.	May be hyperthyroid early in course.
Riedel's thyroiditis	Thyroid replaced by fibrous tissue (hypothyroid). Findings: fixed, hard (rock-like), and painless goiter.	

Hyperthyroidism

Graves' disease	An autoimmune hyperthyroidism with thyroid-stimulating/TSH receptor antibodies. Ophthalmopathy (proptosis, EOM swelling), pretibial myxedema, diffuse goiter. Often presents during stress (e.g., childbirth) (see Image 71).	Graves' is a type II hypersensitivity.
Thyrotoxicosis	Stress-induced catecholamine surge leading to death by arrhythmia. Seen as a serious complication of Graves' and other hyperthyroid disorders.	
Toxic multinodular goiter	Focal patches of hyperfunctioning follicular cells working independently of TSH due to mutation in TSH receptor (see Image 105). ↑ release of T_3 and T_4. Hot nodules are rarely malignant. Jod-Basedow phenomenon—thyrotoxicosis if a patient with iodine deficiency goiter is made iodine replete.	

Thyroid cancer	1. Papillary carcinoma—most common, excellent prognosis, "ground-glass" nuclei (Orphan Annie), psammoma bodies, nuclear grooves. ↑ risk with childhood irradiation. 2. Follicular carcinoma—good prognosis, uniform follicles. 3. Medullary carcinoma—from parafollicular "C cells"; produces calcitonin, sheets of cells in amyloid stroma. Associated with MEN types 2A and 2B. 4. Undifferentiated/anaplastic—older patients; very poor prognosis. 5. Lymphoma—associated with Hashimoto's thyroiditis.

Hyperparathyroidism

Primary
Usually an adenoma. **Hypercalcemia**, hypercalciuria (**renal stones**), hypophosphatemia, ↑ PTH, ↑ alkaline phosphatase, ↑ cAMP in urine. Often asymptomatic, or may present with weakness and constipation ("**groans**").

"**Stones, bones, and groans.**"
Osteitis fibrosa cystica— cystic bone spaces filled with brown fibrous tissue (**bone pain**).

Secondary
2° hyperplasia due to ↓ gut Ca^{2+} absorption and ↑ phosphorus, most often in chronic renal disease (causes hypovitaminosis D → ↓ Ca^{2+} absorption). **Hypocalcemia**, hyperphosphatemia, ↑ alkaline phosphatase, ↑ PTH.

Renal osteodystrophy—bone lesions due to 2° or 3° hyperparathyroidism due in turn to renal disease.

Tertiary
Refractory (autonomous) hyperparathyroidism resulting from chronic renal disease. ↑↑ PTH, ↑ Ca^{2+}.

Hypoparathyroidism

Due to accidental surgical excision (thyroid surgery), autoimmune destruction, or DiGeorge syndrome. Findings: hypocalcemia, tetany.
Chvostek's sign—tapping of facial nerve → contraction of facial muscles.
Trousseau's sign—occlusion of brachial artery with BP cuff → carpal spasm.

Pseudohypoparathyroidism (Albright's hereditary osteodystrophy)— autosomal-dominant kidney unresponsiveness to PTH. Hypocalcemia, shortened 4th/5th digits, short stature.

PTH and calcium pathologies

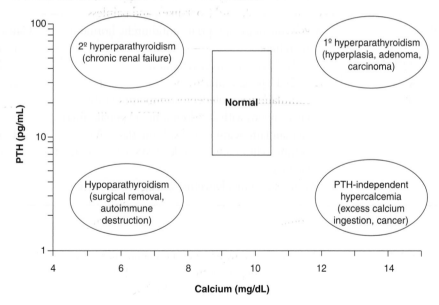

Pituitary adenoma   Most commonly prolactinoma. Findings: amenorrhea, galactorrhea, low libido, infertility (↓ GnRH). Bromocriptine or cabergoline (dopamine agonists) causes shrinkage of prolactinomas. Can impinge on optic chiasm → bitemporal hemianopia.

Acromegaly   Excess GH in adults. Findings: large tongue with deep furrows, deep voice, large hands and feet, coarse facial features, impaired glucose tolerance (insulin resistance). ↑ GH in children → gigantism (↑ linear bone growth). Treatment: pituitary adenoma resection followed by octreotide administration.   ↑ GH is normal in stress, exercise, and hypoglycemia. Diagnosis: ↑ serum IGF-1; failure to suppress serum GH following oral glucose tolerance test.

Diabetes insipidus   Characterized by intense thirst and polyuria together with an inability to concentrate urine owing to lack of ADH (central DI—pituitary tumor, trauma, surgery, histiocytosis X) or to a lack of renal response to ADH (nephrogenic DI—hereditary or 2° to hypercalcemia, lithium, demeclocycline [ADH antagonist]).

Diagnosis   Water deprivation test—urine osmolality doesn't ↑. Response to desmopressin distinguishes between central and nephrogenic.

Findings   Urine specific gravity < 1.006; serum osmolality > 290 mOsm/L.

Treatment   Adequate fluid intake. For central DI—intranasal desmopressin (ADH analog). For nephrogenic DI—hydrochlorothiazide, indomethacin, or amiloride.

SIADH   Syndrome of inappropriate antidiuretic hormone secretion:
1. Excessive water retention
2. Hyponatremia
3. Urine osmolarity > serum osmolarity

Body responds with ↓ aldosterone (hyponatremia) to maintain near-normal volume status. Very low serum sodium levels can lead to seizures (correct slowly).

Treatment: demeclocycline or H_2O restriction.

Causes include:
1. Ectopic ADH (small cell lung cancer)
2. CNS disorders/head trauma
3. Pulmonary disease
4. Drugs (e.g., cyclophosphamide)

Diabetes mellitus

Acute manifestations Polydipsia, polyuria, polyphagia, weight loss, DKA (type 1), hyperosmolar coma (type 2), unopposed secretion of GH and epinephrine (exacerbating hyperglycemia).

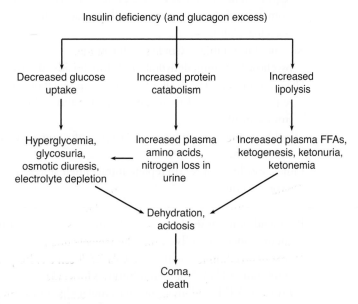

Insulin deficiency (and glucagon excess)

Decreased glucose uptake → Hyperglycemia, glycosuria, osmotic diuresis, electrolyte depletion

Increased protein catabolism → Increased plasma amino acids, nitrogen loss in urine

Increased lipolysis → Increased plasma FFAs, ketogenesis, ketonuria, ketonemia

Dehydration, acidosis

Coma, death

Chronic manifestations

Nonenzymatic glycosylation:
1. Small vessel disease (diffuse thickening of basement membrane) → retinopathy (hemorrhage, exudates, microaneurysms, vessel proliferation), glaucoma, nephropathy (nodular sclerosis, progressive proteinuria, chronic renal failure, arteriosclerosis leading to hypertension, Kimmelstiel-Wilson nodules)
2. Large vessel atherosclerosis, CAD, peripheral vascular occlusive disease, and gangrene → limb loss, cerebrovascular disease

Osmotic damage:
1. Neuropathy (motor, sensory, and autonomic degeneration)
2. Cataracts (sorbitol accumulation)

Tests Fasting serum glucose, glucose tolerance test, HbA_{1c} (measures long-term diabetic control).

Type 1 vs. type 2 diabetes mellitus

Variable	Type 1 (juvenile onset, IDDM)	Type 2 (adult onset, NIDDM)
1° defect	Viral or immune destruction of β cells (see Image 67)	↑ resistance to insulin
Insulin necessary in treatment	Always	Sometimes
Age (exceptions commonly occur)	< 30	> 40
Association with obesity	No	Yes
Genetic predisposition	Weak, polygenic	Strong, polygenic
Association with HLA system	Yes (HLA-DR3 and 4)	No
Glucose intolerance	Severe	Mild to moderate
Insulin sensitivity	High	Low
Ketoacidosis	Common	Rare
β-cell numbers in the islets	↓	Variable (with amyloid deposits)
Serum insulin level	↓	Variable
Classic symptoms of polyuria, polydipsia, thirst, weight loss	Common	Sometimes
Histology	Islet leukocytic infiltrate	Islet amyloid deposit

Diabetic ketoacidosis	One of the most important complications of type 1 diabetes. Usually due to ↑ insulin requirements from ↑ stress (e.g., infection). Excess fat breakdown and ↑ ketogenesis from ↑ free fatty acids, which are then made into ketone bodies (β-hydroxybutyrate > acetoacetate).
Signs/symptoms	Kussmaul respirations (rapid/deep breathing), nausea/vomiting, abdominal pain, psychosis/delirium, dehydration. Fruity breath odor (due to exhaled acetone).
Labs	Hyperglycemia, ↑ H^+, ↓ HCO_3^- (anion gap metabolic acidosis), ↑ blood ketone levels, leukocytosis. Hyperkalemia, but depleted intracellular K^+ due to transcellular shift from ↓ insulin.
Complications	Life-threatening mucormycosis, *Rhizopus* infection, cerebral edema, cardiac arrhythmias, heart failure.
Treatment	Fluids, insulin, and K^+ (to replete intracellular stores); glucose if necessary to prevent hypoglycemia.

Carcinoid syndrome	Rare syndrome caused by carcinoid tumors (neuroendocrine cells), especially metastatic small bowel tumors, which secrete high levels of serotonin (5-HT). Not seen if tumor is limited to GI tract (5-HT undergoes first-pass metabolism in liver). Results in recurrent **diarrhea, cutaneous flushing, asthmatic wheezing,** and **right-sided valvular disease.** Most common tumor of appendix. ↑ 5-HIAA in urine.	Rule of 1/3s: 1/3 metastasize 1/3 present with 2nd malignancy 1/3 multiple Derived from neuroendocrine cells of GI tract. Treatment: octreotide.

Zollinger-Ellison syndrome	Gastrin-secreting tumor of pancreas or duodenum. Stomach shows rugal thickening with acid hypersecretion. Causes recurrent ulcers. May be associated with MEN type 1.

Multiple endocrine neoplasias (MEN)

Subtype	Characteristics	
MEN 1 (Wermer's syndrome)	Parathyroid tumors	MEN 1 = **3 P's** (**P**ancreas, **P**ituitary, and **P**arathyroid).
	Pituitary tumors (prolactin or GH)	
	Pancreatic endocrine tumors—Zollinger-Ellison syndrome, insulinomas, VIPomas, glucagonomas (rare)	MEN 2A = **2 P's** (**P**heochromocytoma and **P**arathyroid).
	Commonly presents with kidney stones and stomach ulcers	MEN 2B = **1 P** (**P**heochromocytoma).
MEN 2A (Sipple's syndrome)	Medullary thyroid carcinoma (secretes calcitonin)	All MEN syndromes have autosomal-dominant inheritance.
	Pheochromocytoma	
	Parathyroid tumors	Associated with *ret* gene in MEN types 2A and 2B.
MEN 2B	Medullary thyroid carcinoma (secretes calcitonin)	
	Pheochromocytoma	
	Oral/intestinal ganglioneuromatosis (associated with marfanoid habitus)	

Diabetes drugs   Treatment strategy for type 1 DM—low-sugar diet, insulin replacement.
Treatment strategy for type 2 DM—dietary modification and exercise for weight loss;
oral hypoglycemics and insulin replacement.

Drug Classes	Action	Clinical Use	Toxicities
Insulin: Lispro (rapid-acting) Aspart (rapid-acting) Regular (rapid-acting) NPH (intermediate) Glargine (long-acting) Detemir (long-acting)	**Bind insulin receptor** (tyrosine kinase activity). Liver: ↑ glucose stored as glycogen. Muscle: ↑ glycogen and protein synthesis, K^+ uptake. Fat: aids TG storage.	Type 1 DM, type 2 DM, gestational diabetes, life-threatening hyperkalemia, and stress-induced hyperglycemia.	Hypoglycemia, hypersensitivity reaction (very rare).

Sulfonylureas:
First generation:
  Tolbutamide
  Chlorpropamide
Second generation:
  Glyburide
  Glimepiride
  Glipizide
	Close K^+ channel in β-cell membrane, so cell depolarizes → **triggering of insulin release** via ↑ Ca^{2+} influx.	Stimulate release of endogenous insulin in type 2 DM. Require some islet function, so useless in type 1 DM.	First generation: disulfiram-like effects.
			Second generation: hypoglycemia.

Biguanides: Metformin	Exact mechanism is unknown. ↓ **gluconeogenesis,** ↑ glycolysis, ↑ peripheral glucose uptake (insulin sensitivity).	Oral. Can be used in patients without islet function.	Most grave adverse effect is lactic acidosis (contraindicated in renal failure).
Glitazones/ thiazolidinediones: Pioglitazone Rosiglitazone	↑ insulin sensitivity in peripheral tissue. Binds to PPAR-γ nuclear transcription regulator.	Used as monotherapy in type 2 DM or combined with above agents.	Weight gain, edema. Hepatotoxicity, CV toxicity.
α-glucosidase inhibitors: Acarbose Miglitol	**Inhibit intestinal brush-border α-glucosidases.** Delayed sugar hydrolysis and glucose absorption lead to ↓ postprandial hyperglycemia.	Used as monotherapy in type 2 DM or in combination with above agents.	GI disturbances.
Mimetics: Pramlintide	↓ glucagon.	Type 2 DM.	Hypoglycemia, nausea, diarrhea.
GLP-1 analogs: Exenatide	↑ insulin, ↓ glucagon release.	Type 2 DM.	Nausea, vomiting; pancreatitis.

Propylthiouracil, methimazole

Mechanism	Inhibit organification of iodide and coupling of thyroid hormone synthesis. Propylthiouracil also ↓ peripheral conversion of T_4 to T_3.
Clinical use	Hyperthyroidism.
Toxicity	Skin rash, agranulocytosis (rare), aplastic anemia. Methimazole is a possible teratogen.

Levothyroxine, triiodothyronine

Mechanism	Thyroxine replacement.
Clinical use	Hypothyroidism, myxedema.
Toxicity	Tachycardia, heat intolerance, tremors, arrhythmias.

Hypothalamic/pituitary drugs

Drug	Clinical use
GH	GH deficiency, Turner syndrome
Somatostatin (octreotide)	Acromegaly, carcinoid, gastrinoma, glucagonoma
Oxytocin	Stimulates labor, uterine contractions, milk let-down; controls uterine hemorrhage
ADH (desmopressin)	Pituitary (central, not nephrogenic) DI

Demeclocycline

Mechanism	ADH antagonist (member of the tetracycline family).
Clinical use	SIADH.
Toxicity	Nephrogenic DI, photosensitivity, abnormalities of bone and teeth.

Glucocorticoids

	Hydrocortisone, prednisone, triamcinolone, dexamethasone, beclomethasone.
Mechanism	↓ the production of leukotrienes and prostaglandins by inhibiting phospholipase A_2 and expression of COX-2.
Clinical use	Addison's disease, inflammation, immune suppression, asthma.
Toxicity	Iatrogenic Cushing's syndrome—buffalo hump, moon facies, truncal obesity, muscle wasting, thin skin, easy bruisability, osteoporosis, adrenocortical atrophy, peptic ulcers, diabetes (if chronic). Adrenal insufficiency when drug stopped after chronic use.

Gastrointestinal

"A good set of bowels is worth more to a man than any quantity of brains."
—Josh Billings

"Man should strive to have his intestines relaxed all the days of his life."
—Moses Maimonides

"The colon is the playing field for all human emotions."
—Cyrus Kapadia, MD

Retroperitoneal structures

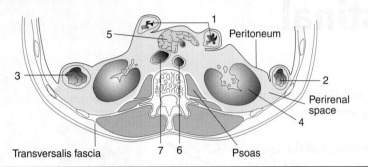

1. Duodenum (2nd, 3rd, 4th parts)
2. Descending colon
3. Ascending colon
4. Kidney and ureters
5. Pancreas (except tail)
6. Aorta
7. IVC

Adrenal glands and rectum (not shown in diagram)

Important GI ligaments

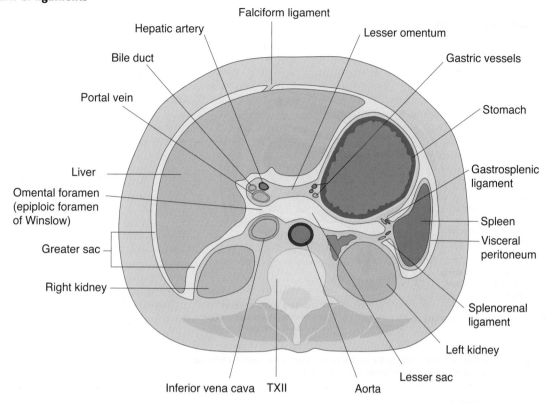

Ligament	Connects	Structures Contained	Notes
Falciform	Liver to anterior abdominal wall	Ligamentum teres	Derivative of fetal umbilical vein
Hepatoduodenal	Liver to duodenum	Portal triad: hepatic artery, portal vein, common bile duct	May be compressed between thumb and index finger placed in omental foramen (epiploic foramen of Winslow) to control bleeding Connects greater and lesser sacs
Gastrohepatic (not shown)	Liver to lesser curvature of stomach	Gastric arteries	Separates right greater and lesser sacs May be cut during surgery to access lesser sac
Gastrocolic (not shown)	Greater curvature and transverse colon	Gastroepiploic arteries	Part of greater omentum
Gastrosplenic	Greater curvature and spleen	Short gastrics	Separates left greater and lesser sacs
Splenorenal	Spleen to posterior abdominal wall	Splenic artery and vein	

Digestive tract anatomy

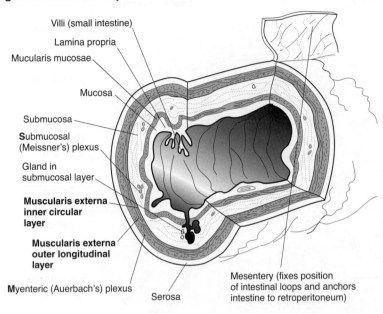

Villi (small intestine)
Lamina propria
Mucularis mucosae
Mucosa
Submucosa
Submucosal (Meissner's) plexus
Gland in submucosal layer
Muscularis externa inner circular layer
Muscularis externa outer longitudinal layer
Myenteric (Auerbach's) plexus
Serosa
Mesentery (fixes position of intestinal loops and anchors intestine to retroperitoneum)

(Adapted, with permission, from McPhee S et al. *Pathophysiology of Disease: An Introduction to Clinical Medicine,* 3rd ed. New York: McGraw-Hill, 2000: 296.)

Layers of gut wall (inside to outside):

1. **Mucosa**—epithelium (absorption), lamina propria (support), muscularis mucosae (motility)
2. **Submucosa**—includes Submucosal nerve plexus (Meissner's)
3. **Muscularis externa**—includes Myenteric nerve plexus (Auerbach's)
4. **Serosa/adventitia**

Frequencies of basal electric rhythm (slow waves):
Stomach—3 waves/min
Duodenum—12 waves/min
Ileum—8–9 waves/min

Digestive tract histology

Organ	Histology
Esophagus	Nonkeratinized stratified squamous epithelium.
Stomach	Gastric glands.
Duodenum	Villi and microvilli ↑ absorptive surface.
	Brunner's glands (submucosa) and crypts of Lieberkühn.
Jejunum	Jejunum has largest number of goblet cells in the small intestine.
	Plicae circulares and crypts of Lieberkühn.
Ileum	Peyer's patches (lamina propria, submucosa), plicae circulares (proximal ileum), and crypts of Lieberkühn.
Colon	Colon has crypts but no villi.

Esophageal anatomy

Upper ⅓	Striated muscle.
Middle ⅓	Striated and smooth muscle.
Lower ⅓	Smooth muscle.

HIGH-YIELD SYSTEMS

GASTROINTESTINAL

Abdominal aorta and branches

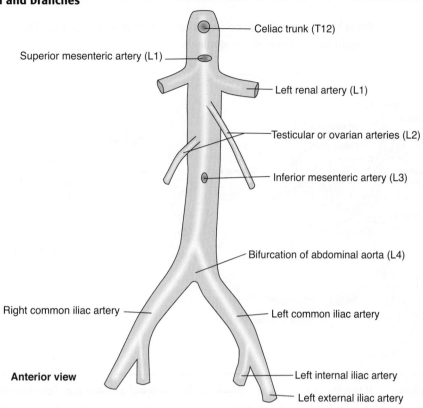

Celiac trunk (T12)

Superior mesenteric artery (L1)

Left renal artery (L1)

Testicular or ovarian arteries (L2)

Inferior mesenteric artery (L3)

Bifurcation of abdominal aorta (L4)

Right common iliac artery

Left common iliac artery

Anterior view

Left internal iliac artery

Left external iliac artery

GI blood supply and innervation

Embryonic gut region	Artery	Parasympathetic innervation	Vertebral level	Structures supplied
Foregut	Celiac	Vagus	T12/L1	Stomach to proximal duodenum; liver, gallbladder, pancreas, spleen (mesoderm)
Midgut	SMA	Vagus	L1	Distal duodenum to proximal ⅔ of transverse colon
Hindgut	IMA	Pelvic	L3	Distal ⅓ of transverse colon to upper portion of rectum; splenic flexure is a watershed region

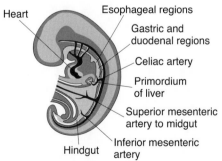

Heart

Esophageal regions

Gastric and duodenal regions

Celiac artery

Primordium of liver

Superior mesenteric artery to midgut

Inferior mesenteric artery

Hindgut

311

Celiac trunk   Branches of celiac trunk: common hepatic, splenic, left gastric. These constitute the main blood supply of the stomach.

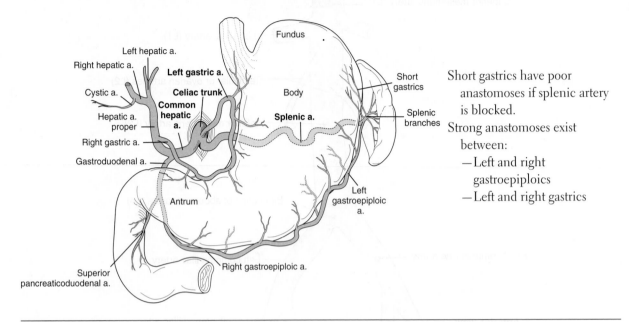

Short gastrics have poor anastomoses if splenic artery is blocked.

Strong anastomoses exist between:
— Left and right gastroepiploics
— Left and right gastrics

Collateral circulation   If the abdominal aorta is blocked, these arterial anastomoses (origin) compensate:

1. Internal thoracic/mammary (subclavian) ↔ superior epigastric (internal thoracic) ↔ inferior epigastric (external iliac)
2. Superior pancreaticoduodenal (celiac trunk) ↔ inferior pancreaticoduodenal (SMA)
3. Middle colic (SMA) ↔ left colic (IMA)
4. Superior rectal (IMA) ↔ middle rectal (internal iliac)

Portosystemic anastomoses

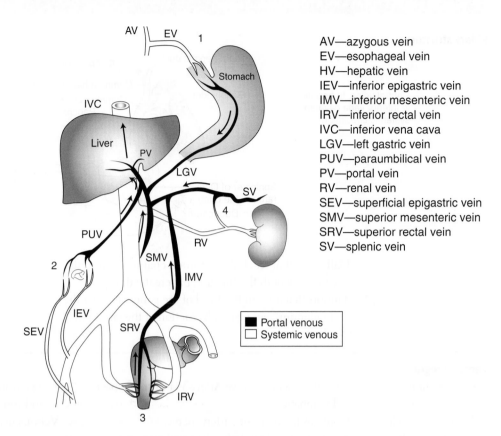

AV—azygous vein
EV—esophageal vein
HV—hepatic vein
IEV—inferior epigastric vein
IMV—inferior mesenteric vein
IRV—inferior rectal vein
IVC—inferior vena cava
LGV—left gastric vein
PUV—paraumbilical vein
PV—portal vein
RV—renal vein
SEV—superficial epigastric vein
SMV—superior mesenteric vein
SRV—superior rectal vein
SV—splenic vein

Site of anastomosis	Clinical sign	Portal ↔ systemic
1. Esophagus	Esophageal varices	Left gastric ↔ esophageal
2. Umbilicus	Caput medusae	Paraumbilical ↔ superficial and inferior epigastric
3. Rectum	Internal hemorrhoids	Superior rectal ↔ middle and inferior rectal

Varices of **gut, butt,** and **caput** (medusae) are commonly seen with portal hypertension. Inserting a transjugular intrahepatic portosystemic shunt (TIPS) between the portal vein and hepatic vein percutaneously relieves portal hypertension by shunting blood to the systemic circulation.

Pectinate line

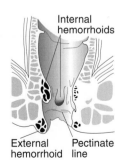

Internal hemorrhoids

External hemorrhoid   Pectinate line

Formed where hindgut meets ectoderm.

Above pectinate line—internal hemorrhoids, adenocarcinoma (endoderm derivation). Arterial supply from superior rectal artery (branch of IMA). Venous drainage is to superior rectal vein → inferior mesenteric vein → portal system.

Below pectinate line—external hemorrhoids, squamous cell carcinoma (ectoderm derivation). Arterial supply from inferior rectal artery (branch of internal pudendal artery). Venous drainage to inferior rectal vein → internal pudendal vein → internal iliac vein → IVC.

Internal hemorrhoids receive visceral innervation and are therefore NOT painful. Can be a sign of portal hypertension.

External hemorrhoids receive somatic innervation and are therefore painful. Innervated by inferior rectal nerve (branch of pudendal nerve).

Biliary structures

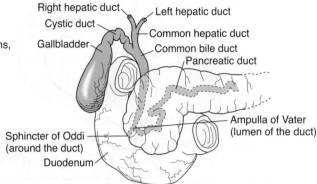

Central veins, to hepatic veins, to inferior vena cava and systemic circulation

Right hepatic duct
Cystic duct
Gallbladder
Left hepatic duct
Common hepatic duct
Common bile duct
Pancreatic duct
Ampulla of Vater (lumen of the duct)
Sphincter of Oddi (around the duct)
Duodenum

Gallstones that reach the common channel at ampulla can block both the bile and pancreatic ducts.

Tumors that arise in the head of the pancreas (near the duodenum) can cause obstruction of the common bile duct.

Femoral region

Organization	Lateral to medial: **N**erve-**A**rtery-**V**ein-**E**mpty space-**L**ymphatics.	You go from lateral to medial to find your **NAVEL.**
Femoral triangle	Contains femoral vein, artery, nerve.	**Venous** near the **penis.**
Femoral sheath	Fascial tube 3–4 cm below inguinal ligament. Contains femoral vein, artery, and canal (deep inguinal lymph nodes) but **not** femoral nerve.	

Sartorius muscle
Femoral triangle
Inguinal ligament
Femoral n.
Empty space
Femoral a.
Femoral v.
Lymphatic
Adductor longus muscle

HIGH-YIELD SYSTEMS

GASTROINTESTINAL

Inguinal canal

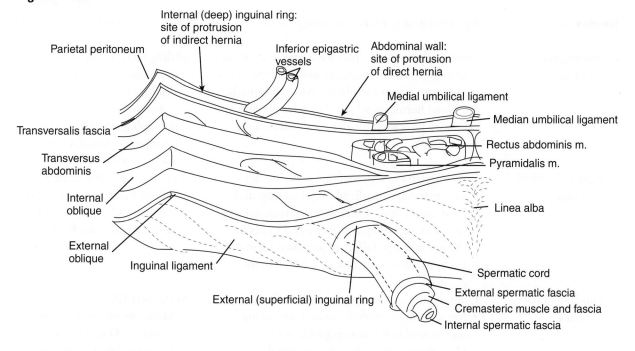

Internal (deep) inguinal ring: site of protrusion of indirect hernia

Parietal peritoneum

Inferior epigastric vessels

Abdominal wall: site of protrusion of direct hernia

Medial umbilical ligament

Median umbilical ligament

Transversalis fascia

Rectus abdominis m.

Transversus abdominis

Pyramidalis m.

Internal oblique

Linea alba

External oblique

Inguinal ligament

Spermatic cord

External (superficial) inguinal ring

External spermatic fascia

Cremasteric muscle and fascia

Internal spermatic fascia

(Adapted, with permission, from White JS. *USMLE Road Map: Gross Anatomy,* 1st ed. New York: McGraw-Hill, 2003: 69.)

Hernias　　　A protrusion of peritoneum through an opening, usually a site of weakness.

Diaphragmatic hernia
Abdominal structures enter the thorax; may occur in infants as a result of defective development of pleuroperitoneal membrane. Most commonly a **hiatal hernia**, in which stomach herniates upward through the esophageal hiatus of the diaphragm.

Sliding hiatal hernia is most common. GE junction is displaced; "hourglass stomach."
Paraesophageal hernia—GE junction is normal. Cardia moves into the thorax.

Indirect inguinal hernia
Goes through the **IN**ternal (deep) inguinal ring, external (superficial) inguinal ring, and **IN**to the scrotum. Enters internal inguinal ring lateral to inferior epigastric artery. Occurs in **IN**fants owing to failure of processus vaginalis to close (can form hydrocele). Much more common in males.

An indirect inguinal hernia follows the path of descent of the testes. Covered by all 3 layers of spermatic fascia.

Direct inguinal hernia
Protrudes through the inguinal (Hesselbach's) triangle. Bulges directly through abdominal wall medial to inferior epigastric artery. Goes through the external (superficial) inguinal ring only. Covered by external spermatic fascia. Usually in older men.

MDs don't **LI**e:
　Medial to inferior epigastric artery = **D**irect hernia.
　Lateral to inferior epigastric artery = **I**ndirect hernia.

Femoral hernia
Protrudes below inguinal ligament through femoral canal below and lateral to pubic tubercle. More common in women.

Leading cause of bowel incarceration.

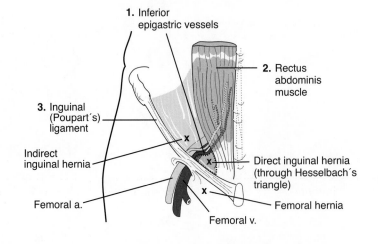

1. Inferior epigastric vessels
2. Rectus abdominis muscle
3. Inguinal (Poupart's) ligament
Indirect inguinal hernia
Femoral a.
Direct inguinal hernia (through Hesselbach's triangle)
Femoral hernia
Femoral v.

Hesselbach's triangle:
　Inferior epigastric artery
　Lateral border of rectus abdominis
　Inguinal ligament

GI hormones

Hormone	Source	Action	Regulation	Notes
Gastrin	G cells (antrum of stomach)	↑ gastric H^+ secretion ↑ growth of gastric mucosa ↑ gastric motility	↑ by stomach distention/ alkalinization, amino acids, peptides, vagal stimulation ↓ by stomach pH < 1.5	↑↑ in Zollinger-Ellison syndrome. Phenylalanine and tryptophan are potent stimulators.
Cholecysto-kinin	I cells (duodenum, jejunum)	↑ pancreatic secretion ↑ gallbladder contraction ↓ gastric emptying, sphincter of Oddi relaxation	↑ by fatty acids, amino acids	CCK acts on neural muscarinic pathways to cause pancreatic secretion.
Secretin	S cells (duodenum)	↑ pancreatic HCO_3^- secretion ↓ gastric acid secretion ↑ bile secretion	↑ by acid, fatty acids in lumen of duodenum	↑ HCO_3^- neutralizes gastric acid in duodenum, allowing pancreatic enzymes to function.
Somatostatin	D cells (pancreatic islets, GI mucosa)	↓ gastric acid and pepsinogen secretion ↓ pancreatic and small intestine fluid secretion ↓ gallbladder contraction ↓ insulin and glucagon release	↑ by acid ↓ by vagal stimulation	Inhibitory hormone. Antigrowth hormone effects (digestion and absorption of substances needed for growth).
Glucose-dependent insulinotropic peptide (also known as gastric inhibitory peptide) (GIP)	K cells (duodenum, jejunum)	Exocrine: ↓ gastric H^+ secretion Endocrine: ↑ insulin release	↑ by fatty acids, amino acids, oral glucose	An oral glucose load is used more rapidly than the equivalent given by IV.
Vasoactive intestinal polypeptide (VIP)	Parasympathetic ganglia in sphincters, gallbladder, small intestine	↑ intestinal water and electrolyte secretion ↑ relaxation of intestinal smooth muscle and sphincters	↑ by distention and vagal stimulation ↓ by adrenergic input	**VIPoma**—non-α, non-β islet cell pancreatic tumor that secretes VIP. Copious diarrhea.
Nitric oxide		↑ smooth muscle relaxation, including lower esophageal sphincter		Loss of NO secretion is implicated in ↑ lower esophageal tone of achalasia.
Motilin	Small intestine	Produces migrating motor complexes (MMCs)	↑ in fasting state	Motilin receptor agonists are used to stimulate intestinal peristalsis.

GI secretory products

Product	Source	Action	Regulation	Notes
Intrinsic factor	Parietal cells (stomach)	Vitamin B_{12} binding protein (required for B_{12} uptake in terminal ileum)		Autoimmune destruction of parietal cells → chronic gastritis and pernicious anemia.
Gastric acid	Parietal cells (stomach)	↓ stomach pH	↑ by histamine, ACh, gastrin ↓ by somatostatin, GIP, prostaglandin, secretin	**Gastrinoma:** gastrin-secreting tumor that causes continuous high levels of acid secretion and ulcers.
Pepsin	Chief cells (stomach)	Protein digestion	↑ by vagal stimulation local acid	Inactive pepsinogen → pepsin by H^+.
HCO_3^-	Mucosal cells (stomach, duodenum, salivary glands, pancreas) and Brunner's glands (duodenum)	Neutralizes acid	↑ pancreatic and biliary secretion with secretin	HCO_3^- is trapped in mucus that covers the gastric epithelium.

Salivary secretion

Source — Parotid (most serous), submandibular, and sublingual (most mucinous) glands.

Serous on the **S**ides (parotids); **M**ucinous in the **M**iddle (sublingual).

Function —
1. α-amylase (ptyalin) begins starch digestion; inactivated by low pH on reaching stomach
2. Bicarbonate neutralizes oral bacterial acids, maintains dental health
3. Mucins (glycoproteins) lubricate food
4. Antibacterial secretory products
5. Growth factors that promote epithelial renewal

Salivary secretion is stimulated by both sympathetic (T1–T3 superior cervical ganglion) and parasympathetic (facial, glossopharyngeal nerve) activity. Low flow rate → hypotonic (more time to reabsorb Na^+ and Cl^-). High flow rate → closer to isotonic (less time to reabsorb Na^+ and Cl^-).

CN VII runs through parotid gland. Can be damaged during surgery.

Locations of GI secretory cells

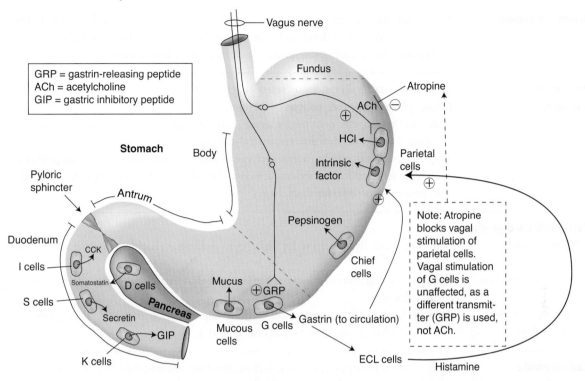

GRP = gastrin-releasing peptide
ACh = acetylcholine
GIP = gastric inhibitory peptide

Note: Atropine blocks vagal stimulation of parietal cells. Vagal stimulation of G cells is unaffected, as a different transmitter (GRP) is used, not ACh.

Gastrin ↑ acid secretion primarily through its effects on ECL cells (leading to histamine release) rather than through its direct effect on parietal cells.

Gastric parietal cell

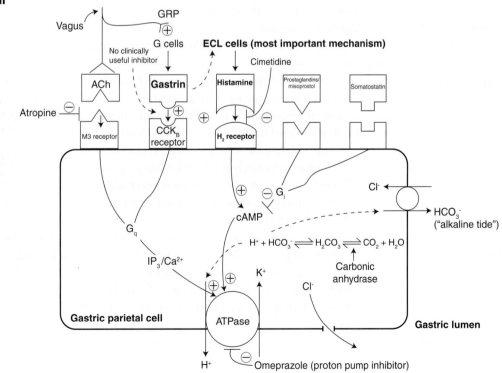

Brunner's glands	Secrete alkaline mucus to neutralize acid contents entering the duodenum from the stomach. Located in **duodenal submucosa** (the only GI submucosal glands). Hypertrophy of Brunner's glands is seen in peptic ulcer disease.
Pancreatic enzymes	α-amylase—starch digestion, secreted in active form. Lipase, phospholipase A, colipase—fat digestion. Proteases (trypsin, chymotrypsin, elastase, carboxypeptidases)—protein digestion, secreted as proenzymes also known as "zymogens." Trypsinogen—converted to active enzyme trypsin by **enterokinase/enteropeptidase**, an enzyme secreted from duodenal mucosa. Trypsin activates other proenzymes and more trypsinogen (positive feedback loop).

Carbohydrate digestion

Salivary amylase	Starts digestion, hydrolyzes α-1,4 linkages to yield disaccharides (maltose and α-limit dextrans).
Pancreatic amylase	Highest concentration in duodenal lumen, hydrolyzes starch to oligosaccharides and disaccharides.
Oligosaccharide hydrolases	At brush border of intestine, the rate-limiting step in carbohydrate digestion, produce monosaccharides from oligo- and disaccharides.

Carbohydrate absorption	Only monosaccharides (glucose, galactose, fructose) are absorbed by enterocytes. Glucose and galactose are taken up by SGLT1 (Na^+ dependent). Fructose is taken up by facilitated diffusion by GLUT-5. All are transported to blood by GLUT-2.

Vitamin/mineral absorption

Iron	Absorbed as Fe^{2+} in duodenum.
Folate	Absorbed in jejunum.
B_{12}	Absorbed in ileum along with bile acids, requires Intrinsic Factor.

Peyer's patches	Unencapsulated lymphoid tissue found in lamina propria and submucosa of small intestine. Contain specialized M cells that take up antigen. B cells stimulated in germinal centers of Peyer's patches differentiate into IgA-secreting plasma cells, which ultimately reside in lamina propria. IgA receives protective secretory component and is then transported across epithelium to gut to deal with intraluminal antigen. Think of **IgA**, the Intra-gut Antibody. And always say "secretory IgA."
Bile	Composed of bile salts (bile acids conjugated to glycine or taurine, making them water soluble), phospholipids, cholesterol, bilirubin, water, and ions. The only significant mechanism for cholesterol excretion. Needed for digestion of triglycerides and micelle formation (required for absorption of non-polar nutrients such as lipids) in small intestine.

Bilirubin	Product of heme metabolism. Bilirubin is removed from blood by liver, conjugated with glucuronate, and excreted in bile. Jaundice (yellow skin/sclerae) results from elevated bilirubin levels.

Direct bilirubin—conjugated with glucuronic acid; water soluble.

Indirect bilirubin—unconjugated; water insoluble.

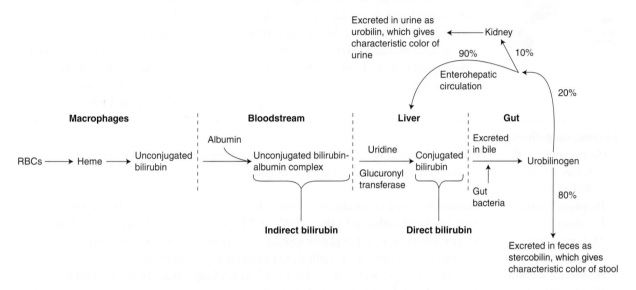

▶ **GASTROINTESTINAL–PATHOLOGY**

Salivary gland tumors	Generally benign and occur in parotid gland. Types include pleomorphic adenoma (most common tumor; painless, movable mass; benign with high rate of recurrence), Warthin's tumor (benign; heterotopic salivary gland tissue trapped in a lymph node, surrounded by lymphatic tissue), and mucoepidermoid carcinoma (most common malignant tumor).

Achalasia

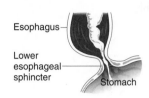

Esophagus

Lower esophageal sphincter

Stomach

Failure of relaxation of lower esophageal sphincter (LES) due to loss of **myenteric (Auerbach's) plexus.** High LES opening pressure and uncoordinated peristalsis → progressive dysphagia to solids and liquids (vs. obstruction—solids only). Barium swallow shows dilated esophagus with an area of distal stenosis. Associated with an ↑ risk of esophageal carcinoma.

A-chalasia = absence of relaxation.
"Bird's beak" on barium swallow.
2° achalasia may arise from Chagas' disease.
Scleroderma (CREST syndrome) is associated with esophageal dysmotility involving low pressure proximal to LES.

Esophageal pathologies

Gastroesophageal reflux disease (GERD)	Commonly presents as heartburn and regurgitation upon lying down. May also present with nocturnal cough and dyspnea.
Esophageal varices	**Painless** bleeding of submucosal veins in lower ⅓ of esophagus (see Image 34).
Esophagitis	Associated with reflux, infection (HSV-1, CMV, *Candida*), or chemical ingestion.
Mallory-Weiss syndrome	Mucosal lacerations at the gastroesophageal junction due to severe vomiting. Leads to hematemesis. Usually found in alcoholics and bulimics.
Boerhaave syndrome	Transmural esophageal rupture due to violent retching. "**B**een-**h**eaving syndrome."
Esophageal strictures	Associated with lye ingestion and acid reflux.
Plummer-Vinson syndrome	Triad of:

1. Dysphagia (due to esophageal webs)
2. Glossitis
3. Iron deficiency anemia

Barrett's esophagus

Glandular metaplasia—replacement of nonkeratinized (stratified) squamous epithelium with intestinal (columnar) epithelium in the distal esophagus. Due to chronic acid reflux (GERD). Associated with esophagitis, esophageal ulcers, and increased risk esophageal cancer.

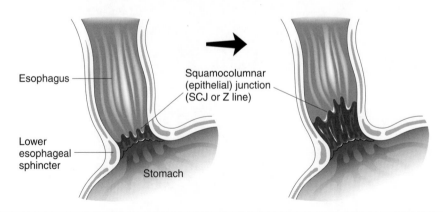

Esophagus

Lower esophageal sphincter

Stomach

Squamocolumnar (epithelial) junction (SCJ or Z line)

Esophageal cancer	Progressive dysphagia (solids → liquids) → weight loss.	
	Risk factors for esophageal cancer are:	
	Alcohol/Achalasia	**ABCDEF.**
	Barrett's esophagus	Worldwide, squamous cell is
	Cigarettes	most common.
	Diverticuli (e.g., Zenker's diverticulum)	In the United States,
	Esophageal web (e.g., Plummer-Vinson)/	adenocarcinoma is
	Esophagitis	most common.
	Familial	Squamous cell—upper and
		middle $\frac{1}{3}$.
		Adenocarcinoma—lower $\frac{1}{3}$.

Malabsorption syndromes	Can cause diarrhea, steatorrhea, weight loss, weakness.	These **W**ill **C**ause **D**evastating **A**bsorption **P**roblems.
Tropical sprue	Probably infectious; responds to antibiotics. Similar to celiac sprue, but can affect entire small bowel.	
Whipple's disease	Infection with *Tropheryma whippelii* (gram positive); PAS-positive macrophages in intestinal lamina propria, mesenteric nodes. Arthralgias, cardiac and neurologic symptoms are common. Most often occurs in older men.	
Celiac sprue	Autoantibodies to gluten (gliadin) in wheat and other grains. Proximal small bowel primarily.	
Disaccharidase deficiency	Most common is lactase deficiency → milk intolerance. Normal-appearing villi. Osmotic diarrhea. Since lactase is located at tips of intestinal villi, self-limited lactase deficiency can occur following injury (e.g., viral diarrhea).	
Abeta-lipoproteinemia	↓ synthesis of apo B → inability to generate chylomicrons → ↓ secretion of cholesterol, VLDL into bloodstream → fat accumulation in enterocytes. Presents in early childhood with malabsorption and neurologic manifestations.	
Pancreatic insufficiency	Due to cystic fibrosis, obstructing cancer, and chronic pancreatitis. Causes malabsorption of fat and fat-soluble vitamins (vitamins A, D, E, K).	

Celiac sprue

Autoimmune-mediated intolerance of gliadin (wheat) leading to steatorrhea. Associated with people of northern European descent. Findings include antibodies to **gliadin** and **tissue transglutaminase,** blunting of villi (see Image 33), and lymphocytes in the lamina propria. ↓ mucosal absorption that primarily affects jejunum. Serum levels of tissue transglutaminase antibodies are used for screening. Associated with dermatitis herpetiformis. Moderately ↑ risk of malignancy (e.g., T-cell lymphoma).

Gastritis

Acute gastritis (erosive)

Disruption of mucosal barrier → inflammation. Can be caused by stress, NSAIDs (↓ PGE_2 → ↓ gastric mucosa protection), alcohol, uremia, burns (**Curling's** ulcer—↓ plasma volume → sloughing of gastric mucosa), and brain injury (**Cush**ing's ulcer— ↑ vagal stimulation → ↑ ACh → ↑ H^+ production).

Burned by the **Curling** iron. Always **Cush**ion the brain. Especially common among alcoholics and patients taking daily NSAIDs (e.g., patients with rheumatoid arthritis).

Chronic gastritis (nonerosive)

Type A (fundus/body)

Autoimmune disorder characterized by **A**utoantibodies to parietal cells, pernicious **A**nemia, and **A**chlorhydria. Associated with other autoimmune disorders.

AB pairing—pernicious **A**nemia affects gastric **B**ody.

Type B (antrum)

Most common type. Caused by *H. pylori* infection. ↑ risk of MALT lymphoma.

H. pylori **B**acterium affects **A**ntrum.

Ménétrier's disease

Gastric hypertrophy with protein loss, parietal cell atrophy, and ↑ mucous cells. Precancerous. Rugae of stomach are so hypertrophied that they look like brain gyri.

Stomach cancer

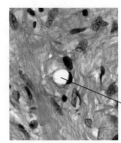

Signet ring cell

(Reproduced, with permission, from USMLERx.com.)

Almost always adenocarcinoma. Early aggressive local spread and node/liver mets. Associated with dietary nitrosamines (smoked foods), achlorhydria, chronic gastritis, type A blood. Signet ring cells, acanthosis nigricans are common features. Termed linitis plastica when diffusely infiltrative (thickened, rigid appearance, "leather bottle").

Virchow's node—involvement of left supraclavicular node by mets from stomach. Krukenberg's tumor—bilateral mets to ovaries. Abundant mucus, signet ring cells. Sister Mary Joseph's nodule—subcutaneous periumbilical metastasis.

Peptic ulcer disease

Gastric ulcer	Pain can be **G**reater with meals—weight loss. Often occurs in older patients. *H. pylori* infection in 70%; positive urease test; chronic NSAID use also implicated. Due to ↓ mucosal protection against gastric acid.
Duodenal ulcer	Pain **D**ecreases with meals—weight gain. Almost 100% have *H. pylori* infection. Due to ↑ gastric acid secretion (e.g., Zollinger-Ellison syndrome) or ↓ mucosal protection. Hypertrophy of Brunner's glands.
	Tend to have clean, "punched-out" margins unlike the raised/irregular margins of carcinoma. Potential complications include bleeding, penetration into pancreas, perforation, and obstruction. Not cancerous.

Inflammatory bowel disease (IBD)

	Crohn's disease	Ulcerative colitis
Possible etiology	Disordered response to intestinal bacteria.	Autoimmune.
Location	Any portion of the GI tract, usually the terminal ileum and colon. **Skip** lesions, **rec**tal sparing.	*Colitis* = colon inflammation. Continuous colonic lesions, always with rectal involvement.
Gross morphology	Transmural inflammation. **Cobblestone** mucosa, creeping **fat**, bowel wall thickening ("string sign" on barium swallow x-ray), linear ulcers, fissures, fistulas.	Mucosal and submucosal inflammation only. Friable mucosal pseudopolyps with freely hanging mesentery. Loss of haustra → "lead pipe" appearance on imaging.
Microscopic morphology	Noncaseating **gran**ulomas and lymphoid aggregates.	Crypt abscesses and ulcers, bleeding, no granulomas.
Complications	Strictures, fistulas, perianal disease, malabsorption, nutritional depletion, colorectal cancer.	Malnutrition, toxic megacolon, **colorectal carcinoma.**
Intestinal manifestation	Diarrhea that may or may not be bloody.	Bloody diarrhea.
Extraintestinal manifestations	Migratory polyarthritis, erythema nodosum, ankylosing spondylitis, uveitis, immunologic disorders.	Pyoderma gangrenosum, 1° sclerosing cholangitis.
Treatment	Corticosteroids, infliximab.	ASA preparations (sulfasalazine), 6-mercaptopurine, infliximab, colectomy.

For **Crohn's,** think of a **fat gran**ny and an old **crone skipping** down a **cobblestone** road away from the **wreck** (rectal sparing).

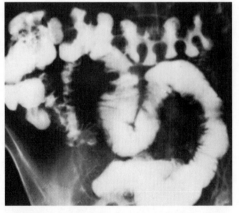

Crohn's disease (note multiple "string sign" lesions)

(Reproduced, with permission, from Way LW, Doherty GM. *Current Surgical Diagnosis & Treatment,* 11th ed. New York: McGraw-Hill, 2003: 691.)

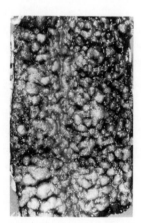

Ulcerative colitis (note pseudopolyps)

Irritable bowel syndrome (IBS)	Recurrent abdominal pain associated with ≥ 2 of the following: 　1. Pain improves with defecation 　2. Change in stool frequency 　3. Change in appearance of stool No structural abnormalities. Chronic symptoms. May present with diarrhea, constipation, or alternating. Pathophysiology is multifaceted. Treat symptoms.

Appendicitis	All age groups; most common indication for emergent abdominal surgery in children. Kids—lymphoid hyperplasia after viral infection. Adults—obstruction, fecalith. Initial diffuse periumbilical pain → localized pain at McBurney's point (⅓ the distance from iliac crest to umbilicus). Nausea, fever; may perforate → peritonitis. Differential: diverticulitis (elderly), ectopic pregnancy (use β-hCG to rule out).	

Diverticular disease

Diverticulum	Blind pouch protruding from the alimentary tract that communicates with the lumen of the gut. Most diverticula (esophagus, stomach, duodenum, colon) are acquired and are termed "false" in that they lack or have an attenuated muscularis externa. Most often in sigmoid colon.	**"True"** diverticulum—all 3 gut wall layers outpouch (e.g., Meckel's). **"False"** diverticulum or pseudodiverticulum—only mucosa and submucosa outpouch. Occur especially where vasa recta perforate muscularis externa.
Diverticulosis	Many diverticula. Common (in ~50% of people > 60 years). Caused by ↑ intraluminal pressure and focal weakness in colonic wall. Associated with low-fiber diets. Most often in sigmoid colon.	Often asymptomatic or associated with vague discomfort and/or painless rectal bleeding.
Diverticulitis	Inflammation of diverticula classically causing LLQ pain, fever, leukocytosis. May perforate → peritonitis, abscess formation, or bowel stenosis (see Image 32). Give antibiotics.	May cause bright red rectal bleeding. May also cause colovesical fistula (fistula with bladder) → pneumaturia. Sometimes called "left-sided appendicitis" due to clinical presentation.

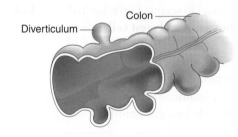

Zenker's diverticulum	False diverticulum. Herniation of mucosal tissue at junction of pharynx and esophagus. Presenting symptoms: halitosis (due to trapped food particles), dysphagia, obstruction.	

Meckel's diverticulum 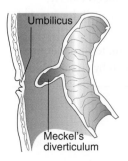	True diverticulum. Persistence of the vitelline duct or yolk stalk. May contain ectopic acid–secreting gastric mucosa and/or pancreatic tissue. **Most common congenital anomaly of the GI tract.** Can cause bleeding, intussusception, volvulus, or obstruction near the terminal ileum. Contrast with omphalomesenteric cyst = cystic dilatation of vitelline duct.	The five 2's: 2 inches long. 2 feet from the ileocecal valve. 2% of population. Commonly presents in first **2** years of life. May have **2** types of epithelia (gastric/ pancreatic). Dx: Pertechnetate. Study for ectopic uptake.

Intussusception and volvulus

Intussusception—"telescoping" of 1 bowel segment into distal segment; can compromise blood supply (see Image 35). Unusual in adults (associated with intraluminal mass or tumor). Majority of cases occur in children (usually idiopathic; may be viral [adenovirus]). Abdominal emergency in early childhood.

Volvulus—twisting of portion of bowel around its mesentery; can lead to obstruction and infarction. May occur at cecum and sigmoid colon, where there is redundant mesentery. Usually in elderly.

Intussusception	Volvulus
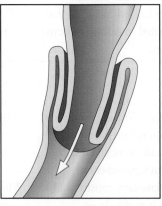	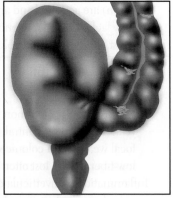

Hirschsprung's disease

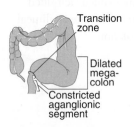
Transition zone
Dilated megacolon
Constricted aganglionic segment

Congenital megacolon characterized by lack of ganglion cells/enteric nervous plexuses (Auerbach's and Meissner's plexuses) in segment on intestinal biopsy. Due to **failure of neural crest cell migration.**

Presents as chronic constipation early in life. Dilated portion of the colon proximal to the aganglionic segment, resulting in a "transition zone." Involves rectum. Usually failure to pass meconium.

Think of a giant spring that has **sprung** in the colon.
Risk ↑ with Down syndrome.

Other intestinal disorders

Duodenal atresia	Causes early bilious vomiting with proximal stomach distention ("double bubble") due to failure of recanalization of small bowel. Associated with Down syndrome.
Meconium ileus	In cystic fibrosis, meconium plug obstructs intestine, preventing stool passage at birth.
Necrotizing enterocolitis	Necrosis of intestinal mucosa and possible perforation. Colon is usually involved, but can involve entire GI tract. In neonates, more common in preemies (↓ immunity).
Ischemic colitis	Reduction in intestinal blood flow causes ischemia. Pain after eating → weight loss. Commonly occurs at splenic flexure and distal colon. Typically affects elderly.
Adhesion	Acute bowel obstruction, commonly from a recent surgery. Can have well-demarcated necrotic zones.
Angiodysplasia	Tortuous dilation of vessels → bleeding. Most often found in cecum, terminal ileum, and ascending colon. More common in older patients. Confirmed by angiography.

Colonic polyps	Masses protruding into gut lumen → sawtooth appearance. 90% are non-neoplastic. Often rectosigmoid.
	Adenomatous polyps are precancerous. Malignant risk is associated with ↑ size, villous histology, ↑ epithelial dysplasia (see Image 31). Precursor to colorectal cancer (CRC). The more villous the polyp, the more likely it is to be malignant (**VILL**ous = **VILL**ain**OUS**).
Hyperplastic	Most common non-neoplastic polyp in colon (> 50% found in rectosigmoid colon).
Juvenile	Mostly sporadic lesions in children < 5 years of age. 80% in rectum. If single, no malignant potential.
	Juvenile polyposis syndrome—multiple juvenile polyps in GI tract, ↑ risk of adenocarcinoma.
Peutz-Jeghers	Single polyps are not malignant.
	Peutz-Jeghers syndrome—autosomal-dominant syndrome featuring multiple nonmalignant hamartomas throughout GI tract, along with hyperpigmented mouth, lips, hands, genitalia. Associated with ↑ risk of CRC and other visceral malignancies.

Colorectal cancer (CRC)

Epidemiology	3rd most common cancer; 3rd most deadly in United States. Most patients are > 50 years of age. ~ 25% have a family history.
Genetics	**Familial adenomatous polyposis (FAP)**—autosomal-dominant mutation of *APC* gene on chromosome 5q. Two-hit hypothesis. 100% progress to CRC. Thousands of polyps; pancolonic; always involves rectum.
	Gardner's syndrome—FAP + osseous and soft tissue tumors, retinal hyperplasia.
	Turcot's syndrome—FAP + malignant CNS tumor. **TUR**cot = **TUR**ban.
	Hereditary nonpolyposis colorectal cancer (HNPCC/Lynch syndrome)—autosomal-dominant mutation of DNA mismatch repair genes. ~ 80% progress to CRC. Proximal colon is always involved.
Additional risk factors	IBD, *Streptococcus bovis* bacteremia, tobacco use, large villous adenomas, juvenile polyposis syndrome, Peutz-Jeghers syndrome.
Presentation	Distal colon—obstruction, colicky pain, hematochezia.
	Proximal colon—dull pain, iron deficiency anemia, fatigue.
Diagnosis	Iron deficiency anemia in older males.
	Screen patients > 50 years of age with stool occult blood test and colonoscopy.
	"Apple core" lesion seen on barium enema x-ray.
	CEA tumor marker.

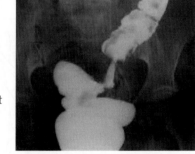

"Apple core" lesion

(Reproduced, with permission, from USMLERx.com.)

Molecular pathogenesis of CRC

There are 2 molecular pathways that lead to CRC:

1. Microsatellite instability pathway (15%): DNA mismatch repair gene mutations → sporadic and HNPCC syndrome. Mutations accumulate, but no defined morphologic correlates.
2. APC/β-catenin (chromosomal instability) pathway (85%):

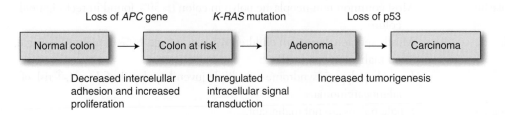

Loss of *APC* gene   *K-RAS* mutation   Loss of p53

Normal colon → Colon at risk → Adenoma → Carcinoma

Decreased intercelullar adhesion and increased proliferation   Unregulated intracellular signal transduction   Increased tumorigenesis

Carcinoid tumor

Tumor of neuro-endocrine cells. Constitute 50% of small bowel tumors. Most common sites are the appendix, ileum, and rectum. Most commonly malignant in the small intestine. "Dense core bodies" seen on EM. Often produce 5-HT, which can lead to carcinoid syndrome. Classic symptoms: wheezing, right-sided heart murmurs, diarrhea, flushing. If tumor is confined to GI system, no carcinoid syndrome is observed, since liver metabolizes 5-HT. If tumor or metastases (usually to liver) exist outside GI system, carcinoid syndrome is observed. Thus, tumor location determines whether the syndrome appears.

Cirrhosis and portal hypertension

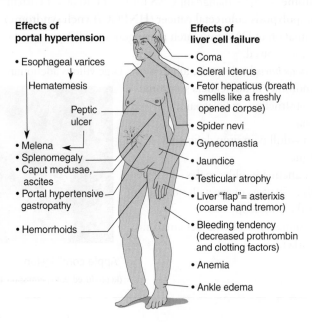

Effects of portal hypertension

• Esophageal varices
    ↓
    Hematemesis

Peptic ulcer

• Melena
• Splenomegaly
• Caput medusae, ascites
• Portal hypertensive gastropathy
• Hemorrhoids

Effects of liver cell failure

• Coma
• Scleral icterus
• Fetor hepaticus (breath smells like a freshly opened corpse)
• Spider nevi
• Gynecomastia
• Jaundice
• Testicular atrophy
• Liver "flap"= asterixis (coarse hand tremor)
• Bleeding tendency (decreased prothrombin and clotting factors)
• Anemia
• Ankle edema

(Adapted, with permission, from Chandrasoma P, Taylor CE. *Concise Pathology,* 3rd ed. Stamford, CT: Appleton & Lange, 1998: 654.)

Cirrho (Greek) = tawny yellow. Diffuse fibrosis of liver, destroys normal architecture. Nodular regeneration.

Micronodular—nodules < 3 mm, uniform size. Due to metabolic insult (e.g., alcohol, hemochromatosis, Wilson's disease).

Macronodular—nodules > 3 mm, varied size. Usually due to significant liver injury leading to hepatic necrosis (e.g., postinfectious or drug-induced hepatitis). ↑ risk of hepatocellular carcinoma.

Shunt between portal and systemic circulation can relieve portal hypertension (see Image 30).

Markers of GI pathology	Serum enzyme	Major diagnostic use
	Aminotransferases (AST and ALT)	Viral hepatitis (ALT > AST)
		Alcoholic hepatitis (AST > ALT)
		Myocardial infarction (AST)
	GGT (γ-glutamyl transpeptidase)	Various liver diseases; ↑ with heavy alcohol consumption
	Alkaline phosphatase	Obstructive liver disease (hepatocellular carcinoma), bone disease, bile duct disease
	Amylase	Acute pancreatitis, mumps
	Lipase	Acute pancreatitis
	Ceruloplasmin (↓)	Wilson's disease

Reye's syndrome

Rare, often fatal childhood hepatoencephalopathy. Findings: mitochondrial abnormalities, fatty liver (microvesicular fatty change), hypoglycemia, coma. Associated with viral infection (especially VZV and influenza B) that has been treated with salicylates. Mechanism: aspirin metabolites ↓ β-oxidation by reversible inhibition of mitochondrial enzyme. **Aspirin is not recommended for children** (use acetaminophen, with caution).

Alcoholic liver disease

Hepatic steatosis	Short-term change with moderate alcohol intake. Macrovesicular fatty change that may be reversible with alcohol cessation (see Image 29).	
Alcoholic hepatitis	Requires sustained, long-term consumption. Swollen and necrotic hepatocytes with neutrophilic infiltration. **Mallory bodies** (intracytoplasmic eosinophilic inclusions) are present.	You're to**AST**ed with alcoholic hepatitis: **AST > ALT** (ratio usually > 1.5).
Alcoholic cirrhosis	Final and irreversible form. Micronodular, irregularly shrunken liver with "hobnail" appearance (see Image 30). Sclerosis around central vein (zone III). Has manifestations of chronic liver disease (e.g., jaundice, hypoalbuminemia).	

Hepatocellular carcinoma/hepatoma

Most common 1° malignant tumor of the liver in adults. ↑ incidence is associated with hepatitis B and C, Wilson's disease, hemochromatosis, α_1-antitrypsin deficiency, alcoholic cirrhosis, and carcinogens (e.g., aflatoxin in peanuts). Findings: jaundice, tender hepatomegaly, ascites, polycythemia, and hypoglycemia.

Commonly spread by hematogenous dissemination. ↑ α-**fetoprotein.** May lead to Budd-Chiari syndrome.

Nutmeg liver

Due to backup of blood into liver. Commonly caused by right-sided heart failure and Budd-Chiari syndrome. The liver appears mottled like a nutmeg. If the condition persists, centrilobular congestion and necrosis can result in cardiac cirrhosis.

Budd-Chiari syndrome	Occlusion of IVC or hepatic veins with centrilobular congestion and necrosis, leading to congestive liver disease (hepatomegaly, ascites, abdominal pain, and eventual liver failure). May develop varices and have visible abdominal and back veins. Absence of JVD. Associated with hypercoaguable state, polycythemia vera, pregnancy, and hepato-cellular carcinoma.
α_1-antitrypsin deficiency	Misfolded gene product protein accumulates in hepatocellular ER. $\downarrow$ elastic tissue in lungs $\rightarrow$ panacinar emphysema. PAS-positive globules in liver. Codominant trait.
Physiologic neonatal jaundice	At birth, immature UDP-glucuronyl transferase $\rightarrow$ unconjugated hyperbilirubinemia $\rightarrow$ jaundice/kernicterus. Treatment: phototherapy (converts UCB to water-soluble form).
Jaundice	Normally, liver cells convert unconjugated (indirect) bilirubin into conjugated (direct) bilirubin. Direct bilirubin is water soluble and can be excreted into urine and by the liver into bile to be converted by gut bacteria to urobilinogen (some of which is reabsorbed). Some urobilinogen is also formed directly from heme metabolism.

Jaundice type	Hyperbilirubinemia	Urine bilirubin	Urine urobilinogen
Hepatocellular	Conjugated/unconjugated	$\uparrow$	Normal/$\downarrow$
Obstructive	Conjugated	$\uparrow$	$\downarrow$
Hemolytic	Unconjugated	Absent (acholuria)	$\uparrow$

HIGH-YIELD SYSTEMS

GASTROINTESTINAL

Hereditary hyperbilirubinemias

Gilbert's syndrome	Mildly ↓ UDP-glucuronyl transferase or ↓ bilirubin uptake. Asymptomatic. Elevated unconjugated bilirubin without overt hemolysis. Bilirubin increases with fasting and stress.	No clinical consequences.
Crigler-Najjar syndrome, type I	Absent UDP-glucuronyl transferase. Presents early in life; patients die within a few years. Findings: jaundice, kernicterus (bilirubin deposition in brain), ↑ unconjugated bilirubin. Treatment: plasmapheresis and phototherapy.	Type II is less severe and responds to phenobarbital, which ↑ liver enzyme synthesis.
Dubin-Johnson syndrome	Conjugated hyperbilirubinemia due to defective liver excretion. Grossly black liver. Benign.	**Rotor's syndrome** is similar but even milder and does not cause black liver.

1. Gilbert's = problem with bilirubin uptake → unconjugated bilirubinemia
2. Crigler-Najjar = problem with bilirubin conjugation → unconjugated bilirubinemia
3. Dubin-Johnson = problem with excretion of conjugated bilirubin → conjugated bilirubinemia

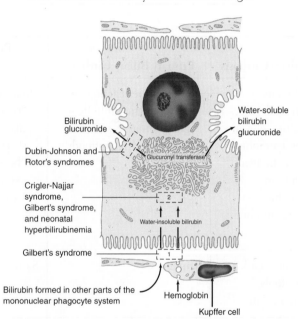

(Adapted, with permission, from Junqueira LC, Carneiro J. *Basic Histology*, 11th ed. New York: McGraw-Hill, 2005: 335.)

Wilson's disease (hepatolenticular degeneration)	Inadequate hepatic copper excretion and failure of copper to enter circulation as ceruloplasmin. Leads to copper accumulation, especially in liver, brain, cornea, kidneys, and joints. Characterized by: Asterixis **B**asal ganglia degeneration (parkinsonian symptoms) **C**eruloplasmin ↓, **C**irrhosis, **C**orneal deposits (Kayser-Fleischer rings—see Image 51), **C**opper accumulation, **C**arcinoma (hepatocellular), **C**horeiform movements **D**ementia **H**emolytic anemia	Treat with penicillamine. Autosomal-recessive inheritance. **ABCD.**

Hemochromatosis

Hemosiderosis is the deposition of hemosiderin (iron); hemochromatosis is the disease caused by this iron deposition (see Image 28). Classic triad of micronodular Cirrhosis, Diabetes mellitus, and skin pigmentation → **"bronze" diabetes.** Results in CHF and ↑ risk of hepatocellular carcinoma. Disease may be 1° (autosomal recessive) or 2° to chronic transfusion therapy (e.g., β-thalassemia major). ↑ ferritin, ↑ iron, ↓ TIBC → ↑ transferrin saturation.

Hemochromatosis Can Cause Deposits.
Total body iron may reach 50 g, enough to set off metal detectors at airports.
Treatment of hereditary hemochromatosis: repeated phlebotomy, deferoxamine.
Associated with HLA-A3.

Biliary tract disease

	Secondary Biliary Cirrhosis	Primary Biliary Cirrhosis	Primary Sclerosing Cholangitis
Pathophysiology/ pathology	Extrahepatic biliary obstruction (gallstone, biliary stricture, chronic pancreatitis, carcinoma of the pancreatic head) → ↑ pressure in intrahepatic ducts → injury/fibrosis and bile stasis.	Autoimmune reaction → lymphocytic infiltrate + granulomas. ↑ serum mitochondrial antibody.	Unknown cause of concentric "onion skin" bile duct fibrosis → alternating strictures and dilation with "beading" of intra- and extrahepatic bile ducts on ERCP.
Presentation	Pruritus, jaundice, dark urine, light stools, hepatosplenomegaly.	Same.	Same.
Labs	↑ conjugated bilirubin, ↑ cholesterol, ↑ alkaline phosphatase.	Same.	Same.
Additional information	Complicated by ascending cholangitis.	↑ **serum mitochondrial antibodies, including IgM.** Associated with other autoimmune conditions (e.g., CREST, rheumatoid arthritis, celiac disease).	Hypergammaglobulinemia (IgM). Associated with ulcerative colitis. Can lead to 2° biliary cirrhosis.

Gallstones (cholelithiasis)

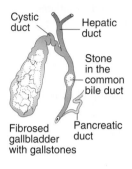

Cystic duct

Hepatic duct

Stone in the common bile duct

Fibrosed gallbladder with gallstones

Pancreatic duct

↑ cholesterol and/or bilirubin, ↓ bile salts, and gallbladder stasis all cause stones.

2 types of stones:
1. **Cholesterol stones** (radiolucent with 10–20% opaque due to calcifications)—80% of stones. Associated with obesity, Crohn's disease, cystic fibrosis, advanced age, clofibrate, estrogens, multiparity, rapid weight loss, and Native American origin.
2. **Pigment stones** (radiopaque)—seen in patients with chronic hemolysis, alcoholic cirrhosis, advanced age, and biliary infection.

Most often causes cholecystitis; also ascending cholangitis, acute pancreatitis, bile stasis.

Can also → **biliary colic**—obstruction of common duct by gallstones causes bile duct contraction—cause bile duct obstruction which results in bile duct contraction. May present without pain (e.g., in diabetics).

Can cause fistula between gallbladder and small intestine leading to air in the biliary tree. If gallstone obstructs ileocecal valve (gallstone ileus), air can be seen in biliary tree on imaging.

Diagnose with ultrasound. Treat with cholecystectomy.

Risk factors (**4 F's**):
1. **F**emale
2. **F**at
3. **F**ertile
4. **F**orty

Charcot's triad of cholangitis:
1. Jaundice
2. Fever
3. RUQ pain

Positive Murphy's sign—inspiratory arrest on deep palpation due to pain.

Cholecystitis

Inflammation of gallbladder. Usually from gallstones; rarely ischemia or infectious (CMV). ↑ alkaline phosphatase if bile duct becomes involved (e.g., ascending cholangitis).

Acute pancreatitis

Autodigestion of pancreas by pancreatic enzymes.

Causes: **G**allstones, **E**thanol, **T**rauma, **S**teroids, **M**umps, **A**utoimmune disease, **S**corpion sting, **H**ypercalcemia/**H**yperlipidemia, **E**RCP, **D**rugs (e.g., sulfa drugs).

Clinical presentation: epigastric abdominal pain radiating to back, anorexia, nausea.

Labs: elevated amylase, lipase (higher specificity).

Can lead to DIC, ARDS, diffuse fat necrosis, hypocalcemia (Ca^{2+} collects in pancreatic calcium soap deposits), pseudocyst formation, hemorrhage, infection, and multiorgan failure.

Chronic pancreatitis can lead to pancreatic insufficiency → steatorrhea, fat-soluble vitamin deficiency, and diabetes mellitus.

Chronic calcifying pancreatitis is strongly associated with alcoholism and smoking, ↑ risk of pancreatic cancer.

GET SMASHED.

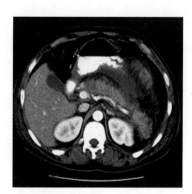

Acute pancreatitis showing pancreatic swelling and peri-pancreatic edema. (Reproduced, with permission, from the PEIR Digital Library.)

Pancreatic adenocarcinoma

Prognosis averages 6 months or less; very aggressive; usually already metastasized at presentation; tumors more common in pancreatic head (→ obstructive jaundice). ↑ risk in Jewish and African-American males. CEA and CA-19-9 tumor markers. Associated with cigarettes and chronic pancreatitis but not EtOH.

Often presents with:

1. Abdominal pain radiating to back
2. Weight loss (due to malabsorption and anorexia)
3. Migratory thrombophlebitis—redness and tenderness on palpation of extremities (Trousseau's syndrome)
4. Obstructive jaundice with palpable gallbladder (Courvoisier's sign)

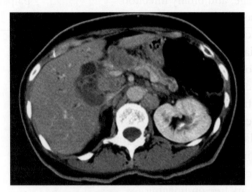

Pancreatic adenocarcinoma (note the large, heterogeneously enhancing mass visible at the neck of the pancreas).

(Reproduced, with permission, from the PEIR Digital Library.)

GI therapy

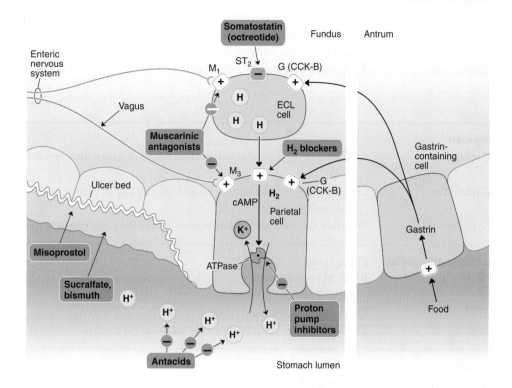

(Adapted, with permission, from Katzung BG, Trevor AJ. *USMLE Road Map: Pharmacology*, 1st ed. New York: McGraw-Hill, 2003: 159.)

H$_2$ blockers	Cimeti**dine**, raniti**dine**, famoti**dine**, nizati**dine**.	Take H$_2$ blockers before you
Mechanism	Reversible block of histamine H$_2$ receptors → ↓ H$^+$ secretion by parietal cells.	**DINE**. Think "**table for 2**" to remember **H$_2$**.
Clinical use	Peptic ulcer, gastritis, mild esophageal reflux.	
Toxicity	Cimetidine is a potent inhibitor of P-450; it also has antiandrogenic effects (prolactin release, gynecomastia, impotence, ↓ libido in males); can cross blood-brain barrier (confusion, dizziness, headaches) and placenta. Both cimetidine and ranitidine ↓ renal excretion of creatinine. Other H$_2$ blockers are relatively free of these effects.	

Proton pump inhibitors	Omeprazole, lansoprazole.
Mechanism	Irreversibly inhibit H$^+$/K$^+$-ATPase in stomach parietal cells.
Clinical use	Peptic ulcer, gastritis, esophageal reflux, Zollinger-Ellison syndrome.

Bismuth, sucralfate

Mechanism	Bind to ulcer base, providing physical protection, and allow HCO_3^- secretion to reestablish pH gradient in the mucous layer.
Clinical use	↑ ulcer healing, traveler's diarrhea.

Triple therapy of *H. pylori* ulcers—**Metronidazole, Amoxicillin** (or **Tetracycline**), **Bismuth.** Can also use PPI—Please **MA**ke Tummy **B**etter.

Misoprostol

Mechanism	A PGE_1 analog. ↑ production and secretion of gastric mucous barrier, ↓ acid production.
Clinical use	Prevention of NSAID-induced peptic ulcers; maintenance of a patent ductus arteriosus. Also used to induce labor.
Toxicity	Diarrhea. Contraindicated in women of childbearing potential (abortifacient).

Muscarinic antagonists Pirenzepine, propantheline.

Mechanism	Block M1 receptors on ECL cells (↓ histamine secretion) and M3 receptors on parietal cells (↓ H^+ secretion).
Clinical use	Peptic ulcer (rarely used).
Toxicity	Tachycardia, dry mouth, difficulty focusing eyes.

Octreotide

Mechanism	Somatostatin analog.
Clinical use	Acute variceal bleeds, acromegaly, VIPoma, and carcinoid tumors.
Toxicity	Nausea, cramps, steatorrhea.

Antacid use

Can affect absorption, bioavailability, or urinary excretion of other drugs by altering gastric and urinary pH or by delaying gastric emptying.
Overuse can also cause the following problems:

1. **Aluminum hydroxide**—constipation and hypophosphatemia; proximal muscle weakness, osteodystrophy, seizures

   Aluminimum amount of feces.

2. **Magnesium hydroxide**—diarrhea, hyporeflexia, hypotension, cardiac arrest

   Mg = **M**ust **g**o to the bathroom.

3. **Calcium carbonate**—hypercalcemia, rebound acid ↑

   Can chelate and ↓ effectiveness of other drugs (e.g., tetracycline).

All can cause hypokalemia.

Infliximab

Mechanism	A monoclonal antibody to TNF, proinflammatory cytokine.
Clinical use	Crohn's disease, rheumatoid arthritis.
Toxicity	Respiratory infection (including reactivation of latent TB), fever, hypotension.

INFLIXimab **INFLIX** pain on TNF.

HIGH-YIELD SYSTEMS

GASTROINTESTINAL

Sulfasalazine

Mechanism	A combination of sulfapyridine (antibacterial) and 5-aminosalicylic acid (anti-inflammatory). Activated by colonic bacteria.
Clinical use	Ulcerative colitis, Crohn's disease.
Toxicity	Malaise, nausea, sulfonamide toxicity, reversible oligospermia.

Ondansetron

Mechanism	5-HT$_3$ antagonist. Powerful central-acting antiemetic.	You will not vomit with **ONDANS**etron, so you can go **ON DANC**ing.
Clinical use	Control vomiting postoperatively and in patients undergoing cancer chemotherapy.	
Toxicity	Headache, constipation.	

Metoclopramide

Mechanism	D$_2$ receptor antagonist. $\uparrow$ resting tone, contractility, LES tone, motility. Does not influence colon transport time.
Clinical use	Diabetic and post-surgery gastroparesis.
Toxicity	$\uparrow$ parkinsonian effects. Restlessness, drowsiness, fatigue, depression, nausea, diarrhea. Drug interaction with digoxin and diabetic agents. Contraindicated in patients with small bowel obstruction.

Hematology and Oncology

"The best blood will at some time get into a fool or a mosquito."
—Austin O'Malley

"A day without blood is like a day without sunshine."
—Joker in *Full Metal Jacket*

▶ Anatomy

▶ Physiology

▶ Pathology

▶ Pharmacology

Study tip: When reviewing oncologic drugs, focus on mechanisms and side effects, rather than details of clinical uses, which may be lower yield.

Blood cell differentiation

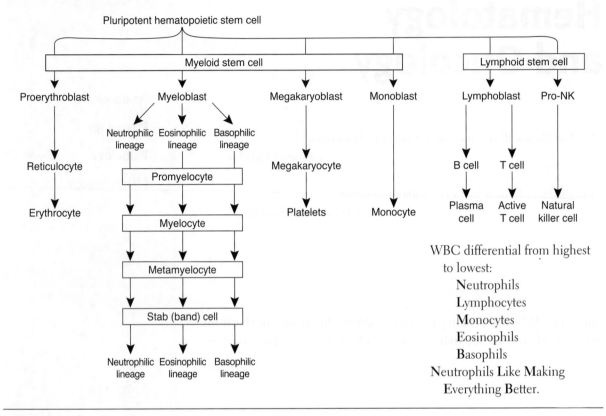

WBC differential from highest to lowest:
  Neutrophils
  Lymphocytes
  Monocytes
  Eosinophils
  Basophils
Neutrophils Like Making Everything Better.

Erythrocyte 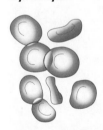	Anucleate, biconcave → large surface area: volume ratio → easy gas exchange (O_2 and CO_2). Source of energy—glucose (90% anaerobically degraded to lactate, 10% by HMP shunt). Membrane contains the chloride-bicarbonate antiport important in the "physiologic chloride shift," which allows the RBC to transport CO_2 from the periphery to the lungs for elimination. Survival time—120 days.	*Eryth* = red; *cyte* = cell. Erythrocytosis = polycythemia = ↑ number of red cells. Anisocytosis = varying sizes. Poikilocytosis = varying shapes. Reticulocyte = immature erythrocyte.
Platelet (thrombocyte) 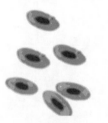	Small cytoplasmic fragment derived from megakaryocytes. Involved in 1° hemostasis. When activated by endothelial injury, aggregates with other platelets and interacts with fibrinogen to form hemostatic plug. Contains dense granules (ADP, calcium) and α-granules (vWF, fibrinogen). Approximately ⅓ of platelet pool is stored in the spleen. Life span of 8–10 days.	Promotes blood clotting and prevents leakage of RBCs from damaged vessels. Thrombocytopenia or platelet dysfunction results in petechiae. vWF receptor: Gplb. Fibrinogen receptor: Gpllb/llla.
Leukocyte	Types: granulocytes (basophils, eosinophils, neutrophils) and mononuclear cells (monocytes, lymphocytes). Responsible for defense against infections. Normally 4000–10,000 per microliter.	*Leuk* = white; *cyte* = cell.

Neutrophil 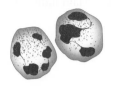	Acute inflammatory response cell. 40–75% WBCs. Phagocytic. Multilobed nucleus. Large, spherical, azurophilic granules (lysosomes) contain hydrolytic enzymes, lysozyme, myeloperoxidase, and lactoferrin.	Hypersegmented polys are seen in vitamin B_{12}/folate deficiency.
Monocyte	2–10% of leukocytes. Large, kidney-shaped nucleus. Extensive "frosted glass" cytoplasm. Differentiates into macrophages in tissues.	*Mono* = one (nucleus); *cyte* = cell. Monocyte: in the blood.
Macrophage 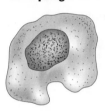	Phagocytoses bacteria, cell debris, and senescent red cells and scavenges damaged cells and tissues. Long life in tissues. Macrophages differentiate from circulating blood monocytes. Activated by γ-interferon. Can function as antigen-presenting cell via MHC II.	*Macro* = large; *phage* = eater. Macrophage: in the tissue.
Eosinophil 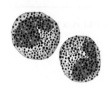	1–6% of all leukocytes. Bilobate nucleus. Packed with large eosinophilic granules of uniform size. Defends against helminthic infections (major basic protein). Highly phagocytic for antigen-antibody complexes. Produces histaminase and arylsulfatase (help limit reaction following mast cell degranulation).	*Eosin* = a dye; *philic* = loving. Causes of eosinophilia = **NAACP:** Neoplastic Asthma Allergic processes Collagen vascular diseases Parasites (invasive)
Basophil	Mediates allergic reaction. < 1% of all leukocytes. Bilobate nucleus. Densely basophilic granules containing heparin (anticoagulant), histamine (vasodilator) and other vasoactive amines, and leukotrienes (LTD-4). Found in the blood.	**Baso**philic—staining readily with **basic** stains.
Mast cell 	Mediates allergic reaction. Degranulation— histamine, heparin, and eosinophil chemotactic factors. Can bind the Fc portion of IgE to membrane. Mast cells resemble basophils structurally and functionally but are not the same cell type. Found in tissue.	Involved in type I hypersensitivity reactions. Cromolyn sodium prevents mast cell degranulation (used to treat asthma).

Dendritic cells

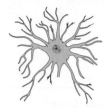

Professional (APCs). Express MHC II and Fc receptor (FcR) on surface. Main inducers of 1° antibody response. Called Langerhans cells on skin.

Lymphocyte

Round, densely staining nucleus. Small amount of pale cytoplasm. B lymphocytes produce antibodies. T lymphocytes manifest the cellular immune response as well as regulate B lymphocytes and macrophages.

B lymphocyte

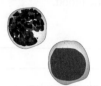

Part of humoral immune response. Arises from stem cells in bone marrow. Matures in marrow. Migrates to peripheral lymphoid tissue (follicles of lymph nodes, white pulp of spleen, unencapsulated lymphoid tissue). When antigen is encountered, B cells differentiate into plasma cells and produce antibodies. Has memory. Can function as an APC via MHC II.

B = **B**one marrow.

Plasma cell

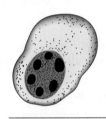

Off-center nucleus, clock-face chromatin distribution, abundant RER and well-developed Golgi apparatus. B cells differentiate into plasma cells, which produce large amounts of antibody specific to a particular antigen.

Multiple myeloma is a plasma cell neoplasm.

T lymphocyte

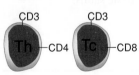

Mediates cellular immune response. Originates from stem cells in the bone marrow, but matures in the thymus. T cells differentiate into cytotoxic T cells (MHC I, CD8), helper T cells (MHC II, CD4), and suppressor T cells. The majority of circulating lymphocytes are T cells (80%).

T is for **T**hymus. **CD** is for **C**luster of **D**ifferentiation. $\mathbf{MHC} \times \mathbf{CD} = 8$ (e.g., MHC 2 × CD4 = 8, and MHC 1 × CD8 = 8).

Blood groups

A	A antigen on RBC surface and B antibody in plasma.	Incompatible blood transfusions can cause immunologic response, hemolysis, renal failure, shock, and death.
B	B antigen on RBC surface and A antibody in plasma.	
AB	A and B antigens on RBC surface; no antibodies in plasma; "universal recipient."	Note: anti-AB antibodies— IgM (do not cross placenta); anti-Rh—IgG (cross placenta).
O	Neither A nor B antigen on RBC surface; both antibodies in plasma; "universal donor."	
Rh	Rh antigen on RBC surface. Rh– mothers exposed to fetal Rh+ blood (often during delivery) may make anti-Rh IgG that can cross placenta during subsequent pregnancies and cause hemolytic disease of the newborn (erythroblastosis fetalis) in the next fetus that is Rh+. Treatment: Rh antigen immunoglobulin (Rhogam) for mother at first delivery to prevent future erythroblastosis.	

Coagulation, complement, and kinin pathways

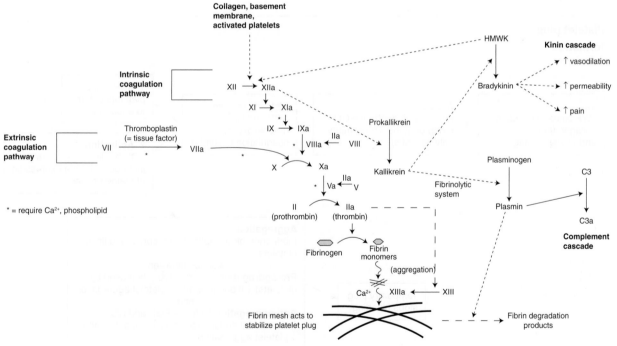

Note: Kallikrein activates bradykinin; ACE inactivates bradykinin.

Hemophilia A: deficiency of factor VIII.
Hemophilia B: deficiency of factor IX.
Vitamin K deficiency: ↓ synthesis of factors II, VII, IX, X, protein C, protein S.
Antithrombin: inhibits thrombin and factors IXa, Xa, XIa, and XIIa. Activated by heparin.

Coagulation cascade components

1. Pro-coagulation:

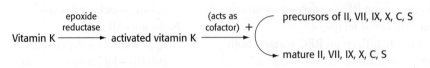

Warfarin inhibits reductase. Neonates lack enteric bacteria, which produce vitamin K.

vWF carries/protects VIII.

2. Anti-coagulation:

Antithrombin inactivates factors II, VII, IX, X, XI, XII.

Heparin-activated antithrombin.

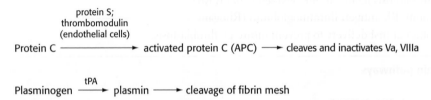

Factor V Leiden mutation produces a factor V resistant to APC's inhibition.

tPA is used clinically as a thrombolytic.

Platelet plug formation

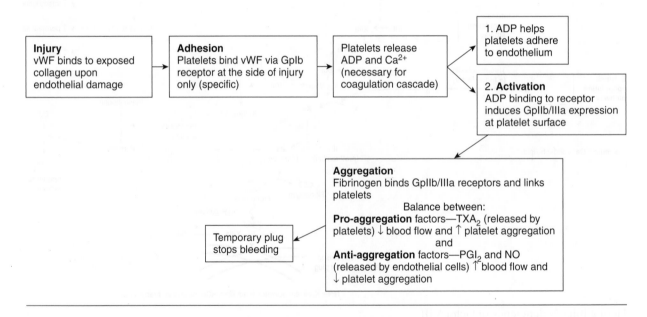

Thrombogenesis

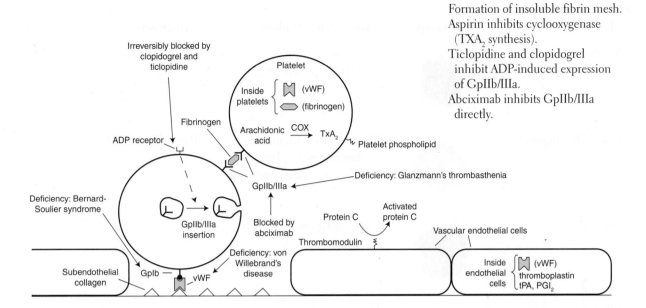

Formation of insoluble fibrin mesh.
Aspirin inhibits cyclooxygenase
  (TXA_2 synthesis).
Ticlopidine and clopidogrel
  inhibit ADP-induced expression
  of GpIIb/IIIa.
Abciximab inhibits GpIIb/IIIa
  directly.

Pathologic RBC forms

Type	Example	Associated pathology	Mnemonic
Acanthocyte (spur cell)		Liver disease, abetalipoproteinemia.	*Acantho* = spiny.
Basophilic stippling		**Tha**lassemias, **A**nemia of chronic disease, **I**ron deficiency, **L**ead poisoning.	**Bas**te the ox **TAIL**.
Bite cell		G6PD deficiency.	
Elliptocyte		Hereditary elliptocytosis.	
Macro-ovalocyte		Megaloblastic anemia (also hypersegmented PMNs), marrow failure.	
Ringed sideroblasts		Sideroblastic anemia.	
Schistocyte, helmet cell		DIC, TTP/HUS, traumatic hemolysis.	
Sickle cell		Sickle cell anemia.	
Spherocyte		Hereditary spherocytosis, autoimmune hemolysis.	
Teardrop cell		Bone marrow infiltration (e.g., myelofibrosis).	
Target cell		**H**bC disease, **A**splenia, **L**iver disease, **T**halassemia.	"**HALT**," said the hunter to his **target**.

Other RBC pathologies

Type	Example	Process	Associated pathology
Heinz bodies		Oxidation of iron from ferrous to ferric form leads to denatured hemoglobin precipitation and damage to RBC membrane. Leads to formation of bite cells.	Seen with α-thalassemia, G6PD deficiency.
Howell-Jolly bodies		Basophilic nuclear remnants found in RBCs.	Seen in patients with functional hyposplenia or asplenia.

Microcytic, hypochromic (MCV < 80) anemia

Iron deficiency	↓ iron due to chronic bleeding, malnutrition/absorption disorders or ↑ demand (e.g., pregnancy) → ↓ heme synthesis (see Image 22). May manifest as Plummer-Vinson syndrome (triad of iron deficiency anemia, esophageal web, and atrophic glossitis).
α-thalassemia	Prevalent in Asian and Africa populations. **Defect:** α-globin gene mutations → ↓ α-globin synthesis. Deletion of 4 genes is incompatible with life → formation of Hb Barts (γ_4), which causes hydrops fetalis. Deletion of 3 genes → HbH disease (β_4). Deletion of 1–2 genes is not associated with significant anemia.

β-thalassemia	Prevalent in Mediterranean populations.
	Defect: point mutations in splicing sites and promoter sequences.
	β-thalassemia minor (heterozygote):
	  1. β chain is underproduced.
	  2. Usually asymptomatic.
	  3. Diagnosis confirmed by ↑ HbA_2 (> 3.5%) on electrophoresis.
	β-thalassemia major (homozygote) (see Image 21):
	  1. β chain is absent → severe anemia requiring blood transfusion (2° hemochromatosis).
	  2. Marrow expansion ("crew cut" on skull x-ray) → skeletal deformities. Chipmunk facies.
	Both major and minor → ↑ HbF ($\alpha_2\gamma_2$).
	HbS/β-thalassemia heterozygote: mild to moderate sickle cell disease depending on amount of β-globin production.

Lead poisoning	Lead inhibits ferrochelatase and ALA dehydratase → ↓ heme synthesis. Also inhibits rRNA degradation, which causes basophilic stippling from the aggregation of ribosomes.
Sideroblastic anemia	**Defect in heme synthesis.** Hereditary: X-linked defect in δ-aminolevulinic acid synthase gene. Treatment: pyridoxine (B_6) therapy. Reversible etiologies: alcohol, lead. ↑ iron, normal TIBC, ↑ ferritin. Ringed sideroblasts (with iron-laden mitochondria).

Lead poisoning	Lead Lines on gingivae (Burton's lines) and on epiphyses of long bones on x-ray. Encephalopathy and Erythrocyte basophilic stippling. Abdominal colic and sideroblastic Anemia. Drops—wrist and foot drop. Dimercaprol and EDTA 1st line of treatment. Succimer for kids.	**LEAD.** High risk in houses with chipped paint. It "sucks" to be a kid who eats lead.

Macrocytic (MCV > 100) anemia	Impaired DNA synthesis → maturation of nucleus delayed relative to maturation of cytoplasm. Ineffective erythropoiesis leads to pancytopenia.
Megaloblastic anemia caused by folate deficiency	Findings: hypersegmented neutrophils, glossitis, ↓ folate, ↑ homocysteine but normal methylmalonic acid. Etiologies: malnutrition (e.g., alcoholics), malabsorption, impaired metabolism (e.g., methotrexate, trimethoprim), ↑ requirement (e.g., hemolytic anemia, pregnancy).

Megaloblastic anemia caused by B_{12} deficiency (cobalamin)	Findings: hypersegmented neutrophils, glossitis, ↓ B_{12}, ↑ homocysteine, ↑ methylmalonic acid.
	Etiologies: insufficient intake (e.g., strict vegans), malabsorption (e.g., Crohn's disease), pernicious anemia, *Diphyllobothrium latum* (fish tapeworm).
	Neurologic symptoms: subacute combined degeneration (due to involvement of B_{12} in fatty acid pathways).
	  1. Peripheral neuropathy with sensorimotor dysfunction
	  2. Posterior columns (vibration/proprioception)
	  3. Lateral corticospinal (spasticity)
	  4. Dementia

Nonmegaloblastic macrocytic anemias	1. Liver disease 2. Alcoholism: macrocytosis and bone marrow suppression can occur in the absence of folate/B_{12} deficiency 3. Reticulocytosis: reticulocytes are bigger than mature RBCs → ↑ MCV 4. Metabolic disorder (e.g., orotic aciduria): congenital deficiencies of purine or pyrimidine synthesis 5. Drugs: 5-FU, AZT, hydroxyurea

Normocytic, normochromic anemia	Normocytic, normochromic anemia may be classified as nonhemolytic vs. hemolytic. The hemolytic anemias are further classified according to the cause of the hemolysis (intrinsic vs. extrinsic to the RBC) and by the location of the hemolysis (intravascular vs. extravascular).
Intravascular hemolysis	Findings: ↓ haptoglobin, ↑ LDH, hemoglobin in urine (e.g., paroxysmal nocturnal hemoglobinuria, mechanical destruction [aortic stenosis, prosthetic valve]).
Extravascular hemolysis	Findings: Macrophage in spleen clears RBC. ↑ LDH plus ↑ UCB, which causes jaundice (e.g., hereditary spherocytosis, G6PD deficiency, sickle cell anemia).

HIGH-YIELD SYSTEMS

HEMATOLOGY AND ONCOLOGY

Nonhemolytic, normocytic anemia

Anemia of chronic disease (ACD)	Inflammation → ↑ hepcidin → ↓ release of iron from macrophages. ↓ iron, ↓ TIBC, ↑ ferritin. Can become microcytic, hypochromic in long-standing disease.
Aplastic anemia	Pathologic features: pancytopenia characterized by severe anemia, neutropenia, and thrombocytopenia. Normal cell morphology, but hypocellular bone marrow with fatty infiltration. Causes: failure or destruction of myeloid stem cells due to: 1. Radiation and drugs (benzene, chloramphenicol, alkylating agents, antimetabolites) 2. Viral agents (parvovirus B19, EBV, HIV, HCV) 3. Fanconi's anemia (inherited defect in DNA repair) 4. Idiopathic (immune mediated, 1° stem cell defect); may follow acute hepatitis Symptoms: fatigue, malaise, pallor, purpura, mucosal bleeding, petechiae, infection. Treatment: withdrawal of offending agent, immunosuppressive regimens (antithymocyte globulin, cyclosporine), allogeneic bone marrow transplantation, RBC and platelet transfusion, G-CSF or GM-CSF.
Kidney disease	↓ erythropoietin → ↓ hematopoiesis.

Intrinsic hemolytic normocytic anemia

E = extravascular; I = intravascular

Hereditary spherocytosis (E)	Defect in proteins interacting with RBC membrane skeleton and plasma membrane (e.g., ankyrin, band 4.1, or spectrin).
	Pathogenesis: less membrane causes small and round RBCs with no central pallor ($\uparrow$ MCHC, $\uparrow$ RDW) $\rightarrow$ premature removal of RBCs by spleen.
	Findings: splenomegaly, aplastic crisis (B19 infection). Howell-Jolly bodies present after splenectomy.
	Labs: positive osmotic fragility test. Treatment: splenectomy.
G6PD deficiency (I)	X-linked. Defect in G6PD $\rightarrow$ $\downarrow$ glutathione $\rightarrow$ $\uparrow$ RBC susceptibility to oxidant stress.
	Findings: hemolytic anemia following oxidant stress (e.g., sulfa drugs, infections, fava beans). Symptoms: back pain, hemoglobinuria a few days later.
	Labs: blood smear shows RBCs with Heinz bodies and bite cells.
Pyruvate kinase deficiency (E)	Autosomal recessive. Defect in pyruvate kinase $\rightarrow$ $\downarrow$ ATP $\rightarrow$ rigid RBCs.
	Presentation: hemolytic anemia in a newborn.
Sickle cell anemia (E)	8% of African-Americans carry the HbS trait; 0.2% have the disease.
	Sickled cells are crescent-shaped RBCs.
	"Crew cut" on skull x-ray due to marrow expansion from $\uparrow$ erythropoiesis (also in thalassemias).
	Newborns are initially asymptomatic owing to $\uparrow$ HbF and $\downarrow$ HbS.
	Mutation: HbS mutation is a single amino acid replacement in β chain (substitution of normal glutamic acid with valine) at position 6. Point mutation.
	Pathogenesis: deoxygenated HbS polymerizes. Low O_2 or dehydration precipitates sickling. Results in anemia and veno-occlusive disease.
	Heterozygotes (sickle cell trait) have resistance to malaria.
	Complications in homozygotes (sickle cell disease):
	1. Aplastic crisis (due to parvovirus B19 infection)
	2. Autosplenectomy $\rightarrow$ $\uparrow$ risk of infection with encapsulated organisms (Howell-Jolly bodies); functional splenic dysfunction occurs in early childhood
	3. *Salmonella* osteomyelitis
	4. Painful crisis (vaso-occlusive)
	5. Renal papillary necrosis (due to low O_2 in papilla) and microhematuria (medullary infarcts)
	6. Splenic sequestration crisis (see Image 23)
	Treatment: hydroxyurea ($\uparrow$ HbF) and bone marrow transplantation.
HbC defect	Glutamic acid–to-lysine mutation at position 6 in chain mutation; patients with HbSC (1 of each mutant gene) have milder disease than do HbSS patients.
Paroxysmal nocturnal hemoglobinuria (I)	Decay-accelerating factor (DAF) inhibits complement on RBC membrane.
	Impaired synthesis of GPI anchor synthesis of GPI anchor, decay accelerating factor and all GPI linked proteins in the RBC membrane.
	Labs: $\uparrow$ urine hemosiderin.

Extrinsic hemolytic normocytic anemia

Autoimmune hemolytic anemia	**Warm** agglutinin (Ig**G**)—chronic anemia seen in SLE, in CLL, or with certain drugs (e.g., α-methyldopa).	**Warm** weather is **GGG**reat.
	Cold agglutinin (Ig**M**)—acute anemia triggered by cold; seen in CLL, *Mycoplasma pneumoniae* infections, or infectious mononucleosis.	**Cold** ice cream—**MMM.**
	For both warm and cold AIHA it should be noted that many cases are idiopathic in etiology.	
	Erythroblastosis fetalis—seen in newborns due to Rh or other blood antigen incompatibility → mother's antibodies attack fetal RBCs.	
	Autoimmune hemolytic anemias are usually Coombs positive.	
	• Direct Coombs' test—anti-Ig antibody added to patient's RBCs agglutinate if RBCs are coated with Ig.	
	• Indirect Coombs' test—normal RBCs added to patient's serum agglutinate if serum has anti-RBC surface Ig.	
Microangiopathic anemia (I)	Pathogenesis: RBCs are damaged when passing through obstructed or narrowed vessel lumina. Seen in DIC, TTP-HUS, SLE, and malignant hypertension.	
	Schistocytes (helmet cells) are seen on blood smear due to mechanical destruction of RBCs.	
Macroangiopathic anemia	**Prosthetic heart valves** and aortic stenosis may also cause hemolytic anemia 2° to mechanical destruction.	
Infections	↑ destruction of RBCs (e.g., malaria, *Babesia*).	

Lab values in anemia

	Iron Deficiency	Chronic Disease	Hemo-chromatosis	Pregnancy/ OCP Use	Lead Poisoning
Serum iron	↓ (1°)	↓	↑ (1°)	—	↑
Transferrin or TIBC (indirectly measures transferrin)	↑	↓*	↓	↑ (1°)	↓
Ferritin	↓	↑ (1°)	↑	—	—
% transferrin saturation (serum Fe/TIBC)	↓↓	—	↑↑	↓	↑

Transferrin—transports iron in blood.
Ferritin—1° iron storage protein of body.
*Evolutionary reasoning—pathogens use circulating iron to thrive. The body has adapted a system in which iron is stored within the cells of the body and prevents pathogens from acquiring circulating iron.

Heme synthesis, porphyrias, and lead poisoning

The porphyrias are conditions of defective heme synthesis that lead to the accumulation of heme precursors. Lead inhibits specific enzymes needed in heme synthesis, leading to a similar condition.

Condition	Affected Enzyme	Accumulated Substrate	Presenting Symptoms
Lead poisoning	Ferrochelatase and ALA dehydratase	Protoporphyrin (blood)	Microcytic anemia, GI and kidney disease. Children—exposure to lead paint → mental deterioration. Adults—environmental exposure (battery/ ammunition/radiator factory) → headache, memory loss, demyelination.
Acute intermittent porphyria	Porphobilinogen deaminase (aka uroporphyrinogen-I-synthase)	Porphobilinogen, δ-ALA, uroporphyrin (urine)	Symptoms Painful abdomen Red wine–colored urine Polyneuropathy Psychological disturbances Precipitated by drugs Treatment: glucose and heme, which inhibit ALA synthase.
Porphyria cutanea tarda	Uroporphyrinogen decarboxylase	Uroporphyrin (tea-colored urine)	Blistering cutaneous photosensitivity. Most common porphyria.

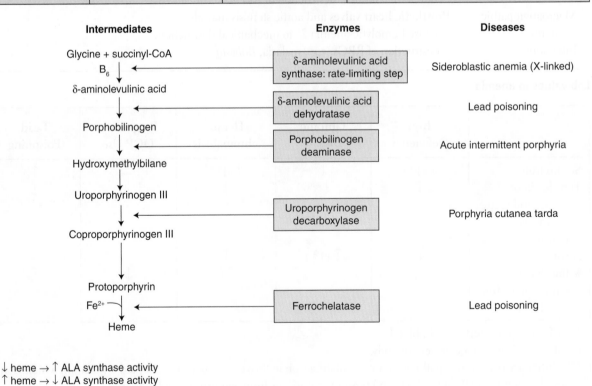

↓ heme → ↑ ALA synthase activity
↑ heme → ↓ ALA synthase activity

Coagulation disorders

PT—tests function of factors I, II, V, VII, and X (extrinsic pathway). Defect → ↑ PT.
PTT—tests function of all factors except VII and XIII (intrinsic pathway).
  Defect → ↑ PTT.

Disorder	PT	PTT	Mechanism and Comments

Hemophilia A or B	—	↑	Intrinsic pathway coagulation defect.
			  A: deficiency of factor VIII → ↑ PTT.
			  B: deficiency of factor IX → ↑ PTT.
			Macrohemorrhage in hemophilia—hemarthroses (bleeding into
			  joints), easy bruising, PTT.

Vitamin K deficiency	↑	↑	General coagulation defect. ↓ synthesis of factors II, VII, IX, X, protein C, protein S.

Platelet disorders

Defects in platelet plug formation → ↑ bleeding time (BT).
Platelet abnormalities → microhemorrhage: mucous membrane bleeding, epistaxis,
  petechiae, purpura, ↑ bleeding time, possible ↓ platelet count (PC).

Disorder	PC	BT	Mechanism and Comments
Bernard-Soulier disease	↓	↑	Defect in platelet plug formation. ↓ Gp1b → defect in platelet-to-collagen adhesion.
Glanzmann's thrombasthenia	—	↑	Defect in platelet plug formation. ↓ GpIIb/IIIa → defect in platelet-to-platelet aggregation. Labs: blood smear shows no platelet clumping.
Idiopathic thrombocytopenic purpura (ITP)	↓	↑	↓ platelet survival. Defect: anti-GpIIb/IIIa antibodies → peripheral platelet destruction. Labs: ↑ megakaryocytes.

Thrombotic thrombocytopenic purpura (TTP)	↓	↑	↓ platelet survival.
			Deficiency of ADAMTS 13 (vWF metalloprotease) → ↓
			  degradation of vWF multimers.
			Pathogenesis: ↑ large vWF multimers → ↑ platelet aggregation
			  and thrombosis.
			Labs: schistocytes, ↑ LDH.
			Symptoms: pentad of neurologic and renal symptoms, fever,
			  thrombocytopenia, and microangiopathic hemolytic anemia.

Mixed platelet and coagulation disorders

Disorder	PC	BT	PT	PTT	Mechanism and Comments
von Willebrand's disease	—	↑	—	— or ↑	Intrinsic pathway coagulation defect: ↓ vWF → normal or ↑ PTT (depends on severity; vWF acts to carry/protect factor VIII). Defect in platelet plug formation: ↓ vWF → defect in platelet-to-collagen adhesion. Mild but most common inherited bleeding disorder autosomal dominant. Treatment: DDAVP (desmopressin), which releases vWF stored in endothelium.
DIC	↓	↑	↑	↑	Widespread activation of clotting leads to a deficiency in clotting factors, which creates a bleeding state. Causes: Sepsis (gram-negative), Trauma, Obstetric complications, acute Pancreatitis, Malignancy, Nephrotic syndrome, Transfusion (**STOP M**aking **N**ew **T**hrombi). Labs: schistocytes, ↑ fibrin split products (D-dimers), ↓ fibrinogen, ↓ factors V and VIII.

Hereditary thrombosis syndromes leading to hypercoagulability

Disease	Description
Factor V Leiden	Production of mutant factor V that cannot be degraded by protein C. Most common cause of inherited hypercoagulability.
Prothrombin gene mutation	Mutation in 3′ untranslated region associated with venous clots.
ATIII deficiency	Inherited deficiency of antithrombin; reduced ↑ in PTT after administration of heparin.
Protein C or S deficiency	↓ ability to inactivate factors V and VIII. ↑ risk of thrombotic skin necrosis with hemorrhage following administration of warfarin.

Leukemia vs. lymphoma	Leukemia—lymphoid neoplasms with widespread involvement of bone marrow. Tumor cells are usually found in peripheral blood.
	Lymphoma—discrete tumor masses arising from lymph nodes.
	Presentations often blur definitions.

Leukemoid reaction	Often confused with leukemia. ↑ WBC count with left shift (e.g., 80% bands) and ↑ leukocyte alkaline phosphatase, usually due to infection.

Hodgkin's vs. Non-Hodgkin's lymphoma

Hodgkin's	Non-Hodgkin's
Presence of Reed-Sternberg cells	May be associated with HIV and immunosuppression
Localized, single group of nodes; extranodal rare; contiguous spread (stage is strongest predictor of prognosis)	Multiple, peripheral nodes; extranodal involvement common; noncontiguous spread
Constitutional ("B") signs/symptoms—low-grade fever, night sweats, weight loss	Majority involve B cells (except those of lymphoblastic T-cell origin)
Mediastinal lymphadenopathy	Fewer constitutional signs/symptoms
50% of cases associated with EBV; bimodal distribution —young and old; more common in men except for nodular sclerosing type	Peak incidence for certain subtypes at 20–40 years of age
Good prognosis = ↑ lymphocytes, ↓ RS	

Reed-Sternberg cells	Distinctive tumor giant cell seen in Hodgkin's disease (see Image 27); binucleate or bilobed with the 2 halves as mirror images ("owl's eyes"). RS cells are CD30+ and CD15+ B-cell origin. Necessary but not sufficient for a diagnosis of Hodgkin's disease. Variants include lacunar cells in nodular sclerosis variant.

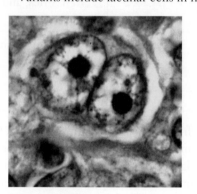

(Reproduced, with permission, from the PEIR Digital Library.)

Hodgkin's lymphoma

Type	RS	Lymphocyte	Prognosis	Comments
Nodular sclerosing (65–75%)	+	+++	Excellent	Most common; collagen banding; lacunar cells; women > men; primarily young adults.
Mixed cellularity (25%)	++++	+++	Intermediate	Numerous RS cells.
Lymphocyte predominant (6%)	+	++++	Excellent	< 35-year-old males.
Lymphocyte depleted (rare)	*	+	Poor	Older males with disseminated disease.

*RS high relative to lymphocytes. Note: ↑ lymphocyte-to-RS ratio roughly correlates with good prognosis.

Non-Hodgkin's lymphoma

Type	Occurs In	Genetics	Comments
Neoplasms of mature B cells			
Burkitt's lymphoma	Adolescents or young adults	t(8;14) c-*myc* gene moves next to heavy-chain Ig gene (14)	"Starry-sky" appearance (sheets of lymphocytes with interspersed macrophages). Associated with EBV. Jaw lesion in endemic form in Africa; pelvis or abdomen in sporadic form (see Image 26).
Diffuse large B-cell lymphoma	Usually older adults, but 20% in children.		Most common adult NHL. May be mature T cell in origin (20%).
Mantle cell lymphoma	Older males	t(11;14)	Poor prognosis, CD5+.
Follicular lymphoma	Adults	t(14;18) *bcl*-2 expression	Difficult to cure; indolent course; *bcl*-2 inhibits apoptosis.
Neoplasms of mature T cells			
Adult T-cell lymphoma	Adults	Caused by HTLV-1	Adults present with cutaneous lesions; especially affects populations in Japan, West Africa, and the Caribbean. Aggressive.
Mycosis fungoides/Sézary syndrome	Adults		Adults present with cutaneous patches/ nodules. Indolent CD4+.

Multiple myeloma

M spike →

Albumin α₁ α₂ β γ

Monoclonal plasma cell ("fried-egg" appearance) cancer that arises in the marrow and produces large amounts of IgG (55%) or IgA (25%). Most common 1° tumor arising within bone in the elderly (> 40–50 years of age).

Associated with:
1. ↑ susceptibility to infection
2. Primary amyloidosis (AL)
3. Punched-out lytic bone lesions on x-ray (see Image 25)
4. M spike on protein electrophoresis
5. Ig light chains in urine (Bence Jones protein)
6. Rouleaux formation (RBCs stacked like poker chips in blood smear)

Distinguish from Waldenström's macroglobulinemia → M spike = IgM (→ hyperviscosity symptoms); no lytic bone lesions.

Think **CRAB**:
hyper**C**alcemia
Renal insufficiency
Anemia
Bone lytic lesions/**B**ack pain

Multiple Myeloma:
Monoclonal **M** protein spike = Ig**M**

MGUS		Monoclonal gammopathy of undetermined significance (MGUS) is monoclonal plasma cell expansion without the symptoms of multiple myeloma.
Leukemias		Unregulated growth of leukocytes in bone marrow → ↑ or ↓ number of circulating leukocytes in blood and marrow failure → anemia (↓ RBCs), infections (↓ mature WBCs), and hemorrhage (↓ platelets); leukemic cell infiltrates in liver, spleen, and lymph nodes are possible (see Image 24).

Type	Occurs In	Comments
Lymphoid neoplasms		
Acute lymphoblastic leukemia/ lymphoma (ALL)	Children	May present with bone marrow involvement in childhood or mediastinal mass in adolescent males. Bone marrow replaced by ↑↑↑ lymphoblasts. TdT+ (marker of pre-T and pre-B cells), CALLA+. Most responsive to therapy. May spread to CNS and testes. t(12;21) → better prognosis.
Small lymphocytic lymphoma (SLL)/chronic lymphocytic leukemia (CLL)	Older adults (> 60 years of age)	Often asymptomatic; smudge cells in peripheral blood smear; warm antibody autoimmune hemolytic anemia. SLL same as CLL except CLL has ↑ peripheral blood lymphocytosis.
Hairy cell leukemia	Elderly	Mature B-cell tumor in the elderly. Cells have filamentous, hairlike projections. Stains TRAP (tartrate-resistant acid phosphatase) positive.
Myeloid neoplasms		
Acute myelogenous leukemia (AML)	Adults	Auer rods; ↑↑↑ circulating myeloblasts on peripheral smear; adults. M3 responds to all-*trans* retinoic acid (vitamin A), inducing differentiation of myeloblasts.
Chronic myelogenous leukemia (CML)		Defined by the Philadelphia chromosome (t[9;22], *bcr-abl*); myeloid stem cell proliferation; presents with ↑ neutrophils, metamyelocytes, basophils; splenomegaly; may accelerate and transform to AML or ALL ("blast crisis"). Very low leukocyte alkaline phosphatase (vs. leukemoid reaction). Responds to imatinib (anti-*bcr-abl* antibody).

Leukemias *(continued)*

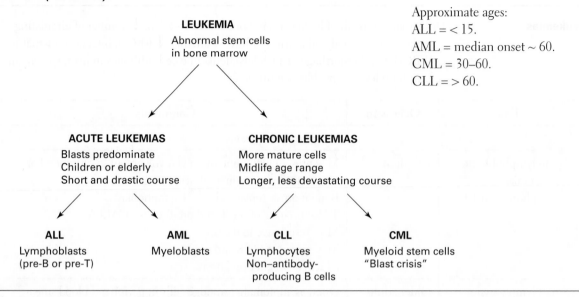

Approximate ages:
ALL = < 15.
AML = median onset ∼ 60.
CML = 30–60.
CLL = > 60.

Auer bodies (rods)	Peroxidase-positive cytoplasmic inclusions in granulocytes and myeloblasts. Commonly seen in acute promyelocytic leukemia (M3). Treatment of AML M3 can release Auer rods → DIC.

Chromosomal translocations

Translocation	Associated disorder	
t(9;22) (**Philadelphia** chromosome)	CML (*bcr-abl* hybrid)	**Philadelphia CreaML** cheese.
t(8;14)	Burkitt's lymphoma (c-*myc* activation)	
t(14;18)	Follicular lymphomas (*bcl-2* activation)	
t(15;17)	M3 type of AML (responsive to all-*trans* retinoic acid)	
t(11;22)	Ewing's sarcoma	
t(11;14)	Mantle cell lymphoma	

Langerhans cell histiocytosis (LCH)	Proliferative disorders of dendritic (Langerhans) cells. Defective cells express S-100 and CD1a. Birbeck granules ("tennis rackets" on EM) are characteristic.

Chronic myeloproliferative disorders

	RBCs	WBCs	Platelets	Philadelphia chromosome	*JAK2* mutations
Polycythemia vera	↑	↑	↑	Negative	Positive
Essential thrombocytosis	–	–	↑	Negative	Positive (30–50%)
Myelofibrosis	↓	Variable	Variable	Negative	Positive (30–50%)
CML	↓	↑	↑	Positive	Negative

The myelofibroproliferative disorders represent an often-overlapping spectrum, but the classic findings are described below.

Polycythemia vera — Abnormal clone of hematopoietic stem cells are increasingly sensitive to growth factors.

Essential thrombocytosis — Similar to polycythemia vera, but specific for megakaryocytes.

Myelofibrosis — Fibrotic obliteration of bone marrow. Teardrop cell. "Bone marrow is crying because it's fibrosed."

CML — *bcr-abl* transformation leads to ↑ cell division and inhibition of apoptosis.

JAK2 is involved in hematopoietic growth factor signaling. Mutations are implicated in myeloproliferative disorders other than CML.

Polycythemia

	Plasma Volume	RBC Mass	O_2 Saturation	EPO	Associated Diseases
Relative	↓	–	–	–	
Appropriate absolute	–	↑	↓	↑	Lung disease, congential heart disease, high altitude.
Inappropriate absolute	–	↑	–	↑	Due to ectopic erythropoietin.
Polycythemia vera	↑	↑↑	–	↓	RCC, Wilms' tumor, cyst, HCC, hydronephrosis.

HIGH-YIELD SYSTEMS

HEMATOLOGY AND ONCOLOGY

Heparin

Mechanism	Cofactor for the activation of antithrombin, ↓ thrombin, and Xa. Short half-life.
Clinical use	Immediate anticoagulation for pulmonary embolism, stroke, acute coronary syndrome, MI, DVT. Used during pregnancy (does not cross placenta). Follow PTT.
Toxicity	Bleeding, thrombocytopenia (HIT), osteoporosis, drug-drug interactions. For rapid reversal (antidote), use **protamine sulfate** (positively charged molecule that binds negatively charged heparin).
Notes	Newer **low-molecular-weight heparins** (e.g., enoxaparin) act more on Xa, have better bioavailability and 2–4 times longer half-life. Can be administered subcutaneously and without laboratory monitoring. Not easily reversible.
	Heparin-induced thrombocytopenia (HIT)—heparin binds to platelet factor IV, causing antibody production that binds to and activates platelets leading to their clearance and resulting in a thrombocytopenic, hypercoagulable state.

Lepirudin, bivalirudin Hirudin derivatives; directly inhibit thrombin. Used as an alternative to heparin for anticoagulating patients with HIT.

Warfarin (Coumadin)

Mechanism	Interferes with normal synthesis and γ-carboxylation of vitamin K–dependent clotting factors II, VII, IX, and X and protein C and S. Metabolized by the cytochrome P-450 pathway. In laboratory assay, has effect on **EX**trinsic pathway and ↑ **PT**. Long half-life.	The **EX-PresidenT** went to **WAR**(farin).
Clinical use	Chronic anticoagulation. Not used in pregnant women (because warfarin, unlike heparin, can cross the placenta). Follow PT/INR values.	For reversal of warfarin overdose, give vitamin K. For rapid reversal of severe warfarin overdose, give fresh frozen plasma.
Toxicity	Bleeding, teratogenic, skin/tissue necrosis, drug-drug interactions.	

Heparin vs. warfarin

	Heparin	Warfarin
Structure	Large anionic, acidic polymer	Small lipid-soluble molecule
Route of administration	Parenteral (IV, SC)	Oral
Site of action	Blood	Liver
Onset of action	Rapid (seconds)	Slow, limited by half-lives of normal clotting factors
Mechanism of action	Activates antithrombin, which ↓ the action of IIa (thrombin) and Xa	Impairs the synthesis of vitamin K–dependent clotting factors II, VII, IX, and X (vitamin K antagonist)
Duration of action	Acute (hours)	Chronic (days)
Inhibits coagulation in vitro	Yes	No
Treatment of acute overdose	Protamine sulfate	IV vitamin K and fresh frozen plasma
Monitoring	PTT (intrinsic pathway)	PT/INR (extrinsic pathway)
Crosses placenta	No	Yes (teratogenic)

Thrombolytics   Streptokinase, urokinase, tPA (alteplase), APSAC (anistreplase).

Mechanism   Directly or indirectly aid conversion of plasminogen to plasmin, which cleaves thrombin and fibrin clots. ↑ PT, ↑ PTT, no change in platelet count.

Clinical use   Early MI, early ischemic stroke.

Toxicity   Bleeding. Contraindicated in patients with active bleeding, history of intracranial bleeding, recent surgery, known bleeding diatheses, or severe hypertension. Treat toxicity with aminocaproic acid, an inhibitor of fibrinolysis.

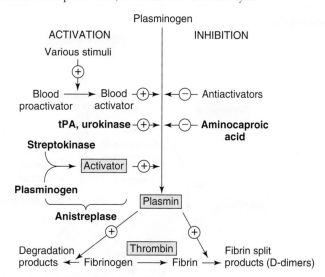

(Adapted, with permission, from Katzung BG. *Basic and Clinical Pharmacology,* 7th ed. Stamford, CT: Appleton & Lange, 1997: 550.)

Aspirin (ASA)

Mechanism   Acetylates and irreversibly inhibits cyclooxygenase (both COX-1 and COX-2) to prevent conversion of arachidonic acid to thromboxane A_2 (TxA_2). ↑ bleeding time. No effect on PT, PTT.

Clinical use   Antipyretic, analgesic, anti-inflammatory, antiplatelet drug.

Toxicity   Gastric ulceration, bleeding, hyperventilation, Reye's syndrome, tinnitus (CN VIII).

Clopidogrel, ticlopidine

Mechanism   Inhibit platelet aggregation by irreversibly blocking ADP receptors. Inhibit fibrinogen binding by preventing glycoprotein IIb/IIIa expression.

Clinical use   Acute coronary syndrome; coronary stenting. ↓ incidence or recurrence of thrombotic stroke.

Toxicity   Neutropenia (ticlopidine).

Abciximab

Mechanism	Monoclonal antibody that binds to the glycoprotein receptor IIb/IIIa on activated platelets, preventing aggregation.
Clinical use	Acute coronary syndromes, percutaneous transluminal coronary angioplasty.
Toxicity	Bleeding, thrombocytopenia.

Cancer drugs–cell cycle

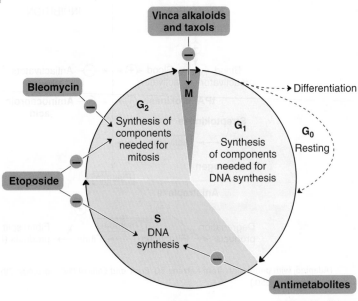

(Adapted, with permission, from Katzung BG, Trevor AJ. *USMLE Road Map: Pharmacology*, 1st ed. New York: McGraw-Hill, 2003: 133.)

Antineoplastics

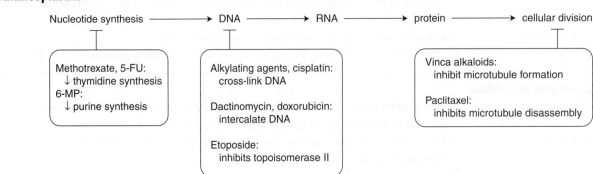

Antimetabolites

Drug	Mechanism*	Clinical Use	Toxicity
Methotrexate (MTX)	**Folic acid analog** that inhibits dihydrofolate reductase → ↓ dTMP → ↓ DNA and ↓ protein synthesis.	**Cancers:** Leukemias, lymphomas, choriocarcinoma, sarcomas. **Non-neoplastic:** Abortion, ectopic pregnancy, rheumatoid arthritis, psoriasis.	1. Myelosuppression, which is reversible with **leucovorin** (folinic acid) "rescue." 2. Macrovesicular fatty change in liver. 3. Mucositis. 4. Teratogenic.
5-fluorouracil (5-FU)	**Pyrimidine analog** bioactivated to 5F-dUMP, which covalently complexes folic acid. This complex **inhibits thymidylate synthase** → ↓ dTMP → ↓ DNA and ↓ protein synthesis.	Colon cancer and other solid tumors, basal cell carcinoma (topical). Synergy with MTX.	1. Myelosuppression, which is **not** reversible with leucovorin. Overdose: "rescue" with **thymidine.** 2. Photosensitivity.
6-mercaptopurine (6-MP)	**Purine** (thiol) analog → ↓ de novo purine synthesis. Activated by HGPRTase.	Leukemias, lymphomas (not CLL or Hodgkin's).	Bone marrow, GI, liver. Metabolized by xanthine oxidase; thus ↑ toxicity with allopurinol.
6-thioguanine (6-TG)	Same as 6-MP.	Acute lymphoid leukemia.	Bone marrow depression, liver. Can be given with allopurinol.
Cytarabine (ara-C)	Pyrimidine antagonist → inhibition of DNA polymerase.	AML, ALL, high-grade non-Hodgkin's lymphoma.	Leukopenia, thrombocytopenia, megaloblastic anemia.

*All are S-phase specific.

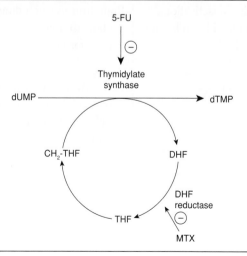

Antitumor antibiotics

Drug	Mechanism	Clinical Use	Toxicity
Dactinomycin (**ACT**inomycin D)	Intercalates in DNA.	Wilms' tumor, Ewing's sarcoma, rhabdomyosarcoma. Used for childhood tumors (children **ACT** out).	Myelosuppression.
Doxorubicin (**Adriamycin**), daunorubicin	Generate free radicals. Noncovalently intercalate in DNA → breaks in DNA → ↓ replication.	Hodgkin's lymphomas; also for myelomas, sarcomas, and solid tumors (breast, ovary, lung).	Cardiotoxicity, myelosuppression, and alopecia. Toxic to tissues with extravasation.
Bleomycin	Induces free radical formation, which causes breaks in DNA strands.	Testicular cancer, Hodgkin's lymphoma.	Pulmonary fibrosis, skin changes. Minimal myelosuppression.
Etoposide (VP-16), teniposide	Inhibits topoisomerase II → ↑ DNA degradation.	Small cell carcinoma of the lung and prostate, testicular carcinoma.	Myelosuppression, GI irritation, alopecia.

Alkylating agents

Drug	Mechanism	Clinical Use	Toxicity
Cyclophosphamide, ifosfamide	Covalently X-link (interstrand) DNA at guanine N-7. Require bioactivation by liver.	Non-Hodgkin's lymphoma, breast and ovarian carcinomas. Also immuno-suppressants.	Myelosuppression; hemorrhagic cystitis, partially prevented with mesna (thiol group of mesna binds toxic metabolite).
Nitrosoureas (carmustine, lomustine, semustine, streptozocin)	Require bioactivation. Cross blood-brain barrier → CNS.	Brain tumors (including glioblastoma multiforme).	CNS toxicity (dizziness, ataxia).
Busulfan	Alkylates DNA.	CML. Also used to ablate patient's bone marrow before bone marrow transplantation.	Pulmonary fibrosis, hyperpigmentation.

Microtubule inhibitors

Drug	Mechanism	Clinical Use	Toxicity
Vincristine, vinblastine	Alkaloids that bind to tubulin in M-phase and block polymerization of microtubules so that mitotic spindle cannot form. Microtubules are the **vines** of your cells.	Hodgkin's lymphoma, Wilms' tumor, choriocarcinoma.	Vincristine—neurotoxicity (areflexia, peripheral neuritis), paralytic ileus. Vin**BLAST**ine **BLAST**s Bone marrow (suppression).
Pacli**TAX**el, other **TAX**ols	Hyperstabilize polymerized microtubules in M-phase so that mitotic spindle cannot break down (anaphase cannot occur). It is **TAX**ing to stay polymerized.	Ovarian and breast carcinomas.	Myelosuppression and hypersensitivity.

Cisplatin, carboplatin

Mechanism	Cross-link DNA.
Clinical use	Testicular, bladder, ovary, and lung carcinomas.
Toxicity	Nephrotoxicity and acoustic nerve damage.

Hydroxyurea

Mechanism	Inhibits **R**ibonucleotide **R**eductase → ↓ DNA **S**ynthesis (**S**-phase specific).
Clinical use	Melanoma, CML, sickle cell disease (↑ HbF).
Toxicity	Bone marrow suppression, GI upset.

Prednisone

Mechanism	May trigger apoptosis. May even work on nondividing cells.
Clinical use	Most commonly used glucocorticoid in cancer chemotherapy. Used in CLL, Hodgkin's lymphomas (part of the MO**PP** regimen). Also an immunosuppressant used in autoimmune diseases.
Toxicity	Cushing-like symptoms; immunosuppression, cataracts, acne, osteoporosis, hypertension, peptic ulcers, hyperglycemia, psychosis.

Tamoxifen, raloxifene

Mechanism	SERMs—receptor antagonists in breast and agonists in bone. Block the binding of estrogen to estrogen receptor–positive cells.
Clinical use	Breast cancer. Also useful to prevent osteoporosis.
Toxicity	Tamoxifen—may ↑ the risk of endometrial carcinoma via partial agonist effects; "hot flashes." Raloxifene—no ↑ in endometrial carcinoma because it is an endometrial antagonist.

Trastuzumab (Herceptin)

Mechanism	Monoclonal antibody against HER-2 (*erb*-B2). Helps kill breast cancer cells that overexpress HER-2, possibly through antibody-dependent cytotoxicity.
Clinical use	Metastatic breast cancer.
Toxicity	Cardiotoxicity.

Imatinib (Gleevec)

Mechanism	Philadelphia chromosome *bcr-abl* tyrosine kinase inhibitor.
Clinical use	CML, GI stromal tumors.
Toxicity	Fluid retention.

Rituximab

Mechanism	Monoclonal antibody against CD20, which is found on most B-cell neoplasms.
Clinical use	Non-Hodgkin's lymphoma, rheumatoid arthritis (with methotrexate).

Musculoskeletal and Connective Tissue

"I just use my muscles like a conversation piece, like someone walking a cheetah down 42nd Street."

—Arnold Schwarzenegger

"Beauty may be skin deep, but ugly goes clear to the bone."

—Redd Foxx

"I try to catch him right on the tip of his nose because I try to punch the bone into the brain."

—Mike Tyson

"The function of muscle is to pull and not to push, except in the case of the genitals and the tongue."

—Leonardo da Vinci

▶ Anatomy and Physiology

▶ Pathology

▶ Pharmacology

Epidermis layers

From surface to base: stratum Corneum, stratum Lucidum, stratum Granulosum, stratum Spinosum, stratum Basalis.

Californians Like Girls in String Bikinis.

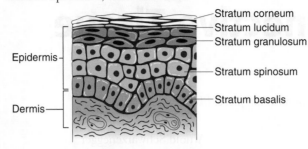

Epidermis
- Stratum corneum
- Stratum lucidum
- Stratum granulosum
- Stratum spinosum
- Stratum basalis

Dermis

Epithelial cell junctions

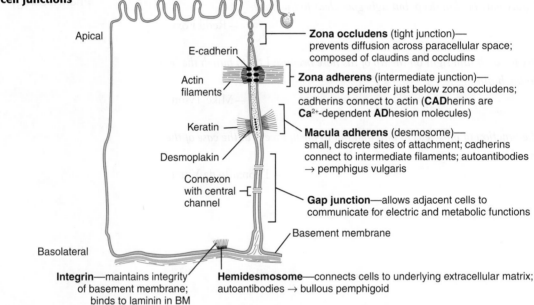

Apical

E-cadherin

Actin filaments

Keratin

Desmoplakin

Connexon with central channel

Basolateral

Integrin—maintains integrity of basement membrane; binds to laminin in BM

Zona occludens (tight junction)—prevents diffusion across paracellular space; composed of claudins and occludins

Zona adherens (intermediate junction)—surrounds perimeter just below zona occludens; cadherins connect to actin (**CAD**herins are **Ca**$^{2+}$-dependent **AD**hesion molecules)

Macula adherens (desmosome)—small, discrete sites of attachment; cadherins connect to intermediate filaments; autoantibodies → pemphigus vulgaris

Gap junction—allows adjacent cells to communicate for electric and metabolic functions

Basement membrane

Hemidesmosome—connects cells to underlying extracellular matrix; autoantibodies → bullous pemphigoid

---

Unhappy triad/ knee injury

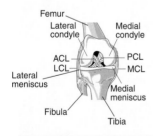

Femur
Lateral condyle
Medial condyle
ACL
LCL
PCL
MCL
Lateral meniscus
Medial meniscus
Fibula
Tibia

Common football injury. Force from the lateral side → damage to the "unhappy triad":
1. Medial collateral ligament (MCL)
2. Anterior cruciate ligament (ACL)
3. Lateral (**not** medial) meniscus

PCL = posterior cruciate ligament.

LCL = lateral collateral ligament.

"Anterior" and "posterior" in ACL and PCL refer to sites of **tibial** attachment.

Positive anterior drawer sign indicates tearing of the ACL.

Abnormal passive abduction indicates a torn MCL.

Clinically important landmarks	Pudendal nerve block (to relieve pain of delivery)—ischial spine.
	Appendix—$^2/_3$ of the way from the umbilicus to the anterior superior iliac spine (McBurney's point).
	Lumbar puncture—iliac crest.

Rotator cuff muscles	Shoulder muscles that form the rotator cuff:	**SItS** (small t is for teres minor).
	Supraspinatus—abducts arm initially (before deltoid); most common rotator cuff injury.	
Acromion Supraspinatus — Coracoid Infra-spinatus — Biceps tendon Teres minor — Sub-scapularis **Posterior ⟶ Anterior**	Infraspinatus—laterally rotates arm; pitching injury. Teres minor—adducts and laterally rotates arm. Subscapularis—medially rotates and adducts arm.	

Upper extremity innervation

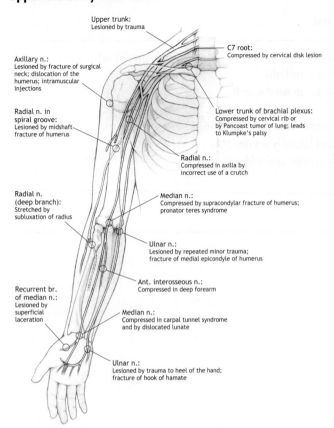

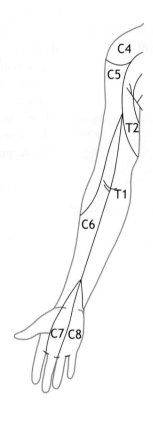

A. Upper limb nerve routes and common lesions

B. Dermatomes of the upper limb/hand

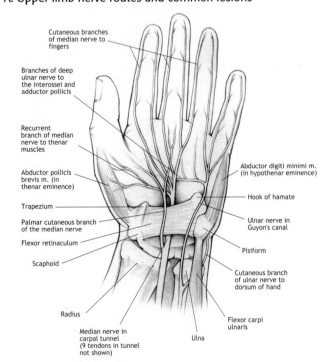

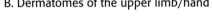

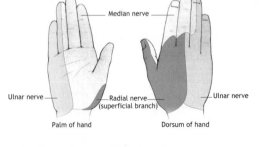

D. Dermatomes of the hand

C. Innervation of the hand

(Adaped, with permission, from White JS. *USMLE Road Map: Gross Anatomy,* 2nd ed. New York: McGraw-Hill, 2005: 145–147.)

Brachial plexus lesions

1. Waiter's tip (Erb's palsy)
2. Total claw hand (Klumpke's palsy)
3. Wrist drop
4. Winged scapula
5. Deltoid paralysis
6. Saturday night palsy (wrist drop)
7. Difficulty flexing elbow, variable sensory loss
8. ↓ thumb function ("ape hand")
9. Intrinsic muscles of hand, claw hand ("Pope's blessing")

LT = long thoracic nerve
Rad = radial nerve
Ax = axillary nerve
MC = musculocutaneous nerve
Med = median nerve
Uln = ulnar nerve

Clavicle fracture is relatively common—brachial plexus is protected from injury by subclavius muscle.

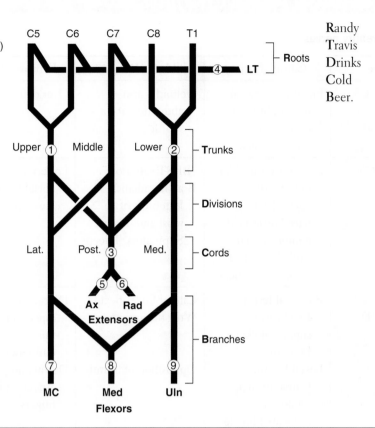

Randy
Travis
Drinks
Cold
Beer.

Roots

Trunks

Divisions

Cords

Branches

Upper extremity nerves

Nerve	Cause of Injury	Motor Deficit	Sensory Deficit	Sign
Axillary (C5, C6)	Fractured surgical neck of humerus, dislocation of humeral head	Deltoid—arm abduction at shoulder	Over deltoid muscle	Flattened deltoid
Radial (C5–C8)	Fracture at midshaft of humerus; "Saturday night palsy" (extended compression of axilla by back of chair or crutches)	"**BEST** extensors" Brachioradialis, Extensors of wrist and fingers, Supinators, Triceps	Posterior arm and dorsal hand and dorsal thumb	Wrist drop
Median (C6–C8, T1)	**Proximal lesion:** Fracture of supracondylar humerus **Distal lesion:** Carpal tunnel syndrome; dislocated lunate	Lateral finger flexion Wrist flexion Opposition of thumb	Dorsal and palmar aspects of lateral 3½ fingers, thenar eminence Dorsal and palmar aspects of lateral 3½ fingers	"Ape hand"; thenar atrophy, loss of opposability of thumb Ulnar deviation of wrist upon wrist flexion
Ulnar (C8, T1)	**Proximal lesion:** Fracture of medial epicondyle of humerus, "funny bone" **Distal lesion:** Fracture of hook of hamate (falling onto outstretched hand)	Medial finger flexion Wrist flexion Abduction and adduction of fingers (interossei) Adduction of thumb Extension of 4th and 5th fingers (lumbricals)	Medial 1½ fingers, hypothenar eminence	Radial deviation of wrist upon wrist flexion Ulnar claw hand (when asked to straighten fingers) —"Pope's blessing/ hand of benediction"
Musculo-cutaneous (C5–C7)	Upper trunk compression	Biceps, Brachialis, Coracobrachialis. Flexion of arm at elbow	Lateral forearm	

Erb-Duchenne palsy ("waiter's tip") 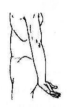	Traction or tear of the upper trunk of the brachial plexus (C5 and C6 roots); follows blow to shoulder or trauma during delivery. Findings: limb hangs by side (paralysis of abductors), medially rotated (paralysis of lateral rotators), forearm is pronated (loss of biceps).	"Waiter's tip" owing to appearance of arm.

Klumpke's palsy and thoracic outlet syndrome

An embryologic or childbirth defect affecting inferior trunk of brachial plexus (C8, T1); a cervical rib can compress subclavian artery and inferior trunk, resulting in thoracic outlet syndrome:

1. Atrophy of the thenar and hypothenar eminences
2. Atrophy of the interosseous muscles
3. Sensory deficits on the medial side of the forearm and hand
4. Disappearance of the radial pulse upon moving the head toward the ipsilateral side

Distortions of the hand

Multiple types: ulnar claw, median claw, "ape hand," and Klumpke's total claw (clawing of all digits). To keep things straight, just remember it's all about the lumbricals, which flex the MCP joints and extend both the DIP and PIP joints.

Ulnar claw

Distal ulnar nerve lesion → loss of medial lumbrical function; 4th and 5th digits are clawed ("Pope's blessing"). Cannot extend 4th and 5th digits. When try to open hand, pinky and ring finger stay clawed. Note: Making fist with **P**roximal median nerve lesion (can't flex lateral fingers) can also look like **P**ope's blessing.

Median claw

Distal median nerve lesion (after branch containing C5–C7 branches off to feed forearm flexors) → loss of lateral lumbrical function; 2nd and 3rd digits are clawed. Cannot extend 2nd and 3rd digit.

"Ape hand"

Proximal median nerve lesion → loss of opponens pollicis muscle function → unopposable thumb (inability to abduct thumb), hence "ape hand."

Klumpke's total claw

Lesion of lower trunk (C8, T1) of brachial plexus → loss of function of all lumbricals; forearm finger flexors (fed by part of median nerve with C5–C7) and finger extensors (fed by radial nerve) are unopposed → clawing of all digits.

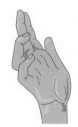

Claw hand of 4th and 5th digits ("Pope's blessing") Distal ulnar nerve lesion

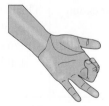

Claw hand of 2nd and 3rd digits Median nerve

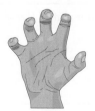

Klumpke's total claw hand Lower trunk (C8, T1)

Long thoracic nerve (C5–C7)

Serratus anterior—connects scapula to thoracic cage. Used for abduction above horizontal position. Can be injured in mastectomy → winged scapula and lymphedema.

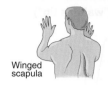

Winged scapula

Hand muscles

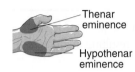

Thenar eminence

Hypothenar eminence

Thenar (median)—Opponens pollicis, Abductor pollicis brevis, Flexor pollicis brevis.
Hypothenar (ulnar)—Opponens digiti minimi, Abductor digiti minimi, Flexor digiti minimi.
Dorsal interosseous muscles—abduct the fingers.
Palmar interosseous muscles—adduct the fingers.
Lumbrical muscles—flex at the MCP joint.

Both groups perform the same functions: Oppose, Abduct, and Flex (OAF).

DAB = Dorsals ABduct.
PAD = Palmars ADduct.

Repetitive elbow trauma

Degenerative injury due to repeated use; leads to tiny tears in tendons and muscles. May be inflammatory—e.g., lateral epicondylitis (tennis elbow), medial epicondylitis (golf elbow).

Lower extremity nerves

Nerve	Cause of Injury	Motor Deficit	Sensory Deficit
Obturator (L2–L4)	Anterior hip dislocation	Thigh adduction	Medial thigh
Femoral (L2–L4)	Pelvic fracture	Thigh flexion and leg extension	Anterior thigh and medial leg
Common peroneal (L4–S2)	Trauma to lateral aspect of leg or fibula neck fracture	Foot eversion and dorsiflexion; toe extension; foot drop, foot slap, steppage gait	Anterolateral leg and dorsal aspect of foot
Tibial (L4–S2)	Knee trauma	Foot inversion and plantarflexion; toe flexion	Sole of foot
Superior gluteal (L4–S1)	Posterior hip dislocation or polio	Thigh abduction (positive Trendelenburg sign—hip drops when standing on opposite foot)	
Inferior gluteal (L5–S2)	Posterior hip dislocation	Can't jump, climb stairs, or rise from seated position; can't push inferiorly (downward)	

PED = Peroneal Everts and Dorsiflexes; if injured, foot dropPED (dorsiflex = extend foot).
TIP = Tibial Inverts and Plantarflexes; if injured, can't stand on TIPtoes.
Sciatic nerve (L4–S2)—posterior thigh, splits into common peroneal and tibial nerve.

Muscle conduction to contraction

A.

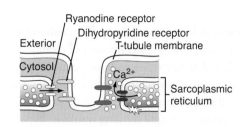

B.

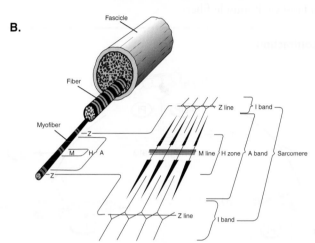

Thin lines along Z line = actin
Triangular structures emanating from M line = myosin

Muscle contraction:

1. Action potential depolarization opens voltage-gated Ca^{2+} channels, inducing neurotransmitter release.
2. Postsynaptic ligand binding leads to muscle cell depolarization in the motor end plate.
3. Depolarization travels along muscle cell and down the T-tubule.
4. Depolarization of the voltage-sensitive dihydropyridine receptor, coupled to the ryanodine receptor on the sarcoplasmic reticulum, induces a conformational change causing Ca^{2+} release from sarcoplasmic reticulum (calcium-induced calcium release).
5. Released Ca^{2+} binds to troponin C, causing a conformational change that moves tropomyosin out of the myosin-binding groove on actin filaments.
6. Myosin releases bound ADP and is displaced on the actin filament (power stroke). Contraction results in H- and I-band shortening, but the A band remains the same length (**A** band is **A**lways the same length; **HIZ** shrinkage).

Types of muscle fibers

Type 1 muscle	Slow twitch; red fibers due to ↑ mitochondria and myoglobin concentration (↑ oxidative phosphorylation) → sustained contraction.
Type 2 muscle	Fast twitch; white fibers due to ↓ mitochondria and myoglobin concentration (↑ anaerobic glycolysis); weight training results in hypertrophy of fast-twitch muscle fibers.

Think "one slow red ox."

Skeletal and cardiac muscle contraction

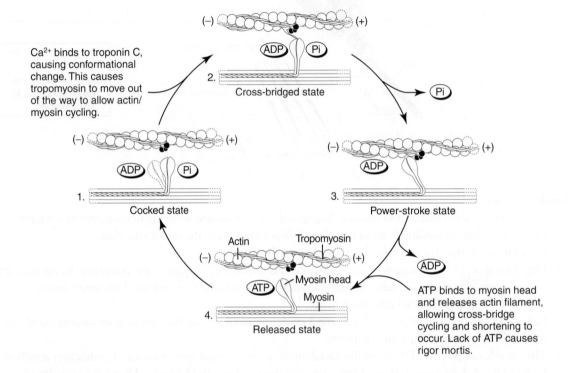

Ca^{2+} binds to troponin C, causing conformational change. This causes tropomyosin to move out of the way to allow actin/myosin cycling.

2. Cross-bridged state

1. Cocked state

3. Power-stroke state

4. Released state

Actin   Tropomyosin

Myosin head
Myosin

ATP binds to myosin head and releases actin filament, allowing cross-bridge cycling and shortening to occur. Lack of ATP causes rigor mortis.

Smooth muscle contraction

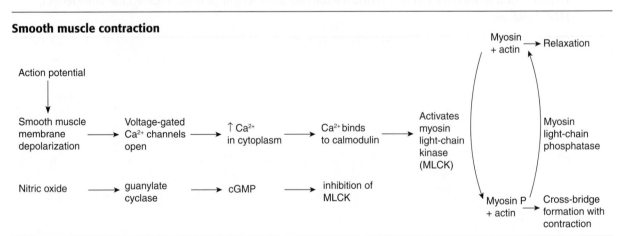

Action potential

Smooth muscle membrane depolarization → Voltage-gated Ca^{2+} channels open → ↑ Ca^{2+} in cytoplasm → Ca^{2+} binds to calmodulin → Activates myosin light-chain kinase (MLCK)

Nitric oxide → guanylate cyclase → cGMP → inhibition of MLCK

Myosin + actin → Relaxation

Myosin light-chain phosphatase

Myosin P + actin → Cross-bridge formation with contraction

Bone formation

Endochondral ossification	Longitudinal bone growth. Cartilaginous model of bone is first made by chondrocytes. Osteoclasts and osteoblasts later replace with woven bone and remodel to lamellar bone.	Osteoblast source— mesenchymal stem cells in periosteum.
Membranous ossification	Flat bone growth (skull, facial bones, and axial skeleton). Woven bone formed directly without cartilage. Later remodeled to lamellar bone.	

► MUSCULOSKELETAL AND CONNECTIVE TISSUE—PATHOLOGY

Achondroplasia	Failure of longitudinal bone growth (endochondrial ossification) → short limbs. Membranous ossification is not affected → large head. Constitutive activation of fibroblast growth factor receptor (FGFR3) actually inhibits chondrocyte proliferation. > 85% of mutations occur sporadically and are associated with advanced paternal age, but the condition also demonstrates autosomal-dominant inheritance. Common cause of dwarfism. Normal life span and fertility.

Osteoporosis	Reduction of primarily trabecular (spongy) bone mass despite normal bone mineralization and lab values.	Vertebral crush fractures— acute back pain, loss of height, kyphosis.
Type I	Postmenopausal; ↑ bone resorption due to ↓ estrogen levels.	Femoral neck fracture, distal radius (Colles') fractures.
Type II	Senile osteoporosis—affects men and women > 70 years of age.	Prophylaxis: exercise and calcium ingestion before age 30. Treatment: estrogen (SERMs) and/or calcitonin; bisphosphonates or pulsatile PTH for severe cases. Glucocorticoids are contraindicated.

Mild compression fracture   Normal vertebra

Osteopetrosis (marble bone disease)	Failure of normal bone resorption → thickened, dense bones that are prone to fracture. Bone defect is due to abnormal function of osteoclasts. Serum calcium, phosphate, and **alkaline phosphatase (ALP)** are **normal**. ↓ marrow space leads to anemia, thrombocytopenia, infection; ↑ extramedullary hematopoiesis. Genetic deficiency of carbonic anhydrase II. X-rays show "Erlenmeyer flask" bones that flare out. Can result in cranial nerve impingement and palsies due to narrowed foramina.
Osteomalacia/rickets	Defective mineralization/calcification of osteoid → soft bones. Vitamin D deficiency in adults → ↓ calcium levels → ↑ secretion of PTH, ↓ in serum phosphate. Reversible when vitamin D is replaced. Vitamin D deficiency in childhood causes rickets.

Paget's disease (osteitis deformans)

Abnormal bone architecture caused by ↑ in both osteoblastic and osteoclastic activity. Possibly viral in origin (paramyxovirus is suspected). Serum calcium, phosphorus, and PTH levels are normal. ↑ **ALP.** Mosaic bone pattern; long bone chalk-stick fractures. ↑ blood flow from ↑ arteriovenous shunts may cause high-output heart failure. Can lead to osteogenic sarcoma.

Hat size can be ↑; hearing loss is common due to auditory foramen narrowing.

Lab values in bone disorders

	Serum Ca^{2+}	Phosphate	ALP	PTH	Comments
Osteoporosis	—	—	—	—	↓ bone mass
Osteopetrosis	—	—	—	—	Thickened, dense bones
Osteomalacia/rickets	↓	↓	—	↑	Soft bones
Osteitis fibrosa cystica	↑	↓	↑	↑	"Brown tumors"
Paget's disease	—	—	↑	—	Abnormal bone architecture

Polyostotic fibrous dysplasia

Bone is replaced by fibroblasts, collagen, and irregular bony trabeculae. Affects many bones. **McCune-Albright syndrome** is a form of polyostotic fibrous dysplasia characterized by multiple unilateral bone lesions associated with endocrine abnormalities (precocious puberty) and unilateral pigmented skin lesions (café-au-lait spots/"coast of Maine" spots).

Primary bone tumors

Benign tumors

Osteoma	Associated with Gardner's syndrome (FAP). New piece of bone grows on another piece of bone, often in the skull.
Osteoid osteoma	Interlacing trabeculae of woven bone surrounded by osteoblasts. < 2 cm and found in proximal tibia and femur. Most common in men < 25 years of age.
Osteoblastoma	Same morphologically as osteoid osteoma, but larger and found in vertebral column.
Giant cell tumor (osteoclastoma)	Occurs most commonly at epiphyseal end of long bones. Peak incidence 20–40 years of age. Locally aggressive benign tumor often around the distal femur, proximal tibial region (knee). Characteristic "double bubble" or "soap bubble" appearance on x-ray. Spindle-shaped cells with multinucleated giant cells.
Osteochondroma (exostosis)	Most common benign bone tumor. Mature bone with cartilaginous cap. Usually in men < 25 years of age. Commonly originates from long metaphysis. Malignant transformation to chondrosarcoma is rare.
Enchondroma	Benign cartilaginous neoplasm found in intramedullary bone. Usually distal extremities (vs. chondrosarcoma).

Malignant tumors

Osteosarcoma (osteogenic sarcoma)	2nd most common 1° malignant tumor of bone (after multiple myeloma). Peak incidence in men 10–20 years of age. Commonly found in the metaphysis of long bones, often around distal femur, proximal tibial region (knee). Predisposing factors include Paget's disease of bone, bone infarcts, radiation, and familial retinoblastoma. Codman's triangle or sunburst pattern (from elevation of periosteum) on x-ray. Poor prognosis.
Ewing's sarcoma	Anaplastic small blue cell malignant tumor. Most common in boys < 15. Extremely aggressive with early mets, but responsive to chemotherapy. Characteristic "**onion**-skin" appearance in bone ("going out for E**wings** and **onion** rings"). Commonly appears in diaphysis of long bones, pelvis, scapula, and ribs. 11;22 translocation. 11 + 22 = 33 (Patrick **Ewing's** jersey number).
Chondrosarcoma	Malignant cartilaginous tumor. Most common in men aged 30–60. Usually located in pelvis, spine, scapula, humerus, tibia, or femur. May be of 1° origin or from osteochondroma. Expansile glistening mass within the medullary cavity.

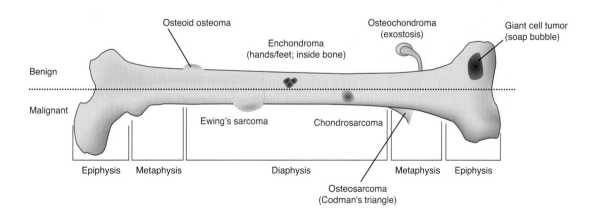

Osteoarthritis

Mechanical—wear and tear of joints leads to destruction of articular cartilage (see Image 119), subchondral cysts, sclerosis, osteophytes (bone spurs), eburnation (polished, ivory-like appearance of bone), Heberden's nodes (DIP), and Bouchard's nodes (PIP). Predisposing factors: age, obesity, joint deformity.

Classic presentation: pain in weight-bearing joints after use (e.g., at the end of the day), improving with rest. In knees, cartilage loss begins on medial aspect ("bowlegged"). Noninflammatory. No systemic symptoms.

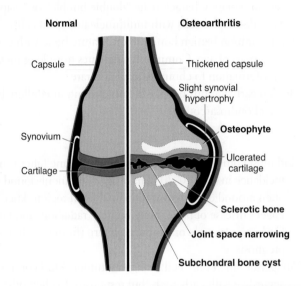

Rheumatoid arthritis	Autoimmune—inflammatory disorder affecting synovial joints, with pannus formation in joints (MCP, PIP), subcutaneous rheumatoid nodules (fibrinoid necrosis surrounded by palisading histiocytes), ulnar deviation, subluxation, Baker's cyst (behind the knee) (see Image 56). No DIP involvement.
	Females > males. Type III hypersensitivity. 80% of RA patients have **positive rheumatoid factor** (anti-IgG antibody); anti-CCP antibody is less sensitive but more specific. Strong association with HLA-DR4.
	Classic presentation: morning stiffness lasting > 30 minutes and improving with use, symmetric joint involvement, systemic symptoms (fever, fatigue, pleuritis, pericarditis).

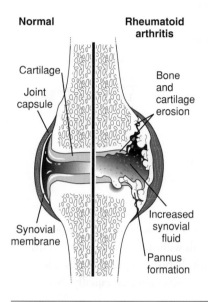

Normal / Rheumatoid arthritis

Cartilage
Joint capsule
Synovial membrane
Bone and cartilage erosion
Increased synovial fluid
Pannus formation

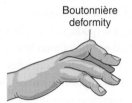

Boutonnière deformity

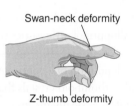

Swan-neck deformity

Z-thumb deformity

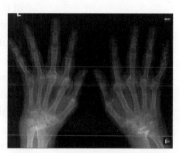

Rheumatoid arthritis (note joint space narrowing of MCP)

(Reproduced, with permission, from USMLERx.com.)

Sjögren's syndrome	Classic triad:	Associated with rheumatoid arthritis.
	1. Xerophthalmia (dry eyes, conjunctivitis, "sand in my eyes")	**Sicca syndrome**—dry eyes, dry mouth, nasal and vaginal dryness, chronic bronchitis, reflux esophagitis. No arthritis.
	2. Xerostomia (dry mouth, dysphagia)	
	3. Arthritis	
	Parotid enlargement, ↑ risk of B-cell lymphoma, dental caries. Autoantibodies to ribonucleoprotein antigens, **SS-A (Ro), SS-B (La).**	
	Predominantly affects females between 40 and 60 years of age.	

Gout

Findings	Precipitation of monosodium urate crystals into joints due to hyperuricemia, which can be caused by Lesch-Nyhan syndrome, PRPP excess, ↓ excretion of uric acid (e.g., thiazide diuretics), ↑ cell turnover, or von Gierke's disease. 90% due to underexcretion; 10% due to overproduction. Crystals are needle shaped and **negatively birefringent** = yellow crystals under parallel light (see Image 54). More common in men.
Symptoms	Asymmetric joint distribution. Joint is swollen, red, and painful. Classic manifestation is painful MTP joint of the big toe (podagra). Tophus formation (often on external ear, olecranon bursa, or Achilles tendon). Acute attack tends to occur after a large meal or alcohol consumption (alcohol metabolites compete for same excretion sites in kidney as uric acid, causing ↓ uric acid secretion and subsequent buildup in blood).
Treatment	Acute: NSAIDs (e.g., indomethacin), colchicine. Chronic: Allopurinol, uricosurics (e.g., probenecid).

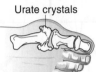

Urate crystals

Pseudogout

Caused by deposition of calcium pyrophosphate crystals within the joint space. Forms basophilic, rhomboid crystals that are **weakly positively birefringent.** Usually affects large joints (classically the knee). > 50 years old; both sexes affected equally. No treatment.

Gout—crystals are yellow when parallel (∥) and blue when perpendicular (⊥) to the light.
Pseudogout—crystals are yellow when perpendicular (⊥) and blue when parallel (∥) to the light.

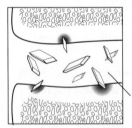

Calcium pyrophosphate crystals

Infectious arthritis

Septic	*S. aureus*, *Streptococcus*, and *Neisseria gonorrhoeae* are common. Gonococcal arthritis is an **STD** that presents as a monoarticular, migratory arthritis with an asymmetrical pattern. Affected joint is swollen, red, and painful. **STD** = **S**ynovitis (e.g., knee), **T**enosynovitis (e.g., hand), and **D**ermatitis (e.g., pustules).
Chronic	TB (from mycobacterial dissemination), Lyme disease.

HIGH-YIELD SYSTEMS

MUSCULOSKELETAL

Seronegative spondylo- arthropathies	Arthritis without rheumatoid factor (no anti-IgG antibody). Strong association with **HLA-B27** (gene that codes for HLA MHC I). Occurs more often in males.	**PAIR**
Psoriatic arthritis	Joint pain and stiffness associated with psoriasis. Asymmetric and patchy involvement. Dactylitis ("sausage fingers"), "pencil-in-cup" deformity on x-ray. Seen in fewer than ⅓ of patients with psoriasis.	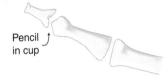 Pencil in cup
Ankylosing spondylitis	Chronic inflammatory disease of spine and sacroiliac joints → ankylosis (stiff spine due to fusion of joints), uveitis, and aortic regurgitation.	Bamboo spine.
Inflammatory bowel disease	Crohn's disease, ulcerative colitis.	
Reactive arthritis (Reiter's syndrome)	Classic triad: 1. Conjunctivitis and anterior uveitis 2. Urethritis 3. Arthritis	"Can't **see**, can't **pee**, can't climb a **tree**." Post-GI or chlamydia infections.

Systemic lupus erythematosus	90% are female and between ages 14 and 45. Most common and severe in black females. Symptoms include fever, fatigue, weight loss, nonbacterial verrucous (Libman-Sacks) endocarditis, hilar adenopathy, and Raynaud's phenomenon (see Image 52). Wire-loop lesions in kidney with immune complex deposition (usually nephritic syndrome); death from renal failure and infections. False positives on syphilis tests (RPR/VDRL) due to antiphospholipid antibodies, which cross-react with cardiolipin used in tests. Lab tests detect presence of: 1. Antinuclear antibodies (ANA)—sensitive, (primary screening) but not specific for SLE 2. Antibodies to double-stranded DNA (anti-dsDNA)—very specific, poor prognosis 3. Anti-Smith antibodies (anti-Sm)— very specific, but not prognostic 4. Antihistone antibodies—drug-induced lupus	**I'M DAMN SHARP:** Immunoglobulins (anti-dsDNA, anti-Sm, antiphospholipid) Malar rash Discoid rash Antinuclear antibody Mucositis (oropharyngeal ulcers) Neurologic disorders Serositis (pleuritis, pericarditis) Hematologic disorders Arthritis Renal disorders Photosensitivity

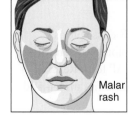

Malar rash

Sarcoidosis

Characterized by immune-mediated, widespread **noncaseating granulomas** and elevated serum ACE levels. Common in black females.

Associated with restrictive lung disease, bilateral hilar lymphadenopathy, erythema nodosum, Bell's palsy, epithelial granulomas containing microscopic Schaumann and asteroid bodies, uveoparotitis, and hypercalcemia (due to elevated 1α-hydroxylase–mediated vitamin D activation in epithelioid macrophages) (see Image 95). Treatment: steroids.

GRAIN:
Gammaglobulinemia
Rheumatoid arthritis
ACE increase
Interstitial fibrosis
Noncaseating granulomas

Polymyalgia rheumatica

Symptoms	Pain and stiffness in shoulders and hips, often with fever, malaise, and weight loss. Does not cause muscular weakness. Occurs in patients > 50 years of age; associated with temporal (giant cell) arteritis.
Findings	↑ ESR, normal CK.
Treatment	Prednisone.

Polymyositis/dermatomyositis

Symptoms	**Polymyositis**—progressive symmetric proximal muscle weakness caused by CD8+ T-cell-induced injury to myofibers. Most often involves shoulders. Muscle biopsy with evidence of perifascicular inflammation is diagnostic.
	Dermatomyositis—similar to polymyositis, but also involves malar rash (similar to SLE), heliotrope rash, "shawl and face" rash, Gottron's papules, "mechanic's hands." ↑ risk of malignancy.
Findings	↑ CK, ↑ aldolase, and **positive ANA, anti-Jo-1**.
Treatment	Steroids.

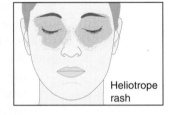

Heliotrope rash

Neuromuscular junction diseases

Myasthenia gravis	Most common NMJ disorder. Autoantibodies to postsynaptic AChR cause ptosis, diplopia, and general weakness. Associated with thymoma. Symptoms worsen with muscle use (diagnose with nerve stimulation/compound muscle AP test). Reversal of symptoms occurs with AChE inhibitors (edrophonium test distinguishes under- and overdosing).
Lambert-Eaton syndrome	Autoantibodies to presynaptic Ca²⁺ channel results in ↓ ACh release leading to proximal muscle weakness. Associated with paraneoplastic diseases (small cell lung cancer). Symptoms improve with muscle use. No reversal of symptoms with AChE inhibitors alone.

Scleroderma (progressive systemic sclerosis—PSS)

Excessive fibrosis and collagen deposition throughout the body. Commonly sclerosis of skin, manifesting as puffy and taut skin with absence of wrinkles (see Image 53). Also sclerosis of renal, pulmonary, cardiovascular, and GI systems. 75% female. 2 major types:

1. Diffuse scleroderma—widespread skin involvement, rapid progression, early visceral involvement. Associated with anti-Scl-70 antibody (anti-DNA topoisomerase I antibody).
2. **CREST** syndrome—**C**alcinosis, **R**aynaud's phenomenon, **E**sophageal dysmotility, **S**clerodactyly, and **T**elangiectasia. Limited skin involvement, often confined to fingers and face. More benign clinical course. Associated with **antiCentromere antibody (C for CREST)**.

Dermatologic terminology

Lesion	Characteristics	Examples
Macule	Flat discoloration < 1 cm	Tinea versicolor
Patch	Macule > 1 cm	
Papule	Elevated skin lesion < 1 cm	Acne vulgaris
Plaque	Papule > 1 cm	Psoriasis
Vesicle	Small fluid-containing blister	Chickenpox
Wheal	Transient vesicle	Hives
Bulla	Large fluid-containing blister	Bullous pemphigoid
Keloid	Irregular, raised lesion resulting from scar tissue hypertrophy (follows trauma to skin, especially in African-Americans)	*T. pertenue* (yaws)
Pustule	Blister containing pus	
Crust	Dried exudates from a vesicle, bulla, or pustule	Impetigo
Hyperkeratosis	↑ thickness of stratum corneum	Psoriasis
Parakeratosis	Hyperkeratosis with retention of nuclei in stratum corneum	Psoriasis
Acantholysis	Separation of epidermal cells	Pemphigus vulgaris
Acanthosis	Epidermal hyperplasia (↑ spinosum)	
Dermatitis	Inflammation of the skin	

Skin disorders

Common disorders

Verrucae	Warts. Soft, tan-colored, cauliflower-like lesions. Epidermal hyperplasia, hyperkeratosis, koilocytosis. Verruca vulgaris on hands; condyloma acuminatum on genitals (caused by HPV).
Nevocellular nevus	Common mole. Benign.
Urticaria	Hives. Intensely pruritic wheals that form after mast cell degranulation.
Ephelis	Freckle. Normal number of melanocytes, ↑ melanin pigment.
Atopic dermatitis (eczema)	Pruritic eruption, commonly on skin flexures. Often associated with other atopic diseases (asthma, allergic rhinitis).
Allergic contact dermatitis	Type IV hypersensitivity reaction that follows exposure to allergen. Lesions occur at site of contact (e.g., nickel, poison ivy).
Psoriasis	Papules and plaques with silvery scaling, especially on knees and elbows (see Image 65). Acanthosis with parakeratotic scaling (nuclei still in stratum corneum). ↑ stratum spinosum, ↓ stratum granulosum. **Auspitz sign** (bleeding spots when scales are scraped off). Can be associated with nail pitting and psoriatic arthritis.
Seborrheic keratosis	Flat, greasy, pigmented squamous epithelial proliferation with keratin-filled cysts (horn cysts). Looks "pasted on." Lesions occur on head, trunk, and extremities. Common benign neoplasm of older persons. Sign of Leser-Trélat—sudden appearance of multiple seborrheic keratoses indicating an underlying malignancy (e.g., GI, lymphoid).

Pigmentation disorders

Albinism	Normal melanocyte number with ↓ melanin production due to ↓ activity of tyrosinase. Can also be caused by failure of neural crest cell migration during development.
Vitiligo	Irregular areas of complete depigmentation. Caused by a ↓ in melanocytes.
Melasma (chloasma)	Hyperpigmentation associated with pregnancy ("mask of pregnancy") or OCP use.

Infectious disorders

Impetigo	Very superficial skin infection. Usually from *S. aureus* or *S. pyogenes*. Highly contagious. **Honey-colored crusting.**
Cellulitis	Acute, painful spreading infection of dermis and subcutaneous tissues. Usually from *S. pyogenes* or *S. aureus*.
Necrotizing fasciitis	Deeper tissue injury, usually from anaerobic bacteria and *S. pyogenes*. Results in crepitus from methane and CO_2 production. "Flesh-eating bacteria."
Staphylococcal scalded skin syndrome (SSSS)	Exotoxin destroys keratinocyte attachments in the stratum granulosum only. Characterized by fever and generalized erythematous rash with sloughing of the upper layers of the epidermis. Seen in newborns and children.
Hairy leukoplakia	White, painless plaques on the tongue that cannot be scraped off. EBV mediated. Occurs in HIV-positive patients.

Blistering disorders

Pemphigus vulgaris	Potentially fatal autoimmune skin disorder with IgG antibody against **desmosomes** (anti-epithelial cell antibody); immunofluorescence reveals antibodies around cells of epidermis in a reticular or netlike pattern. Acantholysis—intraepidermal bullae involving the skin and oral mucosa (see Image 63). Positive Nikolsky's sign (separation of epidermis upon manual stroking of skin).

Skin disorders *(continued)*

Bullous pemphigoid	Autoimmune disorder with IgG antibody against **hemidesmosomes** (epidermal basement membrane; antibodies are **"bullow"** the epidermis); shows linear immunofluorescence. Eosinophils within blisters. Similar to but less severe than pemphigus vulgaris—affects skin but spares oral mucosa (see Image 64). Negative Nikolsky's sign.
Dermatitis herpetiformis	Pruritic papules and vesicles. Deposits of IgA at the tips of dermal papillae. Associated with celiac disease.
Erythema multiforme	Associated with infections (e.g., *Mycoplasma pneumoniae*, HSV), drugs (e.g., sulfa drugs, β-lactams, phenytoin), cancers, and autoimmune disease. Presents with multiple types of lesions—macules, papules, vesicles, and target lesions (red papules with a pale central area).
Stevens-Johnson syndrome	Characterized by fever, bulla formation and necrosis, sloughing of skin, and a high mortality rate. Usually associated with adverse drug reaction. A more severe form of Stevens-Johnson syndrome is known as toxic epidermal necrolysis.

Miscellaneous disorders

Lichen planus	**P**ruritic, **P**urple, **P**olygonal **P**apules. Sawtooth infiltrate of lymphocytes at dermal-epidermal junction. Associated with hepatitis C.
Actinic keratosis	Premalignant lesions caused by sun exposure. Small, rough, erythematous or brownish papules. "Cutaneous horn." Risk of carcinoma is proportional to epithelial dysplasia.
Acanthosis nigricans	Hyperplasia of stratum spinosum. Associated with hyperinsulinemia (e.g., from Cushing's disease, diabetes) and visceral malignancy.
Erythema nodosum	Inflammatory lesions of subcutaneous fat, usually on anterior shins. Associated with coccidioidomycosis, histoplasmosis, TB, leprosy, streptococcal infections, sarcoidosis.
Pityriasis rosea	"Herald patch" followed days later by "Christmas tree" distribution. Multiple papular eruptions; remits spontaneously.
Strawberry hemangioma	First few weeks of life (1/200 births); grows rapidly and regresses spontaneously at 5–8 years of age.
Cherry hemangioma	Appears in 30s–40s; does not regress.

Skin cancer

Squamous cell carcinoma	Very common. Associated with excessive exposure to sunlight and arsenic exposure. Commonly appear on hands and face. Locally invasive, but rarely metastasizes. Ulcerative red lesion. Associated with chronic draining sinuses. Histopathology: keratin "pearls" (see Image 60).	**Actinic keratosis** is a precursor to squamous cell carcinoma. Keratoacanthoma is a variant that grows rapidly (4–6 weeks) and regresses spontaneously (4–8 weeks).
Basal cell carcinoma	Most common in sun-exposed areas of body. Locally invasive, but almost never metastasizes. Rolled edges with central ulceration. Gross pathology: pearly papules, commonly with telangiectasias (see Image 62).	Basal cell tumors have "palisading" nuclei.
Melanoma	Common tumor with significant risk of metastasis. S-100 tumor marker. Associated with sunlight exposure; fair-skinned persons are at ↑ risk. **Depth** of tumor correlates with risk of metastasis. Dark with irregular borders (see Image 61).	Dysplastic nevus (atypical mole) is a precursor to melanoma.

Arachidonic acid products	Lipoxygenase pathway yields Leukotrienes. LTB_4 is a neutrophil chemotactic agent. LTC_4, D_4, and E_4 function in bronchoconstriction, vasoconstriction, contraction of smooth muscle, and ↑ vascular permeability. PGI_2 inhibits platelet aggregation and promotes vasodilation.	L for Lipoxygenase and Leukotriene. Neutrophils arrive "**B4**" others. Platelet-Gathering Inhibitor.

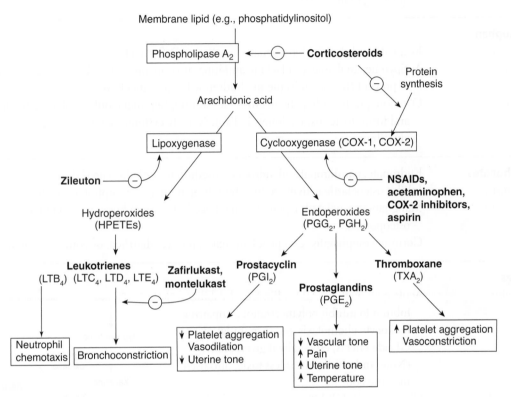

(Adapted, with permission, from Katzung BG, Trevor AJ. *Pharmacology: Examination & Board Review,* 5th ed. Stamford, CT: Appleton & Lange, 1998: 150.)

Aspirin	
Mechanism	Irreversibly inhibits cyclooxygenase by covalent binding, which ↓ synthesis of both thromboxane and prostaglandins. A type of NSAID.
Clinical use	Low dose (< 300 mg/day): ↓ platelet aggregation. Intermediate dose (300–2400 mg/day): antipyretic and analgesic. High dose (2400–4000 mg/day): anti-inflammatory.
Toxicity	Gastric upset. Chronic use can lead to acute renal failure, interstitial nephritis, and upper GI bleeding. Reye's syndrome in children with viral infection.

NSAIDs	Ibuprofen, naproxen, indomethacin, ketorolac.
Mechanism	Reversibly inhibit cyclooxygenase (both COX-1 and COX-2). Block prostaglandin synthesis.
Clinical use	Antipyretic, analgesic, anti-inflammatory. Indomethacin is used to close a PDA.
Toxicity	Renal damage, fluid retention, aplastic anemia, GI distress, ulcers.

HIGH-YIELD SYSTEMS

MUSCULOSKELETAL

COX-2 inhibitors (celecoxib)

Mechanism	Reversibly inhibit specifically the cyclooxygenase (COX) isoform 2, which is found in inflammatory cells and vascular endothelium and mediates inflammation and pain; spares COX-1, which helps maintain the gastric mucosa. Thus, should not have the corrosive effects of other NSAIDs on the GI lining.
Clinical use	Rheumatoid and osteoarthritis; patients with gastritis or ulcers.
Toxicity	↑ risk of thrombosis. Sulfa allergy. Less toxicity to GI mucosa (lower incidence of ulcers, bleeding than NSAIDs).

Acetaminophen

Mechanism	Reversibly inhibits cyclooxygenase, mostly in CNS. Inactivated peripherally.
Clinical use	Antipyretic, analgesic, but lacking anti-inflammatory properties. Used instead of aspirin to prevent Reye's syndrome in children with viral infection.
Toxicity	Overdose produces hepatic necrosis; acetaminophen metabolite depletes glutathione and forms toxic tissue adducts in liver. N-acetylcysteine is antidote—regenerates glutathione.

Bisphosphonates

	Etidronate, pamidronate, alendronate, risedronate, zoledronate (IV).
Mechanism	Inhibit osteoclastic activity; reduce both formation and resorption of hydroxyapatite.
Clinical use	Malignancy-associated hypercalcemia, Paget's disease of bone, postmenopausal osteoporosis.
Toxicity	Corrosive esophagitis (except zoledronate), nausea, diarrhea, osteonecrosis of the jaw.

Gout drugs

Colchicine	Acute gout (with NSAIDs). Binds and stabilizes tubulin to inhibit polymerization, impairing leukocyte chemotaxis and degranulation. GI side effects, especially if given orally. (Note: **indomethacin** is less toxic, also used in acute gout.)
Probenecid	Chronic gout. Inhibits reabsorption of uric acid in PCT (also inhibits secretion of penicillin).
Allopurinol	Chronic gout. Inhibits xanthine oxidase, ↓ conversion of xanthine to uric acid. Also used in lymphoma and leukemia to prevent tumor lysis–associated urate nephropathy. ↑ concentrations of azathioprine and 6-MP (both normally metabolized by xanthine oxidase). Do not give salicylates. All but the highest doses depress uric acid clearance. Even high doses (5–6 g/day) have only minor uricosuric activity.

TNF-α inhibitors

Drug	Mechanism	Clinical Use	Toxicity	Notes
Etanercept	Recombinant form of human TNF receptor that binds TNF	Rheumatoid arthritis, psoriasis, ankylosing spondylitis	—	Etaner**CEPT** is a TNF decoy re**CEPT**or.
Infliximab	Anti-TNF antibody	Crohn's disease, rheumatoid arthritis, ankylosing spondylitis	Predisposes to infections (reactivation of latent TB)	**INFLIX**imab **INFLIX** pain on TNF.
Adalimumab	Anti-TNF antibody	Rheumatoid arthritis, psoriasis, ankylosing spondylitis	—	—

Etanercept
Decoy receptor

Infliximab, Adalimumab
Anti-TNF antibody

Neurology

"Estimated amount of glucose used by an adult human brain each day, expressed in M&Ms: 250."

—Harper's Index

"He has two neurons held together by a spirochete."

—Anonymous

"I never came upon any of my discoveries through the process of rational thinking."

—Albert Einstein

"I like nonsense; it wakes up the brain cells."

—Dr. Seuss

CNS/PNS origins	Neuroectoderm—CNS neurons, ependymal cells (inner lining of ventricles, make CSF), oligodendroglia, astrocytes. Neural crest—Schwann cells, PNS neurons. Mesoderm—**M**icroglia, like **M**acrophages, originate from **M**esoderm.	
Neurons	Compose nervous system. Permanent cells—do not divide in adulthood. Large cells with prominent nucleoli. Nissl substance (RER) in cell body, dendrites, **not** axon.	
Astrocytes 	Physical support, repair, K$^+$ metabolism, removal of excess neurotransmitter, maintenance of blood-brain barrier. Reactive gliosis in response to injury. Astrocyte marker—GFAP.	
Microglia 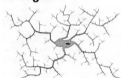	CNS phagocytes. Mesodermal origin. Not readily discernible in Nissl stains. Have small irregular nuclei and relatively little cytoplasm. Scavenger cells of the CNS. Respond to tissue damage by differentiating into large phagocytic cells.	HIV-infected microglia fuse to form multinucleated giant cells in the CNS.
Oligodendroglia 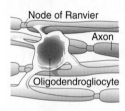	Each oligodendrocyte myelinates multiple CNS axons (up to 30 each). In Nissl stains, they appear as small nuclei with dark chromatin and little cytoplasm. Predominant type of glial cell in white matter.	These cells are destroyed in multiple sclerosis. Look like fried eggs on H&E staining (see Image 49).
Schwann cells	Each Schwann cell myelinates only 1 PNS axon. Also promote axonal regeneration. Derived from neural crest.	These cells are destroyed in Guillain-Barré syndrome. Acoustic neuroma—type of schwannoma. Typically located in internal acoustic meatus (CN VIII).

Sensory corpuscles

Receptor Type	Description	Location	Senses
Free nerve endings	C—slow, unmyelinated fibers; Aδ—fast, myelinated fibers	All skin, epidermis, some viscera	Pain and temperature
Meissner's corpuscles	Large, myelinated fibers	Glabrous (hairless) skin	Position sense, dynamic fine touch (e.g., manipulation), adapt quickly
Pacinian corpuscles	Large, myelinated fibers	Deep skin layers, ligaments, and joints	Vibration, pressure
Merkel's disks	Large, myelinated fibers	Hair follicles	Position sense, static touch (e.g., shapes, edges, textures), adapt slowly

Peripheral nerve layers

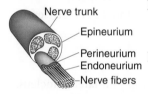

Nerve trunk
Epineurium
Perineurium
Endoneurium
Nerve fibers

Endoneurium—invests single nerve fiber (inflammatory infiltrate in Guillain-Barré)

Perineurium (**P**ermeability barrier)—surrounds a fascicle of nerve fibers. Must be rejoined in microsurgery for limb reattachment.

Epineurium—dense connective tissue that surrounds entire nerve (fascicles and blood vessels).

Endo = inner.
Peri = around.
Epi = outer.

Neurotransmitters

Type	Change in disease	Locations of synthesis*
NE	↑ in anxiety, ↓ in depression	Locus ceruleus
Dopamine	↑ in schizophrenia, ↓ in Parkinson's and depression	Ventral tegmentum and SNc
5-HT	↓ in anxiety, depression	Raphe nucleus
ACh	↓ in Alzheimer's, Huntington's, REM sleep	Basal nucleus of Meynert
GABA	↓ in anxiety, Huntington's	Nucleus accumbens

*Locus ceruleus—stress and panic. Nucleus accumbens and septal nucleus—reward center, pleasure, addiction, fear.

Blood-brain barrier

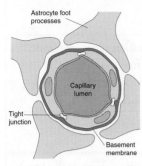

Astrocyte foot processes

Capillary lumen

Tight junction

Basement membrane

Formed by 3 structures:
1. Tight junctions between nonfenestrated capillary endothelial cells
2. Basement membrane
3. Astrocyte processes

Glucose and amino acids cross slowly by carrier-mediated transport mechanism.

Nonpolar/lipid-soluble substances cross rapidly via diffusion.

A few specialized brain regions with fenestrated capillaries and no blood-brain barrier allow molecules in the blood to affect brain function (e.g., area postrema—vomiting after chemo, OVLT—osmotic sensing) or neurosecretory products to enter circulation (e.g., neurohypophysis—ADH release).

Other barriers include:
1. Blood-testis barrier
2. Maternal-fetal blood barrier of placenta

Infarction destroys endothelial cell tight junctions → vasogenic edema.

Hypothalamic inputs and outputs permeate the BBB.

Hypothalamus

The hypothalamus wears **TAN HATS**—**T**hirst and water balance, **A**denohypophysis control, **N**eurohypophysis releases hormones from hypothalamus, **H**unger, **A**utonomic regulation, **T**emperature regulation, **S**exual urges. Inputs: OVLT (senses change in osmolarity), area postrema (responds to emetics).

Supraoptic nucleus makes ADH.

Paraventricular nucleus makes oxytocin.

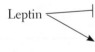
Leptin

Lateral area—hunger. Destruction → anorexia, failure to thrive (infants). Inhibited by leptin.

Ventromedial area—satiety. Destruction (e.g., craniopharyngioma) → hyperphagia. Stimulated by leptin.

Anterior hypothalamus—cooling, p**A**rasympathetic.

Posterior hypothalamus—heating, sympathetic.

Suprachiasmatic nucleus—circadian rhythm.

If you zap your **lateral** nucleus, you shrink **laterally.**

If you zap your **ventromedial** nucleus, you grow **ventrally** and **medially.**

Anterior nucleus = cool off (cooling, parasympathetic). A/C = anterior cooling.

Posterior nucleus = get fired up (heating, sympathetic). If you zap your **P**osterior hypothalamus, you become a **P**oikilotherm (cold-blooded, like a snake).

You need **sleep** to be **charismatic** (chiasmatic).

Posterior pituitary (neurohypophysis)

Receives hypothalamic axonal projections from supraoptic (ADH) and paraventricular (oxytocin) nuclei.

Oxytocin: *oxys* = quick; *tocos* = birth.

Adenohypophysis = **A**nterior pituitary.

	Nucleus	Input	Info	Destination
Thalamus		Major relay for ascending sensory information.		
	VPL	Spinothalamic and dorsal columns/ medial lemniscus.	Pain and temperature; position and proprioception.	1° somatosensory cortex.
	VPM	Trigeminal and gustatory pathway.	Face sensation and taste.	1° somatosensory cortex.
	LGN	CN II.	Vision.	Calcarine sulcus.
	MGN	Superior olive and inferior colliculus of pons.	Hearing.	Auditory cortex of temporal lobe.

Makeup goes on the face (VPM).
Lateral = Light.
Medial = Music.

Limbic system

Includes cingulate gyrus, hippocampus, fornix, mammillary bodies, and septal nucleus. Responsible for **F**eeding, **F**leeing, **F**ighting, **F**eeling, and sex.

The famous 5 F's.

Cerebellum

Receives contralateral cortical input via middle cerebellar peduncle and ipsilateral proprioceptive information via inferior cerebellar peduncle. Input nerves = climbing and mossy fibers.

Provides stimulatory feedback to contralateral cortex to modulate movement. Output nerves = Purkinje fibers output to deep nuclei of cerebellum, which in turn output to cortex via superior cerebellar peduncle.

Deep nuclei (L → M)—**D**entate, **E**mboliform, **G**lobose, **F**astigial ("**D**on't **E**at **G**reasy **F**oods").

Lateral—voluntary movement of extremities.

Medial—balance, truncal coordination, ataxia, propensity to fall toward injured (ipsilateral) side.

Basal ganglia

Important in voluntary movements and making postural adjustments.
Receives cortical input, provides negative feedback to cortex to modulate movement.
Striatum = putamen + caudate.
Lentiform = putamen + globus pallidus.

■ stimulatory
■ inhibitory
SNc   Substantia nigra pars compacta
SNr   Substantia nigra pars reticulata
GPe   Globus pallidus externus
GPi   Globus pallidus internus
STN   Subthalamic nucleus
D1   Dopamine D1 receptor (excitatory)
D2   Dopamine D2 receptor (inhibitory)

D1-R = D1Rect pathway.
Indirect = Inhibitory.

D1 (+) = excitatory
D2 (+) = inhibit inhibitory = excitatory

Excitatory pathway—SNc's dopamine binds to D1 receptors in the excitatory pathway, stimulating the
   excitatory pathway (↑ motion). Therefore, loss of dopamine in Parkinson's inhibits the excitatory pathway
   (↓ motion).
Inhibitory pathway—SNc's dopamine binds to D2 receptors in the inhibitory pathway, inhibiting the
   inhibitory pathway (↑ motion). Therefore, loss of dopamine in Parkinson's excites (i.e., disinhibits) the inhibitory
   pathway (↓ motion).

Parkinson's disease	Degenerative disorder of CNS associated with Lewy bodies (composed of α-synuclein—intracellular inclusion) and depigmentation of the substantia nigra pars compacta (loss of dopaminergic neurons).	**TRAP** = **T**remor (at rest—e.g., pill-rolling tremor), cogwheel **R**igidity, **A**kinesia, and **P**ostural instability (you are **TRAP**ped in your body).
Hemiballismus	Sudden, wild flailing of 1 arm +/− leg. Characteristic of contralateral subthalamic nucleus lesion (e.g., lacunar stroke in a patient with a history of hypertension). Loss of inhibition of thalamus through globus pallidus.	Half ballistic (as in throwing a baseball).
Huntington's disease	Autosomal-dominant trinucleotide repeat disorder. Characterized by chorea, aggression, depression, and dementia (sometimes initially mistaken for substance abuse). Neuronal death via NMDA-R binding and glutamate toxicity. Atrophy of striatal nuclei (main inhibitors of movement) can be seen on imaging.	Expansion of **CAG** repeats (anticipation). Caudate loses ACh and GABA.
Chorea	Sudden, jerky, purposeless movements. Characteristic of basal ganglia lesion (e.g., Huntington's disease).	*Chorea* = dancing (Greek). Think choral dancing or choreography.
Athetosis	Slow, writhing movements, especially of fingers. Characteristic of basal ganglia lesion (e.g., Huntington's disease).	*Athetos* = not fixed (Greek). Think snakelike.
Myoclonus	Sudden, brief muscle contraction.	Jerks, hiccups.
Dystonia	Sustained, involuntary muscle contractions.	Writer's cramp.

Tremor

Essential/postural tremor—action tremor (worsens when holding posture), autosomal dominant. Essential tremor patients often self-medicate with alcohol, which ↓ tremor. Treatment: β-blockers.

Resting tremor—most noticeable distally. Seen in Parkinson's (pill-rolling tremor).

Intention tremor—slow, zigzag motion when pointing toward a target; associated with cerebellar dysfunction.

Cerebral cortex functions

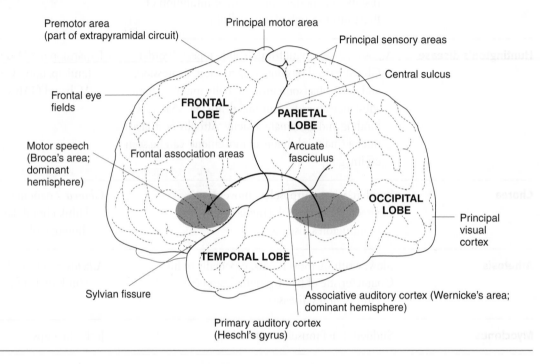

Homunculus

Topographical representation of sensory and motor areas in the cerebral cortex. Used to localize lesion (e.g., in blood supply) leading to specific defects.

For example, lower extremity deficit in sensation or movement may indicate involvement of the anterior cerebral artery.

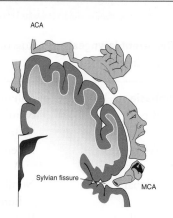

Motor homunculus

Brain lesions

Area of lesion	Consequence	Notes
Amygdala (bilateral)	Klüver-Bucy syndrome (hyperorality, hypersexuality, disinhibited behavior)	
Frontal lobe	Disinhibition and deficits in concentration, orientation, and judgment; may have reemergence of primitive reflexes	
Right parietal lobe	Spatial neglect syndrome (agnosia of the contralateral side of the world)	
Reticular activating system (midbrain)	Reduced levels of arousal and wakefulness (e.g., coma)	
Mammillary bodies (bilateral)	Wernicke-Korsakoff syndrome (Wernicke—confusion, ophthalmoplegia, ataxia; Korsakoff—memory loss, confabulation, personality changes)	
Basal ganglia	May result in tremor at rest, chorea, or athetosis	
Cerebellar hemisphere	Intention tremor, limb ataxia; damage to the cerebellum results in ipsilateral deficits; fall toward side of lesion (cerebellum → SCP → contralateral cortex → corticospinal decussation = ipsilateral)	Cerebellar hemispheres are **laterally** located—affect **lateral** limbs.
Cerebellar vermis	Truncal ataxia, dysarthria	Vermis is **centrally** located—affects **central** body.
Subthalamic nucleus	Contralateral hemiballismus	
Hippocampus	Anterograde amnesia—inability to make new memories	
Paramedian pontine reticular formation (PPRF)	Eyes look away from side of lesion	
Frontal eye fields	Eyes look toward lesion	

Central pontine myelinolysis

Acute paralysis, dysarthria, dysphagia, diplopia, and loss of consciousness. Commonly caused by very rapid correction of hyponatremia. Arrow in axial T1-weighted MRI shows abnormal increased signal in the pons.

Recurrent laryngeal nerve injury	Loss of all laryngeal muscles except cricothyroid. Hoarseness.	
Aphasia	Aphasia = higher-order inability to speak. Dysarthria = motor inability to speak.	
Broca's	Nonfluent aphasia with intact comprehension. Broca's area—inferior frontal gyrus.	**Broca's Bro**ken **Boca.** Wernicke's is **W**ordy but makes no sense.
Wernicke's	Fluent aphasia with impaired comprehension. Wernicke's area—superior temporal gyrus.	**W**ernicke's = "**W**hat?"
Global	Nonfluent aphasia with impaired comprehension. Both Broca's and Wernicke's areas affected.	
Conduction	Poor repetition but fluent speech, intact comprehension. Arcuate fasciculus—connects Broca's, Wernicke's areas.	Can't repeat phrases such as, "No ifs, ands, or buts."

Cerebral arteries—cortical distribution

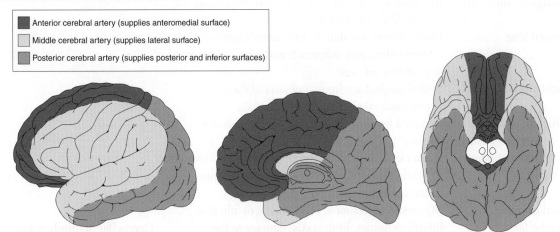

■ Anterior cerebral artery (supplies anteromedial surface)
□ Middle cerebral artery (supplies lateral surface)
■ Posterior cerebral artery (supplies posterior and inferior surfaces)

Circle of Willis

Right anterior cerebral artery
Middle cerebral artery
Posterior communicating artery
Basilar artery
Vertebral artery
Anterior spinal artery

Anterior communicating artery
Optic chiasm
Internal carotid artery (ICA)
Lateral striate
CN III
Posterior cerebral artery
Anterior inferior cerebellar artery (AICA)
Posterior inferior cerebellar artery (PICA)

Region	Associated area/deficit
Anterior spinal artery (medial medullary syndrome)	Contralateral hemiparesis (lower extremities), medial lemniscus (↓ contralateral proprioception), ipsilateral paralysis of hypoglossal nerve.
PICA (lateral medullary syndrome, aka Wallenberg's)	Contralateral loss of pain and temperature, ipsilateral dysphagia, hoarseness, ↓ gag reflex, vertigo, diplopia, nystagmus, vomiting, ipsilateral Horner's, ipsilateral facial pain and temperature, trigeminal nucleus (spinal tract and nucleus), ipsilateral ataxia.
AICA (lateral inferior pontine syndrome)	Ipsilateral facial paralysis, ipsilateral cochlear nucleus, vestibular (nystagmus), ipsilateral facial pain and temperature, ipsilateral dystaxia (MCP, ICP).
Posterior cerebral artery	Contralateral hemianopia with macular sparing; supplies occipital cortex.
Middle cerebral artery	Contralateral face and arm paralysis and sensory loss, aphasia (dominant sphere), left-sided neglect.
Anterior cerebral artery	Supplies medial surface of the brain, leg-foot area of motor and sensory cortices.
Anterior communicating artery	Most common site of circle of Willis aneurysm; lesions may cause visual field defects.
Posterior communicating artery	Common area of aneurysm; causes CN III palsy.
Lateral striate	Divisions of middle cerebral artery; supply internal capsule, caudate, putamen, globus pallidus. "Arteries of stroke"; infarct of the posterior limb of the internal capsule causes pure motor hemiparesis.
Watershed zones	Between anterior cerebral/middle cerebral, posterior cerebral/middle cerebral arteries. Damage in severe hypotension → upper leg/upper arm weakness, defects in higher-order visual processing.
Basilar artery	Infarct causes "locked-in syndrome" (CN III is typically intact).
In general, stroke of anterior circle	General sensory and motor dysfunction, aphasia.
In general, stroke of posterior circle	Cranial nerve deficits (vertigo, visual deficits), coma, cerebellar deficits (ataxia). Dominant hemisphere (ataxia), nondominant (neglect).

Aneurysms

Berry aneurysms—occur at the bifurcations in the circle of Willis. Most common site is bifurcation of the anterior communicating artery. Rupture (most common complication) leads to hemorrhagic stroke/subarachnoid hemorrhage. Associated with adult polycystic kidney disease, Ehlers-Danlos syndrome, and Marfan's syndrome. Other risk factors: advanced age, hypertension, smoking, race (higher risk in blacks) (see Image 46).

Charcot-Bouchard microaneurysms—associated with chronic hypertension; affects small vessels (e.g., in basal ganglia, thalamus).

Intracranial hemorrhage

Epidural hematoma

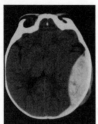

(Reproduced, with permission, from the PEIR Digital Library.)

Rupture of middle meningeal artery (branch of maxillary artery), often 2° to fracture of temporal bone (see Image 44). Lucid interval. Rapid expansion under systemic arterial pressure → transtentorial herniation, CN III palsy.

CT shows "biconvex disk" not crossing suture lines. Can cross falx, tentorium.

Subdural hematoma

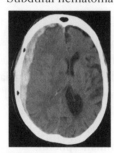

(Reproduced, with permission, from Chen MY et al. *Basic Radiology*, 1st ed. New York: McGraw-Hill, 2005, Fig. 12-32.)

Rupture of bridging veins. Slow venous bleeding (less pressure = hematoma develops over time) with delayed onset of symptoms. Seen in elderly individuals, alcoholics, blunt trauma, shaken baby (predisposing factors—brain atrophy, shaking, whiplash) (see Image 43).

Crescent-shaped hemorrhage that crosses suture lines. Gyri are preserved, since pressure is distributed equally. Cannot cross falx, tentorium.

Subarachnoid hemorrhage

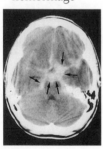

Rupture of an aneurysm (usually berry aneurysm in Marfan's, Ehlers-Danlos, APCKD) or an AVM. Patients complain of "worst headache of my life." Bloody or yellow (xanthochromic) spinal tap. 2–3 days afterward, there is a risk of vasospasm due to blood breakdown products, which irritate vessels (treat with calcium channel blockers).

Parenchymal hematoma

Caused by hypertension, amyloid angiopathy—lobar strokes all over brain, diabetes mellitus, and tumor. Typically occurs in basal ganglia and internal capsule.

Ischemic brain disease	Irreversible damage after 5 minutes. Most vulnerable—hippocampus, neocortex, cerebellum, watershed areas. Irreversible neuronal injury—red neurons (12–48 hours), necrosis + neutrophils (24–72 hours), macrophages (3–5 days), reactive gliosis + vascular proliferation (1–2 weeks), glial scar (> 2 weeks).
	Atherosclerosis—thrombi lead to ischemic stroke with subsequent necrosis. Form cystic cavity with reactive gliosis.
	Hemorrhagic stroke—intracerebral bleeding, often due to aneurysm rupture. May be 2° to ischemic stroke followed by reperfusion (↑ vessel fragility).
	Ischemic stroke—emboli block large vessels; etiologies include atrial fibrillation, carotid dissection, patent foramen ovale, endocarditis. Lacunar strokes block small vessels, may be 2° to hypertension. Treatment: tPA within 3 hours.
	Transient ischemic attack (TIA)—brief, reversible episode of neurologic dysfunction due to focal ischemia. Typically, symptoms last for < 24 hours.
	Stroke imaging: bright on diffusion-weighted MRI in 3–30 minutes and remains bright for 10 days, dark on noncontrast CT in ~ 24 hours. Bright areas on noncontrast CT indicate hemorrhage (tPA contraindicated).

Dural venous sinuses	Venous sinuses run in the dura mater where its meningeal and periosteal layers separate. Cerebral veins → venous sinuses → internal jugular vein.

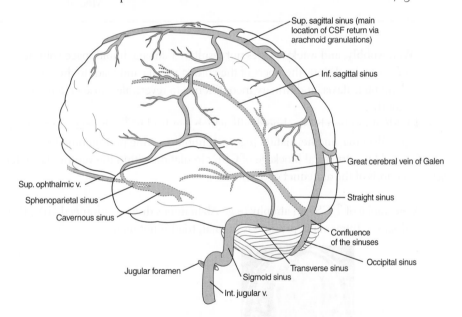

(Adapted, with permission, from White JS. *USMLE Road Map: Gross Anatomy,* 2nd ed. New York: McGraw-Hill, 2006, Fig. 8-3.)

Ventricular system

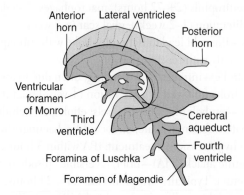

CSF is made by the choroid plexus; it is reabsorbed by venous sinus arachnoid granulations.

Lateral ventricle → 3rd ventricle via foramen of Monro.

3rd ventricle → 4th ventricle via cerebral aqueduct.

4th ventricle → subarachnoid space via:
Foramina of Luschka = Lateral.
Foramen of Magendie = Medial.

Hydrocephalus

Normal pressure hydrocephalus	"Wet, wobbly, and wacky." Does **not** result in ↑ subarachnoid space volume. Expansion of ventricles distorts the fibers of the corona radiata and leads to the clinical triad of dementia, ataxia, and urinary incontinence (a reversible cause of dementia in the elderly).
Communicating hydrocephalus	↓ CSF absorption by arachnoid villi, which can lead to ↑ intracranial pressure, papilledema, and herniation (e.g., arachnoid scarring post-meningitis).
Obstructive (noncommunicating) hydrocephalus	Caused by a structural blockage of CSF circulation within the ventricular system (e.g., stenosis of the aqueduct of Sylvius).
Hydrocephalus ex vacuo	Appearance of ↑ CSF in atrophy (e.g., Alzheimer's disease, advanced HIV, Pick's disease). Intracranial pressure is normal; triad is not seen.

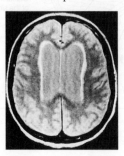

(Reproduced, with permission, from Ropper AH et al. *Adams and Victor's Principles of Neurology,* 8th ed. New York: McGraw-Hill, 2005, Fig. 30-2.)

Spinal nerves	There are 31 spinal nerves altogether: 8 cervical, 12 thoracic, 5 lumbar, 5 sacral, 1 coccygeal.	31, just like 31 flavors!
	Nerves C1–C7 exit via intervertebral foramina above the corresponding vertebra. All other nerves exit below.	Vertebral disk herniation (nucleus pulposus herniates through annulus fibrosus) usually occurs between L5 and S1.

| **Spinal cord—lower extent** | In adults, spinal cord extends to lower border of L1–L2; subarachnoid space extends to lower border of S2. Lumbar puncture is usually performed in L3–L4 or L4–L5 interspaces, at level of cauda equina. | To keep the cord **alive**, keep the spinal needle between **L3 and L5.** |

Spinal cord and associated tracts

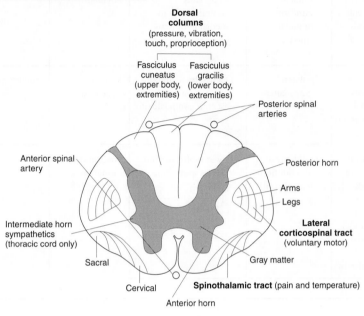

Legs are Lateral in Lateral corticospinal, spinothalamic tracts.

Dorsal column is organized as you are, with hands at sides. Arms outside, legs inside.

Spinal tract anatomy and functions

Remember, ascending tracts synapse and **then** cross.

Tract and Function	1st-Order Neuron	Synapse 1	2nd-Order Neuron	Synapse 2	3rd-Order Neuron
Dorsal column—medial lemniscal pathway (ascending pressure, vibration, touch, and proprioceptive sensation)	Sensory nerve ending → cell body in dorsal root ganglion → enters spinal cord, ascends ipsilaterally in dorsal column	Ipsilateral nucleus cuneatus or gracilis (medulla)	**Decussates** in medulla → ascends contralaterally in medial lemniscus	VPL of thalamus	Sensory cortex
Spinothalamic tract (ascending pain and temperature sensation)	Sensory nerve ending (A-delta and C fibers) (cell body in dorsal root ganglion) → enters spinal cord	Ipsilateral gray matter (spinal cord)	**Decussates** at anterior white commissure → ascends contralaterally	VPL of thalamus	Sensory cortex
Lateral corticospinal tract (descending voluntary movement of contralateral limbs)	**Upper motor neuron:** cell body in 1° motor cortex → descends ipsilaterally (through internal capsule) until **decussating** at caudal medulla (pyramidal decussation) → descends contralaterally	Cell body of anterior horn (spinal cord)	**Lower motor neuron:** Leaves spinal cord	Neuromuscular junction	

Motor neuron signs

Sign	UMN lesion	LMN lesion
Weakness	+	+
Atrophy	−	+
Fasciculation	−	+
Reflexes	↑	↓
Tone	↑	↓
Babinski	+	−
Spastic paralysis	+	−
Clasp knife spasticity	+	−

Lower MN = everything **lowered** (less muscle mass, ↓ muscle tone, ↓ reflexes, downgoing toes).

Upper MN = everything **up** (tone, DTRs, toes).

Upgoing Babinski is normal in infants.

Fasciculation = muscle twitching.

Spinal cord lesions

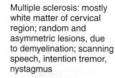

Poliomyelitis and Werdnig-Hoffmann disease: lower motor neuron lesions only, due to destruction of anterior horns; flaccid paralysis

Multiple sclerosis: mostly white matter of cervical region; random and asymmetric lesions, due to demyelination; scanning speech, intention tremor, nystagmus

ALS: combined upper and lower motor neuron deficits with no sensory deficit; both upper and lower motor neuron signs

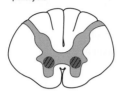 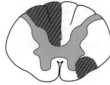 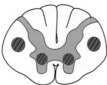

Complete occlusion of anterior spinal artery; spares dorsal columns and tract of Lissauer; upper thoracic ASA territory is a watershed area, as artery of Adamkiewicz supplies ASA below ~ T8

Tabes dorsalis (3° syphilis): degeneration of dorsal roots and dorsal columns; impaired proprioception, locomotor ataxia

Syringomyelia: damages anterior white commissure of spinothalamic tract (2nd-order neurons), resulting in bilateral loss of pain and temperature sensation (usually C8–T1); seen with Chiari I types 1 and 2; can expand and affect other tracts

Vitamin B_{12} neuropathy, vitamin E deficiency, and Friedreich's ataxia: demyelination of dorsal columns, lateral corticospinal tracts, and spinocerebellar tracts; ataxic gait, hyperreflexia, impaired position and vibration sense

Posterior spinal arteries

 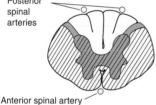 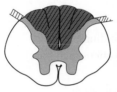 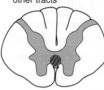 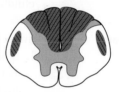

Anterior spinal artery

Poliomyelitis	Caused by poliovirus, which is transmitted by the fecal-oral route. Replicates in the oropharynx and small intestine before spreading through the bloodstream to the CNS, where it leads to the destruction of cells in the anterior horn of the spinal cord, leading in turn to LMN destruction.
Symptoms	Malaise, headache, fever, nausea, abdominal pain, sore throat. Signs of LMN lesions—muscle weakness and atrophy, fasciculations, fibrillation, and hyporeflexia.
Findings	CSF with lymphocytic pleocytosis with slight elevation of protein (with no change in CSF glucose). Virus recovered from stool or throat.
Werdnig-Hoffman disease	Also known as infantile spinal muscular atrophy. Autosomal-recessive inheritance; presents at birth as a "floppy baby," tongue fasciculations; median age of death 7 months. Associated with degeneration of anterior horns. LMN involvement only.

Amyotrophic lateral sclerosis

Associated with **both** LMN and UMN signs; no sensory, cognitive, or oculomotor deficits. Can be caused by defect in superoxide dismutase 1 (SOD1). Commonly presents as fasciculations and eventual atrophy; progressive and fatal. Riluzole treatment modestly lengthens survival by decreasing presynaptic glutamate release.

Commonly known as Lou Gehrig's disease. Stephen Hawking is a well-known living patient (highlighting the lack of cognitive deficit).

Tabes dorsalis

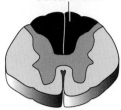

Dorsal column

Degeneration of dorsal columns and dorsal roots due to 3° syphilis, resulting in impaired proprioception and locomotor ataxia. Associated with Charcot's joints, shooting (lightning) pain (see Image 12), Argyll Robertson pupils (reactive to accommodation but not to light), absence of DTRs, positive Romberg, and sensory ataxia at night.

Argyll Robertson pupils are also known as "prostitute's pupils" because they accommodate but do not react.

Friedreich's ataxia

Autosomal-recessive trinucleotide repeat disorder (GAA) in gene that encodes frataxin. Leads to impairment in mitochondrial functioning. Staggering gait, frequent falling, nystagmus, dysarthria, pes cavus, hammer toes, hypertrophic cardiomyopathy (cause of death). Presents in childhood with kyphoscoliosis.

Friedreich is Fratastic (**frataxin**): he's your favorite frat brother, always stumbling, staggering, and falling.

Brown-Séquard syndrome

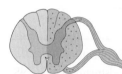

Lesion

Hemisection of spinal cord. Findings:
1. Ipsilateral UMN signs (corticospinal tract) below lesion
2. Ipsilateral loss of tactile, vibration, proprioception sense (dorsal column) below lesion
3. Contralateral pain and temperature loss (spinothalamic tract) below lesion
4. Ipsilateral loss of all sensation at level of lesion
5. LMN signs (e.g., flaccid paralysis) at level of lesion

If lesion occurs above T1, presents with Horner's syndrome.

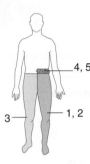

Horner's syndrome

Sympathectomy of face:
1. **P**tosis (slight drooping of eyelid: superior tarsal muscle)
2. **A**nhidrosis (absence of sweating) and flushing (rubor) of affected side of face
3. **M**iosis (pupil constriction)

Associated with lesion of spinal cord above T1 (e.g., Pancoast's tumor, Brown-Séquard syndrome [cord hemisection], late-stage syringomyelia).

PAM is **horny** (Horner's).

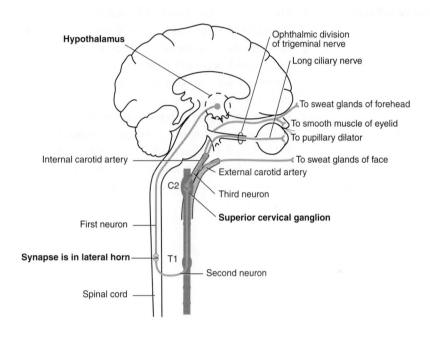

The 3-neuron oculosympathetic pathway projects from the hypothalamus to the intermediolateral column of the spinal cord, then to the superior cervical (sympathetic) ganglion, and finally to the pupil, the smooth muscle of the eyelids, and the sweat glands of the forehead and face. Interruption of any of these pathways results in Horner's syndrome.

Landmark dermatomes

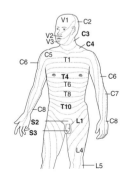

C2—posterior half of a skull "cap."
C3—high turtleneck shirt.
C4—low-collar shirt.

T4—at the nipple.
T7—at the xiphoid process.
T10—at the umbilicus (important for early appendicitis pain referral).
L1—at the inguinal ligament.
L4—includes the kneecaps.
S2, S3, S4—erection and sensation of penile and anal zones.

Diaphragm and gallbladder pain referred to the right shoulder via the phrenic nerve.

T4 at the **teat pore.**

T10 at the belly but**TEN.**

L1 is **IL** (Inguinal Ligament).
Down on **L4s** (**all fours**).
"**S2, 3, 4** keep the penis off the floor."

Clinical reflexes

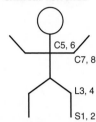

Biceps = C5 nerve root.
Triceps = C7 nerve root.
Patella = L4 nerve root.
Achilles = S1 nerve root.
Babinski—dorsiflexion of the big toe and fanning of other toes; sign of UMN lesion, but normal reflex in 1st year of life.

Reflexes count up in order:
S1, 2
L3, 4
C5, 6
C7, 8

Primitive reflexes

1. Moro reflex—"hang on for life" reflex—abduct/extend limbs when startled, and then draw together
2. Rooting reflex—movement of head toward one side if cheek or mouth is stroked (nipple seeking)
3. Sucking reflex—sucking response when roof of mouth is touched
4. Palmar and plantar reflexes—curling of fingers/toes if palms of hands/feet are stroked
5. Babinski reflex—dorsiflexion of large toe and fanning of other toes with plantar stimulation

Normally disappear within 1st year of life. May reemerge following frontal lobe lesion.

Brain stem—ventral view

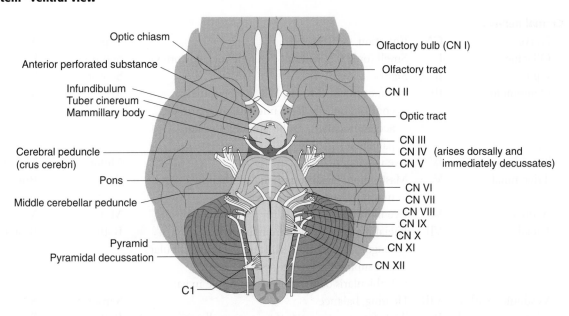

- Optic chiasm
- Anterior perforated substance
- Infundibulum
- Tuber cinereum
- Mammillary body
- Cerebral peduncle (crus cerebri)
- Pons
- Middle cerebellar peduncle
- Pyramid
- Pyramidal decussation
- C1

- Olfactory bulb (CN I)
- Olfactory tract
- CN II
- Optic tract
- CN III
- CN IV (arises dorsally and immediately decussates)
- CN V
- CN VI
- CN VII
- CN VIII
- CN IX
- CN X
- CN XI
- CN XII

CNs that lie medially at brain stem: III, VI, XII. 3(×2) = 6(×2) = 12 (**M**otor = **M**edial).

Brain stem—dorsal view (cerebellum removed)

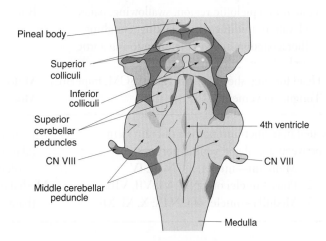

- Pineal body
- Superior colliculi
- Inferior colliculi
- Superior cerebellar peduncles
- CN VIII
- Middle cerebellar peduncle

- 4th ventricle
- CN VIII
- Medulla

Pineal gland—melatonin secretion, circadian rhythms.

Superior colliculi—conjugate vertical gaze center.

Inferior colliculi—auditory.

Parinaud syndrome—paralysis of conjugate vertical gaze due to lesion in superior colliculi (e.g., pinealoma).

Your eyes are **above** your ears, and the superior colliculus (visual) is **above** the inferior colliculus (auditory).

HIGH-YIELD SYSTEMS

NEUROLOGY

Cranial nerves

Nerve	CN	Function	Type	Mnemonic
Olfactory	I	Smell (only CN without thalamic relay to cortex)	Sensory	Some
Optic	II	Sight	Sensory	Say
Oculomotor	III	Eye movement (SR, IR, MR, IO), pupillary constriction (PS: E-W nucleus, muscarinic-R), accommodation, eyelid opening (levator palpebrae)	Motor	Marry
Trochlear	IV	Eye movement (SO)	Motor	Money
Trigeminal	V	Mastication, facial sensation (ophthalmic, maxillary, mandibular divisions)	Both	But
Abducens	VI	Eye movement (LR)	Motor	My
Facial	VII	Facial movement, taste from anterior $2/3$ of tongue, lacrimation, salivation (submandibular and sublingual glands), eyelid closing (orbicularis oculi), stapedius muscle in ear	Both	Brother
Vestibulocochlear	VIII	Hearing, balance	Sensory	Says
Glossopharyngeal	IX	Taste from posterior $1/3$ of tongue, swallowing, salivation (parotid gland), monitoring carotid body and sinus chemo- and baroreceptors, and stylopharyngeus (elevates pharynx, larynx)	Both	Big
Vagus	X	Taste from epiglottic region, swallowing, palate elevation, midline uvula, talking, coughing, thoracoabdominal viscera, monitoring aortic arch chemo- and baroreceptors	Both	Brains
Accessory	XI	Head turning, shoulder shrugging (SCM, trapezius)	Motor	Matter
Hypoglossal	XII	Tongue movement	Motor	Most

Cranial nerve nuclei	Located in tegmentum portion of brain stem (between dorsal and ventral portions). 1. Midbrain—nuclei of CN III, IV 2. Pons—nuclei of CN V, VI, VII, VIII 3. Medulla—nuclei of CN IX, X, XI, XII	Lateral nuclei = sensory (alar plate). — Sulcus limitans — Medial nuclei = Motor (basal plate).

Cranial nerve reflexes

Reflex	Afferent	Efferent
Corneal	V_1 ophthalmic (nasociliary branch: levator palpebrae)	VII (temporal branch: orbicularis oculi)
Lacrimation	V_1 (loss of reflex does not preclude emotional tears)	VII
Jaw jerk	V_3 (sensory—muscle spindle from masseter)	V_3 (motor—masseter)
Pupillary	II	III
Gag	IX	IX, X

Vagal nuclei

Nucleus Solitarius	Visceral **S**ensory information (e.g., taste, baroreceptors, gut distention).	VII, IX, X.
Nucleus a**M**biguus	**M**otor innervation of pharynx, larynx, and upper esophagus (e.g., swallowing, palate elevation).	IX, X, XI.
Dorsal motor nucleus	Sends autonomic (parasympathetic) fibers to heart, lungs, and upper GI.	

Cranial nerve and vessel pathways

Cribriform plate (CN I).

Middle cranial fossa (CN II–VI)—through sphenoid bone:
1. Optic canal (CN II, ophthalmic artery, central retinal vein)
2. Superior orbital fissure (CN III, IV, V_1, VI, ophthalmic vein, sympathetic fibers)
3. Foramen **R**otundum (CN V_2)
4. Foramen **O**vale (CN V_3)
5. Foramen spinosum (middle meningeal artery)

Posterior cranial fossa (CN VII–XII)—through temporal or occipital bone:
1. Internal auditory meatus (CN VII, VIII)
2. Jugular foramen (CN IX, X, XI, jugular vein)
3. Hypoglossal canal (CN XII)
4. Foramen magnum (spinal roots of CN XI, brain stem, vertebral arteries)

Divisions of CN V exit owing to **S**tanding **R**oom **O**nly.

Cavernous sinus

A collection of venous sinuses on either side of the pituitary. Blood from eye and superficial cortex → cavernous sinus → internal jugular vein.

CN III, IV, V_1, V_2, and VI and postganglionic sympathetic fibers en route to the orbit all pass through the cavernous sinus. Cavernous portion of internal carotid artery is also here.

The nerves that control extraocular muscles (plus V_1 and V_2) pass through the cavernous sinus.

Cavernous sinus syndrome (e.g., due to mass effect)— ophthalmoplegia, ophthalmic and maxillary sensory loss.

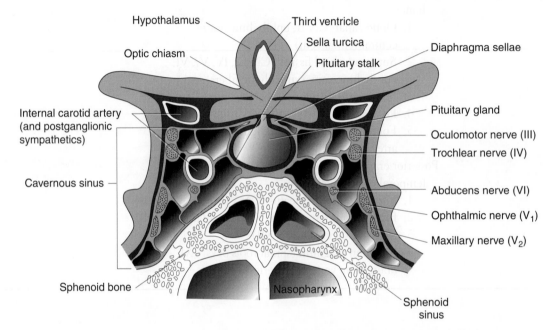

Hypothalamus · Third ventricle · Sella turcica · Optic chiasm · Pituitary stalk · Diaphragma sellae · Internal carotid artery (and postganglionic sympathetics) · Pituitary gland · Oculomotor nerve (III) · Trochlear nerve (IV) · Cavernous sinus · Abducens nerve (VI) · Ophthalmic nerve (V_1) · Maxillary nerve (V_2) · Sphenoid bone · Nasopharynx · Sphenoid sinus

(Adapted, with permission, from Stobo J et al. *The Principles and Practice of Medicine,* 23rd ed. Stamford, CT: Appleton & Lange, 1996: 277.)

Cranial nerve lesions

CN XII lesion (LMN)—tongue deviates **toward** side of lesion (lick your wounds). Decussates before medulla and synapse on contralateral hypoglossal nucleus.

CN V motor lesion—jaw deviates **toward** side of lesion. Bilateral cortical input to lateral pterygoid muscle.

CN X lesion—uvula deviates **away** from side of lesion. Weak side collapses and uvula points away.

CN XI lesion—weakness turning head to contralateral side of lesion (SCM). Shoulder droop on side of lesion (trapezius).

Facial lesions

UMN lesion — Lesion of motor cortex or connection between cortex and facial nucleus. Contralateral paralysis of lower face only, since upper face receives bilateral UMN innervation.

LMN lesion — Ipsilateral paralysis of upper **and** lower face.

Bell's palsy — Complete destruction of the facial nucleus itself or its branchial efferent fibers (facial nerve proper).

Peripheral ipsilateral facial paralysis with inability to close eye on involved side.

Can occur idiopathically; gradual recovery in most cases.

Seen as a complication in **A**IDS, **L**yme disease, **H**erpes simplex, **S**arcoidosis, **T**umors, **D**iabetes (**AL**exander gra**H**am **Bell** with **STD**).

Face area of motor cortex

Cortico-bulbar tract (UMN lesion = **central facial**)

Facial nucleus

Upper division
Lower division

LMN lesion *Cannot wrinkle forehead.

CN VII (LMN lesion = **Bell's palsy**)

KLM sounds: kuh, la, mi

Kuh-kuh-kuh tests palate elevation (CN X—vagus).
La-la-la tests tongue (CN XII—hypoglossal).
Mi-mi-mi tests lips (CN VII—facial).

Say it aloud.
It would be a **K**a**L**a**M**ity to lose CN X, XII, and VII.

Mastication muscles

3 muscles close jaw: **M**asseter, te**M**poralis, **M**edial pterygoid. 1 opens: lateral pterygoid. All are innervated by the trigeminal nerve (V_3).

M's **M**unch.
Lateral **L**owers (when speaking of pterygoids with respect to jaw motion).
"It takes more muscle to keep your mouth shut."

Eye and retina

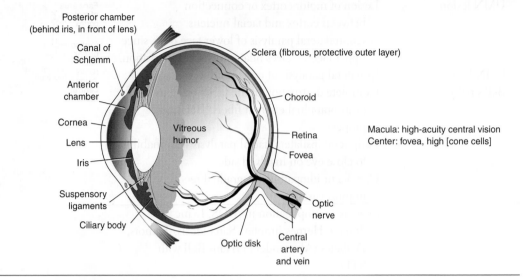

Posterior chamber
(behind iris, in front of lens)

Canal of Schlemm

Anterior chamber

Cornea

Lens

Iris

Suspensory ligaments

Ciliary body

Sclera (fibrous, protective outer layer)

Choroid

Vitreous humor

Retina

Fovea

Optic nerve

Optic disk

Central artery and vein

Macula: high-acuity central vision
Center: fovea, high [cone cells]

Eye pathology

Retinitis	Retinal necrosis + edema → atrophic scar.
Iritis	Systemic inflammation (e.g., Reiter's).
Near vision	Ciliary muscle contracts (zonular fibers relax → lens relaxes → more convex).
Distant vision	Ciliary muscle relaxes (lens flattens).
Aging	Sclerosis and ↓ elasticity cause lens shape to change.
Retinal artery occlusion	Acute, painless monocular loss of vision; pale retina and cherry-red macula (has its own blood supply—choroid artery).

Aqueous humor pathway

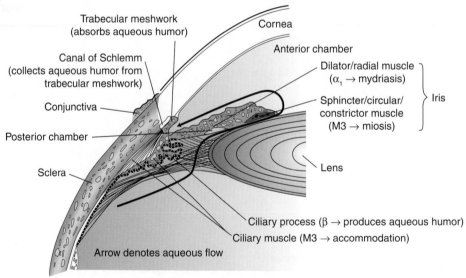

Trabecular meshwork
(absorbs aqueous humor)

Canal of Schlemm
(collects aqueous humor from
trabecular meshwork)

Conjunctiva

Posterior chamber

Sclera

Cornea

Anterior chamber

Dilator/radial muscle
(α_1 → mydriasis)

Sphincter/circular/
constrictor muscle
(M3 → miosis)

Iris

Lens

Ciliary process (β → produces aqueous humor)

Ciliary muscle (M3 → accommodation)

Arrow denotes aqueous flow

Glaucoma   Impaired flow of aqueous humor → ↑ intraocular pressure → optic disk atrophy with cupping.

Open/wide angle—obstructed outflow (e.g., canal of Schlemm); associated with myopia, ↑ age, African-American race. More common, "silent," painless.

Closed/narrow angle—obstruction of flow between iris and lens → pressure buildup behind iris. Very painful, ↓ vision, rock-hard eye, frontal headache. An ophthalmologic emergency. Do not give epinephrine.

Closed/narrow-angle glaucoma

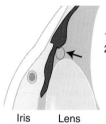

1. Iris and lens stick together
2. Pressure buildup behind iris

Iris   Lens

Open/wide-angle glaucoma

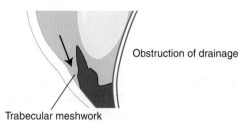

Obstruction of drainage

Trabecular meshwork

Cataract   Painless, bilateral opacification of lens → ↓ in vision. Risk factors: age, smoking, EtOH, sunlight, classic galactosemia, galactokinase deficiency, diabetes (sorbitol), trauma, infection.

Papilledema   ↑ in intracranial pressure → elevated optic disk with blurred margins, bigger blind spot (can be seen in hydrocephalus).

Extraocular muscles and nerves

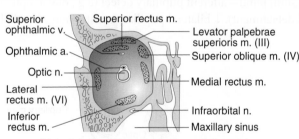

Superior ophthalmic v.
Ophthalmic a.
Optic n.
Lateral rectus m. (VI)
Inferior rectus m.
Superior rectus m.
Levator palpebrae superioris m. (III)
Superior oblique m. (IV)
Medial rectus m.
Infraorbital n.
Maxillary sinus

(Note: inferior oblique not in plane of diagram)

CN III damage—eye looks down and out; ptosis, pupillary dilation, loss of accommodation.

CN IV damage—eye drifts upward causing vertical diplopia (problems reading newspaper or going down stairs).

CN VI damage—medially directed eye.

CN VI innervates the Lateral Rectus.
CN IV innervates the Superior Oblique.
CN III innervates the Rest.
The "chemical formula"
$LR_6SO_4R_3$.
The superior oblique abducts, intorts, and depresses while adducted.

Testing extraocular muscles

To test the function of each muscle, have the patient look in the following directions (e.g., to test SO, have patient depress eye from adducted position):

IOU: to test **I**nferior **O**blique, have patient look **U**p.

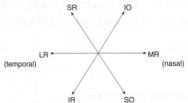

Pupillary control

1. Constriction (miosis)—Pupillary sphincter muscle (aka circular muscle). Parasympathetic. Innervation—CN III from Edinger-Westphal nucleus → ciliary ganglion.
2. Dilation (my**D**riasis)—radial muscle (aka pupillary dilator muscle), sympathetic. Innervation—T1 preganglionic sympathetic → superior cervical ganglion → postganglionic sympathetic → long ciliary nerve.

Pupillary light reflex

Light in either retina sends a signal via CN II to pretectal nuclei (dashed lines) in midbrain that activate bilateral Edinger-Westphal nuclei; pupils contract bilaterally (consensual reflex).

Result: illumination of 1 eye results in bilateral pupillary constriction.

Marcus Gunn pupil—afferent pupillary defect (e.g., due to optic nerve damage or retinal detachment). ↓ bilateral pupillary constriction when light is shone in affected eye.

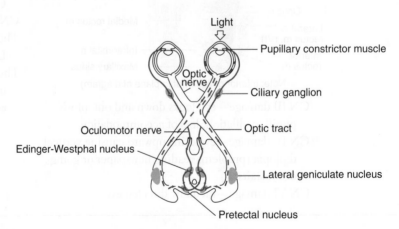

(Adapted, with permission, from Simon RP et al. *Clinical Neurology,* 3rd ed. Stamford, CT: Appleton & Lange, 1996.)

Cranial nerve III in cross section

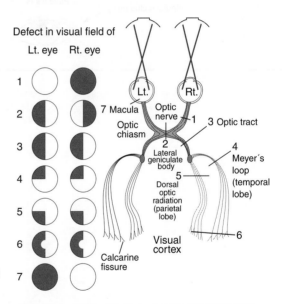

CN III

Output to ocular muscles—affected primarily by vascular disease (e.g., diabetes: glucose → sorbitol) due to ↑ diffusion to interior.

Parasympathetic output—affected 1st by compression (e.g., PCA berry aneurysm, uncal herniation); use pupillary light reflex in assessment, "blown pupil."

Retinal detachment	Separation of neurosensory layer of retina from pigment epithelium → degeneration of photoreceptors → vision loss. May be 2° to trauma, diabetes.
Age-related macular degeneration (ARMD)	Degeneration of macula (central area of retina). Causes loss of central vision (scotomas). "Dry"/atrophic ARMD is slow, due to fat deposits and causes gradual ↓ in vision. "Wet" ARMD is rapid, due to neovascularization.

Visual field defects

1. Right anopia
2. Bitemporal hemianopia
3. Left homonymous hemianopia
4. Left upper quadrantic anopia (right temporal lesion, MCA)
5. Left lower quadrantic anopia (right parietal lesion, MCA)
6. Left hemianopia with macular sparing (PCA), macula → bilateral projection to occiput
7. Central scotoma (macular degeneration)

Defect in visual field of

Lt. eye Rt. eye

7 Macula
Optic nerve — 1
Optic chiasm
3 Optic tract
2
Lateral geniculate body
4 Meyer's loop (temporal lobe)
5
Dorsal optic radiation (parietal lobe)
Visual cortex
6
Calcarine fissure

Note: When an image hits 1° visual cortex, it is upside down and left-right reversed.

Meyer's loop—inferior retina; loops around inferior horn of lateral ventricle. Dorsal optic radiation—superior retina; takes shortest path via internal capsule.

Internuclear ophthalmoplegia (MLF syndrome)

Lesion in the medial longitudinal fasciculus (MLF) → medial rectus palsy on attempted lateral gaze. Nystagmus in abducting eye. Convergence is normal. Syndrome is seen in many patients with multiple sclerosis.

MLF = MS.
When looking left, the left nucleus of CN VI fires, which contracts the left lateral rectus and stimulates the contralateral (right) nucleus of CN III via the right MLF to contract the right medial rectus.

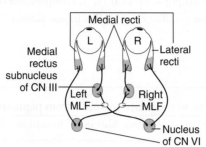

Looking to the left with right MLF damage

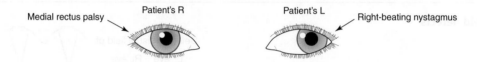

Dementia

A ↓ in cognitive ability, memory, or function with intact consciousness.

Disease	Description	Histologic/Gross Findings
Alzheimer's disease	Most common cause in elderly. Down syndrome patients have an ↑ risk of developing Alzheimer's. Familial form (10%) associated with the following genes (see Image 41): 　■ **Early onset:** APP (21), presenilin-1 (14), presenilin-2 (1) 　■ **Late onset:** ApoE4 (19) ApoE2 (19) is protective.	■ Widespread cortical atrophy ■ ↓ ACh ■ Senile plaques (extracellular β-amyloid core): may cause amyloid angiopathy → intracranial hemorrhage (Aβ-amyloid synthesized by cleaving amyloid protein) ■ Neurofibrillary tangles (intracellular, abnormally phosphorylated tau protein = insoluble cytoskeletal elements; tangles correlate with degree of dementia)
Pick's disease (frontotemporal dementia)	Dementia, aphasia, parkinsonian aspects; change in personality. Spares parietal lobe and posterior ⅔ of superior temporal gyrus.	■ Pick bodies (intracellular, aggregated tau protein) ■ Frontotemporal atrophy
Lewy body dementia	Parkinsonism with dementia and hallucinations.	■ α-synuclein defect
Creutzfeldt-Jakob disease (CJD)	Rapidly progressive (weeks to months) dementia with myoclonus.	■ Spongiform cortex ■ Prions (α helix → β sheet [resistant to proteases])
Other causes	**Multi-infarct** (2nd most common in elderly), **syphilis, HIV, vitamin B$_{12}$ deficiency, Wilson's disease.**	

Multiple sclerosis

Autoimmune inflammation and demyelination of CNS (brain and spinal cord). Patients can present with optic neuritis (sudden loss of vision), MLF syndrome (internuclear ophthalmoplegia), hemiparesis, hemisensory symptoms, or bladder/bowel incontinence. Relapsing and remitting course. Most often affects women in their 20s and 30s; more common in whites.

Findings: ↑ protein (IgG) in CSF. Oligoclonal bands are diagnostic. MRI is gold standard. Periventricular plaques (areas of oligodendrocyte loss and reactive gliosis) with preservation of axons (see Image 47).

Charcot's classic triad of **MS** is a **SIN:**

　Scanning speech
　Intention tremor,
　　Incontinence,
　　Internuclear ophthalmoplegia
　Nystagmus

Treatment: β-interferon or immunosuppressant therapy. Symptomatic treatment for neurogenic bladder, spasticity, pain.

Guillain-Barré syndrome (acute inflammatory demyelinating polyradiculopathy)	Inflammation and demyelination of peripheral nerves and motor fibers of ventral roots (sensory effect less severe than motor), causing symmetric ascending muscle weakness beginning in distal lower extremities. Facial paralysis in 50% of cases. Autonomic function may be severely affected (e.g., cardiac irregularities, hypertension, or hypotension). Almost all patients survive; the majority recover completely after weeks to months. Findings: ↑ CSF protein with normal cell count (albuminocytologic dissociation). ↑ protein → papilledema.	Associated with infections → autoimmune attack of peripheral myelin due to molecular mimicry (e.g., *Campylobacter jejuni* or herpesvirus infection), inoculations, and stress, but no definitive link to pathogens. Respiratory support is critical until recovery. Additional treatment: plasmapheresis, IV immune globulins.
Other demyelinating and dysmyelinating diseases	**Progressive multifocal leukoencephalopathy (PML)**—demyelination of CNS due to destruction of oligodendrocytes. Associated with JC virus and seen in 2–4% of AIDS patients (reactivation of latent viral infection). Rapidly progressive, usually fatal. **Acute disseminated (postinfectious) encephalomyelitis**—multifocal perivenular inflammation and demyelination after infection (e.g., chickenpox, measles) or certain vaccinations (e.g., rabies, smallpox). **Metachromatic leukodystrophy**—autosomal-recessive lysosomal storage disease, most commonly due to arylsulfatase A deficiency. Buildup of sulfatides leads to impaired production of myelin sheath. **Charcot-Marie-Tooth disease**—also known as hereditary motor and sensory neuropathy (HMSN). Group of progressive hereditary nerve disorders related to the defective production of proteins involved in the structure and function of peripheral nerves or the myelin sheath.	

Seizures	Seizure—characterized by synchronized, high-frequency neuronal firing. Variety of forms.
	Partial seizures—1 area of the brain. Most commonly originates in mesial temporal lobe. Often preceded by seizure aura; can secondarily generalize.
	  1. Simple partial (consciousness intact)— motor, sensory, autonomic, psychic
	  2. Complex partial (impaired consciousness)
	Generalized seizures—diffuse.
	  1. Absence (petit mal, 3 Hz, no postictal confusion)—blank stare
	  2. Myoclonic—quick, repetitive jerks
	  3. Tonic-clonic (grand mal)—alternating stiffening and movement
	  4. Tonic—stiffening
	  5. Atonic—"drop" seizures (falls to floor); commonly mistaken for fainting
		Epilepsy—a disorder of recurrent seizures (febrile seizures are not epilepsy).
		Causes of seizures by age:
		  Children—genetic, infection (febrile), trauma, congenital, metabolic.
		  Adults—tumors, trauma, stroke, infection.
		  Elderly—stroke, tumor, trauma, metabolic, infection.

HIGH-YIELD SYSTEMS

NEUROLOGY

Headache	Pain due to irritation of structures such as dura, cranial nerves, or extracranial structures, not brain parenchyma itself.

Migraine—unilateral; 4–72 hours of pulsating pain with nausea, photophobia, or phonophobia. +/– "aura" of neurologic symptoms before headache, including visual, sensory, speech disturbances. Due to irritation of CN V and release of substance P, CGRP, vasoactive peptides. Treatment: propranolol; NSAIDs; sumatriptan for acute migraines.

Tension headache—bilateral; > 30 minutes of steady pain. Not aggravated by light or noise; no aura.

Cluster headache—unilateral; repetitive brief headaches characterized by periorbital pain associated with ipsilateral lacrimation, rhinorrhea, Horner's syndrome. Much more common in males. Treatment: sumatriptan.

Other causes of headache include subarachnoid hemorrhage ("worst headache of life"), meningitis, hydrocephalus, neoplasia, arteritis.

Vertigo	Illusion of movement, not to be confused with dizziness or lightheadedness.

Peripheral vertigo—more common. Inner ear etiology (e.g., semicircular canal debris, vestibular nerve infection, Ménière's disease). Positional testing → delayed horizontal nystagmus.

Central vertigo—brain stem or cerebellar lesion (e.g., vestibular nuclei, posterior fossa tumor). Positional testing → immediate nystagmus in any direction; may change directions.

Neurocutaneous disorders

Sturge-Weber syndrome

Congenital disorder with port-wine stains (aka nevus flammeus), typically in V_1 ophthalmic distribution; ipsilateral leptomeningeal angiomas, pheochromocytomas.

Can cause glaucoma, seizures, hemiparesis, and mental retardation. Occurs sporadically.

Tuberous sclerosis

Hamartomas in CNS, skin, organs; cardiac rhabdomyoma, renal angiomyolipoma, subependymal giant cell astrocytoma, mental retardation, seizures, hypopigmented "ash leaf spots," sebaceous adenoma, shagreen patch. Autosomal dominant.

Neurofibromatosis type I (von Recklinghausen's disease)

Café-au-lait spots, Lisch nodules (pigmented iris hamartomas), neurofibromas in skin, optic gliomas, pheochromocytomas. Autosomal dominant. Mutated NF-1 gene on chromosome 17.

von Hippel–Lindau disease

Cavernous hemangiomas in skin, mucosa, organs; bilateral renal cell carcinoma, hemangioblastoma in retina, brain stem, cerebellum; pheochromocytomas. Autosomal dominant; mutated tumor suppressor VHL on chromosome 3.

Primary brain tumors	Clinical presentation due to mass effects (e.g., seizures, dementia, focal lesions); 1° brain tumors rarely undergo metastasis. The majority of adult 1° tumors are supratentorial, while the majority of childhood 1° tumors are infratentorial. Note: half of adult brain tumors are metastases (well circumscribed; usually present at the gray-white junction).	

Adult peak incidence

Glioblastoma multiforme (grade IV astrocytoma)	Most common 1° brain tumor. Prognosis grave; < 1-year life expectancy. Found in cerebral hemispheres. Can cross corpus callosum ("butterfly glioma") (see Image 48). Stain astrocytes for GFAP.	"Pseudopalisading" pleomorphic tumor cells—border central areas of necrosis and hemorrhage.
Meningioma	2nd most common 1° brain tumor. Most often occurs in convexities of hemispheres and parasagittal region. Arises from arachnoid cells external to brain. Resectable.	Spindle cells concentrically arranged in a whorled pattern; **psammoma bodies** (laminated calcifications).
Schwannoma	3rd most common 1° brain tumor. Schwann cell origin; often localized to CN VIII → acoustic schwannoma. Resectable. Usually found at cerebellopontine angle; S-100 positive.	Bilateral schwannoma found in neurofibromatosis type 2.
Oligodendro-glioma	Relatively rare, slow growing. Most often in frontal lobes. Chicken-wire capillary pattern (see Image 49).	Oligodendrocytes = "fried egg" cells—round nuclei with clear cytoplasm. Often calcified in oligodendroglioma.
Pituitary adenoma	Most commonly prolactinoma. Bitemporal hemianopia (due to pressure on optic chiasm) and hyper- or hypopituitarism are sequelae.	Rathke's pouch.

Childhood peak incidence

Pilocytic (low-grade) astrocytoma	Usually well circumscribed. In children, most often found in posterior fossa. May be supratentorial. GFAP positive. Benign; good prognosis.	Rosenthal fibers—eosinophilic, corkscrew fibers. Cystic + solid (gross).
Medullo-blastoma	Highly malignant cerebellar tumor. A form of primitive neuroectodermal tumor (PNET). Can compress 4th ventricle, causing hydrocephalus.	Rosettes or perivascular pseudorosette pattern of cells. Solid (gross), small blue cells (histology). Radiosensitive.
Ependymoma	Ependymal cell tumors most commonly found in 4th ventricle. Can cause hydrocephalus. Poor prognosis.	Characteristic perivascular pseudorosettes. Rod-shaped blepharoplasts (basal ciliary bodies) found near nucleus.
Hemangio-blastoma	Most often cerebellar; associated with von Hippel–Lindau syndrome when found with retinal angiomas. Can produce EPO → 2° polycythemia.	Foamy cells and high vascularity are characteristic.
Craniopharyn-gioma	Benign childhood tumor, confused with pituitary adenoma (can also cause bitemporal hemianopia). Most common childhood supratentorial tumor.	Derived from remnants of Rathke's pouch. Calcification is common (tooth enamel–like).

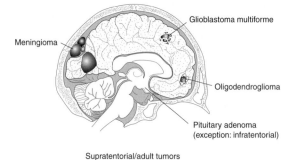

Supratentorial/adult tumors

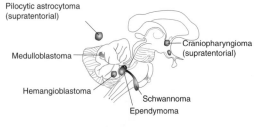

Infratentorial/childhood tumors

Herniation syndromes

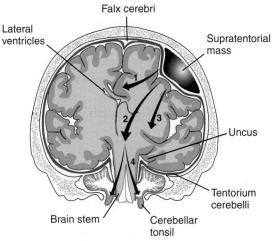

1. Cingulate (subfalcine) herniation under falx cerebri
2. Downward transtentorial (central) herniation
3. Uncal herniation
4. Cerebellar tonsillar herniation into the foramen magnum

Can compress anterior cerebral artery.
Coma and death result when these herniations compress the brain stem.
Uncus = medial temporal lobe.

(Adapted, with permission, from Simon RP et al. *Clinical Neurology*, 4th ed. Stamford, CT: Appleton & Lange, 1999: 314.)

Uncal herniation

Clinical signs	Cause
Ipsilateral dilated pupil/ptosis	Stretching of CN III (innervates levator palpebrae)
Contralateral homonymous hemianopia	Compression of ipsilateral posterior cerebral artery
Ipsilateral paresis	Compression of contralateral crus cerebri (Kernohan's notch)
Duret hemorrhages— paramedian artery rupture	Caudal displacement of brain stem

Differential diagnosis of brain lesions

Ring-enhancing lesion	Metastases, abscesses, toxoplasmosis, AIDS lymphoma.
Uniformly enhancing lesion	Lymphoma, meningioma, metastases (usually ring enhancing).
Heterogeneously enhancing lesion	Glioblastoma multiforme.

Glaucoma drugs

Drug	Mechanism	Side effects
α-agonists		
Epinephrine	↓ aqueous humor synthesis due to vasoconstriction	Mydriasis, stinging; do not use in closed-angle glaucoma
Brimonidine	↓ aqueous humor synthesis	No pupillary or vision changes
β-blockers		
Timolol, betaxolol, carteolol	↓ aqueous humor secretion	No pupillary or vision changes
Diuretics		
Acetazolamide	↓ aqueous humor secretion due to ↓ HCO_3^- (via inhibition of carbonic anhydrase)	No pupillary or vision changes
Cholinomimetics		
Direct (pilocarpine, carbachol), indirect (physostigmine, echothiophate)	↑ outflow of aqueous humor; contract ciliary muscle and open trabecular meshwork; use pilocarpine in emergencies; very effective at opening meshwork into canal of Schlemm	Miosis, cyclospasm
Prostaglandin		
Latanoprost ($PGF_{2\alpha}$)	↑ outflow of aqueous humor	Darkens color of iris (browning)

Opioid analgesics — Morphine, fentanyl, codeine, heroin, methadone, meperidine, dextromethorphan.

Mechanism	Act as agonists at opioid receptors (mu = morphine, delta = enkephalin, kappa = dynorphin) to modulate synaptic transmission—open K^+ channels, close Ca^{2+} channels → ↓ synaptic transmission. Inhibit release of ACh, NE, 5-HT, glutamate, substance P.
Clinical use	Pain, cough suppression (dextromethorphan), diarrhea (loperamide and diphenoxylate), acute pulmonary edema, maintenance programs for addicts (methadone).
Toxicity	Addiction, **respiratory depression,** constipation, miosis (**pinpoint pupils**), additive **CNS depression** with other drugs. Tolerance does not develop to miosis and constipation. Toxicity treated with naloxone or naltrexone (opioid receptor antagonist).

Butorphanol

Mechanism	Partial agonist at opioid mu receptors, agonist at kappa receptors.
Clinical use	Pain; causes less respiratory depression than full agonists.
Toxicity	Causes withdrawal if on full opioid agonist.

Tramadol

Mechanism	Very weak opioid agonist; also inhibits serotonin and NE reuptake (works on multiple neurotransmitters—"**tram it all**" in).
Clinical use	Chronic pain.
Toxicity	Similar to opioids. Decreases seizure threshold.

Epilepsy drugs

	PARTIAL		GENERALIZED			Mechanism	Notes
	Simple	Complex	Tonic-Clonic	Absence	Status		
Phenytoin	✓	✓	1st line		1st line for prophylaxis	↑ Na⁺ channel inactivation	Fosphenytoin for parenteral use
Carbamazepine	✓	✓	1st line			↑ Na⁺ channel inactivation	1st line for trigeminal neuralgia
Lamotrigine	✓	✓	✓			Blocks voltage-gated Na⁺ channels	
Gabapentin	✓	✓	✓			Designed as GABA analog, but primarily inhibits HVA Ca²⁺ channels	Also used for peripheral neuropathy, bipolar disorder
Topiramate	✓	✓	✓			Blocks Na⁺ channels, ↑ GABA action	
Phenobarbital	✓	✓	✓			↑ GABA$_A$ action	1st line in pregnant women, children
Valproic acid	✓	✓	1st line	✓		↑ Na⁺ channel inactivation, ↑ GABA concentration	Also used for myoclonic seizures
Ethosuximide				1st line		Blocks thalamic T-type Ca²⁺ channels	
Benzodiazepines (diazepam or lorazepam)					1st line for acute	↑ GABA$_A$ action	Also used for seizures of eclampsia (1st line is MgSO$_4$)
Tiagabine	✓	✓				Inhibits GABA reuptake	
Vigabatrin	✓	✓				Irreversibly inhibits GABA transaminase → ↑ GABA	
Levetiracetam	✓	✓	✓			Unknown; may modulate GABA and glutamate release	

Epilepsy drug toxicities

Benzodiazepines	Sedation, tolerance, dependence.	
Carbamazepine	Diplopia, ataxia, blood dyscrasias (agranulocytosis, aplastic anemia), liver toxicity, teratogenesis, induction of cytochrome P-450, SIADH, Stevens-Johnson syndrome.	
Ethosuximide	GI distress, fatigue, headache, urticaria, Stevens-Johnson syndrome.	**EFGH**—Ethosuximide, Fatigue, GI, Headache.
Phenobarbital	Sedation, tolerance, dependence, induction of cytochrome P-450.	Stevens-Johnson syndrome—prodrome of malaise and fever followed by rapid onset of erythematous/purpuric macules (oral, ocular, genital). Skin lesions progress to epidermal necrosis and sloughing.
Phenytoin	Nystagmus, diplopia, ataxia, sedation, gingival hyperplasia, hirsutism, megaloblastic anemia, teratogenesis (fetal hydantoin syndrome), SLE-like syndrome, induction of cytochrome P-450.	
Valproic acid	GI distress, rare but fatal hepatotoxicity (measure LFTs), neural tube defects in fetus (spina bifida), tremor, weight gain. Contraindicated in pregnancy.	
Lamotrigine	Stevens-Johnson syndrome.	
Gabapentin	Sedation, ataxia.	
Topiramate	Sedation, mental dulling, kidney stones, weight loss.	

Phenytoin

Mechanism	Use-dependent blockade of Na^+ channels; ↑ refractory period; inhibition of glutamate release from excitatory presynaptic neuron.
Clinical use	Tonic-clonic seizures. Also a class IB antiarrhythmic.
Toxicity	Nystagmus, ataxia, diplopia, sedation, SLE-like syndrome, induction of cytochrome P-450. Chronic use produces gingival hyperplasia in children, peripheral neuropathy, hirsutism, megaloblastic anemia (↓ folate absorption). Teratogenic (fetal hydantoin syndrome).

Barbiturates

	Phenobarbital, pentobarbital, thiopental, secobarbital.	
Mechanism	Facilitate $GABA_A$ action by ↑ **duration** of Cl^- channel opening, thus ↓ neuron firing.	BarbiDURATe (↑ **DURAT**ion). Contraindicated in porphyria.
Clinical use	Sedative for anxiety, seizures, insomnia, induction of anesthesia (thiopental).	
Toxicity	Dependence, additive CNS depression effects with alcohol, respiratory or cardiovascular depression (can lead to death), drug interactions owing to induction of liver microsomal enzymes (cytochrome P-450).	
	Treat overdose with symptom management (assist respiration, ↑ BP).	

Benzodiazepines	Diazepam, lorazepam, triazolam, temazepam, oxazepam, midazolam, chlordiazepoxide, alprazolam.	
Mechanism	Facilitate GABA$_A$ action by ↑ **frequency** of Cl$^-$ channel opening. ↓ REM sleep. Most have long half-lives and active metabolites.	**FRE**nzodiazepines (↑ **FRE**quency). Short acting = **TOM** Thumb = **T**riazolam, **O**xazepam, **M**idazolam. Highest addictive potential. Benzos, barbs, and EtOH all bind GABA(A)-R, which is a ligand-gated chloride channel.
Clinical use	Anxiety, spasticity, status epilepticus (lorazepam and diazepam), detoxification (especially alcohol withdrawal–DTs), night terrors, sleepwalking, general anesthetic (amnesia, muscle relaxation), hypnotic (insomnia).	
Toxicity	Dependence, additive CNS depression effects with alcohol. Less risk of respiratory depression and coma than with barbiturates. Treat overdose with flumazenil (competitive antagonist at GABA benzodiazepine receptor).	

Nonbenzodiazepine hypnotics	Zolpidem (Ambien), zaleplon, eszopiclone.
Mechanism	Act via the BZ1 receptor subtype and is reversed by flumazenil.
Clinical use	Insomnia.
Toxicity	Ataxia, headaches, confusion. Short duration because of rapid metabolism by liver enzymes. Unlike older sedative-hypnotics, cause only modest day-after psychomotor depression and few amnestic effects. Lower dependence risk than benzodiazepines.

Anesthetics—general principles	CNS drugs must be lipid soluble (cross the blood-brain barrier) or be actively transported.
	Drugs with ↓ solubility in blood = rapid induction and recovery times.
	Drugs with ↑ solubility in lipids = ↑ potency = $\dfrac{1}{MAC}$ where MAC = minimal alveolar concentration at which 50% of the population is anesthetized. Varies with age.
	Examples: N$_2$O has low blood and lipid solubility, and thus fast induction and low potency. Halothane, in contrast, has ↑ lipid and blood solubility, and thus high potency and slow induction.

Organ	Mechanism of Action
Lungs	↑ rate + depth of ventilation = ↑ gas tension
Blood	↑ blood solubility = ↑ blood/gas partition coefficient = ↑ solubility = ↑ gas required to saturate blood = **slower** onset of action
Tissue (e.g., brain)	AV concentration gradient ↑ = ↑ solubility = ↑ gas required to saturate tissue = **slower** onset of action

Inhaled anesthetics	Halothane, enflurane, isoflurane, sevoflurane, methoxyflurane, nitrous oxide.
Mechanism	Mechanism unknown.
Effects	Myocardial depression, respiratory depression, nausea/emesis, ↑ cerebral blood flow (↓ cerebral metabolic demand).
Toxicity	Hepatotoxicity (halothane), nephrotoxicity (methoxyflurane), proconvulsant (enflurane), malignant hyperthermia (rare), expansion of trapped gas (nitrous oxide).

Intravenous anesthetics

Barbiturates	Thiopental—high potency, high lipid solubility, rapid entry into brain. Used for induction of anesthesia and short surgical procedures. Effect terminated by rapid redistribution into tissue and fat. ↓ cerebral blood flow.	**B. B. K**ing on **OPIATES PROPO**ses **FOOL**ishly.
Benzodiazepines	Midazolam most common drug used for endoscopy; used adjunctively with gaseous anesthetics and narcotics. May cause severe postoperative respiratory depression, ↓ BP (treat overdose with flumazenil), and amnesia.	
Arylcyclohexylamines (**K**etamine)	PCP analogs that act as dissociative anesthetics. Block NMDA receptors. Cardiovascular stimulants. Cause disorientation, hallucination, and bad dreams. ↑ cerebral blood flow.	
Opiates	Morphine, fentanyl used with other CNS depressants during general anesthesia.	
Propofol	Used for rapid anesthesia induction and short procedures. Less postoperative nausea than thiopental. Potentiates $GABA_A$.	Not recommended for home use by pop stars.

Local anesthetics Esters—procaine, cocaine, tetracaine; amides—l**I**doca**I**ne, mep**I**vaca**I**ne, bup**I**vaca**I**ne (am**I**des have 2 **I**'s in name).

Mechanism	Block Na^+ channels by binding to specific receptors on inner portion of channel. Preferentially bind to activated Na^+ channels, so most effective in rapidly firing neurons. 3° amine local anesthetics penetrate membrane in uncharged form, then bind to ion channels as charged form.
Principle	1. In infected (acidic) tissue, alkaline anesthetics are charged and cannot penetrate membrane effectively. More anesthetic is needed in these cases. 2. Order of nerve blockade—small-diameter fibers > large diameter. Myelinated fibers > unmyelinated fibers. Overall, size factor predominates over myelination such that small myelinated fibers > small unmyelinated fibers > large myelinated fibers > large unmyelinated fibers. Order of loss—pain (lose first) > temperature > touch > pressure (lose last). 3. Except for cocaine, given with vasoconstrictors (usually epinephrine) to enhance local action—↓ bleeding, ↑ anesthesia by ↓ systemic concentration.
Clinical use	Minor surgical procedures, spinal anesthesia. If allergic to esters, give amides.
Toxicity	CNS excitation, severe cardiovascular toxicity (bupivacaine), hypertension, hypotension, and arrhythmias (cocaine).

Neuromuscular blocking drugs	Used for muscle paralysis in surgery or mechanical ventilation. Selective for motor (vs. autonomic) nicotinic receptor.
Depolarizing	Succinylcholine (complications include hypercalcemia and hyperkalemia). Reversal of blockade:
	Phase I (prolonged depolarization)—no antidote. Block potentiated by cholinesterase inhibitors.
	Phase II (repolarized but blocked)—antidote consists of cholinesterase inhibitors (e.g., neostigmine).
Nondepolarizing	Tubocurarine, atracurium, mivacurium, pancuronium, vecuronium, rocuronium. Competitive—compete with ACh for receptors.
	Reversal of blockade—neostigmine, edrophonium, and other cholinesterase inhibitors.

Dantrolene	Used in the treatment of **malignant hyperthermia**, which is caused by inhalation anesthetics (except N_2O) and succinylcholine. Also used to treat **neuroleptic malignant syndrome** (a toxicity of antipsychotic drugs).
	Mechanism: prevents the release of Ca^{2+} from the sarcoplasmic reticulum of skeletal muscle.

Parkinson's disease drugs

Parkinsonism is due to loss of dopaminergic neurons and excess cholinergic activity.

Strategy	Agents	
Agonize dopamine receptors	Bromocriptine, pramipexole, ropinirole (non-ergot); non-ergots are preferred	**BALSA:**
↑ dopamine	Amantadine (may ↑ dopamine release); also used as an antiviral against influenza A and rubella; toxicity = ataxia	**B**romocriptine **A**mantadine **L**evodopa (with carbidopa) **S**elegiline (and COMT inhibitors) **A**ntimuscarinics
	L-dopa/carbidopa (converted to dopamine in CNS)	
Prevent dopamine breakdown	Selegiline (selective MAO type B inhibitor); entacapone, tolcapone (COMT inhibitors—prevent L-dopa degradation, thereby increasing dopamine availability)	
Curb excess cholinergic activity	**Benz**tropine (**A**ntimuscarinic; improves tremor and rigidity but has little effect on bradykinesia)	**Park** your Mercedes-**Benz.**
	For essential or familial tremors, use a β-blocker (e.g., propranolol).	

L-dopa (levodopa)/carbidopa

Mechanism	↑ level of dopamine in brain. Unlike dopamine, L-dopa can cross blood-brain barrier and is converted by dopa decarboxylase in the CNS to dopamine.
Clinical use	Parkinsonism.
Toxicity	Arrhythmias from peripheral conversion to dopamine. Long-term use can → dyskinesia following administration, akinesia between doses. Carbidopa, a peripheral decarboxylase inhibitor, is given with L-dopa in order to ↑ the bioavailability of L-dopa in the brain and to limit peripheral side effects.

Selegiline

Mechanism	Selectively inhibits MAO-B, which preferentially metabolizes dopamine over NE and 5-HT, thereby increasing the availability of dopamine.
Clinical use	Adjunctive agent to L-dopa in treatment of Parkinson's disease.
Toxicity	May enhance adverse effects of L-dopa.

Alzheimer's drugs

Memantine

Mechanism	NMDA receptor antagonist; helps prevent excitotoxicity (mediated by Ca^{2+}).
Toxicity	Dizziness, confusion, hallucinations.

Donepezil, galantamine, rivastigmine

Mechanism	Acetylcholinesterase inhibitors.
Toxicity	Nausea, dizziness, insomnia.

Huntington's drugs

Disease—↑ dopamine, ↓ GABA + ACh.
Reserpine + tetrabenazine—amine depleting.
Haloperidol—dopamine receptor antagonist.

Sumatriptan

Mechanism	$5\text{-}HT_{1B/1D}$ agonist. Causes vasoconstriction, inhibition of trigeminal activation and vasoactive peptide release. Half-life < 2 hours.
Clinical use	Acute migraine, cluster headache attacks.
Toxicity	Coronary vasospasm (contraindicated in patients with CAD or Prinzmetal's angina), mild tingling.

A **SUM**o wrestler **TRIP**s **AN**d falls on your **head.**

Psychiatry

"A Freudian slip is when you say one thing but mean your mother."
> —Anonymous

"Men will always be mad, and those who think they can cure them are the maddest of all."
> —Voltaire

"Anyone who goes to a psychiatrist ought to have his head examined."
> —Samuel Goldwyn

Intelligence quotient	Stanford-Binet—calculates IQ as mental age/ chronological age × 100. Mean is defined at 100, with standard deviation of 15. IQ < 70 is one of the criteria for diagnosis of mental retardation (MR). IQ < 40—severe MR. IQ < 20—profound MR.	Standard-Binet IQ test.
Simple learning	Habituation—repeated stimulation leads to ↓ response. Sensitization—repeated stimulation leads to ↑ response.	
Classical conditioning	Learning in which a natural response (salivation) is elicited by a conditioned, or learned, stimulus (bell) that previously was presented in conjunction with an unconditioned stimulus (food).	Pavlov's classical experiments with dogs—ringing the bell provoked salivation.
Operant conditioning	Learning in which a particular action is elicited because it produces a reward. Positive reinforcement—desired reward produces action (mouse presses button to get food). Negative reinforcement—removal of aversive stimulus elicits behavior (mouse presses button to avoid shock). Punishment—application of aversive stimulus extinguishes unwanted behavior. Extinction—discontinuation of reinforcement eliminates behavior.	
Reinforcement schedules	Pattern of reinforcement determines how quickly a behavior is learned or extinguished.	
Continuous	Reward received after every response. Rapidly extinguished.	Think vending machine—stop using it if it does not deliver.
Variable ratio	Reward received after random number of responses. Slowly extinguished.	Think slot machine—continue to play even if it rarely rewards.

Transference and countertransference

Transference	Patient projects feelings about formative or other important persons onto physician (e.g., psychiatrist = parent).
Countertransference	Doctor projects feelings about formative or other important persons onto patient.

Freud's structural theory of the mind

The central goal of Freudian psychoanalysis is to make the patient aware of what is hidden in his/her unconscious.

Id	Primal urges, food, sex, and aggression. The id "drives"; Instinct. Entirely subconscious.	"I want it."
Ego	Mediator between primal urges and behavior accepted in reality.	"Take it and you will get in trouble."
Superego	Moral values, conscience; can lead to self-blame and attacks on ego.	"You know you can't have it. Taking it is wrong."

Social learning

Shaping—behavior achieved following reward of closer and closer approximations of desired behavior.

Modeling—behavior acquired by watching others and assimilating actions into one's own repertoire.

Ego defenses — Unconscious mental processes of the ego uses to resolve conflict and prevent feelings of anxiety and depression.

Immature—more primitive

Acting out	Unacceptable feelings and thoughts are expressed through actions.	Tantrums.
Dissociation	Temporary, drastic change in personality, memory, consciousness, or motor behavior to avoid emotional stress.	Extreme forms can result in dissociative identity disorder (multiple personality disorder).
Denial	Avoidance of awareness of some painful reality.	A common reaction in newly diagnosed AIDS and cancer patients.
Displacement	Process whereby avoided ideas and feelings are transferred to some neutral person or object (vs. projection).	Mother places blame on child because she is angry at her husband.
Fixation	Partially remaining at a more childish level of development (vs. regression).	Men fixating on sports games.
Identification	Modeling behavior after another person who is more powerful (though not necessarily admired).	Abused child identifies himself/herself as an abuser.
Isolation of affect	Separation of feelings from ideas and events.	Describing murder in graphic detail with no emotional response.
Projection	An unacceptable internal impulse is attributed to an external source.	A man who wants another woman thinks his wife is cheating on him.
Rationalization	Proclaiming logical reasons for actions actually performed for other reasons, usually to avoid self-blame.	After getting fired, claiming that the job was not important anyway.
Reaction formation	Process whereby a warded-off idea or feeling is replaced by an (unconsciously derived) emphasis on its opposite.	A patient with libidinous thoughts enters a monastery.
Regression	Turning back the maturational clock and going back to earlier modes of dealing with the world.	Seen in children under stress (e.g., bedwetting) and in patients on dialysis (e.g., crying).
Repression	Involuntary withholding of an idea or feeling from conscious awareness.	Not remembering a conflictual or traumatic experience; pressing bad thoughts into the unconscious.
Splitting	Belief that people are either all good or all bad at different times due to intolerance of ambiguity. Seen in borderline personality disorder.	A patient says that all the nurses are cold and insensitive but that the doctors are warm and friendly.

Mature—less primitive

Altruism	Guilty feelings alleviated by unsolicited generosity toward others.	Mafia boss makes large donation to charity.
Humor	Appreciating the amusing nature of an anxiety-provoking or adverse situation.	Nervous medical student jokes about the boards.
Sublimation	Process whereby one replaces an unacceptable wish with a course of action that is similar to the wish but does not conflict with one's value system.	Actress uses experience of abuse to enhance her acting.
Suppression	Voluntary withholding of an idea or feeling from conscious awareness (vs. repression).	Choosing not to think about the USMLE until the week of the exam.

Mature women wear a **SASH**: Sublimation, Altruism, Suppression, Humor.

Infant deprivation effects	Long-term deprivation of affection results in: 1. ↓ muscle tone 2. Poor language skills 3. Poor socialization skills 4. Lack of basic trust 5. Anaclitic depression 6. Weight loss 7. Physical illness Severe deprivation can result in infant death.	The **4 W's: W**eak, **W**ordless, **W**anting (socially), **W**ary. Deprived babies say **W**ah, **W**ah, **W**ah, **W**ah. Deprivation for > 6 months can lead to irreversible changes.

Anaclitic depression (hospitalism)	Depression in an infant attributable to continued separation from caregiver. Infant becomes withdrawn and unresponsive. Reversible, but prolonged separation can result in failure to thrive or other developmental disturbances (e.g., delayed speech).	

Child abuse

	Physical abuse	**Sexual abuse**
Evidence	Healed fractures on x-ray, cigarette burns, subdural hematomas, multiple bruises, retinal hemorrhage or detachment	Genital/anal trauma, STDs, UTIs
Abuser	Usually female and the 1° caregiver	Known to victim, usually male
Epidemiology	~3000 deaths/year in the United States	Peak incidence 9–12 years of age

Child neglect	Failure to provide a child with adequate food, shelter, supervision, education, and/or affection. Most common form of child maltreatment. Evidence: poor hygiene, malnutrition, withdrawal, impaired social/emotional development, failure to thrive. As with child abuse, child neglect must be reported to local child protective services.

Regression in children	Children regress to younger patterns of behavior under conditions of stress such as physical illness, punishment, birth of a new sibling, or fatigue (e.g., bedwetting in a previously toilet-trained child when hospitalized).

HIGH-YIELD PRINCIPLES

PSYCHIATRY

441

Childhood and early-onset disorders	Attention-deficit hyperactivity disorder (ADHD)—limited attention span and poor impulse control. Onset before age 7. Characterized by hyperactivity, motor impairment, and emotional lability. Normal intelligence, but commonly coexists with difficulties in school. May continue into adulthood in as many as 50% of individuals. Associated with ↓ frontal lobe volumes. Treatment: methylphenidate (Ritalin), amphetamines (Dexedrine), atomoxetine (nonstimulant SNRI).
	Conduct disorder—repetitive and pervasive behavior violating social norms (physical aggression, destruction of property, theft). After 18 years of age, diagnosed as antisocial personality disorder.
	Oppositional defiant disorder—enduring pattern of hostile, defiant behavior toward authority figures in the absence of serious violations of social norms.
	Tourette's syndrome—characterized by sudden, rapid, recurrent, nonrhythmic, stereotyped motor movements or vocalizations (tics) that persist for > 1 year. Lifetime prevalence of 0.1–1.0% in the general population. Coprolalia (obscene speech) found in only 20% of patients. Associated with OCD. Onset at < 18 years of age. Treatment: antipsychotics (e.g., haloperidol).
	Separation anxiety disorder—overwhelming fear of separation from home or loss of attachment figure. May lead to factitious physical complaints to avoid going to school. Common onset at 7–9 years of age.
Pervasive developmental disorders	Characterized by difficulties with language and failure to acquire, or early loss of, social skills.
	Autistic disorder—severe language impairment and poor social interactions. Greater focus on objects than on people. Characterized by repetitive behavior and usually below-normal intelligence. Rarely, may have unusual abilities (savants). More common in boys. Treatment: behavioral and supportive therapy to improve communication and social skills.
	Asperger's disorder—a milder form of autism. Characterized by all-absorbing interests, repetitive behavior, and problems with social relationships. Children are of normal intelligence and lack verbal or cognitive deficits. No language impairment.
	Rett's disorder—X-linked disorder seen almost exclusively in girls (affected males die in utero or shortly after birth). Symptoms usually become apparent starting at ages 1–4, followed by regression characterized by loss of development, mental retardation, loss of verbal abilities, ataxia, and stereotyped hand-wringing.
	Childhood disintegrative disorder—marked regression in multiple areas of functioning after at least 2 years of apparently normal development. Significant loss of expressive or receptive language skills, social skills or adaptive behavior, bowel or bladder control, play, or motor skills. Common onset between 3 and 4 years of age. More common in boys.
Neurotransmitter changes with disease	Anxiety—↑ NE, ↓ GABA, ↓ serotonin (5-HT).
	Depression—↓ NE, ↓ serotonin (5-HT), ↓ dopamine.
	Alzheimer's dementia—↓ ACh.
	Huntington's disease—↓ GABA, ↓ ACh.
	Schizophrenia—↑ dopamine.
	Parkinson's disease—↓ dopamine, ↑ serotonin, ↑ ACh.

Orientation	Patient's ability to know who he or she is, what date and time it is, and what his or her present circumstances are. Common causes of loss of orientation: alcohol, drugs, fluid/electrolyte imbalance, head trauma, hypoglycemia, nutritional deficiencies.	Order of loss: 1st—time; 2nd—place; last—person.
Amnesia types	*Retro*grade amnesia—inability to remember things that occurred before a CNS insult. *Antero*grade amnesia—inability to remember things that occurred after a CNS insult (no new memory). Korsakoff's amnesia—classic anterograde amnesia caused by thiamine deficiency. Leads to bilateral destruction of mammillary bodies. May also lead to some retrograde amnesia. Seen in alcoholics, and associated with confabulations. Dissociative amnesia—inability to recall important personal information, usually subsequent to severe trauma or stress.	
Delirium	**Waxing and waning level of consciousness with acute onset;** rapid ↓ in attention span and level of arousal. Characterized by acute changes in mental status, disorganized thinking, hallucinations (often visual), illusions, misperceptions, disturbance in sleep-wake cycle, cognitive dysfunction. Usually secondary to other illness (e.g., CNS disease, infection, trauma, substance abuse/withdrawal). Most common psychiatric illness on medical and surgical floors. Abnormal EEG.	Deli**RIUM** = changes in senso**RIUM**. Check for drugs with anticholinergic effects. Often reversible.
Dementia	**Gradual ↓ in cognition with no change in level of consciousness.** Characterized by memory deficits, aphasia, apraxia, agnosia, loss of abstract thought, behavioral/personality changes, impaired judgment. Patient is alert. No psychotic symptoms. ↑ incidence with age. More often gradual onset. Normal EEG. Caused by Alzheimer's disease, vascular thrombosis/hemorrhage (may have acute/subacute onset), HIV, Pick's disease, substance abuse, CJD.	De**MEM**tia is characterized by **MEM**ory loss. Usually irreversible. In elderly patients, depression may present like dementia (pseudodementia).
Hallucination vs. illusion vs. delusion vs. loose association	Hallucinations—perceptions in the absence of external stimuli (e.g., seeing a light that is not actually present). Illusions—misinterpretations of actual external stimuli (e.g., seeing a light and thinking that it is the sun). Delusions—false beliefs not shared with other members of culture/subculture that are firmly maintained in spite of obvious proof to the contrary (e.g., thinking the CIA is spying on you). Loose associations—disorders in the form of thought (the way ideas are tied together).	

Hallucination types

Visual hallucinations—common in delirium.
Auditory hallucinations—common in schizophrenia.
Olfactory hallucination—often occurs as an aura of psychomotor epilepsy and in brain tumors.
Gustatory hallucination—rare.
Tactile hallucinations—common in alcohol withdrawal (e.g., formication—the sensation of ants crawling on one's skin). Also seen in cocaine abusers ("cocaine bugs").
Hypna**GO**gic hallucination—occurs while **GO**ing to sleep.
Hypno**POMP**ic hallucination—occurs while waking from sleep (**POMP**ous upon awakening).

Schizophrenia

Chronic mental disorder with periods of psychosis, disturbed behavior and thought, and decline in functioning that lasts > 6 months. Associated with ↑ dopaminergic activity, ↓ dendritic branching. Marijuana use is a risk factor for schizophrenia in teens.

Diagnosis requires 2 or more of the following (1–4 are "positive symptoms"):
1. Delusions
2. Hallucinations—often auditory
3. Disorganized speech (loose associations)
4. Disorganized or catatonic behavior
5. "Negative symptoms"—flat affect, social withdrawal, lack of motivation, lack of speech or thought

Brief psychotic disorder—< 1 month, usually stress related.
Schizophreniform disorder—1–6 months.
Schizoaffective disorder—at least 2 weeks of stable mood with psychotic symptoms, plus a major depressive, manic, or mixed (both) episode. 2 subtypes: bipolar or depressive.

5 subtypes:
1. Paranoid (delusions)
2. Disorganized (with regard to speech, behavior, and affect)
3. Catatonic (automatisms)
4. Undifferentiated (elements of all types)
5. Residual

Genetic factors outweigh environmental factors in the etiology of schizophrenia.
Lifetime prevalence—1.5% (males = females, blacks = whites). Presents earlier in men (late teens to early 20s vs. late 20s to early 30s in women). Patients are at ↑ risk for suicide.

Delusional disorder

Fixed, persistent, nonbizarre belief system lasting > 1 month. Functioning otherwise not impaired. Often self-limited.
Shared psychotic disorder (folie à deux)—development of delusions in a person in a close relationship with someone with delusional disorder. Often resolves upon separation.

Dissociative disorders

Dissociative identity disorder—formerly known as multiple personality disorder. Presence of 2 or more distinct identities or personality states. More common in women. Associated with history of sexual abuse.
Depersonalization disorder—persistent feelings of detachment or estrangement from one's own body, a social situation, or the environment.
Dissociative fugue—abrupt change in geographic location with inability to recall past, confusion about personal identity, or assumption of a new identity. Associated with traumatic circumstances (e.g., natural disasters, wartime, trauma). Leads to significant distress or impairment. Not the result of substance abuse or general medical condition.

Manic episode	Distinct period of abnormally and persistently elevated, expansive, or irritable mood lasting at least 1 week. Often disturbing to patient. Diagnosis requires 3 or more of the following are present during mood disturbance:	
	1. **D**istractibility	Maniacs **DIG FAST.**
	2. **I**rresponsibility—seeks pleasure without regard to consequences (hedonistic)	
	3. **G**randiosity—inflated self-esteem	
	4. **F**light of ideas—racing thoughts	
	5. ↑ in goal-directed **A**ctivity/psychomotor **A**gitation	
	6. ↓ need for **S**leep	
	7. **T**alkativeness or pressured speech	
Hypomanic episode	Like manic episode except mood disturbance is not severe enough to cause marked impairment in social and/or occupational functioning or to necessitate hospitalization. No psychotic features.	
Bipolar disorder	Defined by the presence of at least 1 manic (bipolar I) or hypomanic (bipolar II) episode. Depressive symptoms always occur eventually. Patient's mood and functioning usually return to normal between episodes. Use of antidepressants can lead to ↑ mania. High suicide risk. Treatment: mood stabilizers (e.g., lithium, valproic acid, carbamazepine), atypical antipsychotics. Cyclothymic disorder—dysthymia and hypomania; milder form of bipolar disorder lasting at least 2 years.	
Major depressive episode	Self-limited disorder, with each episode usually lasting 6–12 months. Characterized by at least 5 of the following 9 symptoms for 2 or more weeks (symptoms must include patient-reported depressed mood or anhedonia):	
	1. **S**leep disturbance	**SIG E CAPS.**
	2. Loss of **I**nterest (anhedonia)	Commonly used mnemonic for depression screening.
	3. **G**uilt or feelings of worthlessness	Historically used by physicians in prescription writing. **SIG** is short for *signatura* (Latin for "directions"). Depressed patients were **directed** to take **E**nergy **CAPS**ules.
	4. Loss of **E**nergy	
	5. Loss of **C**oncentration	
	6. **A**ppetite/weight changes	
	7. **P**sychomotor retardation or agitation	
	8. **S**uicidal ideations	
	9. Depressed mood	
	Major depressive disorder, recurrent—requires 2 or more major depressive episodes with a symptom-free interval of 2 months.	Lifetime prevalence of major depressive episode: 5–12% male, 10–25% female.
	Dysthymia—milder form of depression lasting at least 2 years.	
	Seasonal affective disorder—associated with winter season; improves in response to full-spectrum light exposure.	

Atypical depression	Differs from classical forms of depression. Characterized by hypersomnia, overeating, and mood reactivity (the ability to experience improved mood in response to positive events vs. persistent sadness). Associated with weight gain and sensitivity to rejection. Most common subtype of depression. Treatment: MAO inhibitors, SSRIs.	
Postpartum mood disturbances	Maternal (postpartum) blues: 50–85% incidence rate. Characterized by depressed affect, tearfulness, and fatigue. Usually resolves within 10 days. Treatment: supportive. Follow-up to assess for possible postpartum depression.	
	Postpartum depression: 10–15% incidence rate. Characterized by depressed affect, anxiety, and poor concentration. Lasts 2 weeks to 2 months. Treatment: antidepressants, psychotherapy.	
	Postpartum psychosis: 0.1–0.2% incidence rate. Characterized by delusions, confusion, unusual behavior, and possible homicidal/suicidal ideations or attempts. Usually lasts days to 4–6 weeks. Treatment: antipsychotics, antidepressants, possible inpatient hospitalization.	
Electroconvulsive therapy (ECT)	Treatment option for major depressive disorder refractory to other treatment. Produces a painless seizure in an anesthetized patient. Major adverse effects are disorientation and temporary anterograde/retrograde amnesia usually fully resolving in 6 months.	
Risk factors for suicide completion	**S**ex (male), **A**ge (teenager or elderly), **D**epression, **P**revious attempt, **E**thanol or drug use, loss of **R**ational thinking, **S**ickness (medical illness, 3 or more prescription medications), **O**rganized plan, **N**o spouse (divorced, widowed, or single, especially if childless), **S**ocial support lacking. Women try more often; men succeed more often.	**SAD PERSONS**.
Panic disorder	Defined by the presence of recurrent periods of intense fear and discomfort peaking in 10 minutes with at least 4 of the following: **P**alpitations, **P**aresthesias, **A**bdominal distress, **N**ausea, **I**ntense fear of dying or losing control, l**I**ght-headedness, **C**hest pain, **C**hills, **C**hoking, dis**C**onnectedness, **S**weating, **S**haking, **S**hortness of breath. Strong genetic component. Treatment: cognitive behavioral therapy (CBT), SSRIs, TCAs, benzodiazepines.	**PANICS**. Described in context of occurrence (e.g., panic disorder with agoraphobia). Associated with persistent fear of having another attack.
Specific phobia	Fear that is excessive or unreasonable and interferes with normal function. **Cued** by presence or anticipation of a specific object or situation. Person recognizes fear is excessive. Can treat with systematic desensitization.	
	Social phobia (social anxiety disorder)—exaggerated fear of embarrassment in social situations (e.g., public speaking, using public restrooms). Treatment: SSRIs.	

Obsessive-compulsive disorder (OCD)	Recurring, intrusive thoughts, feelings, or sensations (obsessions) that cause severe distress; relieved in part by the performance of repetitive actions (compulsions). Ego dystonic: behavior inconsistent with one's own beliefs and attitudes (vs. obsessive-compulsive personality disorder). Associated with Tourette's disorder. Treatment: SSRIs, clomipramine.
Post-traumatic stress disorder	Persistent reexperiencing of a previous traumatic event (e.g., war, rape, robbery, serious accident, fire). May involve nightmares or flashbacks, intense fear, helplessness, or horror. Leads to avoidance of stimuli associated with the trauma and persistently ↑ arousal. **Disturbance lasts > 1 month,** with onset of symptoms beginning anytime after event, and causes significant distress and/or impaired functioning. Treatment: psychotherapy, SSRIs. Acute stress disorder—lasts between 2 days and 1 month.
Generalized anxiety disorder	Pattern of uncontrollable anxiety for at least 6 months that is unrelated to a specific person, situation, or event. Associated with sleep disturbance, fatigue, GI disturbance, and difficulty concentrating. Treatment: benzodiazepines, buspirone, SSRIs. Adjustment disorder—emotional symptoms (anxiety, depression) causing impairment following an identifiable psychosocial stressor (e.g., divorce, illness) and lasting < 6 months (> 6 months in presence of chronic stressor).
Malingering	Patient consciously fakes or claims to have a disorder in order to attain a specific 2° gain (e.g., avoiding work, obtaining drugs). Avoids treatment by medical personnel; complaints cease after gain (vs. factitious disorder).
Factitious disorder	Patient consciously creates physical and/or psychological symptoms in order to assume "sick role" and to get medical attention (1° gain). Munchausen's syndrome—**chronic** factitious disorder with predominantly physical signs and symptoms. Characterized by a history of multiple hospital admissions and willingness to receive invasive procedures. Munchausen's syndrome by proxy—when illness in a child is caused by the caregiver. Motivation is to assume a sick role by proxy. Form of child abuse.
Somatoform disorders	Category of disorders characterized by physical symptoms with no identifiable physical cause. Both illness production and motivation are unconscious drives. Symptoms not intentionally produced or feigned. More common in women. Several types: 1. Somatization disorder—variety of complaints in multiple organ systems (at least 4 pain, 2 GI, 1 sexual, 1 pseudoneurologic) over a period of years 2. Conversion—sudden loss of sensory or motor function (e.g., paralysis, blindness, mutism), often following an acute stressor; patient is aware of but indifferent toward symptoms ("la belle indifférence"); more common in adolescents and young adults 3. Hypochondriasis—preoccupation with and fear of having a serious illness despite medical evaluation and reassurance 4. Body dysmorphic disorder—preoccupation with minor or imagined defect in appearance, leading to significant emotional distress or impaired functioning; patients often repeatedly seek cosmetic surgery 5. Pain disorder—prolonged pain with no physical findings. Pain is the predominant focus of clinical presentation and psychological factors play an important role in severity, exacerbation, or maintenance of the pain.

Personality	Personality trait—an enduring, repetitive pattern of perceiving, relating to, and thinking about the environment and oneself. Personality disorder—inflexible, maladaptive, and rigidly pervasive pattern of behavior causing subjective distress and/or impaired functioning; person is usually not aware of problem. Usually presents by early adulthood.	
Cluster A personality disorders	Odd or eccentric; inability to develop meaningful social relationships. No psychosis; genetic association with schizophrenia. Types: 1. Paranoid—pervasive distrust and suspiciousness; projection is major defense mechanism 2. Schizoid—voluntary social withdrawal, limited emotional expression, content with social isolation (vs. avoidant) 3. Schizotypal—eccentric appearance, odd beliefs or magical thinking, interpersonal awkwardness	"Weird" (**A**ccusatory, **A**loof, **A**wkward). Schizoi**D** = **D**istant. Schizo**T**ypal = magical **T**hinking.
Cluster B personality disorders	Dramatic, emotional, or erratic; genetic association with mood disorders and substance abuse. Types: 1. Antisocial—disregard for and violation of rights of others, criminality; males > females; conduct disorder if < 18 years 2. Borderline—unstable mood and interpersonal relationships, impulsiveness, self-mutilation, boredom, sense of emptiness; females > males; splitting is a major defense mechanism 3. Histrionic—excessive emotionality and excitability, attention seeking, sexually provocative, overly concerned with appearance 4. Narcissistic—grandiosity, sense of entitlement; lacks empathy and requires excessive admiration; often demands the "best" and reacts to criticism with rage	"Wild" (**B**ad to the **B**one). Anti**SOC**ial = **SOC**iopath.
Cluster C personality disorders	Anxious or fearful; genetic association with anxiety disorders. Types: 1. Avoidant—hypersensitive to rejection, socially inhibited, timid, feelings of inadequacy, desires relationships with others (vs. schizoid) 2. Obsessive-compulsive—preoccupation with order, perfectionism, and control; ego syntonic: behavior consistent with one's own beliefs and attitudes (vs. OCD) 3. Dependent—submissive and clinging, excessive need to be taken care of, low self-confidence	"Worried" (**C**owardly, **C**ompulsive, **C**lingy).

HIGH-YIELD PRINCIPLES

PSYCHIATRY

Keeping "schizo-" straight	Schizoid	<	Schizotypal (schizoid + odd thinking)	<	Schizophrenic (greater odd thinking than schizotypal)	<	Schizoaffective (schizophrenic psychotic symptoms + bipolar or depressive mood disorder)

Schizophrenia time course:
   < 1 mo—brief psychotic disorder, usually stress related.
   1–6 mo—schizophreniform disorder.
   > 6 mo—schizophrenia.

Eating disorders	**Anorexia nervosa**—excessive dieting +/– purging; intense fear of gaining weight, body image distortion, and ↑ exercise, leading to body weight < 85% of ideal body weight. Associated with ↓ bone density. Severe weight loss, metatarsal stress fractures, amenorrhea, anemia, and electrolyte disturbances. Seen primarily in adolescent girls. Commonly coexists with depression. **Bulimia nervosa**—binge eating +/– purging; followed by self-induced vomiting or use of laxatives, diuretics, or emetics. Body weight often maintained within normal range. Associated with parotitis, enamel erosion, electrolyte disturbances, alkalosis, dorsal hand calluses from inducing vomiting (Russell's sign).
Gender identity disorder	Strong, persistent cross-gender identification. Characterized by persistent discomfort with one's sex, causing significant distress and/or impaired functioning. Trans**sexual**ism—desire to live as the opposite **sex**, often through surgery or hormone treatment. Trans**vest**ism—paraphilia; wearing clothes (**vest**) of the opposite sex (cross-dressing).

Substance dependence	Maladaptive pattern of substance use defined as 3 or more of the following signs in 1 year:
	  1. Tolerance—need more to achieve same effect
	  2. Withdrawal
	  3. Substance taken in larger amounts or over longer time than desired
	  4. Persistent desire or unsuccessful attempts to cut down
	  5. Significant energy spent obtaining, using, or recovering from substance
	  6. Important social, occupational, or recreational activities reduced because of substance use
	  7. Continued use in spite of knowing the problems that it causes

Substance abuse	Maladaptive pattern leading to clinically significant impairment or distress.
	  1. Recurrent use resulting in failure to fulfill major obligations at work, school, or home
	  2. Recurrent use in physically hazardous situations
	  3. Recurrent substance-related legal problems
	  4. Continued use in spite of persistent problems caused by use

Substance withdrawal	Behavioral, physiologic, and cognitive state caused by cessation or reduction of heavy and prolonged substance use. Signs and symptoms often opposite to those seen in intoxication.

Stages of change in overcoming substance addiction

1. Precontemplation–not yet acknowledging that there is a problem.
2. Contemplation–acknowledging that there is a problem, but not yet ready or willing to make a change.
3. Preparation/Determination–getting ready to change behavior.
4. Action/Willpower–changing behaviors.
5. Maintenance–maintaining the behavior change.
6. Relapse–returning to old behaviors and abandoning new changes.

Signs and symptoms of substance abuse

Drug	Intoxication	Withdrawal
Depressants	Nonspecific: mood elevation, ↓ anxiety, sedation, behavioral disinhibition, respiratory depression.	Nonspecific: anxiety, tremor, seizures, insomnia.
Alcohol	Emotional lability, slurred speech, ataxia, coma, blackouts. Serum. γ-glutamyltransferase (**GGT**)—sensitive indicator of alcohol use Lab AST value is twice ALT value. Treatment: naltrexone.	Mild alcohol withdrawal: symptoms similar to other depressants. Severe alcohol withdrawal: DTs. Treatment for DTs: benzodiazepines.
Opioids (e.g., morphine, heroin, methadone)	CNS depression, nausea and vomiting, constipation, pupillary constriction (**pinpoint pupils**), seizures (overdose is life-threatening). Treatment: naloxone, naltrexone.	Sweating, dilated pupils, piloerection ("cold turkey"), fever, rhinorrhea, nausea, stomach cramps, diarrhea ("flulike" symptoms). Treatment: symptomatic.
Barbiturates	Low safety margin, **marked respiratory depression.** Treatment: symptom management (assist respiration, ↑ BP).	Delirium, life-threatening cardiovascular collapse.
Benzodiazepines	Greater safety margin. Ataxia, minor respiratory depression. Treatment: flumazenil (competitive GABA antagonist).	
Stimulants	Nonspecific: mood elevation, psychomotor agitation, insomnia, cardiac arrhythmias, tachycardia, anxiety.	Nonspecific: post-use "crash," including depression, lethargy, weight gain, headache.
Amphetamines	Impaired judgment, pupillary dilation, prolonged wakefulness and attention, delusions, hallucinations, fever.	Stomach cramps, hunger, hypersomnolence.
Cocaine	Impaired judgment, pupillary dilation, hallucinations (including tactile), paranoid ideations, angina, sudden cardiac death. Treatment: benzodiazepines.	Suicidality, hypersomnolence, malaise, severe psychological craving.
Caffeine	Restlessness, ↑ diuresis, muscle twitching.	
Nicotine	Restlessness.	Irritability, anxiety, craving. Treatment: nicotine patch, gum, or lozenges; bupropion/varenicline.

Hallucinogens

PCP	Belligerence, impulsiveness, fever, psychomotor agitation, vertical and horizontal nystagmus, tachycardia, homicidality, psychosis, delirium.	Depression, anxiety, irritability, restlessness, anergia, disturbances of thought and sleep.
LSD	Marked anxiety or depression, delusions, visual hallucinations, **flashbacks,** pupillary dilation.	
Marijuana	Euphoria, anxiety, paranoid delusions, perception of slowed time, impaired judgment, social withdrawal, ↑ appetite, dry mouth, hallucinations.	Irritability, depression, insomnia, nausea, anorexia. Most symptoms peak in 48 hours and last for 5–7 days. Can be detected in urine up to 1 month after last use.

Heroin addiction	Users at ↑ risk for hepatitis, abscesses, overdose, hemorrhoids, AIDS, and right-sided endocarditis. Look for track marks (needle sticks in veins). Methadone—long-acting oral opiate; used for heroin detoxification or long-term maintenance. Suboxone—naloxone + buprenorphine (partial agonist); long acting with fewer withdrawal symptoms than methadone. Naloxone is not active when taken orally, so withdrawal symptoms occur only if injected (lower abuse potential).
Alcoholism	Physiologic tolerance and dependence with symptoms of withdrawal (tremor, tachycardia, hypertension, malaise, nausea, DTs) when intake is interrupted. Complications: alcoholic cirrhosis, hepatitis, pancreatitis, peripheral neuropathy, testicular atrophy. Wernicke-Korsakoff syndrome—caused by thiamine deficiency. Triad of confusion, ophthalmoplegia, and ataxia (Wernicke's encephalopathy). May progress to irreversible memory loss, confabulation, personality change (Korsakoff's psychosis). Associated with periventricular hemorrhage/necrosis of mammillary bodies. Treatment: IV vitamin B_1 (thiamine). Mallory-Weiss syndrome—longitudinal lacerations at the gastroesophageal junction caused by excessive vomiting. Often presents with hematemesis. Associated with pain (vs. esophageal varices). Treatment: disulfiram (to condition the patient to abstain from alcohol use), supportive care. Alcoholics Anonymous and other peer support groups are helpful in sustaining abstinence.
Delirium tremens (DTs)	Life-threatening alcohol withdrawal syndrome that peaks 2–5 days after last drink. Symptoms in order of appearance: autonomic system hyperactivity (tachycardia, tremors, anxiety, seizures), psychotic symptoms (hallucinations, delusions), confusion. Treatment: benzodiazepines.

Treatment for selected psychiatric conditions

Psychiatric condition	Drug
Alcohol withdrawal	Benzodiazepines
Anorexia/bulimia	SSRIs
Anxiety	Benzodiazepines
	Buspirone
	SSRIs
ADHD	Methylphenidate (Ritalin)
	Amphetamines (Dexedrine)
Atypical depression	MAO inhibitors
	SSRIs
Bipolar disorder	"Mood stabilizers":
	Lithium
	Valproic acid
	Carbamazepine
	Atypical antipsychotics
Depression	SSRIs, SNRIs
	TCAs
Depression with insomnia	Mirtazapine
Obsessive-compulsive disorder	SSRIs
	Clomipramine
Panic disorder	SSRIs
	TCAs
	Benzodiazepines
PTSD	SSRIs
Schizophrenia	Antipsychotics
Tourette's syndrome	Antipsychotics (haloperidol)
Social phobias	SSRIs

CNS stimulants	Methylphenidate, dextroamphetamine, mixed amphetamine salts.
Mechanism	↑ catecholamines at the synaptic cleft, especially NE and dopamine.
Clinical use	ADHD, narcolepsy, appetite control.

Antipsychotics (neuroleptics)	Haloperidol, trifluoperazine, fluphenazine, thioridazine, chlorpromazine (haloperidol + "-azine"s).	
Mechanism	All typical antipsychotics block dopamine D_2 receptors ($\uparrow$ [cAMP]$_1$).	High potency: haloperidol, trifluoperazine, fluphenazine —neurologic side effects (extrapyramidal symptoms).
Clinical use	Schizophrenia (primarily positive symptoms), psychosis, acute mania, Tourette's syndrome.	Low potency: thioridazine, chlorpromazine— non-neurologic side effects (anticholinergic, antihista- mine, and α blockade effects)
Toxicity	1. Highly lipid soluble and stored in body fat; thus, very slow to be removed from body 2. Extrapyramidal system (EPS) side effects 3. Endocrine side effects (e.g., dopamine receptor antagonism $\rightarrow$ hyperprolactinemia $\rightarrow$ galactorrhea) 4. Side effects arising from blocking muscarinic (dry mouth, constipation), α (hypotension), and histamine (sedation) receptors **Other toxicities: Neuroleptic malignant syndrome (NMS)**—rigidity, myoglobinuria, autonomic instability, hyperpyrexia. Treatment: dantrolene, agonists (e.g., bromocriptine). **Tardive dyskinesia**—stereotypic oral-facial movements due to long-term antipsychotic use. Often irreversible.	Chlorpromazine— Corneal deposits; Thioridazine— reTinal deposits. Evolution of EPS side effects: 4 h acute dystonia (muscle spasm, stiffness, oculogyric crisis) 4 d akinesia (parkinsonian symptoms) 4 wk akathisia (restlessness) 4 mo tardive dyskinesia For NMS, think **FEVER:** **F**ever **E**ncephalopathy **V**itals unstable **E**levated enzymes **R**igidity of muscles
Atypical antipsychotics	Olanzapine, clozapine, quetiapine, risperidone, aripiprazole, ziprasidone.	It's **atypical** for **old closets** to **quietly risper** from **A** to **Z**.
Mechanism	Block 5-HT$_2$, dopamine, α, and H1 receptors.	
Clinical use	Schizophrenia—both positive and negative symptoms. **Olanzapine** is also used for OCD, anxiety disorder, depression, mania, Tourette's syndrome.	
Toxicity	Fewer extrapyramidal and anticholinergic side effects than traditional antipsychotics. Olanzapine/clozapine may cause significant weight gain. **Clozapine** may cause agranulocytosis (requires weekly WBC monitoring).	Must watch **clozapine clozely!**

Lithium

Mechanism	Not established; possibly related to inhibition of phosphoinositol cascade.
Clinical use	Mood stabilizer for bipolar disorder; blocks relapse and acute manic events. Also SIADH.
Toxicity	Tremor, sedation, edema, heart block, hypothyroidism, polyuria (ADH antagonist causing nephrogenic diabetes insipidus), teratogenesis. Fetal cardiac defects include Ebstein anomaly and malformation of the great vessels. Narrow therapeutic window requires close monitoring of serum levels. Almost exclusively excreted by the kidneys; most is reabsorbed at the proximal convoluted tubules following Na^+ reabsorption.

LMNOP:
Lithium side effects—
Movement (tremor)
Nephrogenic diabetes insipidus
Hyp**O**thyroidism
Pregnancy problems

Buspirone

Mechanism	Stimulates 5-HT$_{1A}$ receptors
Clinical use	Generalized anxiety disorder. Does not cause sedation, addiction, or tolerance. Does not interact with alcohol (vs. barbiturates, benzodiazepines).

I'm always anxious if the **BUS** will be **ON** time, so I take **BUS**pir**ON**e.

Antidepressants

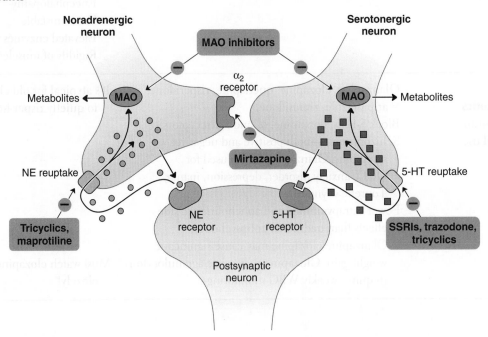

(Adapted, with permission, from Katzung BG, Trevor AJ. *USMLE Road Map: Pharmacology*, 2nd ed. New York: McGraw-Hill, 2006: Fig. 5-7.)

Tricyclic antidepressants	Imipramine, amitriptyline, desipramine, nortriptyline, clomipramine, doxepin, amoxapine.	
Mechanism	Block reuptake of NE and serotonin.	
Clinical use	Major depression, bedwetting (imipramine), OCD (clomipramine), fibromyalgia.	
Side effects	Sedation, α-blocking effects, atropine-like (anticholinergic) side effects (tachycardia, urinary retention). 3° TCAs (amitriptyline) have more anticholinergic effects than do 2° TCAs (nortriptyline). Desipramine is the least sedating and has lower seizure threshold.	
Toxicity	**Tri-C's: Convulsions, Coma, Cardiotoxicity** (arrhythmias); also respiratory depression, hyperpyrexia. Confusion and hallucinations in elderly due to anticholinergic side effects (use nortriptyline). Treatment: $NaHCO_3$ for CV toxicity.	

SSRIs	Fluoxetine, paroxetine, sertraline, citalopram.	
Mechanism	Serotonin-specific reuptake inhibitors.	It normally takes 2–4 weeks for antidepressants to have an effect.
Clinical use	Depression, OCD, bulimia, social phobias.	
Toxicity	Fewer than TCAs. GI distress, sexual dysfunction (anorgasmia). **"Serotonin syndrome"** with any drug that ↑ serotonin (e.g., MAO inhibitors) —hyperthermia, muscle rigidity, cardiovascular collapse, flushing, diarrhea, seizures. Treatment: cyproheptadine (5-HT_2 receptor antagonist).	

SNRIs	Venlafaxine, duloxetine.
Mechanism	Inhibit serotonin and NE reuptake.
Clinical use	Depression. Venlafaxine is also used in generalized anxiety disorder; duloxetine is also indicated for diabetic peripheral neuropathy. Duloxetine has greater effect on NE.
Toxicity	↑ BP most common; also stimulant effects, sedation, nausea.

Monoamine oxidase (MAO) inhibitors	Phenelzine, tranylcypromine, isocarboxazid, selegiline (selective MAO-B inhibitor).
Mechanism	Nonselective MAO inhibition ↑ levels of amine neurotransmitters (NE, serotonin, dopamine).
Clinical use	Atypical depression, anxiety, hypochondriasis.
Toxicity	Hypertensive crisis with tyramine ingestion (in many foods, such as wine and cheese) and β-agonists; CNS stimulation. Contraindicated with SSRIs or meperidine (to prevent serotonin syndrome).

Atypical antidepressants

Bupropion	Also used for smoking cessation. ↑ NE and dopamine via unknown mechanism. Toxicity: stimulant effects (tachycardia, insomnia), headache, seizure in bulimic patients. No sexual side effects.	
Mirtazapine	α_2 antagonist (↑ release of NE and serotonin) and potent 5-HT$_2$ and 5-HT$_3$ receptor antagonist. Toxicity: sedation, ↑ appetite, weight gain, dry mouth.	
Maprotiline	Blocks NE reuptake. Toxicity: sedation, orthostatic hypotension.	
Trazodone	Primarily inhibits serotonin reuptake. Used for insomnia, as high doses are needed for antidepressant effects. Toxicity: sedation, nausea, priapism, postural hypotension.	Called Trazo**BONE** due to male-specific side effects.

Renal

"But I know all about love already. I know precious little about kidneys."
—Aldous Huxley, *Antic Hay*

"This too shall pass. Just like a kidney stone."

—Hunter Madsen

"When the patient dies the kidneys may go to the pathologist, but while he lives the urine is ours."

—Thomas Addis

▶ Anatomy

▶ Physiology

▶ Pathology

▶ Pharmacology

Kidney anatomy and glomerular structure

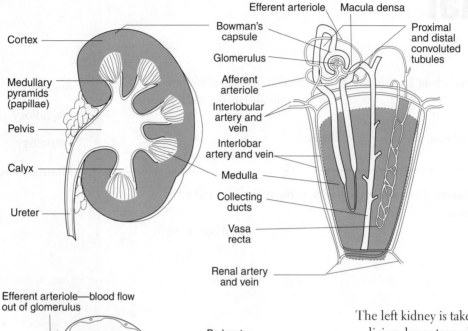

The left kidney is taken during living donor transplantation because it has a longer renal vein.

(Adapted, with permission, from McPhee S et al. *Pathophysiology of Disease: An Introduction to Clinical Medicine,* 3rd ed. New York: McGraw-Hill, 2000: 284.)

Ureters: course	Ureters pass **under** uterine artery and **under** ductus deferens (retroperitoneal).	Water (ureters) **under** the bridge (artery, ductus deferens).

Fluid compartments

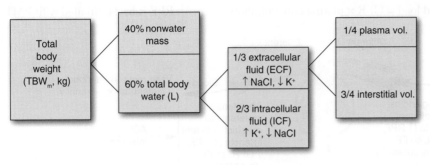

HIKIN': HIgh K
INtracellular.
60–40–20 rule (% of body weight):
  60% total body water
  40% ICF
  20% ECF
Plasma volume measured by
  radiolabeled albumin.
Extracellular volume measured
  by inulin.
Osmolarity = 290 mOsm.

Glomerular filtration barrier	Responsible for filtration of plasma according to size and net charge. Composed of: 1. Fenestrated capillary endothelium (size barrier) 2. Fused basement membrane with heparan sulfate (negative charge barrier) 3. Epithelial layer consisting of podocyte foot processes	The charge barrier is lost in **nephrotic syndrome,** resulting in albuminuria, hypoproteinemia, generalized edema, and hyperlipidemia.
Renal clearance	$C_x = U_x V / P_x$ = volume of plasma from which the substance is completely cleared per unit time. $C_x < GFR$: net tubular reabsorption of X. $C_x > GFR$: net tubular secretion of X. $C_x = GFR$: no net secretion or reabsorption.	Be familiar with calculations. C_x = clearance of X. Units are mL/min. U_x = urine concentration of X. P_x = plasma concentration of X. V = urine flow rate.
Glomerular filtration rate (GFR)	Inulin can be used to calculate GFR because it is freely filtered and is neither reabsorbed nor secreted. $GFR = U_{inulin} \times V / P_{inulin} = C_{inulin}$ $= K_f [(P_{GC} - P_{BS}) - (\pi_{GC} - \pi_{BS})]$. (GC = glomerular capillary; BS = Bowman's space.) π_{BS} normally equals zero.	Normal GFR ≈ 100 mL/min. Creatinine clearance is an approximate measure of GFR. Slightly overestimates GFR because creatinine is moderately secreted by the renal tubules.
Effective renal plasma flow (ERPF)	ERPF can be estimated using PAH clearance because it is both filtered and actively secreted in the proximal tubule. All PAH entering the kidney is excreted. $ERPF = U_{PAH} \times V / P_{PAH} = C_{PAH}$. $RBF = RPF / (1 - Hct)$. ERPF underestimates true RPF by ~10%.	

Filtration

Filtration fraction (FF) = GFR/RPF.
Normal FF = 20%.
Filtered load = GFR × plasma concentration.

GFR can be estimated with creatinine.
RPF is best estimated with PAH.

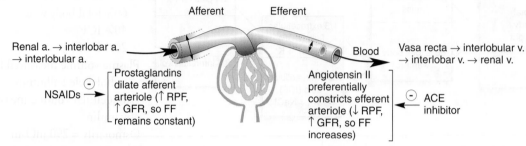

Renal a. → interlobar a. → interlobular a.

NSAIDs ⊖→ Prostaglandins dilate afferent arteriole (↑ RPF, ↑ GFR, so FF remains constant)

Afferent   Efferent

Blood

Angiotensin II preferentially constricts efferent arteriole (↓ RPF, ↑ GFR, so FF increases) ⊖ ACE inhibitor

Vasa recta → interlobular v. → interlobar v. → renal v.

Changes in glomerular dynamics

Effect	RPF	GFR	FF (GFR/RPF)
Afferent arteriole constriction	↓	↓	NC
Efferent arteriole constriction	↓	↑	↑
↑ plasma protein concentration	NC	↓	↓
↓ plasma protein concentration	NC	↑	↑
Constriction of ureter	NC	↓	↓

Calculation of reabsorption and secretion rate

Filtered load = GFR × P_x.
Excretion rate = V × U_x.
Reabsorption = filtered – excreted.
Secretion = excreted – filtered.

Glucose clearance

Glucose at a normal plasma level is completely reabsorbed in proximal tubule by Na^+/glucose cotransport.
At plasma glucose of 160–200 mg/dL, glucosuria begins (threshold). At 350 mg/dL, all transporters are fully saturated (T_m).

Glucosuria is an important clinical clue to diabetes mellitus.

Amino acid clearance

Sodium-dependent transporters in proximal tubule reabsorb amino acids by at least 3 distinct carrier systems, with competitive inhibition within each group.
Hartnup's disease—deficiency of neutral amino acid (tryptophan) transporter; results in pellagra.

Nephron physiology

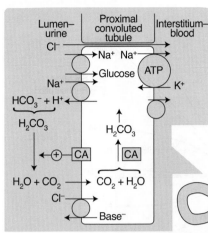

Early proximal tubule—contains brush border.
Reabsorbs all of the glucose and amino acids
and most of the bicarbonate, sodium, chloride,
and water. Isotonic absorption. Generates and
secretes ammonia, which acts as a buffer for
secreted H^+.

PTH—inhibits Na^+/phosphate cotransport →
phosphate excretion.

AT II—stimulates Na^+/H^+ exchange → ↑ Na^+
and H_2O reabsorption (permitting contraction
alkalosis).

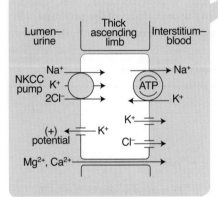

Thick ascending loop of Henle—actively
reabsorbs Na^+, K^+, and Cl^- and indirectly
induces the paracellular reabsorption of Mg^{2+}
and Ca^{2+}. Impermeable to H_2O. Makes urine
less concentrated as it ascends.

Thin descending loop of
Henle—passively reabsorbs
water via medullary hypertonicity (impermeable to sodium).
Concentrating segment. Makes
urine hypertonic.

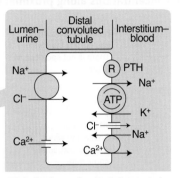

Early distal convoluted tubule—actively
reabsorbs Na^+, Cl^-. Diluting segment.
Makes urine hypotonic.

PTH—↑ Ca^{2+}/Na^+ exchange → Ca^{2+}
reabsorption.

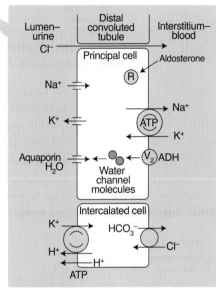

Collecting tubules—reabsorb Na^+ in exchange for
secreting K^+ and H^+ (regulated by aldosterone).

Aldosterone—leads to insertion of Na^+ channel on
luminal side.

ADH—acts at V_2 receptors → insertion of
aquaporin H_2O channels on luminal side.

Relative concentrations along proximal tubule

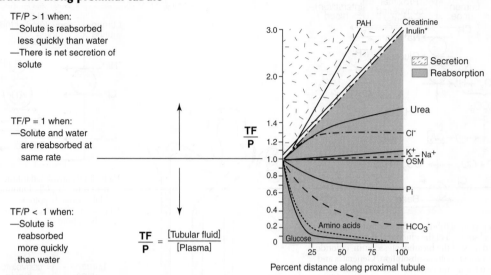

TF/P > 1 when:
—Solute is reabsorbed less quickly than water
—There is net secretion of solute

TF/P = 1 when:
—Solute and water are reabsorbed at same rate

TF/P < 1 when:
—Solute is reabsorbed more quickly than water

$$\frac{TF}{P} = \frac{[Tubular\ fluid]}{[Plasma]}$$

* Neither secreted nor reabsorbed; concentration increases as water is reabsorbed.

(Adapted, with permission, from Ganong WF. *Review of Medical Physiology*, 22nd ed. New York: McGraw-Hill, 2005.)

Tubular creatinine and inulin ↑ in concentration (but not amount) along the proximal tubule due to water reabsorption.

Cl^- reabsorption occurs at a slower rate than Na^+ in the proximal ⅓ of the proximal tubule and then matches the rate of Na^+ reabsorption more distally. Thus, its relative concentration ↑ before it plateaus.

Na^+ reabsorption drives H_2O reabsorption, so it nearly matches osm.

Renin-angiotensin-aldosterone system

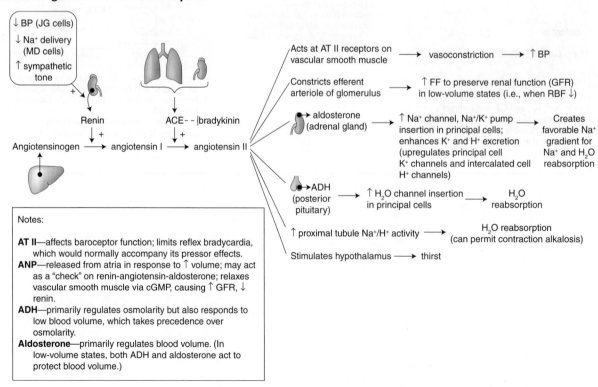

Notes:

AT II—affects baroceptor function; limits reflex bradycardia, which would normally accompany its pressor effects.
ANP—released from atria in response to ↑ volume; may act as a "check" on renin-angiotensin-aldosterone; relaxes vascular smooth muscle via cGMP, causing ↑ GFR, ↓ renin.
ADH—primarily regulates osmolarity but also responds to low blood volume, which takes precedence over osmolarity.
Aldosterone—primarily regulates blood volume. (In low-volume states, both ADH and aldosterone act to protect blood volume.)

Juxtaglomerular apparatus (JGA)	JGA—JG cells (modified smooth muscle of afferent arteriole) and macula densa (Na^+ sensor, part of the distal convoluted tubule). JG cells secrete renin in response to ↓ renal blood pressure, ↓ Na^+ delivery to distal tubule, and ↑ sympathetic tone (β_1).	JGA defends glomerular filtration rate via renin-angiotensin-aldosterone system. *Juxta* = close by.
Kidney endocrine functions	1. **Erythropoietin**—released in response to hypoxia from endothelial cells of peritubular capillaries. 2. **1,25-(OH)$_2$ vitamin D**—proximal tubule cells convert 25-OH vitamin D to 1,25-(OH)$_2$ vitamin D, which ↑ intestinal reabsorption of both calcium and phosphate. Parathyroid hormone (PTH) acts directly on the kidney to ↑ renal calcium reabsorption and ↓ renal phosphate reabsorption. However, PTH also acts indirectly, stimulating proximal tubule cells to make 1,25-(OH)$_2$ vitamin D, which ↑ intestinal absorption of both **calcium** and **phosphate**.	NSAIDs can cause acute renal failure by inhibiting the renal production of prostaglandins, which keep the afferent arterioles vasodilated to maintain GFR.

$$25\text{-OH vitamin D} \xrightarrow{\text{1}\alpha\text{-hydroxylase}} \text{1,25-(OH)}_2 \text{ vitamin D}$$

$$\oplus$$

$$\text{PTH}$$

3. **Renin**—secreted by JG cells in response to ↓ renal arterial pressure and ↑ renal sympathetic discharge (β_1 effect).
4. **Prostaglandins** (e.g., PGE$_2$)—paracrine secretion vasodilates the afferent arterioles to ↑ GFR.

Hormones acting on kidney

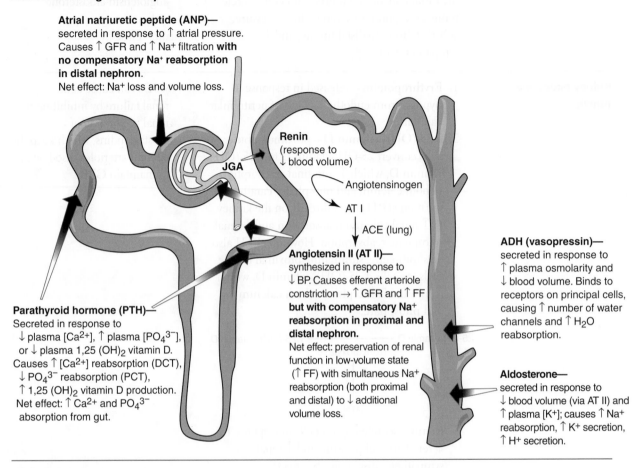

Atrial natriuretic peptide (ANP)—
secreted in response to ↑ atrial pressure.
Causes ↑ GFR and ↑ Na⁺ filtration **with
no compensatory Na⁺ reabsorption
in distal nephron.**
Net effect: Na⁺ loss and volume loss.

Renin
(response to
↓ blood volume)

JGA

Angiotensinogen

AT I

ACE (lung)

Angiotensin II (AT II)—
synthesized in response to
↓ BP. Causes efferent arteriole
constriction → ↑ GFR and ↑ FF
**but with compensatory Na⁺
reabsorption in proximal and
distal nephron.**
Net effect: preservation of renal
function in low-volume state
(↑ FF) with simultaneous Na⁺
reabsorption (both proximal
and distal) to ↓ additional
volume loss.

Parathyroid hormone (PTH)—
Secreted in response to
↓ plasma [Ca²⁺], ↑ plasma [PO₄³⁻],
or ↓ plasma 1,25 (OH)₂ vitamin D.
Causes ↑ [Ca²⁺] reabsorption (DCT),
↓ PO₄³⁻ reabsorption (PCT),
↑ 1,25 (OH)₂ vitamin D production.
Net effect: ↑ Ca²⁺ and PO₄³⁻
absorption from gut.

ADH (vasopressin)—
secreted in response to
↑ plasma osmolarity and
↓ blood volume. Binds to
receptors on principal cells,
causing ↑ number of water
channels and ↑ H₂O
reabsorption.

Aldosterone—
secreted in response to
↓ blood volume (via AT II) and
↑ plasma [K⁺]; causes ↑ Na⁺
reabsorption, ↑ K⁺ secretion,
↑ H⁺ secretion.

Potassium shifts

Shift out of cell (causing hyperkalemia):
1. Insulin deficiency (↓ Na⁺/K⁺ ATPase)
2. β-adrenergic antagonists (↓ Na⁺/K⁺ ATPase)
3. Acidosis, severe exercise (↑ K⁺/H⁺ exchanger)
4. Hyperosmolarity
5. Digitalis (blocks Na⁺/K⁺ ATPase)
6. Cell lysis

Shift into cell (causing hypokalemia):
1. Insulin (↑ Na⁺/K⁺ ATPase)
2. β-adrenergic agonists (↑ Na⁺/K⁺ ATPase)
3. Alkalosis (↑ K⁺/H⁺ exchanger)
4. Hypo-osmolarity

Electrolyte disturbances

Electrolyte	Low serum concentration	High serum concentration
Na⁺	Disorientation, stupor, coma	Neurologic: irritability, delirium, coma
Cl⁻	2° to metabolic alkalosis, hypokalemia, hypovolemia, ↑ aldosterone	2° to non–anion gap acidosis
K⁺	U waves on ECG, flattened T waves, arrhythmias, paralysis	Peaked T waves, wide QRS, arrhythmias
Ca²⁺	Tetany, neuromuscular irritability	Delirium, renal stones, abdominal pain, not necessarily calciuria
Mg²⁺	Neuromuscular irritability, arrhythmias	Delirium, ↓ DTRs, cardiopulmonary arrest
PO₄³⁻	Low-mineral ion product causes bone loss, osteomalacia	High-mineral ion product causes renal stones, metastatic calcifications

Acid-base physiology

	pH	PCO₂	[HCO₃⁻]	Compensatory response
Metabolic acidosis	↓	↓	**↓**	Hyperventilation (immediate)
Metabolic alkalosis	↑	↑	**↑**	Hypoventilation (immediate)
Respiratory acidosis	↓	**↑**	↑	↑ renal [HCO₃⁻] reabsorption (delayed)
Respiratory alkalosis	↑	**↓**	↓	↓ renal [HCO₃⁻] reabsorption (delayed)

Key: **↑ ↓** = 1° disturbance; ↓ ↑ = compensatory response.

Henderson-Hasselbalch equation: $pH = pKa + \log\dfrac{[HCO_3^-]}{0.03\ P_{CO_2}}$

Respiratory compensation in response to metabolic acidosis can be quantified with Winter's formula:

$$P_{CO_2} = 1.5\ (HCO_3^-) + 8 +\!/\!- 2$$

P_{CO_2} ↑ 0.7 mmHg for every ↑ 1 mEq/L HCO_3^-

Acidosis/alkalosis

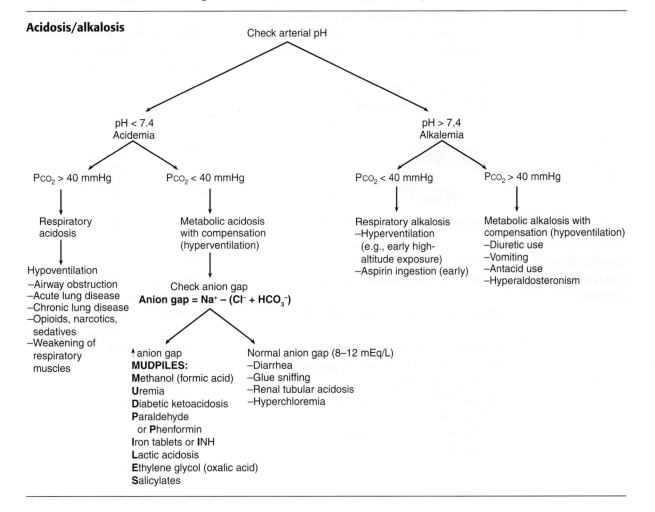

Renal tubular acidosis (RTA)

Type 1 ("distal")	Defect in collecting tubule's ability to excrete H^+. Associated with hypokalemia and risk for calcium-containing kidney stones.
Type 2 ("proximal")	Defect in proximal tubule HCO_3^- reabsorption. Associated with hypokalemia and hypophosphatemic rickets.
Type 4 ("hyperkalemic")	Hypoaldosteronism or lack of collecting tubule response to aldosterone. Associated with hyperkalemia and inhibition of ammonium excretion in proximal tubule. Leads to ↓ urine pH due to ↓ buffering capacity.

Casts in urine

RBC casts—glomerulonephritis, ischemia, or malignant hypertension.
WBC casts—tubulointerstitial inflammation, acute pyelonephritis, transplant rejection.
Granular ("muddy brown") casts—acute tubular necrosis.
Waxy casts—advanced renal disease/CRF.
Hyaline casts—nonspecific.

Presence of casts indicates that hematuria/pyuria is of renal origin.
Bladder cancer, kidney stones → hematuria, no casts.
Acute cystitis → pyuria, no casts.

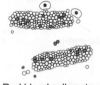

| Red blood cell casts | White blood cell casts | Hyaline casts | Granular casts |

Nomenclature of glomerular disorders

Type	Example
Focal → few glomeruli are involved	Focal segmental glomerulosclerosis
Diffuse → all glomeruli are involved	Diffuse proliferative glomerulonephritis
Proliferative → hypercellular glomeruli	Mesangial proliferative
Membranous → thickening of glomerular basement membrane	Membranous glomerulonephritis
1° glomerular disease → involves only glomeruli	Minimal change
2° glomerular disease → involves glomeruli and other organs	SLE

Nephritic syndrome	NephrItic syndrome = an Inflammatory process. When it involves glomeruli, it leads to hematuria and RBC casts in urine. Associated with azotemia, oliguria, hypertension, and proteinuria (< 3.5 g/day).	
Acute poststreptococcal glomerulonephritis	LM—glomeruli enlarged and hypercellular, neutrophils, "lumpy-bumpy" appearance. EM—subepithelial immune complex (IC) humps. IF—granular.	Most frequently seen in children. Peripheral and periorbital edema. Resolves spontaneously.
Rapidly progressive (crescentic) glomerulonephritis (RPGN)	LM and IF—crescent-moon shape. Crescents consist of fibrin and plasma proteins (e.g., C3b) with glomerular function parietal cells, monocytes, and macrophages. Several disease processes may result in this pattern, including:	Poor prognosis. Rapidly deteriorating renal function (days to weeks).
	1. **Goodpasture syndrome**—type II hypersensitivity; antibodies to GBM and alveolar basement membrane → linear IF	Hematuria/hemoptysis.
	2. **Wegener's granulomatosis**	c-ANCA.
	3. **Microscopic polyangiitis**	p-ANCA.
Diffuse proliferative glomerulonephritis (due to SLE or MPGN)	LM—"wire looping" of capillaries (see Image 86). EM—subendothelial DNA-anti-DNA ICs. IF—granular.	Most common cause of death in SLE. SLE and MPGN can present as nephrotic syndrome (see below).
Berger's disease (IgA glomerulopathy)	↑ synthesis of IgA. LM and IF—ICs deposit in mesangium.	Often presents/flares with a URI or acute gastroenteritis.
Alport's syndrome	Mutation in type IV collagen → split basement membrane.	Nerve disorders, ocular disorders, deafness X-linked dominant.

(LM = light microscopy; EM = electron microscopy; IF = immunofluorescence.)

Nephrotic syndrome	NephrOtic syndrome presents with massive prOteinuria (> 3.5g/day, frothy urine), hyperlipidemia, fatty casts, edema. Associated with thromboembolism and ↑ risk of infection (loss of immunoglobulins).	
Membranous glomerulonephritis (diffuse membranous glomerulopathy)	LM—diffuse capillary and GBM thickening. EM—"spike and dome" appearance with subepithelial deposits. IF—granular. SLE's nephrotic presentation (see Image 86).	Caused by drugs, infections, SLE, solid tumors. Most common cause of adult nephrotic syndrome.
Minimal change disease (lipoid nephrosis)	LM—normal glomeruli. EM—foot process effacement (see Image 85). Selective loss of albumin, not globulins, due to GBM polyanion loss.	May be triggered by a recent infection or an immune stimulus. Most common in children. Responds to corticosteroids.
Amyloidosis	LM—Congo red stain, apple-green birefringence.	Associated with chronic conditions (e.g., multiple myeloma, TB, RA).
Diabetic glomerulo-nephropathy	Nonenzymatic glycosylation (NEG) of GBM → ↑ permeability, thickening. NEG of efferent arterioles → ↑ GFR → mesangial expansion. LM—mesangial expansion, GBM thickening, nodular glomerulosclerosis (Kimmelstiel-Wilson lesion) (see Image 87).	
Focal segmental glomerulosclerosis	LM—segmental sclerosis and hyalinosis.	Most common glomerular disease in HIV patients.
Membrano-proliferative glomerulonephritis	Subendothelial ICs with granular IF. Type I EM—"tram-track" appearance due to GBM splitting caused by mesangial ingrowth. Type II EM—"dense deposits."	Can also present as nephritic syndrome. Type I is associated with HBV, HCV. Type II is associated with C3 nephritic factor.

Glomerular histopathology

EP = epithelium with foot processes
US = urinary space
GBM = glomerular basement membrane
EN = fenestrated endothelium
MC = mesangial cells
EM = extracellular matrix

1 = effacement of epithelial foot processes (common in all forms of glomerular injury with proteinuria)
2 = large irregular subepithelial deposits or "lumpy-bumpy" appearance (acute glomerulonephritis)
3 = subendothelial deposits in lupus glomerulonephritis
4 = mesangial deposits (IgA nephropathy)
5 = antibody binding to GBM—smooth linear pattern on immunofluorescence (Goodpasture's)

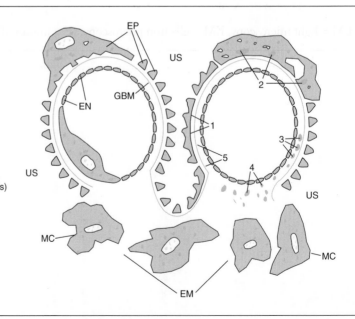

Kidney stones   Can lead to severe complications, such as hydronephrosis and pyelonephritis. Treat and prevent by encouraging fluid intake.

Content	Frequency	X-ray	Notes
Calcium	75–85%	Radiopaque	Calcium oxalate (see Image 88), calcium phosphate, or both. Conditions that cause hypercalcemia (cancer, ↑ PTH) can → hypercalciuria and stones. Oxalate crystals can result from ethylene glycol (antifreeze) or vitamin C abuse.
Ammonium magnesium phosphate	15%	Radiopaque	Caused by infection with urease-positive magnesium or radiolucent bugs (*Proteus mirabilis*, *Staphylococcus*, phosphate *Klebsiella*). Can form **staghorn calculi** that can be a nidus for UTIs. Worsened by alkaluria.
Uric acid	5%	RadiolUcent	Strong association with hyperuricemia (e.g., gout). Often seen in diseases with ↑ cell turnover, such as leukemia.
Cystine	1%	Radiopaque	Most often 2° to cystinuria. Hexagonal. Treat with alkalinization of urine.

Renal cell carcinoma   Originates in renal tubular cells → polygonal clear cells (see Image 89). Most common in men 50–70 years of age. ↑ incidence with smoking and obesity. Manifests clinically with hematuria, palpable mass, 2° polycythemia, flank pain, fever, and weight loss. Associated with paraneoplastic syndromes (ectopic EPO, ACTH, PTHrP, and prolactin). Invades IVC and spreads hematogenously; metastasizes to lung and bone.

Most common renal malignancy. Associated with von Hippel-Lindau syndrome and gene deletion in chromosome 3 (3p).

Wilms' tumor (nephroblastoma)   Most common renal malignancy of early childhood (ages 2–4). Contains embryonic glomerular structures. Presents with huge, palpable flank mass and/or hematuria.

Deletion of tumor suppressor gene *WT1* on chromosome 11 (11p). May be part of **WAGR** complex: Wilms' tumor, Aniridia, Genitourinary malformation, and mental-motor Retardation.

Transitional cell carcinoma	Most common tumor of urinary tract system (can occur in renal calyces, renal pelvis, ureters, and bladder). Painless hematuria suggests bladder cancer.	Associated with problems in your **P**ee **SAC**: **P**henacetin, **S**moking **A**niline dyes, and **C**yclophosphamide (see Image 82).
Pyelonephritis		
Acute	Affects cortex with relative sparing of glomeruli/vessels. Presents with fever, CVA tenderness, nausea, and vomiting.	White cell casts in urine are classic (see Image 81A).
Chronic	Coarse, asymmetric corticomedullary scarring, blunted calyx. Tubules can contain eosinophilic casts (thyroidization of kidney) (see Image 81B).	
Drug-induced interstitial nephritis	Acute interstitial renal inflammation. Pyuria (typically eosinophils) and azotemia occurring 1–2 weeks after administration of drugs (e.g., diuretics, NSAIDs, penicillin derivatives, sulfonamides, rifampin), which act as haptens, inducing hypersensitivity.	Associated with fever, rash, hematuria, and CVA tenderness.
Diffuse cortical necrosis	Acute generalized cortical infarction of both kidneys. Likely due to a combination of vasospasm and DIC.	Associated with obstetric catastrophes (e.g., abruptio placentae) and septic shock.
Acute tubular necrosis	Most common cause of acute renal failure in hospital. Self-reversible, but fatal if left untreated. Death most often occurs during initial oliguric phase. 3 stages: inciting event → maintenance (low urine output) → recovery (2–3 weeks).	Associated with renal ischemia (e.g., shock, sepsis), crush injury (myoglobinuria), toxins. Key finding: granular ("muddy brown") casts.
Renal papillary necrosis	Sloughing of renal papillae → gross hematuria, proteinuria. May be triggered by a recent infection or immune stimulus. Associated with: 1. Diabetes mellitus 2. Acute pyelonephritis 3. Chronic phenacetin use (acetaminophen is phenacetin derivative) 4. Sickle cell anemia	

Acute renal failure (acute kidney injury)

In normal nephron, BUN is reabsorbed (for countercurrent multiplication), but creatinine is not.

Acute renal failure is defined as an abrupt decline in renal function with ↑ creatinine and ↑ BUN over a period of several days.

1. Prerenal azotemia— due to ↓ RBF (e.g., hypotension) → ↓ GFR. Na^+/H_2O and urea retained by kidney in an attempt to conserve volume, so BUN/creatinine ratio ↑.

2. Intrinsic renal—generally due to acute tubular necrosis or ischemia/toxins; less commonly due to acute glomerulonephritis (e.g., RPGN). Patchy necrosis leads to debris obstructing tubule and fluid backflow across necrotic tubule → ↓ GFR. Urine has epithelial/granular casts. BUN reabsorption is impaired → ↓ BUN/creatinine ratio.

3. Postrenal—due to outflow obstruction (stones, BPH, neoplasia, congenital anomalies). Develops only with bilateral obstruction.

Variable	Prerenal	Renal	Postrenal
Urine osmolality	> 500	< 350	< 350
Urine Na	< 10	> 20	> 40
Fe_{Na}	< 1%	> 2%	> 4%
Serum BUN/Cr	> 20	< 15	> 15

Consequences of renal failure

Inability to make urine and excrete nitrogenous wastes.

Consequences:

1. Na^+/H_2O retention (CHF, pulmonary edema, hypertension)
2. Hyperkalemia
3. Metabolic acidosis
4. Uremia—clinical syndrome marked by ↑ BUN and ↑ creatinine
   a. Nausea and anorexia
   b. Pericarditis
   c. Asterixis
   d. Encephalopathy
   e. Platelet dysfunction
5. Anemia (failure of erythropoietin production)
6. Renal osteodystrophy (failure of vitamin D hydroxylation); Ca^{2+} wasting and PO_4^{3-} retention → 2° hyperparathyroidism
7. Dyslipidemia (especially ↑ triglycerides)
8. Growth retardation and developmental delay (in children)

2 forms of renal failure— acute (e.g., ATN) and chronic (e.g., hypertension and diabetes).

Renal cysts

ADPKD (formerly adult polycystic kidney disease)	Multiple, large, bilateral cysts that ultimately destroy the kidney parenchyma. Presents with flank pain, hematuria, hypertension, urinary infection, progressive renal failure. **A**utosomal-**d**ominant mutation in *APKD1* or *APKD2*. Death from complications of chronic kidney disease or hypertension (due to ↑ renin production). Associated with polycystic liver disease, berry aneurysms, mitral valve prolapse.

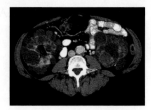

(Reproduced, with permission, from the PEIR Digital Library.)

ARPKD (formerly infantile polycystic kidney disease)	Infantile presentation in parenchyma. **A**utosomal **r**ecessive. Associated with congenital hepatic fibrosis. Significant renal failure in utero can lead to Potter's. Concerns beyond neonatal period include hypertension, portal hypertension, and progressive renal insufficiency.
Dialysis cysts	Cortical and medullary cysts resulting from long-standing dialysis.
Simple cysts	Benign, common (occurs in more than 40% of elderly), incidental finding. Thin, nonenhancing, cortical, fluid filled.
Medullary cystic disease	Medullary cysts sometimes lead to fibrosis and progressive renal insufficiency with urinary concentrating defects. Ultrasound shows small kidney. Poor prognosis.

Diuretics: site of action

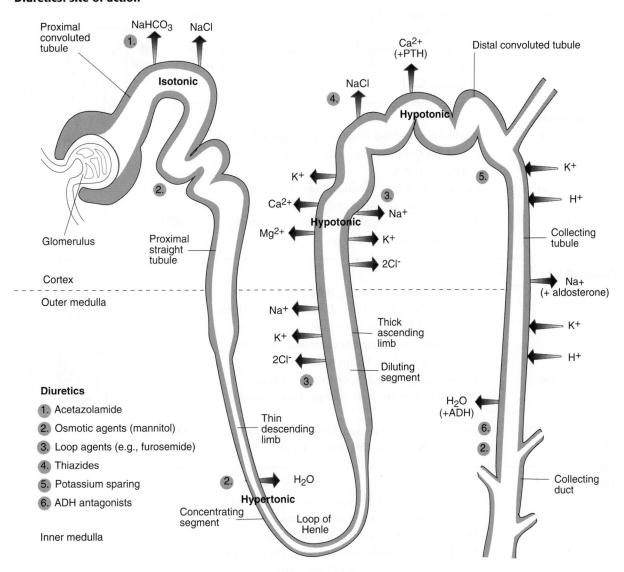

Proximal convoluted tubule

NaHCO$_3$ NaCl

1.

Isotonic

Glomerulus

2.

Proximal straight tubule

Cortex

Outer medulla

Ca^{2+} (+PTH)

Distal convoluted tubule

NaCl

4.

Hypotonic

K$^+$

Ca^{2+}

Mg^{2+}

Hypotonic

3.

Na$^+$

K$^+$

2Cl$^-$

5.

K$^+$

H$^+$

Collecting tubule

Na+ (+ aldosterone)

Na$^+$

K$^+$

2Cl$^-$

Thick ascending limb

Diluting segment

3.

K$^+$

H$^+$

H$_2$O (+ADH)

6.

2.

Collecting duct

Thin descending limb

Diuretics

1. Acetazolamide
2. Osmotic agents (mannitol)
3. Loop agents (e.g., furosemide)
4. Thiazides
5. Potassium sparing
6. ADH antagonists

Inner medulla

2.   H$_2$O

Hypertonic

Concentrating segment

Loop of Henle

(Adapted, with permission, from Katzung BG. *Basic and Clinical Pharmacology*, 7th ed. Stamford, CT: Appleton & Lange, 1997: 243.)

HIGH-YIELD SYSTEMS

RENAL

Mannitol

Mechanism   Osmotic diuretic, ↑ tubular fluid osmolarity, producing ↑ urine flow.

Clinical use   Shock, drug overdose, ↑ intracranial/intraocular pressure.

Toxicity   Pulmonary edema, dehydration. Contraindicated in anuria, CHF.

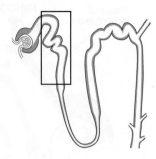

Acetazolamide

Mechanism   Carbonic anhydrase inhibitor. Causes self-limited $NaHCO_3$ diuresis and reduction in total-body HCO_3^- stores.

Clinical use   Glaucoma, urinary alkalinization, metabolic alkalosis, altitude sickness.

Toxicity   Hyperchloremic metabolic acidosis, neuropathy, NH_3 toxicity, sulfa allergy.

ACIDazolamide causes **ACID**osis.

Furosemide

Mechanism   Sulfonamide loop diuretic. Inhibits cotransport system (Na^+, K^+, $2\ Cl^-$) of thick ascending limb of loop of Henle. Abolishes hypertonicity of medulla, preventing concentration of urine. ↑ Ca^{2+} excretion. Loops Lose calcium.

Clinical use   Edematous states (CHF, cirrhosis, nephrotic syndrome, pulmonary edema), hypertension, hypercalcemia.

Toxicity   **O**totoxicity, **H**ypokalemia, **D**ehydration, **A**llergy (sulfa), **N**ephritis (interstitial), **G**out.

OH DANG!

Ethacrynic acid

Mechanism   Phenoxyacetic acid derivative (NOT a sulfonamide). Essentially same action as furosemide.

Clinical use   Diuresis in patients allergic to sulfa drugs.

Toxicity   Similar to furosemide; can be used in hyperuricemia, acute gout (never used to treat gout).

Hydrochlorothiazide

Mechanism   Thiazide diuretic. Inhibits NaCl reabsorption in early distal tubule, reducing diluting capacity of the nephron. ↓ Ca^{2+} excretion.

Clinical use   Hypertension, CHF, idiopathic hypercalciuria, nephrogenic diabetes insipidus.

Toxicity   Hypokalemic metabolic alkalosis, hyponatremia, hyper**G**lycemia, hyper**L**ipidemia, hyper**U**ricemia, and hyper**C**alcemia. Sulfa allergy.

HyperGLUC.

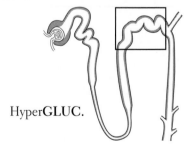

K+-sparing diuretics	Spironolactone, **T**riamterene, **A**miloride, eplerenone.	The K+ **STA**ys.
Mechanism	Spironolactone is a competitive aldosterone receptor antagonist in the cortical collecting tubule. Triamterene and amiloride act at the same part of the tubule by blocking Na+ channels in the CCT.	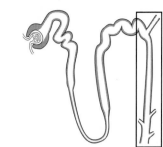
Clinical use	Hyperaldosteronism, K+ depletion, CHF.	
Toxicity	Hyperkalemia (can lead to arrhythmias), endocrine effects with aldosterone antagonists (e.g., spironolactone causes gynecomastia, antiandrogen effects).	

Diuretics: electrolyte changes

Urine NaCl	$\uparrow$ (all diuretics—carbonic anhydrase inhibitors, loop diuretics, thiazides, K+-sparing diuretics). Serum NaCl may $\downarrow$ as a result.
Urine K+	$\uparrow$ (all except K+-sparing diuretics). Serum K+ may $\downarrow$ as a result.
Blood pH	$\downarrow$ (**acidemia**): Carbonic anhydrase inhibitors— $\downarrow$ HCO_3^- reabsorption. K+ sparing— aldosterone blockade prevents K+ secretion and H+ secretion. Additionally, hyperkalemia leads to K+ entering all cells (via H^+/K^+ exchanger) in exchange for H+ exiting cells.
	$\uparrow$ (**alkalemia**): Loop diuretics and thiazides cause alkalemia through several mechanisms:
	1. Volume contraction $\rightarrow$ $\uparrow$ AT II $\rightarrow$ $\uparrow$ Na^+/H^+ exchange in proximal tubule $\rightarrow$ $\uparrow$ HCO_3^- ("contraction alkalosis")
	2. K+ loss leads to K+ exiting all cells (via H^+/K^+ exchanger) in exchange for H+ entering cells
	3. In low K+ state, H+ (rather than K+) is exchanged for Na+ in cortical collecting tubule, leading to alkalosis and "paradoxical aciduria"
Urine Ca2+	$\uparrow$ **loop diuretics**: Abolish lumen-positive potential in thick ascending limb of loop of Henle $\rightarrow$ $\downarrow$ paracellular Ca+ reabsorption $\rightarrow$ hypocalcemia, $\uparrow$ urinary Ca2+.
	$\downarrow$ **thiazides**: Volume depletion $\rightarrow$ upregulation of sodium reabsorption $\rightarrow$ enhanced paracellular Ca2+ reabsorption in proximal tubule and loop of Henle. Thiazides also block luminal Na^+/Cl^- cotransport in distal convoluted tubule $\rightarrow$ $\uparrow$ Na+ gradient $\rightarrow$ $\uparrow$ interstitial Na^+/Ca^{2+} exchange $\rightarrow$ hypercalcemia.

ACE inhibitors	Captopril, enalapril, lisinopril.	
Mechanism	Inhibit angiotensin-converting enzyme, reducing levels of angiotensin II and preventing inactivation of bradykinin, a potent vasodilator. **Renin release is** $\uparrow$ due to loss of feedback inhibition.	**Losartan** is an angiotensin II receptor antagonist. It is **not** an ACE inhibitor and does not cause cough.
Clinical use	Hypertension, CHF, diabetic renal disease.	
Toxicity	**C**ough, **A**ngioedema, **P**roteinuria, **T**aste changes, hyp**O**tension, **P**regnancy problems (fetal renal damage), **R**ash, **I**ncreased renin, **L**ower angiotensin II. Also **hyperkalemia**. Avoid with bilateral renal artery stenosis because ACE inhibitors significantly $\downarrow$ GFR by preventing constriction of efferent arterioles.	**CAPTOPRIL**.

Reproductive

"Artificial insemination is when the farmer does it to the cow instead of the bull."

—Student essay

"Whoever called it necking was a poor judge of anatomy."

—Groucho Marx

"See, the problem is that God gives men a brain and a penis, and only enough blood to run one at a time."

—Robin Williams

▶ Anatomy

▶ Physiology

▶ Pathology

▶ Pharmacology

Gonadal drainage

Venous drainage	Left ovary/testis → left gonadal vein → left renal vein → IVC.	Just as the left adrenal vein drains to the left renal vein before the IVC.
	Right ovary/testis → right gonadal vein → IVC.	
Lymphatic drainage	Ovaries/testes → para-aortic lymph nodes.	As a result, varicocele is more common on left.
	Distal ⅓ of vagina/vulva/scrotum → superficial inguinal nodes.	
	Proximal ⅔ of vagina/uterus → obturator, external iliac and hypogastric nodes.	

Female reproductive anatomy

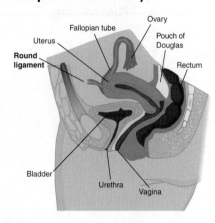
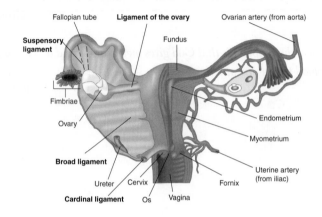

Ligament	Connects	Structures contained	Notes
Suspensory ligament of the ovaries	Ovaries to lateral pelvic wall	Ovarian vessels	Right ovarian vein → IVC.
Cardinal ligament	Cervix to side wall of pelvis	Uterine vessels	Left ovarian vein → left renal vein.
Round ligament of the uterus	Uterine fundus to labia majora	0	**Round** like the number 0. Derivative of gubernaculum. Travels through **round** inguinal canal.
Broad ligament	Uterus, fallopian tubes, and ovaries to pelvic side wall	Ovaries, fallopian tubes, and round ligaments of uterus	
Ligament of the ovary	Ovary to lateral uterus		Don't confuse with the suspensory ligament of the ovaries.

Female reproductive histology

Ovary	Simple cuboidal epithelium
Fallopian tube	Simple columnar epithelium, ciliated
Uterus	Simple columnar epithelium, pseudostratified, tubular glands
Endocervix	Simple columnar epithelium
Ectocervix	Stratified squamous epithelium
Vagina	Stratified squamous epithelium, nonkeratinized

Male reproductive anatomy

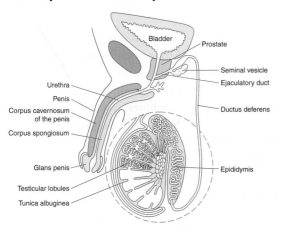

(Reproduced, with permission, from Junqueira LC et al. *Basic Histology,* 9th ed. New York: McGraw-Hill, 1998.)

Pathway of sperm during ejaculation—SEVEN UP:

Seminiferous tubules
Epididymis
Vas deferens
Ejaculatory ducts
(**N**othing)
Urethra
Penis

Autonomic innervation of the male sexual response	Erection—**P**arasympathetic nervous system (pelvic nerve): 1. NO → ↑ cGMP → smooth muscle relaxation → vasodilation → proerectile. 2. NE → ↑ $[Ca^2]_{in}$ → smooth muscle contraction → vasoconstriction → antierectile. Emission—**S**ympathetic nervous system (hypogastric nerve). Ejaculation—visceral and somatic nerves (pudendal nerve).	**P**oint and **S**hoot. Sildenafil and vardenafil inhibit cGMP breakdown.
Derivation of sperm parts	Occurs during final phase of spermatogenesis (spermiogenesis): spermatid → spermatozoa. Acrosome is derived from the Golgi apparatus and flagellum (tail) from one of the centrioles. **M**iddle piece (neck) has **M**itochondria. **F**eeds on **F**ructose. Tail forms from centrioles.	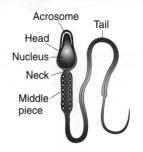

Seminiferous tubules

Cell	Function	Location/notes
Spermatogonia (germ cells)	Maintain germ pool and produce 1° spermatocytes	Line seminiferous tubules
Sertoli cells (non–germ cells)	Secrete inhibin → inhibit FSH	Line seminiferous tubules
	Secrete androgen-binding protein (ABP) → maintain levels of testosterone	**S**ertoli cells **S**upport **S**perm **S**ynthesis
	Tight junctions between adjacent Sertoli cells form blood-testis barrier → isolate gametes from autoimmune attack	
	Support and nourish developing spermatozoa	
	Regulate spermatogenesis	
	Produce anti-müllerian hormone	
Leydig cells (endocrine cells)	Secrete testosterone	Interstitium

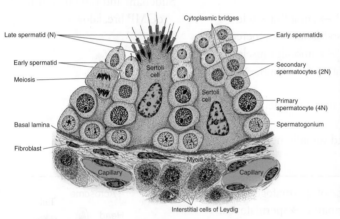

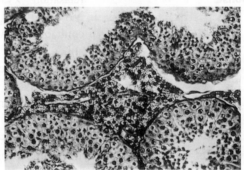

(Reproduced, with permission, from Junqueira LC, Carneiro J. *Basic Histology*, 11th ed. New York: McGraw-Hill, 2005: 420.)

Spermatogenesis

Spermatogenesis begins at puberty with spermatogonia. Full development takes 2 months. Occurs in seminiferous tubules. Produces spermatids that undergo spermiogenesis (loss of cytoplasmic contents, gain of acrosomal cap) to form mature spermatozoan.

"**Gonium**" is **going** to be a sperm; "**Z**oan" is "**Z**ooming" out of cell.

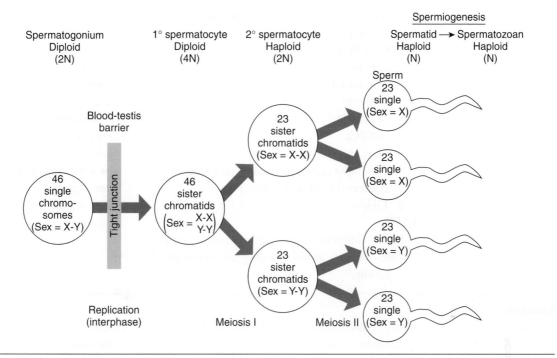

Regulation of spermatogenesis

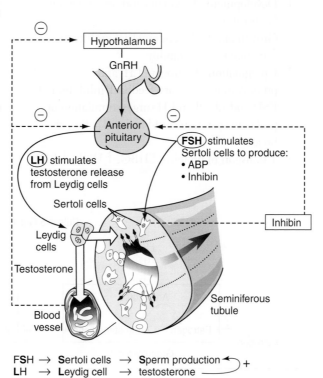

FSH → **S**ertoli cells → **S**perm production ⤶ +
LH → **L**eydig cell → testosterone ⤵

Androgens   Testosterone, dihydrotestosterone (DHT), androstenedione.

Source   DHT and testosterone (testis), androstenedione (adrenal).

Potency—DHT > testosterone > androstenedione.

Function   **Testosterone:**
1. Differentiation of epididymis, vas deferens, seminal vesicles (internal genitalia, except prostate)
2. Growth spurt
   —Penis
   —Seminal vesicles
   —Sperm
   —Muscle
   —RBCs
3. Deepening of voice
4. Closing of epiphyseal plates (via estrogen converted from testosterone)
5. Libido

DHT:
Early—differentiation of penis, scrotum, prostate.
Late—prostate growth, balding, sebaceous gland activity.

Testosterone is converted to DHT by the enzyme 5α-reductase, which is inhibited by finasteride.

Testosterone and androstenedione are converted to estrogen in adipose tissue and Sertoli cells by enzyme aromatase.

Exogenous testosterone → inhibition of HPG axis → ↓ intratesticular testosterone → ↓ testicular size → azoospermia.

Estrogen

Source   Ovary (17β-estradiol), placenta (estriol), blood (aromatization).

Potency—estradiol > estrone > estriol.

Function
1. Development of genitalia and breast, female fat distribution
2. Growth of follicle, endometrial proliferation, ↑ myometrial excitability
3. Upregulation of estrogen, LH, and progesterone receptors; feedback inhibition of FSH and LH, then LH surge; stimulation of prolactin secretion (**but** blocks its action at breast)
4. ↑ transport of proteins, SHBG; ↑ HDL; ↓ LDL

Pregnancy:
50-fold ↑ in estradiol and estrone
1000-fold ↑ in estriol (indicator of fetal well-being)

Estrogen receptors expressed in the cytoplasm; translocate to the nucleus when bound by ligand.

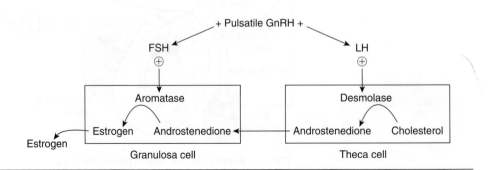

Progesterone

Source   Corpus luteum, placenta, adrenal cortex, testes.

Function

1. Stimulation of endometrial glandular secretions and spiral artery development
2. Maintenance of pregnancy
3. ↓ myometrial excitability
4. Production of thick cervical mucus, which inhibits sperm entry into the uterus
5. ↑ body temperature
6. Inhibition of gonadotropins (LH, FSH)
7. Uterine smooth muscle relaxation (preventing contractions)
8. ↓ estrogen receptor expressivity

Elevation of progesterone is indicative of ovulation.
PROGESTerone is **PRO-GEST**ation.

Menstrual cycle

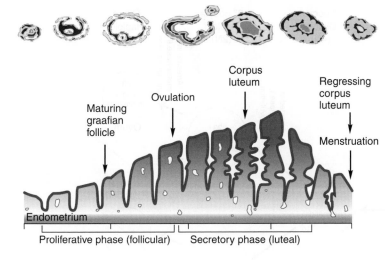

Maturing graafian follicle

Ovulation

Corpus luteum

Regressing corpus luteum

Menstruation

Endometrium

Proliferative phase (follicular)   Secretory phase (luteal)

Follicular growth is fastest during 2nd week of proliferative phase.
Estrogen stimulates endometrial proliferation.
Progesterone maintains endometrium to support implantation.
↓ progesterone leads to ↓ fertility.
Follicular phase can vary in length. Luteal phase is usually a constant 14 days. Ovulation day + 14 days = menstruation.
Oligomenorrhea: > 35-day cycle.
Polymenorrhea: < 21-day cycle.
Metrorrhagia: frequent but irregular menstruation.
Menometrorrhagia: heavy, irregular menstruation at irregular intervals.

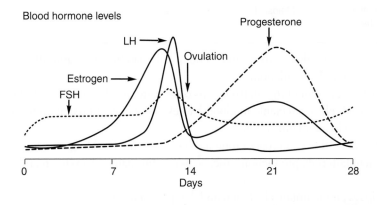

Blood hormone levels

LH

Progesterone

Ovulation

Estrogen

FSH

0   7   14   21   28

Days

Estrogen
↓
LH surge
↓
Ovulation
↓
Progesterone (from corpus luteum)
↓
Menstruation (via apoptosis of endometrial cells)

Ovulation | ↑ estrogen, ↑ GnRH receptors on anterior pituitary. Estrogen surge then stimulates LH release, causing ovulation (rupture of follicle). ↑ temperature (progesterone induced). | Mittelschmerz—blood from ruptured follicle causes peritoneal irritation that can mimic appendicitis.

Oogenesis | 1° oocytes begin meiosis I during fetal life and complete meiosis I just prior to ovulation.
Meiosis I is arrested in pr**O**phase for years until **O**vulation (1° oocytes).
Meiosis II is arrested in **MET**aphase until fertilization (2° oocytes).
If fertilization does not occur, the 2° oocyte degenerates. | An egg **MET** a sperm.

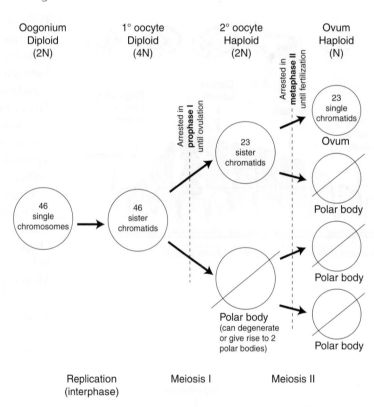

Pregnancy | Fertilization most commonly occurs in upper end of fallopian tube (the ampulla). Occurs within 1 day after ovulation.
Implantation within the wall of the uterus occurs 6 days after fertilization. Trophoblasts secrete β-hCG, which is detectable in blood 1 week after conception and on home test in urine 2 weeks after conception.
Lactation—after labor, the ↓ in progesterone induces lactation. Suckling is required to maintain milk production, since ↑ nerve stimulation ↑ oxytocin and prolactin.
Prolactin—induces and maintains lactation and ↓ reproductive function.
Oxytocin—appears to help with milk letdown and may be involved with uterine contractions (function not yet entirely known).

hCG

  Source   Syncytiotrophoblast of placenta.

  Function

1. Maintains the corpus luteum (and thus progesterone) for the 1st trimester by acting like LH (otherwise no luteal cell stimulation, and abortion results). In the 2nd and 3rd trimester, the placenta synthesizes its own estriol and progesterone and the corpus luteum degenerates.
2. Used to detect pregnancy because it appears early in the urine (see above).
3. Elevated hCG in pathologic states (e.g., hydatidiform moles, choriocarcinoma, gestational trophoblastic tumors).

| **Menopause** | ↓ estrogen production due to age-linked decline in number of ovarian follicles. Average age of onset is 51 years (earlier in smokers).

 Usually preceded by 4–5 years of abnormal menstrual cycles. Source of estrogen (estrone) after menopause becomes peripheral conversion of androgens. ↑ androgens cause hirsutism.

 ↑↑ FSH is the best test to confirm menopause (loss of negative feedback for FSH due to ↓ estrogen). | Hormonal changes:
 ↓ estrogen, ↑↑ FSH, ↑ LH (no surge), ↑ GnRH.
 Menopause causes **HHAVOC**: **H**irsutism, **H**ot flashes, **A**trophy of the **V**agina, **O**steoporosis, **C**oronary artery disease.
 Early menopause can indicate premature ovarian failure. |

Sex chromosome disorders

Klinefelter's syndrome [male] (XXY), 1:850 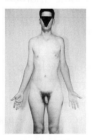	Testicular atrophy, eunuchoid body shape, tall, long extremities, gynecomastia, female hair distribution. May present with developmental delay. Presence of inactivated X chromosome (Barr body). Common cause of hypogonadism seen in infertility workup.	Dysgenesis of seminiferous tubules → ↓ inhibin → ↑ FSH. Abnormal Leydig cell function → ↓ testosterone → ↑ LH → ↑ estrogen.
Turner syndrome [female] (XO) 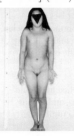	Short stature (if left untreated, < 5 feet), ovarian dysgenesis (streak ovary with infertility), shield chest, bicuspid aortic valve, webbing of neck (cystic hygroma), preductal coarctation of the aorta, most common cause of 1° amenorrhea. No Barr body.	"Hugs and kisses" **(XO)** from Tina **Turner** (female). ↓ estrogen leads to ↑ LH and FSH.
Double Y males [male] (XYY), 1:1000	Phenotypically normal, very tall, severe acne, antisocial behavior (seen in 1–2% of XYY males). Normal fertility.	

Diagnosing disorders of sex hormones

Testosterone	LH	Diagnosis
↑	↑	Defective androgen receptor
↑	↓	Testosterone-secreting tumor, exogenous steroids
↓	↑	1° hypogonadism
↓	↓	**H**ypo**g**onadotropic **h**ypo**g**onadism

Pseudo-hermaphroditism	Disagreement between the phenotypic (external genitalia) and gonadal (testes vs. ovaries) sex.
Female pseudo-hermaphrodite (XX)	Ovaries present, but external genitalia are virilized or ambiguous. Due to excessive and inappropriate exposure to androgenic steroids during early gestation (e.g., congenital adrenal hyperplasia or exogenous administration of androgens during pregnancy).
Male pseudo-hermaphrodite (XY)	Testes present, but external genitalia are female or ambiguous. Most common form is androgen insensitivity syndrome (testicular feminization).

True hermaphrodite (46,XX or 47,XXY)	Both ovary and testicular tissue present (ovotestis); ambiguous genitalia. Very rare.

Androgen insensitivity syndrome (46,XY)	Defect in androgen receptor resulting in normal-appearing female; female external genitalia with rudimentary vagina; uterus and uterine tubes generally absent; presents with no sexual hair; develops testes (often found in labia majora; surgically removed to prevent malignancy). ↑ **testosterone, estrogen,** LH (vs. sex chromosome disorders).

5α-reductase deficiency	Autosomal recessive; sex limited to genetic males. Inability to convert testosterone to DHT. Ambiguous genitalia until puberty, when ↑ testosterone causes masculinization/↑ growth of external genitalia. Testosterone/estrogen levels are normal; LH is normal or ↑. "Penis at 12." Internal genitalia are normal.

Kallmann syndrome	↓ synthesis of gonadotropin in the anterior pituitary; anosmia; lack of secondary sexual characteristics.

SRY gene

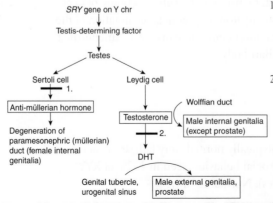

1. No Sertoli cell or lack of anti-müllerian hormone: develop both male and female internal genitalia and male external genitalia

2. 5α-reductase deficiency: male internal genitalia, ambiguous external genitalia until puberty

Hydatidiform mole   Cystic swelling of chorionic villi and proliferation of chorionic epithelium (trophoblast) that presents with abnormal vaginal bleeding. Most common precursor of choriocarcinoma. ↑ β-hCG. "Honeycombed uterus," "cluster of grapes" appearance, abnormally enlarged uterus (see Image 74). Complete moles classically have "snowstorm" appearance with no fetus during 1st sonogram. Moles can lead to uterine rupture. Treatment: dilatation and curettage and methotrexate. Monitor β-hCG.

	Complete Mole	Partial Mole
Karyotype	46,XX (46,XY)	69,XXY
hCG	↑↑↑↑	↑
Uterine size	↑	—
Convert to choriocarcinoma	2%	Rare
Fetal parts	No	Yes (**partial** = fetal **parts**)
Components	2 sperm + empty egg	2 sperm + 1 egg
Risk of complications	15-20% malignant trophoblastic disease	Low risk of malignancy (< 5%)

Common causes of recurrent miscarriages   1st weeks—low progesterone levels (no response to β-hCG).
1st trimester—chromosomal abnormalities (e.g., robertsonian translocation).
2nd trimester—bicornuate uterus (incomplete fusion of paramesonephric ducts).

Pregnancy-induced hypertension (preeclampsia-eclampsia)   Preeclampsia—hypertension, proteinuria, and edema. Eclampsia—preeclampsia + seizures. Occurs in 7% of pregnant women from 20 weeks' gestation to 6 weeks postpartum (before 20 weeks suggests molar pregnancy). ↑ incidence in patients with preexisting hypertension, diabetes, chronic renal disease, and autoimmune disorders. Caused by **placental ischemia** due to impaired vasodilation of spiral arteries, resulting in ↑ vascular tone. Can be associated with **HELLP syndrome** (Hemolysis, Elevated LFTs, Low Platelets). Mortality due to cerebral hemorrhage and ARDS.

Clinical features   Headache, blurred vision, abdominal pain, edema of face and extremities, altered mentation, hyperreflexia; lab findings may include thrombocytopenia, hyperuricemia.

Treatment   Delivery of fetus as soon as viable. Otherwise bed rest, salt restriction, and monitoring and treatment of hypertension. Treatment: IV magnesium sulfate and diazepam to prevent and treat seizures of eclampsia.

Pregnancy complications	Abruptio placentae—premature detachment of placenta from implantation site. Fetal death. May be associated with DIC. ↑ risk with smoking, hypertension, cocaine use.	Painful bleeding in 3rd trimester. **Abrupt** detachment/death.
	Placenta accreta—defective decidual layer allows placenta to attach to myometrium. No separation of placenta after birth. Prior C-section, inflammation, and placenta previa predispose.	Massive bleeding after delivery. Accreta = "encased in" → encased in myometrium.
	Placenta previa—attachment of placenta to lower uterine segment. May occlude internal os. Multiparity and prior C-section predispose.	Painless bleeding in any trimester.
	Ectopic pregnancy—most often in fallopian tubes. Suspect with ↑ hCG and sudden lower abdominal pain; confirm with ultrasound. Often clinically mistaken for appendicitis.	Pain with or without bleeding. Risk factors: —History of infertility —Salpingitis (PID) —Ruptured appendix —Prior tubal surgery
	Retained placental tissue—may cause postpartum hemorrhage.	

Amniotic fluid abnormalities

Polyhydramnios	> 1.5–2 L of amniotic fluid; associated with esophageal/duodenal atresia, causing inability to swallow amniotic fluid, and with anencephaly.
Oligohydramnios	< 0.5 L of amniotic fluid; associated with placental insufficiency, bilateral renal agenesis, or posterior urethral valves (in males) and resultant inability to excrete urine. Can give rise to Potter's syndrome.

Cervical pathology

Dysplasia and carcinoma in situ	Disordered epithelial growth; begins at basal layer of squamo-columnar junction and extends outward. Classified as CIN 1, CIN 2, or CIN 3 (carcinoma in situ), depending on extent of dysplasia. Associated with HPV **16, 18.** Vaccine available. May progress slowly to invasive carcinoma if left untreated. Risk factors: multiple sexual partners (#1), smoking, early sexual intercourse, HIV infection.	Koilocytic change typical of HPV infection 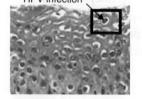 **HPV cell** (Reproduced, with permission, from Kantarjian HM et al. *MD Anderson Manual of Medical Oncology.* New York: McGraw-Hill, 2006, Fig. 24-4B.)
Invasive carcinoma	Often squamous cell carcinoma. Pap smear can catch cervical dysplasia (koilocytes) before it progresses to invasive carcinoma. Lateral invasion can block ureters, causing renal failure.	

Endometriosis	Non-neoplastic endometrial glands/stroma in abnormal locations outside the uterus. Characterized by **cyclic bleeding** (menstrual type) from ectopic endometrial tissue resulting in blood-filled "**chocolate cysts.**" In ovary or on peritoneum. Manifests clinically as severe menstrual-related pain. Often results in infertility. Can be due to retrograde menstrual flow or ascending infection. Adenomyosis—endometrium within the myometrium.

Endometrial proliferation

Endometrial hyperplasia	Abnormal endometrial gland proliferation usually caused by excess estrogen stimulation. ↑ risk for endometrial carcinoma. Clinically manifests as postmenopausal vaginal bleeding. Risk factors include anovulatory cycles, hormone replacement therapy, polycystic ovarian syndrome, and granulosa cell tumor.
Endometrial carcinoma	**Most common gynecologic malignancy.** Peak occurrence at 55–65 years of age. Clinically presents with vaginal bleeding. Typically preceded by endometrial hyperplasia. Risk factors include prolonged use of estrogen without progestins, obesity, diabetes, hypertension, nulliparity, and late menopause. ↑ myometrial invasion → ↓ prognosis.

Myometrial tumors

Leiomyoma (fibroid)	**Most common of all tumors** in females. Often presents with multiple tumors with well-demarcated borders. ↑ incidence in blacks. Benign smooth muscle tumor; malignant transformation is rare. Estrogen sensitive—tumor size ↑ with pregnancy and ↓ with menopause. Peak occurrence at 20–40 years of age. May be asymptomatic, cause abnormal uterine bleeding, or result in miscarriage. Severe bleeding may lead to iron deficiency anemia. Does not progress to leiomyosarcoma. **Whorled pattern of smooth muscle bundles.**

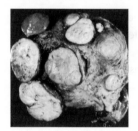

Leiomyosarcoma	Bulky, irregularly shaped tumor with areas of necrosis and hemorrhage, typically arising de novo (not from leiomyoma). ↑ incidence in blacks. Highly aggressive tumor with tendency to recur. May protrude from cervix and bleed. Most commonly seen in middle-aged women.

Gynecologic tumor epidemiology	Incidence—endometrial > ovarian > cervical (data pertain to the United States; cervical cancer is most common worldwide). Worst prognosis—ovarian > cervical > endometrial.

Premature ovarian failure	Premature atresia of ovarian follicles in women of reproductive age. Patients present with signs of menopause after puberty but before age 40.	↓ estrogen, ↑ LH, FSH.

Most common causes of anovulation	Polycystic ovarian syndrome, obesity, Asherman's syndrome (adhesions), HPO axis abnormalities, premature ovarian failure, hyperprolactinemia, thyroid disorders, eating disorders, Cushing's syndrome, adrenal insufficiency.

Polycystic ovarian syndrome

↑ LH production leads to anovulation, hyperandrogenism due to deranged steroid synthesis by theca cells. Enlarged, bilateral cystic ovaries manifest clinically with amenorrhea, infertility, obesity, and hirsutism. Associated with insulin resistance. ↑ risk of endometrial cancer. Treatment: weight loss, OCPs, gonadotropin analogs, clomiphene, spironolactone (to treat hirsutism), or surgery.

↑ LH, ↓ FSH, ↑ testosterone.

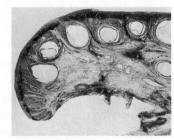

(Reproduced, with permission, from DeCherney AH, Nathan L. *Current Diagnosis & Treatment: Obstetrics & Gynecology,* 10th ed. New York, McGraw-Hill, 2007, Fig. 40-3.)

Ovarian cysts

Follicular cyst	Distention of unruptured graafian follicle. May be associated with hyperestrinism and endometrial hyperplasia.
Corpus luteum cyst	Hemorrhage into persistent corpus luteum. Commonly regresses spontaneously.
Theca-lutein cyst	Often bilateral/multiple. Due to gonadotropin stimulation. Associated with choriocarcinoma and moles.
"Chocolate cyst"	Blood-containing cyst from ovarian endometriosis. Varies with menstrual cycle.

HIGH-YIELD SYSTEMS

REPRODUCTIVE

Ovarian germ cell tumors Most common in adolescents.

Type	Characteristics	Tumor markers
Dysgerminoma	Malignant, equivalent to male seminoma but rarer (1% of germ cell tumors in females vs. 30% in males). Sheets of uniform cells.	hCG, LDH.
Choriocarcinoma	Rare but malignant; can develop during pregnancy in mother or baby. Large, hyperchromatic syncytiotrophoblastic cells. ↑ frequency of theca-lutein cysts. Along with moles, comprise spectrum of gestational trophoblastic neoplasia.	hCG.
Yolk sac (endodermal sinus) tumor	Aggressive malignancy in ovaries (testes in boys) and sacrococcygeal area of young children. Yellow, friable, solid masses. 50% have Schiller-Duval bodies (resemble glomeruli).	AFP.
Teratoma	90% of ovarian germ cell tumors. Contain cells from 2 or 3 germ layers. Mature teratoma ("dermoid cyst")—most frequent benign ovarian tumor. Immature teratoma—aggressively malignant. Struma ovarii—contains functional thyroid tissue. Can present as hyperthyroidism.	

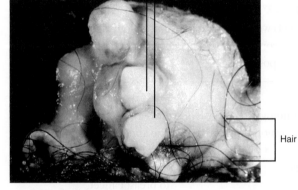

Teratoma of the ovary

Teeth

Hair

Glial tissue

Stratified squamous epithelium

Respiratory epithelium and glands

Ovarian non–germ cell tumors

Serous cystadenoma	20% of ovarian tumors. Frequently bilateral, lined with fallopian tube–like epithelium. Benign.	↑ CA-125 is general ovarian cancer marker.
Serous cystadenocarcinoma	50% of ovarian tumors, malignant and frequently bilateral.	Risk factors—BRCA-1, HNPCC. Significant genetic
Mucinous cystadenoma	Multilocular cyst lined by mucus-secreting epithelium. Benign. Intestine-like tissue.	predisposition makes family history the most important
Mucinous cystadenocarcinoma	Malignant. Pseudomyxoma peritonei—intraperitoneal accumulation of mucinous material from ovarian or appendiceal tumor.	risk factor.
Brenner tumor	**B**enign. Looks like **B**ladder.	
Fibromas	Bundles of spindle-shaped fibroblasts. Meigs' syndrome—triad of ovarian fibroma, ascites, and hydrothorax. Pulling sensation in groin.	
Granulosa cell tumor	Secretes estrogen → precocious puberty (kids). Can cause endometrial hyperplasia or carcinoma in adults. Call-Exner bodies—small follicles filled with eosinophilic secretions. Abnormal uterine bleeding.	
Krukenberg tumor	GI malignancy that metastasizes to ovaries, causing a mucin-secreting signet cell adenocarcinoma.	

Vaginal carcinoma

1. Squamous cell carcinoma (SCC)—2° to cervical SCC.
2. Clear cell adenocarcinoma—affects women who had exposure to DES in utero.
3. Sarcoma botryoides (rhabdomyosarcoma variant)—affects girls < 4 years of age; spindle-shaped tumor cells that are desmin positive.

Benign breast tumors

Type	Characteristics	Epidemiology	Notes
Fibroadenoma	**Small**, mobile, firm mass with sharp edges.	Most common tumor in those < 25 years of age.	↑ size and tenderness with ↑ estrogen (e.g., pregnancy, menstruation). Not a precursor to breast cancer.
Intraductal papilloma	Small tumor that grows in lactiferous ducts. Typically beneath areola.		Serous or bloody nipple discharge. Slight (1.5–2 ×) ↑ in risk for carcinoma.
Phyllodes tumor	**Large** bulky mass of connective tissue and cysts. "Leaf-like" projections.	Most common in 6th decade.	Some may become malignant.

Malignant breast tumors

Common postmenopause. Arise from mammary duct epithelium or lobular glands. Overexpression of estrogen/progesterone receptors or *erb*-B2 (HER-2, an EGF receptor) is common; affects therapy and prognosis. Axillary lymph node involvement is the single most important prognostic factor.

Risk factors: ↑ estrogen exposure, ↑ total number of menstrual cycles, older age at 1st live birth, obesity (adipose tissue serves as major source of estrogen in postmenopausal women by converting androstenedione to estrone; therefore, obesity is associated with ↑ estrogen exposure).

Type	Characteristics	Notes
Ductal carcinoma in situ (DCIS)	Fills ductal lumen. Arises from ductal hyperplasia.	Early malignancy without basement membrane penetration.
Invasive ductal	Firm, fibrous, "rock-hard" mass with sharp margins and small, glandular, duct-like cells.	Worst and most invasive. Most common (76% breast cancer).
Invasive lobular	Orderly row of cells.	Often multiple. Bilateral.
Medullary	Fleshy, cellular, lymphocytic infiltrate.	Good prognosis.
Comedocarcinoma	Ductal, caseous necrosis. Subtype of DCIS.	
Inflammatory	Dermal lymphatic invasion by breast carcinoma. Peau d'orange (breast skin resembles orange peel); neoplastic cells block lymphatic drainage.	50% survival at 5 years.
Paget's disease	Eczematous patches on nipple. Paget cells = large cells in epidermis with clear halo.	Suggests underlying carcinoma. Also seen on vulva.

Common breast conditions

Fibrocystic disease	Most common cause of "breast lumps" from age 25 to menopause. Presents with premenstrual breast pain and multiple lesions, often bilateral. Fluctuation in size of mass. Usually does not indicate ↑ risk of carcinoma. Histologic types: 1. Fibrosis—hyperplasia of breast stroma. 2. Cystic—fluid filled, blue dome. Ductal dilation. 3. Sclerosing adenosis—↑ acini and intralobular fibrosis. Associated with calcifications. 4. Epithelial hyperplasia—↑ in number of epithelial cell layers in terminal duct lobule. ↑ risk of carcinoma with atypical cells. Occurs in women > 30 years of age.	
Acute mastitis	Breast abscess; during breast-feeding, ↑ risk of bacterial infection through cracks in the nipple; *S. aureus* is the most common pathogen.	
Fat necrosis	A benign painless lump; forms as a result of injury to breast tissue. Up to 50% of patients may not report trauma.	
Gynecomastia	Results from hyperestrogenism (cirrhosis, testicular tumor, puberty, old age), Klinefelter's syndrome, or drugs (estrogen, marijuana, heroin, psychoactive drugs, **S**pironolactone, **D**igitalis, **C**imetidine, **A**lcohol, **K**etoconazole).	**S**ome **D**rugs **C**reate **A**wesome **K**nockers.

Breast pathology

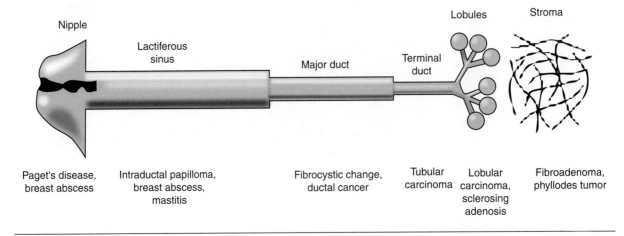

| Paget's disease, breast abscess | Intraductal papilloma, breast abscess, mastitis | Fibrocystic change, ductal cancer | Tubular carcinoma | Lobular carcinoma, sclerosing adenosis | Fibroadenoma, phyllodes tumor |

Prostate pathology

Prostatitis—dysuria, frequency, urgency, low back pain. Acute: bacterial (e.g., *E. coli*); chronic: bacterial or abacterial (most common).

Benign prostatic hyperplasia (BPH)

Common in men > 50 years of age. Hyperplasia (**not** hypertrophy) of the prostate gland. May be due to an age-related ↑ in estradiol with possible sensitization of the prostate to the growth-promoting effects of DHT. Characterized by a nodular enlargement of the periurethral (lateral and middle) lobes, which compress the urethra into a vertical slit. Often presents with ↑ frequency of urination, nocturia, difficulty starting and stopping the stream of urine, and dysuria. May lead to distention and hypertrophy of the bladder, hydronephrosis, and UTIs. Not considered a premalignant lesion. ↑ **free prostate-specific antigen (PSA).** Treatment: α_1-antagonists (terazosin, tamsulosin), which cause relaxation of smooth muscle; finasteride.

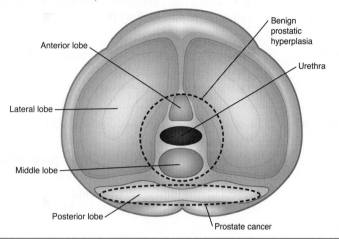

Prostatic adenocarcinoma

Common in men > 50 years of age. Arises most often from the posterior lobe (peripheral zone) of the prostate gland and is most frequently diagnosed by digital rectal examination (hard nodule) and prostate biopsy. Prostatic acid phosphatase (PAP) and PSA are useful tumor markers (↑ total PSA, with ↓ **fraction of free PSA).** Osteoblastic metastases in bone may develop in late stages, as indicated by lower back pain and an ↑ in serum alkaline phosphatase and PSA.

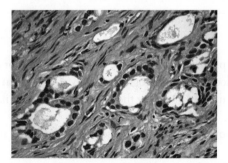

Prostatic adenocarcinoma: small infiltrating glands with prominent nucleoli

(Reproduced, with permission, from USMLERx.com.)

Cryptorchidism

Undescended testis (one or both); lack of spermatogenesis due to ↑ body temperature; associated with ↑ risk of germ cell tumors. Prematurity ↑ the risk of cryptorchidism.

Testicular germ cell tumors	~95% of all testicular tumors. Can present as a mixed germ cell tumor.
Seminoma	Malignant; painless, homogenous testicular enlargement; most common testicular tumor, mostly affecting males age 15–35. Large cells in lobules with watery cytoplasm and a "fried egg" appearance. Radiosensitive. Late metastasis, excellent prognosis.
Embryonal carcinoma	Malignant; painful; worse prognosis than seminoma. Often glandular/papillary morphology. Can differentiate to other tumors. May be associated with ↑ AFP, hCG.
Yolk sac (endodermal sinus) tumor	Yellow, mucinous. Analogous to ovarian yolk sac tumor. Schiller-Duval bodies resemble primitive glomeruli (↑ AFP).
Choriocarcinoma	Malignant, ↑ hCG. Disordered syncytiotrophoblastic and cytotrophoblastic elements. Hematogenous metastases.
Teratoma	Unlike in females, mature teratoma in males is most often malignant.

Testicular non–germ cell tumors	5% of all testicular tumors. Mostly benign.
Leydig cell	Contains Reinke crystals; usually androgen producing, gynecomastia in men, precocious puberty in boys. Golden brown color.
Sertoli cell	Androblastoma from sex cord stroma.
Testicular lymphoma	Most common testicular cancer in older men.

Tunica vaginalis lesions	Lesions in the serous covering of testis—present as testicular masses that can be transilluminated (vs. testicular tumors). 1. Varicocele—dilated vein in pampiniform plexus; can cause infertility; "bag of worms" 2. Hydrocele—↑ fluid 2° to incomplete fusion of processus vaginalis 3. Spermatocele—dilated epididymal duct

Penile pathology	
Carcinoma in situ	
Bowen's disease	Gray, solitary, crusty plaque, usually on the shaft of the penis or on the scrotum; peak incidence in 5th decade of life; progresses to invasive SCC in < 10% of cases.
Erythroplasia of Queyrat	Red velvety plaques, usually involving the glans; otherwise similar to Bowen's disease.
Bowenoid papulosis	Multiple papular lesions; affects younger age group than other subtypes; usually does not become invasive.
Squamous cell carcinoma (SCC)	More common in Asia, Africa, and South America. Commonly associated with HPV, lack of circumcision.
Peyronie's disease	Bent penis due to acquired fibrous tissue formation.

Control of reproductive hormones

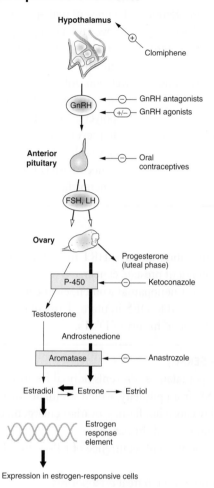

Control of female hormones

(Adapted, with permission, from Katzung BG. *Basic & Clinical Pharmacology,* 10th ed. New York: McGraw-Hill, 2006, Fig. 40-5.)

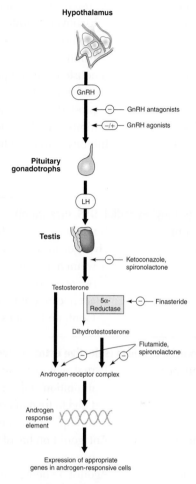

Control of androgen secretion

(Adapted, with permission, from Katzung BG. *Basic & Clinical Pharmacology,* 10th ed. New York: McGraw-Hill, 2006, Fig. 40-6.)

Leuprolide

Mechanism	GnRH analog with agonist properties when used in pulsatile fashion; antagonist properties when used in continuous fashion.	**Leu**prolide can be used in **lieu** of GnRH.
Clinical use	Infertility (pulsatile), prostate cancer (continuous—use with flutamide), uterine fibroids.	
Toxicity	Antiandrogen, nausea, vomiting.	

Testosterone (methyltestosterone)

Mechanism	Agonist at androgen receptors.
Clinical use	Treat hypogonadism and promote development of 2° sex characteristics; stimulation of anabolism to promote recovery after burn or injury; treat ER-positive breast cancer (exemestane).
Toxicity	Causes masculinization in females; reduces intratesticular testosterone in males by inhibiting release of LH (via negative feedback), leading to gonadal atrophy. Premature closure of epiphyseal plates. ↑ LDL, ↓ HDL.

Antiandrogens

Testosterone $\xrightarrow{5\alpha\text{-reductase}}$ DHT (more potent).

Finasteride (Propecia)
: A 5α-reductase inhibitor (↓ conversion of testosterone to dihydrotestosterone). Useful in BPH. Also promotes hair growth—used to treat male-pattern baldness.

Flutamide
: A nonsteroidal competitive inhibitor of androgens at the testosterone receptor. Used in prostate carcinoma.

Ketoconazole
: Inhibits steroid synthesis (inhibits desmolase).

Spironolactone
: Inhibits steroid binding.

To prevent male-pattern hair loss, give a drug that will encourage female breast growth.

Ketoconazole and spironolactone are used in the treatment of polycystic ovarian syndrome to prevent hirsutism. Both have side effects of gynecomastia and amenorrhea.

Estrogens (ethinyl estradiol, DES, mestranol)

Mechanism
: Bind estrogen receptors.

Clinical use
: Hypogonadism or ovarian failure, menstrual abnormalities, HRT in postmenopausal women; use in men with androgen-dependent prostate cancer.

Toxicity
: ↑ risk of endometrial cancer, bleeding in postmenopausal women, clear cell adenocarcinoma of vagina in females exposed to DES in utero, ↑ risk of thrombi. Contraindications—ER-positive breast cancer, history of DVTs.

Estrogen partial agonists (selective estrogen receptor modulators—SERMs)

Clomiphene
: Partial agonist at estrogen receptors in hypothalamus. Prevents normal feedback inhibition and ↑ release of LH and FSH from pituitary, which stimulates ovulation. Used to treat infertility and PCOS. May cause hot flashes, ovarian enlargement, multiple simultaneous pregnancies, and visual disturbances.

Tamoxifen
: Antagonist on breast tissue; used to treat and prevent recurrence of ER-positive breast cancer.

Raloxifene
: Agonist on bone; reduces resorption of bone; used to treat osteoporosis.

Hormone replacement therapy (HRT)

Used for relief or prevention of menopausal symptoms (e.g., hot flashes, vaginal atrophy) and osteoporosis (↑ estrogen, ↓ osteoclast activity).

Unopposed estrogen replacement therapy (ERT) ↑ the risk of endometrial cancer, so progesterone is added. Possible ↑ CV risk.

Anastrozole/ exemestane

Aromatase inhibitors used in postmenopausal women with breast cancer.

Progestins

Mechanism
: Bind progesterone receptors, reduce growth, and ↑ vascularization of endometrium.

Clinical use
: Used in oral contraceptives and in the treatment of endometrial cancer and abnormal uterine bleeding.

Mifepristone (RU-486)

Mechanism
: Competitive inhibitor of progestins at progesterone receptors.

Clinical use
: Termination of pregnancy. Administered with misoprostol (PGE$_1$).

Toxicity
: Heavy bleeding, GI effects (nausea, vomiting, anorexia), abdominal pain.

Oral contraception (synthetic progestins, estrogen)	Oral contraceptives prevent estrogen surge, LH surge does not occur → ovulation does not occur.	
	Advantages	**Disadvantages**
	Reliable (< 1% failure)	Taken daily
	↓ risk of endometrial and ovarian cancer	No protection against STDs
		↑ triglycerides
	↓ incidence of ectopic pregnancy	Depression, weight gain, nausea, hypertension
	↓ pelvic infections	
	Regulation of menses	Hypercoagulable state
	Contraindications—smokers > 35 years of age (↑ risk of cardiovascular events), patients with history of thromboembolism and stroke or history of estrogen-dependent tumor.	
Dinoprostone	PGE_2 analog causing cervical dilation and uterine contraction, inducing labor.	
Ritodrine/terbutaline	β_2-agonists that relax the uterus; reduce premature uterine contractions.	**Ritodrine** allows the fetus to "**return to dreams**" by preventing early delivery.
Tamsulosin	α_1-antagonist used to treat BPH by inhibiting smooth muscle contraction. Selective for $\alpha_{1A,D}$ receptors (found on prostate) vs. vascular α_{1B} receptors.	
Sildenafil, vardenafil		
Mechanism	Inhibit cGMP phosphodiesterase, causing ↑ cGMP, smooth muscle relaxation in the corpus cavernosum, ↑ blood flow, and penile erection.	Sildena**fil** and vardena**fil** **fill** the penis.
Clinical use	Treatment of erectile dysfunction.	
Toxicity	Headache, flushing, dyspepsia, impaired blue-green color vision. Risk of life-threatening hypotension in patients taking nitrates.	"**H**ot and sweaty," but then **H**eadache, **H**eartburn, **H**ypotension.

Respiratory

"There's so much pollution in the air now that if it weren't for our lungs, there'd be no place to put it all."

—Robert Orben

"Mars is essentially in the same orbit. Somewhat the same distance from the Sun, which is very important. We have seen pictures where there are canals, we believe, and water. If there is water, that means there is oxygen. If there is oxygen, that means we can breathe."

—Former Vice President Dan Quayle

▶ Anatomy

▶ Physiology

▶ Pathology

▶ Pharmacology

Respiratory tree

Conducting zone
Consists of nose, pharynx, trachea, bronchi, bronchioles, and terminal bronchioles. Cartilage is present only in the trachea and bronchi. Brings air in and out. Warms, humidifies, filters air. Anatomic dead space. Walls of conducting airways contain smooth muscle.

Respiratory zone
Consists of respiratory bronchioles, alveolar ducts, and alveoli. Participates in gas exchange.

Pneumocytes

Pseudostratified ciliated columnar cells extend to the respiratory bronchioles (macrophages clear debris in alveoli); goblet cells extend only to the bronchi.

Type I cells (97% of alveolar surfaces) line the alveoli. Squamous; thin for optimal gas diffusion.

Type II cells (3%) secrete pulmonary surfactant (dipalmitoyl phosphatidylcholine), which ↓ the alveolar surface tension. Cuboidal and clustered. Also serve as precursors to type I cells and other type II cells. Type II cells proliferate during lung damage.

Clara cells—nonciliated; columnar with secretory granules. Secrete component of surfactant; degrade toxins; act as reserve cells.

Mucus secretions are swept out of the lungs toward the mouth by ciliated cells.

A lecithin-to-sphingomyelin ratio of > 2.0 in amniotic fluid indicates fetal lung maturity.

Gas exchange barrier

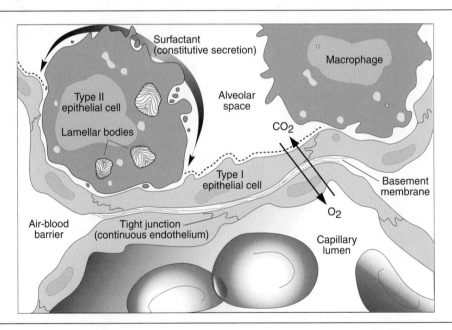

Bronchopulmonary segments	Each bronchopulmonary segment has a 3° (segmental) bronchus and 2 arteries (bronchial and pulmonary) in the center; veins and lymphatics drain along the borders.	Arteries run with Airways.
	Pulmonary arteries carry deoxygenated blood from the right side of the heart. Elastic walls maintain pulmonary arterial pressure at relatively constant levels throughout cardiac cycle.	

Lung relations	Right lung has 3 lobes; **L**eft has 2 lobes and **L**ingula (homologue of right middle lobe). Right lung is more common site for inhaled foreign body because the right main stem bronchus is wider and more vertical than the left.	Instead of a middle lobe, the left lung has a space occupied by the heart. The relation of the pulmonary artery to the bronchus at each lung hilus is described by **RALS**—**R**ight **A**nterior; **L**eft **S**uperior.
	Aspirate a peanut:	
	While upright—lower portion of right inferior lobe.	
	While supine—superior portion of right inferior lobe.	

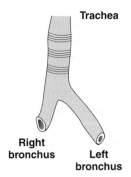

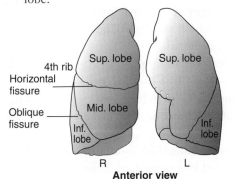

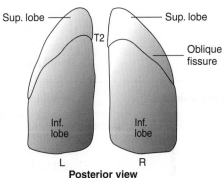

Diaphragm structures	Structures perforating diaphragm:	Number of letters = T level:
	At T8: IVC.	**T8**: vena cava
	At T10: esophagus, vagus (2 trunks).	**T10**: (o)esophagus
	At T12: aorta (red), thoracic duct (white), azygous vein (blue).	**T12**: aortic hiatus
	Diaphragm is innervated by **C3, 4, and 5** (phrenic nerve). Pain from the diaphragm can be referred to the shoulder.	"I (IVC) ate (8) ten (10) eggs (esophagus) at (aorta) twelve (12)."
		"C3, 4, 5 keeps the diaphragm alive."

Central tendon
Inferior vena cava (T8)
Esophagus (T10)
Descending aorta (T12)
Rib
Vertebrae
Inferior view

Muscles of respiration	Quiet breathing:
	    Inspiration—diaphragm.
	    Expiration—passive.
	Exercise:
	    InSpiration—external intercostals, Scalene muscles, Sternomastoids.
	    Expiration—rectus abdominis, internal and external obliques, transversus abdominis, internal intercostals.

▶ **RESPIRATORY—PHYSIOLOGY**

Important lung products	1. Surfactant—produced by type II pneumocytes, ↓ alveolar surface tension, ↑ compliance, ↓ work of inspiration 2. Prostaglandins 3. Histamine ↑ bronchoconstriction 4. Angiotensin-converting enzyme (ACE)— angiotensin I → angiotensin II; inactivates bradykinin (ACE inhibitors ↑ bradykinin and cause cough, angioedema) 5. Kallikrein—activates bradykinin	**Surfactant**—dipalmitoyl phosphatidylcholine (lecithin) deficient in neonatal RDS. Collapsing pressure = $$P = \dfrac{2\ (\text{surface tension})}{\text{radius}}$$ Tendency to collapse on expiration as radius ↓ (law of Laplace).
Lung volumes	1. Residual volume (RV)—air in lung after maximal expiration; cannot be measured on spirometry 2. Expiratory reserve volume (ERV)—air that can still be breathed out after normal expiration 3. Tidal volume (TV)—air that moves into lung with each quiet inspiration, typically 500 mL 4. Inspiratory reserve volume (IRV)—air in excess of tidal volume that moves into lung on maximum inspiration 5. Vital capacity (VC): TV + IRV + ERV 6. Functional residual capacity (FRC): RV + ERV (volume in lungs after normal expiration) 7. Inspiratory capacity (IC): IRV + TV 8. Total lung capacity: TLC = IRV + TV + ERV + RV	Vital capacity is everything but the residual volume. A capacity is a sum of ≥ 2 volumes.

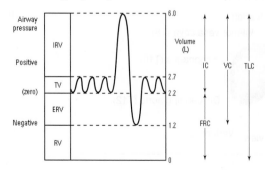

Determination of physiologic dead space

$$V_D = V_T \times \frac{(Pa_{CO_2} - Pe_{CO_2})}{Pa_{CO_2}}$$

V_D = physiologic dead space = anatomical dead space of conducting airways plus functional dead space in alveoli; apex of healthy lung is largest contributor of functional dead space. Volume of inspired air that does not take part in gas exchange.

V_T = tidal volume.

Pa_{CO_2} = arterial P_{CO_2}, Pe_{CO_2} = expired air P_{CO_2}.

Lung and chest wall

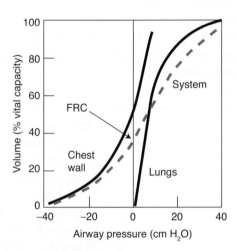

Relaxation pressure-volume curve

Tendency for lungs to collapse inward and chest wall to spring outward.

At FRC, inward pull of lung is balanced by outward pull of chest wall, and system pressure is atmospheric.

Elastic properties of both chest wall and lungs determine their combined volume.

At FRC, airway and alveolar pressure are 0, and intra-pleural pressure is negative (prevents pneumothorax).

Compliance—change in lung volume for a given change in pressure; decreased in pulmonary fibrosis, insufficient surfactant, and pulmonary edema.

Hemoglobin

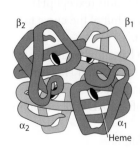

Hemoglobin is composed of 4 polypeptide subunits (2 α and 2 β) and exists in 2 forms:

1. T (taut) form has low affinity for O_2.
2. R (relaxed) form has high affinity for O_2 (300×). Hemoglobin exhibits positive cooperativity and negative allostery (accounts for the sigmoid-shaped O_2 dissociation curve for hemoglobin), unlike myoglobin.

↑ Cl^-, H^+, CO_2, 2,3-BPG, and temperature favor T form over **R** form (shifts dissociation curve to right, leading to ↑ O_2 unloading).

Fetal hemoglobin (2α and 2γ subunits) has lower affinity for 2,3-BPG than adult hemoglobin (HbA) and thus has higher affinity for O_2.

When you're **R**elaxed, you do your job better (carry O_2).

Hemoglobin modifications

Lead to tissue hypoxia from ↓ O_2 saturation and ↓ O_2 content.

Methemoglobin

Oxidized form of hemoglobin (ferric, Fe^{3+}) that does not bind O_2 as readily, but has ↑ affinity for CN^-.

Iron in hemoglobin is normally in a reduced state (ferrous, Fe^{2+}).

To treat cyanide poisoning, use nitrites to oxidize hemoglobin to methemoglobin, which binds cyanide, allowing cytochrome oxidase to function. Use thiosulfate to bind this cyanide, forming thiocyanate, which is renally excreted.

METHemoglobinemia can be treated with **METH**ylene blue.

Carboxyhemoglobin

Form of hemoglobin bound to CO in place of O_2. Causes ↓ oxygen-binding capacity with a left shift in the oxygen-hemoglobin dissociation curve. ↓ oxygen unloading in tissues.

CO has 200 × greater affinity than O_2 for hemoglobin.

Oxygen-hemoglobin dissociation curve

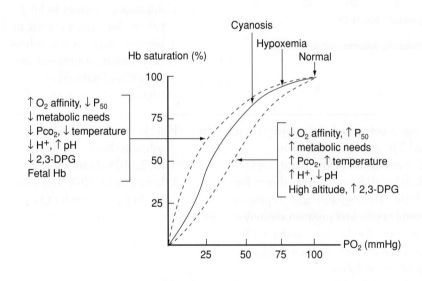

↑ O_2 affinity, ↓ P_{50}
↓ metabolic needs
↓ Pco_2, ↓ temperature
↓ H^+, ↑ pH
↓ 2,3-DPG
Fetal Hb

↓ O_2 affinity, ↑ P_{50}
↑ metabolic needs
↑ Pco_2, ↑ temperature
↑ H^+, ↓ pH
High altitude, ↑ 2,3-DPG

Sigmoidal shape due to positive cooperativity, i.e., hemoglobin can bind 4 oxygen molecules and has higher affinity for each subsequent oxygen molecule bound.

When curve shifts to the right, ↓ affinity of hemoglobin for O_2 (facilitates unloading of O_2 to tissue).

An ↑ in all factors (except pH) causes a shift of the curve to the right.

A ↓ in all factors (except pH) causes a shift of the curve to the left.

Fetal Hb has a higher affinity for oxygen than adult Hb, so its dissociation curve is shifted left.

Right shift—CADET face **right**:
CO_2
Acid/Altitude
DPG (2,3-DPG)
Exercise
Temperature

Pulmonary circulation	Normally a low-resistance, high-compliance system. P_{O_2} and P_{CO_2} exert opposite effects on pulmonary and systemic circulation. A ↓ in PA_{O_2} causes a hypoxic vasoconstriction that shifts blood away from poorly ventilated regions of lung to well-ventilated regions of lung.	A consequence of pulmonary hypertension is cor pulmonale and subsequent right ventricular failure (jugular venous distention, edema, hepatomegaly).
	1. Perfusion limited—O_2 (normal health), CO_2, N_2O. Gas equilibrates early along the length of the capillary. Diffusion can be ↑ only if blood flow ↑.	Diffusion: $V_{gas} = A/T \times D_k(P_1 - P_2)$ where A = area, T = thickness, and $D_k(P_1 - P_2) \approx$ difference in partial pressures.
	2. Diffusion limited—O_2 (emphysema, fibrosis), CO. Gas does not equilibrate by the time blood reaches the end of the capillary.	A ↓ in emphysema. T ↑ in pulmonary fibrosis.

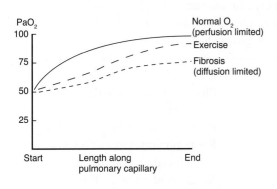

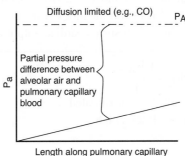

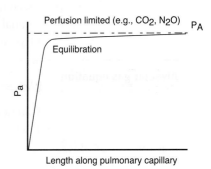

P_a = partial pressure of gas in pulmonary capillary blood
P_A = partial pressure of gas in alveolar air

Pulmonary hypertension	Normal pulmonary artery pressure = 10–14 mmHg; pulmonary hypertension ≥ 25 mmHg or > 35 mmHg during exercise. Results in atherosclerosis, medial hypertrophy, and intimal fibrosis of pulmonary arteries.
	1°—due to an inactivating mutation in the *BMPR2* gene (normally functions to inhibit vascular smooth muscle proliferation); poor prognosis.
	2°—due to COPD (destruction of lung parenchyma); mitral stenosis (↑ resistance → ↑ pressure); recurrent thromboemboli (↓ cross-sectional area of pulmonary vascular bed); autoimmune disease (e.g., systemic sclerosis; inflammation → intimal fibrosis → medial hypertrophy); left-to-right shunt (↑ shear stress → endothelial injury); sleep apnea or living at high altitude (hypoxic vasoconstriction).
	Course: severe respiratory distress → cyanosis and RVH → death from decompensated cor pulmonale.

| Pulmonary vascular resistance (PVR) | $PVR = \dfrac{P_{pulm\ artery} - P_{L\ atrium}}{Cardiac\ output}$

 Remember: $\Delta P = Q \times R$, so $R = \Delta P / Q$.
 $R = 8\eta l / \pi r^4$ | $P_{pulm\ artery}$ = pressure in pulmonary artery.
 $P_{L\ atrium}$ = pulmonary wedge pressure.
 η = the viscosity of blood;
 l = vessel length;
 r = vessel radius. |

| Oxygen content of blood | O_2 content = (O_2 binding capacity $\times$ % saturation) + dissolved O_2.
 Normally 1 g Hb can bind 1.34 mL O_2; normal Hb amount in blood is 15 g/dL.
    Cyanosis results when deoxygenated Hb > 5 g/dL.
 O_2 binding capacity $\approx$ 20.1 mL O_2 / dL.
 O_2 content of arterial blood ↓ as Hb falls, but O_2 saturation and arterial P_{O_2} do not.
 Arterial P_{O_2} ↓ with chronic lung disease because physiologic shunt ↓ O_2 extraction ratio.
 Oxygen delivery to tissues = cardiac output $\times$ oxygen content of blood. |

| Alveolar gas equation | $PA_{O_2} = PI_{O_2} - \dfrac{PA_{CO_2}}{R}$
 Can normally be approximated:
 $PA_{O_2} = 150 - PA_{CO_2} / 0.8$ | PA_{O_2} = alveolar P_{O_2} (mmHg).
 PI_{O_2} = P_{O_2} in inspired air (mmHg).
 PA_{CO_2} = alveolar P_{CO_2} (mmHg).
 R = respiratory quotient = CO_2 produced/O_2 consumed.
 A-a gradient = $PA_{O_2} - Pa_{O_2}$ = 10–15 mmHg.
 ↑ A-a gradient may occur in hypoxemia; causes include shunting, V/Q mismatch, fibrosis (diffusion block). |

Oxygen deprivation

Hypoxemia (↓ Pa_{O_2})	Hypoxia (↓ O_2 delivery to tissue)	Ischemia (loss of blood flow)
High altitude (normal A-a gradient) Hypoventilation (normal A-a gradient) V/Q mismatch (↑ A-a gradient) Diffusion limitation (↑ A-a gradient) Right-to-left shunt (↑ A-a gradient)	↓ cardiac output Hypoxemia Anemia Cyanide poisoning CO poisoning	Impeded arterial flow Reduced venous drainage

V/Q mismatch

Ideally, ventilation is matched to perfusion (i.e., $V/Q = 1$) in order for adequate gas exchange to occur. Lung zones:

1. Apex of the lung—$V/Q = 3$ (wasted ventilation)
2. Base of the lung—$V/Q = 0.6$ (wasted perfusion)

Both ventilation and perfusion are greater at the base of the lung than at the apex of the lung.

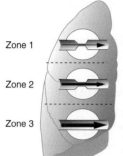

Zone 1

Apex: $P_A > P_a > P_v \rightarrow V/Q = 3$ (wasted ventilation, ↑ dead space); NOTE: high alveolar pressure compresses capillaries

Zone 2

$P_a > P_A > P_v$

Zone 3

Base: $P_a > P_v > P_A \rightarrow V/Q = 0.6$ (wasted perfusion); NOTE: both ventilation and perfusion are greater at the base of the lung than at the apex

With exercise (↑ cardiac output), there is vasodilation of apical capillaries, resulting in a V/Q ratio that approaches 1.

Certain organisms that thrive in high O_2 (e.g., TB) flourish in the apex.

$V/Q \rightarrow 0$ = airway obstruction (shunt). In shunt, 100% O_2 does not improve P_{O_2}.

$V/Q \rightarrow \infty$ = blood flow obstruction (physiologic dead space). Assuming < 100% dead space, 100% O_2 improves P_{O_2}.

CO_2 transport

Carbon dioxide is transported from tissues to the lungs in 3 forms:

1. **Bicarbonate (90%)**

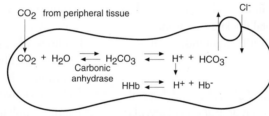

CO_2 from peripheral tissue

$CO_2 + H_2O \rightleftarrows H_2CO_3 \rightleftarrows H^+ + HCO_3^-$

Carbonic anhydrase

$HHb \rightleftarrows H^+ + Hb^-$

Cl^-

(Figure modified, with permission, from Ganong WF. *Review of Medical Physiology*, 22nd ed. New York: McGraw-Hill, 2005: 670.)

2. Bound to hemoglobin at N terminus of globin (**not** heme) as carbaminohemoglobin (5%). CO_2 binding favors taut form (O_2 unloaded).
3. Dissolved CO_2 (5%).

In lungs, oxygenation of Hb promotes dissociation of H^+ from Hb. This shifts equilibrium toward CO_2 formation; therefore, CO_2 is released from RBCs (Haldane effect).

In peripheral tissue, ↑ H^+ from tissue metabolism shifts curve to right, unloading O_2 (Bohr effect).

Response to high altitude

1. Acute ↑ in ventilation
2. Chronic ↑ in ventilation
3. ↑ erythropoietin → ↑ hematocrit and hemoglobin (chronic hypoxia)
4. ↑ 2,3-DPG (binds to hemoglobin so that hemoglobin releases more O_2)
5. Cellular changes (↑ mitochondria)
6. ↑ renal excretion of bicarbonate (e.g., can augment by use of acetazolamide) to compensate for the respiratory alkalosis
7. Chronic hypoxic pulmonary vasoconstriction results in RVH

Response to exercise

1. ↑ CO_2 production
2. ↑ O_2 consumption
3. ↑ ventilation rate to meet O_2 demand
4. V/Q ratio from apex to base becomes more uniform
5. ↑ pulmonary blood flow due to ↑ cardiac output
6. ↓ pH during strenuous exercise (2° to lactic acidosis)
7. No change in Pa_{O_2} and Pa_{CO_2}, but ↑ in venous CO_2 content

Embolus types	**F**at, **A**ir, **T**hrombus, **B**acteria, **A**mniotic fluid, **T**umor. Fat emboli are associated with long bone fractures and liposuction. Amniotic fluid emboli can lead to DIC, especially postpartum. Pulmonary embolus—chest pain, tachypnea, dyspnea.	An embolus moves like a **FAT BAT**. Approximately 95% of pulmonary emboli arise from deep leg veins. CT angiography is the imaging test of choice for a PE.
Deep venous thrombosis	Predisposed by Virchow's triad: 1. Stasis 2. Hypercoagulability (e.g., defect in coagulative cascade proteins) 3. Endothelial damage (exposed collagen provides impetus for clotting cascade)	Can lead to pulmonary embolus. Homans' sign— dorsiflexion of foot → tender calf muscle. Prevent with heparin.

Obstructive lung disease (COPD)

Obstruction of air flow resulting in air trapping in the lungs. Airways close prematurely at high lung volumes, resulting in ↑ RV and ↓ FVC. PFTs: ↓↓ FEV_1, ↓ FVC → ↓ FEV_1/FVC ratio (hallmark), V/Q mismatch.

Type	Pathology	Other
Chronic **B**ronchitis ("**B**lue **B**loater")	Hypertrophy of mucus-secreting glands in the bronchioles → Reid index = gland depth / total thickness of bronchial wall; in COPD, Reid index > 50%.	Productive cough for > 3 consecutive months in ≥ 2 years. Disease of small airways. Findings: wheezing, crackles, cyanosis (early-onset hypoxemia due to shunting), late-onset dyspnea.
Emphysema ("pink puffer," barrel-shaped chest)	Enlargement of air spaces and ↓ recoil resulting from destruction of alveolar walls; ↑ compliance. Centriacinar—caused by smoking. Panacinar—α_1-antitrypsin deficiency (also liver cirrhosis). Paraseptal emphysema—associated with bullae → can rupture → spontaneous pneumothorax; often in young, otherwise healthy males.	↑ elastase activity. ↑ lung compliance due to loss of elastic fibers. Exhale through pursed lips to ↑ airway pressure and prevent airway collapse during exhalation. Findings: dyspnea, ↓ breath sounds, tachycardia, late-onset hypoxemia due to eventual loss of capillary beds (occurs with loss of alveolar walls), early-onset dyspnea.
Asthma	Bronchial hyperresponsiveness causes reversible bronchoconstriction. Smooth muscle hypertrophy and Curschmann's spirals (shed epithelium from mucous plugs).	Can be triggered by viral URIs, allergens, and stress. Test with methacholine challenge. Findings: cough, wheezing, dyspnea, tachypnea, hypoxemia, ↓ I/E ratio, pulsus paradoxus, mucus plugging.
Bronchiectasis	Chronic necrotizing infection of bronchi → permanently dilated airways, purulent sputum, recurrent infections, hemoptysis.	Associated with bronchial obstruction, CF, poor ciliary motility, Kartagener's syndrome. Can develop aspergillosis.

Restrictive lung disease	Restricted lung expansion causes ↓ lung volumes (↓ FVC and TLC). PFTs—FEV_1/FVC ratio > 80%.

Types:

1. Poor breathing mechanics (extrapulmonary, peripheral hypoventilation):
   a. Poor muscular effort—polio, myasthenia gravis
   b. Poor structural apparatus—scoliosis, morbid obesity
2. Interstitial lung diseases (pulmonary, lowered diffusing capacity):
   a. Acute respiratory distress syndrome (ARDS)
   b. Neonatal respiratory distress syndrome (hyaline membrane disease)
   c. Pneumoconioses (coal miner's, silicosis, asbestosis)
   d. Sarcoidosis: bilateral hilar lymphadenopathy, noncaseating granuloma; ↑ ACE and calcium.
   e. Idiopathic pulmonary fibrosis (repeated cycles of lung injury and wound healing with ↑ collagen)
   f. Goodpasture's syndrome
   g. Wegener's granulomatosis
   h. Eosinophilic granuloma (histiocytosis X)
   i. Drug toxicity (bleomycin, busulfan, amiodarone)

Pneumoconioses

Coal miner's	Associated with coal mines. Can result in cor pulmonale, Caplan's syndrome.	Affects upper lobes.
Silicosis	Associated with foundries, sandblasting, and mines. Macrophages respond to silica and release fibrogenic factors, leading to fibrosis. It is thought that silica may disrupt phagolysosomes and impair macrophages, increasing susceptibility to TB.	Affects upper lobes. "Eggshell" calcification of hilar lymph nodes.
Asbestosis	Associated with shipbuilding, roofing, and plumbing. Results in "ivory white," calcified pleural plaques. Associated with an ↑ incidence of bronchogenic carcinoma and mesothelioma (see Image 42).	Affects lower lobes. Asbestos bodies are golden-brown fusiform rods resembling dumbbells, located inside macrophages.

Neonatal respiratory distress syndrome	Surfactant deficiency leading to ↑ surface tension, resulting in alveolar collapse. Surfactant is made by type II pneumocytes most abundantly after 35th week of gestation. The lecithin-to-sphingomyelin ratio in the amniotic fluid, a measure of lung maturity, is usually < 1.5 in neonatal respiratory distress syndrome. Persistently low O_2 tension → risk of PDA. Therapeutic supplemental O_2 can result in retinopathy of prematurity. Surfactant—dipalmitoyl phosphatidylcholine. Risk factors: prematurity, maternal diabetes (due to elevated insulin), cesarean delivery (↓ release of fetal glucocorticoids). Treatment: maternal steroids before birth; artificial surfactant for infant; thyroxine.

Acute respiratory distress syndrome (ARDS)	May be caused by trauma, sepsis, shock, gastric aspiration, uremia, acute pancreatitis, or amniotic fluid embolism. Diffuse alveolar damage → ↑ alveolar capillary permeability → protein-rich leakage into alveoli. Results in formation of intra-alveolar hyaline membrane. Initial damage due to neutrophilic substances toxic to alveolar wall, activation of coagulation cascade, or oxygen-derived free radicals (see Image 39).

Obstructive vs. restrictive lung disease

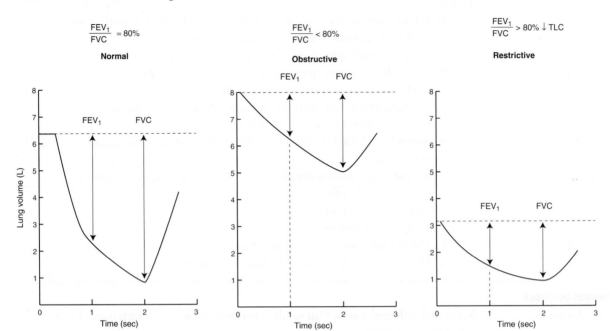

Note: Obstructive lung volumes > normal (↑ TLC, ↑ FRC, ↑ RV); restrictive lung volumes < normal. In both obstructive and restrictive, FEV_1 and FVC are reduced, but in obstructive, FEV_1 is more dramatically reduced, resulting in a ↓ FEV_1/FVC ratio.

| Sleep apnea | Person stops breathing for at least 10 seconds repeatedly during sleep. **Central sleep apnea**—no respiratory effort. **Obstructive sleep apnea**—respiratory effort against airway obstruction. Associated with obesity, loud snoring, systemic/pulmonary hypertension, arrhythmias, and possibly sudden death. Individuals may become chronically tired. | Treatment: weight loss, CPAP, surgery. Hypoxia → ↑ EPO release → ↑ erythrocytosis. |

Lung—physical findings

Abnormality	Breath Sounds	Resonance	Fremitus	Tracheal Deviation
Bronchial obstruction	Absent/↓ over affected area	↓	↓	Toward side of lesion
Pleural effusion	↓ over effusion	Dullness	↓	—
Pneumonia (lobar)	May have bronchial breath sounds over lesion	Dullness	↑	—
Tension pneumothorax	↓	Hyperresonant	Absent	Away from side of lesion (see Image 40)

Lung cancer

Lung cancer is the leading cause of cancer death. Presentation: cough, hemoptysis, bronchial obstruction, wheezing, pneumonic "coin" lesion on x-ray film or noncalcified nodule on CT. Metastases to lung is most common, often from breast, colon, prostate, and bladder cancer. Sites of metastases—adrenals, brain (epilepsy), bone (pathologic fracture), liver (jaundice, hepatomegaly).

SPHERE of complications:
Superior vena cava syndrome
Pancoast's tumor
Horner's syndrome
Endocrine (paraneoplastic)
Recurrent laryngeal symptoms (hoarseness)
Effusions (pleural or pericardial)

Type	Location	Characteristics	Histology
Squamous cell carcinoma (Squamous Sentral Smoking)	Central	Hilar mass arising from bronchus; Cavitation; Clearly linked to Smoking; parathyroid-like activity → PTHrP.	Keratin pearls and intercellular bridges.
Adenocarcinoma: Bronchial Bronchioloalveolar	Peripheral	Develops in site of prior pulmonary inflammation or injury (most common lung cancer in nonsmokers and females). Not linked to smoking; grows along airways; can present like pneumonia. Can result in hypertrophic osteoarthropathy.	Both types: Clara cells → type II pneumocytes; multiple densities on x-ray of chest.
Small cell (oat cell) carcinoma	Central	Undifferentiated → very aggressive; often associated with ectopic production of ACTH or ADH; may lead to Lambert-Eaton syndrome (autoantibodies against calcium channels). Responsive to chemotherapy. Inoperable.	Neoplasm of neuroendocrine Kulchitsky cells → small dark blue cells (see Image 37).
Large cell carcinoma	Peripheral	Highly anaplastic undifferentiated tumor; poor prognosis; less responsive to chemotherapy. Removed surgically.	Pleomorphic giant cells with leukocyte fragments in cytoplasm.
Carcinoid tumor	—	Secretes serotonin, can cause carcinoid syndrome (flushing, diarrhea, wheezing, salivation). Fibrous deposits in right heart valves may lead to tricuspid insufficiency, pulmonary stenosis, and right heart failure.	—
Mesothelioma	Pleural	Malignancy of the pleura associated with asbestosis. Results in hemorrhagic pleural effusions and pleural thickening.	Psammoma bodies.

Pancoast's tumor

Carcinoma that occurs in apex of lung and may affect cervical sympathetic plexus, causing Horner's syndrome.

Horner's syndrome—ptosis, miosis, anhidrosis.

Pneumonia

Type	Organism(s)	Characteristics
Lobar	Pneumococcus most frequently, *Klebsiella*	Intra-alveolar exudate → consolidation; may involve entire lung
Bronchopneumonia	*S. aureus, H. flu, Klebsiella, S. pyogenes*	Acute inflammatory infiltrates from bronchioles into adjacent alveoli; patchy distribution involving ≥ 1 lobes (see Image 107).
Interstitial (atypical) pneumonia	Viruses (RSV, adenoviruses), *Mycoplasma, Legionella, Chlamydia*	Diffuse patchy inflammation localized to interstitial areas at alveolar walls; distribution involving ≥ 1 lobes. Generally follows a more indolent course than bronchopneumonia.

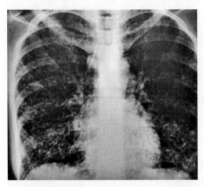

Interstitial pneumonia

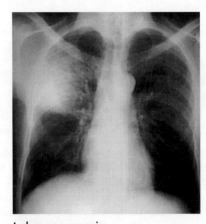

Lobar pneumonia

Lung abscess	Localized collection of pus within parenchyma, usually resulting from bronchial obstruction (e.g., cancer) or aspiration of oropharyngeal contents (especially in patients predisposed to loss of consciousness, e.g., alcoholics or epileptics). Often due to *S. aureus* or anaerobes.

Pleural effusions

Transudate	↓ protein content. Due to CHF, nephrotic syndrome, or hepatic cirrhosis.
Exudate	↑ protein content, cloudy. Due to malignancy, pneumonia, collagen vascular disease, trauma (occurs in states of ↑ vascular permeability). Must be drained in light of risk of infection.
Lymphatic	Milky fluid; ↑ triglycerides.

▶ RESPIRATORY–PHARMACOLOGY

H₁ blockers	Reversible inhibitors of H_1 histamine receptors.
1st generation	Diphenhydramine, dimenhydrinate, chlorpheniramine.
Clinical uses	Allergy, motion sickness, sleep aid.
Toxicity	Sedation, antimuscarinic, anti-α-adrenergic.
2nd generation	Loratadine, fexofenadine, desloratadine, cetirizine.
Clinical uses	Allergy.
Toxicity	Far less sedating than 1st generation because of ↓ entry into CNS.

Asthma drugs	Bronchoconstriction is mediated by (1) inflammatory processes and (2) sympathetic tone; therapy is directed at these 2 pathways.
Nonspecific β-agonists	**Isoproterenol**—relaxes bronchial smooth muscle (β_2). Adverse effect is tachycardia (β_1).
β_2-agonists	**Albuterol**—relaxes bronchial smooth muscle (β_2). Use during acute exacerbation.
	Salmeterol—long-acting agent for prophylaxis. Adverse effects are tremor and arrhythmia.
Methylxanthines	**Theophylline**—likely causes bronchodilation by inhibiting phosphodiesterase, thereby ↓ cAMP hydrolysis. Usage is limited because of narrow therapeutic index (cardiotoxicity, neurotoxicity); metabolized by P-450. Blocks actions of adenosine.
Muscarinic antagonists	**Ipratropium**—competitive block of muscarinic receptors, preventing bronchoconstriction. Also used for COPD.
Cromolyn	Prevents release of mediators from mast cells. Effective only for the prophylaxis of asthma. Not effective during an acute asthmatic attack. Toxicity is rare.
Corticosteroids	**Beclomethasone, prednisone**—inhibit the synthesis of virtually all cytokines. Inactivate NF-κB, the transcription factor that induces the production of TNF-α, among other inflammatory agents. 1st-line therapy for chronic asthma.
Antileukotrienes	**Zileuton**—A 5-lipoxygenase pathway inhibitor. Blocks conversion of arachidonic acid to leukotrienes.
	Zafirlukast, montelukast—block leukotriene receptors. Especially good for aspirin-induced asthma.

Treatment strategies in asthma

(Adapted, with permission, from Katzung BG, Trevor AJ. *Pharmacology: Examination & Board Review,* 5th ed. Stamford, CT: Appleton & Lange, 1998: 159 and 161.)

Expectorants

Guaifenesin — Expectorant—removes excess sputum; does not suppress cough reflex.

N-acetylcysteine — Mucolytic—can loosen mucous plugs in CF patients. Also used as an antidote for acetaminophen overdose.

Bosentan — Used to treat pulmonary hypertension. Competitively antagonizes endothelin-1 receptors, decreasing pulmonary vascular resistance.

Rapid Review

The following tables represent a collection of high-yield associations of diseases with their clinical findings and pathophysiology. They serve as a quick review before the exam to tune your senses to commonly tested cases and "buzzwords."

▶ Classic Presentations

▶ Classic Labs/Findings

▶ Key Associations

▶ Equation Review

Clinical presentation	Diagnosis/disease
Abdominal pain, ascites, hepatomegaly	Budd-Chiari syndrome (posthepatic venous thrombosis)
Achilles tendon xanthoma	Familial hypercholesterolemia
Adrenal hemorrhage, hypotension, DIC	Waterhouse-Friderichsen syndrome (meningococcemia)
Arachnodactyly, lens dislocation, aortic dissection, hyperflexible joints	Marfan's syndrome (fibrillin defect)
Athlete with polycythemia	Erythropoietin injection
Back pain, fever, night sweats, weight loss	Pott's disease (vertebral tuberculosis)
Bilateral hilar adenopathy, uveitis	Sarcoidosis (noncaseating granulomas)
Blue sclera	Osteogenesis imperfecta (collagen defect)
Bluish line on gingiva	Burton's line (lead poisoning)
Bone pain, bone enlargement, arthritis	Paget's disease of bone ($\uparrow$ osteoblastic and osteoclastic activity)
Bounding pulses, diastolic heart murmur, head bobbing	Aortic regurgitation
Café-au-lait spots, Lisch nodules (iris hamartoma)	Neurofibromatosis type I (+ pheochromocytoma, optic gliomas) Neurofibromatosis type II (+ bilateral acoustic neuromas)
Café-au-lait spots, polyostotic fibrous dysplasia, precocious puberty	McCune-Albright syndrome (mosaic G-protein signaling mutation)
Calf pseudohypertrophy	Muscular dystrophy (most commonly Duchenne's)
"Cherry-red spot" on macula	Tay-Sachs (ganglioside accumulation) or Niemann-Pick (sphingomyelin accumulation), central retinal artery occlusion
Chest pain, pericardial effusion/friction rub, persistent fever following MI	Dressler's syndrome (autoimmune-mediated post-MI fibrinous pericarditis, 1–12 weeks after acute episode)
Child uses arms to stand up from squat	Gowers' sign (Duchenne muscular dystrophy: X-linked recessive deleted dystrophin gene)
Child with fever develops red rash on face that spreads to body	"Slapped cheeks" (erythema infectiosum/fifth disease: parvovirus B19)
Chorea, dementia, caudate degeneration	Huntington's disease (autosomal-dominant CAG repeat expansion)
Chronic exercise intolerance with myalgia, fatigue, painful cramps	McArdle's disease (muscle phosphorylase deficiency)
Cold intolerance	Hypothyroidism
Conjugate lateral gaze palsy, horizontal diplopia	Internuclear ophthalmoplegia (damage to MLF; bilateral [multiple sclerosis], unilateral [stroke])
Continuous "machinery" heart murmur	PDA (close with indomethacin; open with misoprostol)
Cutaneous/dermal edema due to connective tissue deposition	Myxedema (hypothyroidism, Graves' disease)
Dark purple skin/mouth nodules	Kaposi's sarcoma (usually AIDS patients [gay men]: associated with HHV-8)

Deep, labored breathing/hyperventilation	Kussmaul breathing (diabetic ketoacidosis)
Dermatitis, dementia, diarrhea	Pellagra (niacin [vitamin B_3] deficiency)
Dilated cardiomyopathy, edema, polyneuropathy	Wet beriberi (thiamine [vitamin B_1] deficiency)
Dog or cat bite resulting in infection	*Pasteurella multocida* (cellulitis at inoculation site)
Dry eyes, dry mouth, arthritis	Sjögren's syndrome (autoimmune destruction of exocrine glands)
Dysphagia (esophageal webs), glossitis, iron deficiency anemia	Plummer-Vinson syndrome (may progress to esophageal squamous cell carcinoma)
Elastic skin, hypermobility of joints	Ehlers-Danlos syndrome (collagen defect, usually type III)
Enlarged, hard left supraclavicular node	Virchow's node (abdominal metastasis)
Erythroderma, lymphadenopathy, hepatosplenomegaly, atypical T cells	Sézary syndrome (cutaneous T-cell lymphoma) or mycosis fungoides
Facial muscle spasm upon tapping	Chvostek's sign (hypocalcemia)
Fat, female, forty, and fertile	Acute cholecystitis (bile duct blockage)
Fever, chills, headache, myalgia following antibiotic treatment for syphilis	Jarisch-Herxheimer reaction (rapid lysis of spirochetes results in toxin release)
Fever, cough, conjunctivitis, coryza, diffuse rash	Measles (Morbillivirus)
Fever, night sweats, weight loss	B symptoms (lymphoma)
Fibrous plaques in soft tissue of penis	Peyronie's disease (connective tissue disorder)
Gout, mental retardation, self-mutilating behavior in a boy	Lesch-Nyhan syndrome (HGPRT deficiency, X-linked recessive)
Green-yellow rings around peripheral cornea	Kayser-Fleischer rings (copper accumulation from Wilson's disease)
Hamartomatous GI polyps, hyperpigmentation of mouth/feet/hands	Peutz-Jeghers syndrome (genetic benign polyposis can cause bowel obstruction; ↑ cancer risk)
Hepatosplenomegaly, osteoporosis, neurologic symptoms	Gaucher's disease (glucocerebrosidase deficiency)
Hereditary nephritis, sensorineural hearing loss, cataracts	Alport's syndrome (type IV collagen mutation)
Hypercoagulability (leading to migrating DVTs and vasculitis)	Trousseau's sign (adenocarcinoma of pancreas or lung)
Hyperphagia, hypersexuality, hyperorality, hyperdocility	Klüver-Bucy syndrome (bilateral amygdala lesion)
Hypertension, hypokalemia, metabolic acidosis	Conn's syndrome (1° hyperaldosteronism)
Hypoxemia, polycythemia, hypercapnia	"Blue bloater" (chronic bronchitis: hyperplasia of mucous cells)
Indurated, ulcerated genital lesion	Nonpainful: chancre (1° syphilis, *Treponema pallidum*) Painful, with exudate: chancroid (*Haemophilus ducreyi*)

Infant with failure to thrive, hepatosplenomegaly, neurodegeneration	Niemann-Pick disease (genetic sphingomyelinase deficiency)
Infant with hypoglycemia, failure to thrive, and hepatomegaly	Cori's disease (debranching enzyme deficiency)
Infant with microcephaly, rocker-bottom feet, clenched hands, and structural heart defect	Edwards' syndrome (trisomy 18)
Jaundice, RUQ pain, fever	Charcot's triad 2 (ascending cholangitis)
Keratin pearls on a skin biopsy	Squamous cell carcinoma
Large rash with bull's-eye appearance	Erythema chronicum migrans from *Ixodes* tick bite (Lyme disease: *Borrelia*)
Lucid interval after traumatic brain injury	Epidural hematoma (middle meningeal artery rupture)
Male child, recurrent infections, no mature B cells	Bruton's disease (X-linked agammaglobulinemia)
Mucosal bleeding and prolonged bleeding time	Glanzmann's thrombasthenia (defect in platelet aggregation due to lack of GpIIb/IIIa)
Multiple colon polyps, osteomas/soft tissue tumors, impacted/supernumerary teeth	Gardner's syndrome (subtype of FAP)
Necrotizing vasculitis (lungs) and necrotizing glomerulonephritis	Wegener's (c-ANCA positive) and Goodpasture's syndromes (anti–basement membrane antibodies)
Neonate with arm paralysis following difficult birth	Erb-Duchenne palsy (superior trunk [C5–C6] brachial plexus injury: "waiter's tip")
No lactation postpartum, absent menstruation, cold intolerance	Sheehan's syndrome (pituitary infarction)
Nystagmus, intention tremor, scanning speech, bilateral internuclear ophthalmoplegia	Multiple sclerosis
Oscillating slow/fast breathing	Cheyne-Stokes respirations (central apnea in CHF or ↑ intracranial pressure)
Painful blue fingers/toes, hemolytic anemia	Cold agglutinin disease (autoimmune hemolytic anemia caused by *Mycoplasma pneumoniae,* infectious mononucleosis)
Painful, pale, cold fingers/toes	Raynaud's syndrome (vasospasm in extremities)
Painful, raised red lesions on palms and soles	Osler's node (infective endocarditis)
Painless erythematous lesions on palms and soles	Janeway lesions (infective endocarditis)
Painless jaundice	Cancer of the pancreatic head obstructing bile duct
Palpable purpura, joint pain, abdominal pain (child)	Henoch-Schönlein purpura (IgA vasculitis affecting skin and kidneys)
Pancreatic, pituitary, parathyroid tumors	Wermer's syndrome (MEN 1)

Pink complexion, dyspnea, hyperventilation	"Pink puffer" (emphysema: centroacinar [smoking], panacinar [α_1-antitrypsin deficiency])
Polyuria, acidosis, growth failure, electrolyte imbalances	Fanconi's syndrome (proximal tubular reabsorption defect)
Positive anterior "drawer sign"	Anterior cruciate ligament (ACL) injury
Ptosis, miosis, anhidrosis	Horner's syndrome (sympathetic chain lesion)
Pupil accommodates but doesn't react	Argyll Robertson pupil (neurosyphilis)
Rapidly progressive leg weakness that ascends (following GI/upper respiratory infection)	Guillain-Barré syndrome (autoimmune acute inflammatory demyelinating polyneuropathy)
Rash on palms and soles	2° syphilis, Rocky Mountain spotted fever
Recurrent colds, unusual eczema, high serum IgE	Job's syndrome (hyper-IgE syndrome: neutrophil chemotaxis abnormality)
Red "currant jelly" sputum in alcoholic or diabetic patients	*Klebsiella pneumoniae*
Red, itchy, swollen rash of nipple/areola	Paget's disease of the breast (represents underlying neoplasm)
Red urine in the morning, fragile RBCs	Paroxysmal nocturnal hemoglobinuria
Renal cell carcinoma, hemangioblastomas, angiomatosis, pheochromocytoma	von Hippel–Lindau disease (dominant tumor suppressor gene mutation)
Resting tremor, rigidity, akinesia, postural instability	Parkinson's disease (nigrostriatal dopamine depletion)
Restrictive cardiomyopathy (juvenile form: cardiomegaly), exercise intolerance	Pompe's disease (lysosomal glucosidase deficiency)
Retinal hemorrhages with pale centers	Roth's spots (bacterial endocarditis)
Severe jaundice in neonate	Crigler-Najjar syndrome (congenital unconjugated hyperbilirubinemia)
Severe RLQ pain with rebound tenderness	McBurney's sign (appendicitis)
Short stature, ↑ incidence of tumors/leukemia, aplastic anemia	Fanconi's anemia (genetically inherited; often progresses to AML)
Single palm crease	Simian crease (Down syndrome)
Situs inversus, chronic sinusitis, bronchiectasis	Kartagener's syndrome (dynein defect affecting cilia)
Skin hyperpigmentation	Addison's disease (1° adrenocortical insufficiency of autoimmune or infectious etiology)
Slow, progressive muscle weakness in boys	Becker's muscular dystrophy (X-linked, defective dystrophin; less severe than Duchenne's)
Small, irregular red spots on buccal/lingual mucosa with blue-white centers	Koplik spots (measles)
Smooth, flat, moist white lesions on genitals	Condylomata lata (2° syphilis)
Splinter hemorrhages in fingernails	Bacterial endocarditis
"Strawberry tongue"	Scarlet fever, Kawasaki disease, toxic shock syndrome

Streak ovaries, congenital heart disease, horseshoe kidney	Turner syndrome (XO, short stature, webbed neck, lymphedema)
Sudden swollen/painful big toe joint, tophi	Gout/podagra (hyperuricemia)
Swollen gums, mucous bleeding, poor wound healing, spots on skin	Scurvy (vitamin C deficiency: can't hydroxylate proline/lysine for collagen synthesis)
Swollen, hard, painful finger joints	Osteoarthritis (osteophytes on PIP [Bouchard's nodes], DIP [Heberden's nodes])
Systolic ejection murmur (crescendo-decrescendo)	Aortic valve stenosis
Thyroid and parathyroid tumors, pheochromocytoma	Sipple's syndrome (MEN 2A)
Toe extension/fanning upon plantar scrape	Babinski's sign (UMN lesion)
Unilateral facial drooping involving forehead	Bell's palsy (LMN CN VII palsy)
Urethritis, conjunctivitis, arthritis in a male	Reiter's syndrome (reactive arthritis associated with HLA-B27)
Vascular birthmark (port-wine stain)	Hemangioma (benign, but associated with Sturge-Weber syndrome)
Vasculitis from exposure to endotoxin causing glomerular thrombosis	Shwartzman reaction (following second exposure to endotoxin)
Vomiting blood following esophagogastric lacerations	Mallory-Weiss syndrome (alcoholic and bulimic patients)
"Waxy" casts with very low urine flow	Chronic end-stage renal disease
WBC casts in urine	Acute pyelonephritis
Weight loss, diarrhea, arthritis, fever, adenopathy	Whipple's disease (*Tropheryma whippelii*)
"Worst headache of my life"	Subarachnoid hemorrhage

Lab/diagnostic finding	Diagnosis/disease
Anticentromere antibodies	Scleroderma (CREST)
Antidesmoglein (epithelial) antibodies	Pemphigus vulgaris (blistering)
Anti–glomerular basement membrane antibodies	Goodpasture's syndrome (glomerulonephritis and hemoptysis)
Antihistone antibodies	Drug-induced SLE (hydralazine, isoniazid, phenytoin, procainamide)
Anti-IgG antibodies	Rheumatoid arthritis (systemic inflammation, joint pannus, boutonnière deformity)
Antimitochondrial antibodies (AMAs)	1° biliary cirrhosis (female, cholestasis, portal hypertension)
Antineutrophil cytoplasmic antibodies (ANCAs)	Vasculitis (c-ANCA: Wegener's; p-ANCA: microscopic polyangiitis, Churg-Strauss syndrome)
Antinuclear antibodies (ANAs: anti-Smith and anti-dsDNA)	SLE (type III hypersensitivity)
Antiplatelet antibodies	Idiopathic thrombocytopenic purpura (ITP) (bleeding diathesis)
Anti-topoisomerase antibodies	Diffuse systemic scleroderma
Anti-transglutaminase/antigliadin/anti-endomysial antibodies	Celiac disease (diarrhea, distention, weight loss)
Azurophilic granular needles in leukemic blasts	Auer rods (acute myelogenous leukemia: especially the promyelocytic type)
"Bamboo spine" on x-ray	Ankylosing spondylitis (chronic inflammatory arthritis: HLA-B27)
Basophilic nuclear remnants in RBCs	Howell-Jolly bodies (due to splenectomy or nonfunctional spleen)
Basophilic stippling of RBCs	Lead poisoning or sideroblastic anemia
Bloody tap on LP	Subarachnoid hemorrhage
"Boot-shaped" heart on x-ray	Tetralogy of Fallot, RVH
Branching gram-positive rods with sulfur granules	*Actinomyces israelii*
Bronchogenic apical lung tumor	Pancoast's tumor (can compress sympathetic ganglion and cause Horner's syndrome)
"Brown" tumor of bone	Hemorrhage (hemosiderin) causes brown color of osteolytic cysts. Due to: 1. Hyperparathyroidism 2. Osteitis fibrosa cystica
Cardiomegaly with apical atrophy	Chagas' disease (*Trypanosoma cruzi*)
Cellular crescents in Bowman's capsule	Rapidly progressive crescentic glomerulonephritis
"Chocolate cyst" of ovary	Endometriosis (frequently involves both ovaries)
Circular grouping of dark tumor cells surrounding pale neurofibrils	Homer Wright rosettes (neuroblastoma, medulloblastoma, retinoblastoma)
Colonies of mucoid *Pseudomonas* in lungs	Cystic fibrosis (CFTR mutation in Caucasians resulting in fat-soluble vitamin deficiency and mucous plugs)

Degeneration of dorsal column nerves	Tabes dorsalis (3° syphilis)
Depigmentation of neurons in substantia nigra	Parkinson's disease (basal ganglia disorder: rigidity, resting tremor, bradykinesia)
Desquamated epithelium casts in sputum	Curschmann's spirals (bronchial asthma; can result in whorled mucous plugs)
Disarrayed granulosa cells in eosinophilic fluid	Call-Exner bodies (granulosa-theca cell tumor of the ovary)
Dysplastic squamous cervical cells with nuclear enlargement and hyperchromasia	Koilocytes (HPV: predisposes to cervical cancer)
Enlarged cells with intranuclear inclusion bodies	"Owl's-eye" appearance of CMV
Enlarged thyroid cells with ground-glass nuclei	"Orphan Annie" eye nuclei (papillary carcinoma of the thyroid)
Eosinophilic cytoplasmic inclusion in liver cell	Mallory bodies (alcoholic liver disease)
Eosinophilic cytoplasmic inclusion in nerve cell	Lewy body (Parkinson's disease)
Eosinophilic globule in liver	Councilman body (toxic or viral hepatitis, often yellow fever)
Eosinophilic inclusion bodies in cytoplasm of hippocampal nerve cells	Rabies virus (Lyssavirus)
Extracellular amyloid deposition in gray matter of brain	Senile plaques (Alzheimer's disease)
Giant B cells with bilobed nuclei with prominent inclusions ("owl's eye")	Reed-Sternberg cells (Hodgkin's lymphoma)
Glomerulus-like structure surrounding vessel in germ cells	Schiller-Duval bodies (yolk sac tumor)
"Hair-on-end" (crew-cut) appearance on x-ray	β-thalassemia, sickle cell anemia (extramedullary hematopoiesis)
hCG elevated	Choriocarcinoma, hydatidiform mole (occurs with and without embryo)
Heart nodules (inflammatory)	Aschoff bodies (rheumatic fever)
Heterophile antibodies	Infectious mononucleosis (EBV)
Hexagonal, double-pointed, needle-like crystals in bronchial secretions	Bronchial asthma (Charcot-Leyden crystals: eosinophilic granules)
High level of D-dimers	DVT, pulmonary embolism, DIC
Hilar lymphadenopathy, peripheral granulomatous lesion in middle or lower lung lobes (can calcify)	Ghon focus (1° TB: *Mycobacterium* bacilli)
"Honeycomb lung" on x-ray	Interstitial fibrosis
Hypersegmented neutrophils	Megaloblastic anemia (B_{12}, folate deficiency)

Hypochromic, microcytic anemia	Iron deficiency anemia, lead poisoning, thalassemia (HbF sometimes present)
Increased α-fetoprotein in amniotic fluid/ maternal serum	Anencephaly, spina bifida (neural tube defects)
Increased uric acid levels	Gout, Lesch-Nyhan syndrome, tumor lysis syndrome, loop and thiazide diuretics
Intranuclear eosinophilic droplet-like bodies	Cowdry type A bodies (HSV or yellow fever)
Iron-containing nodules in alveolar septum	Ferruginous bodies (asbestosis: ↑ chance of mesothelioma)
Large lysosomal vesicles in phagocytes, immunodeficiency	Chédiak-Higashi disease (congenital failure of phagolysosome formation)
Low serum ceruloplasmin	Wilson's disease (hepatolenticular degeneration)
"Lumpy-bumpy" appearance of glomeruli on immunofluorescence	Poststreptococcal glomerulonephritis (immune complex deposition of IgG and C3b)
Lytic ("hole-punched") bone lesions on x-ray	Multiple myeloma
Mammary gland ("blue-domed") cyst	Fibrocystic change of the breast
Monoclonal antibody spike	1. Multiple myeloma (called the M protein; usually IgG or IgA) 2. Monoclonal gammopathy of undetermined significance (MGUS; normal consequence of aging) 3. Waldenström's (M protein = IgM) macroglobulinemia 4. Primary amyloidosis
Monoclonal globulin protein in blood/urine	Bence Jones proteins (multiple myeloma [kappa or lambda Ig light chains in urine]), Waldenström's macroglobulinemia (IgM)
Mucin-filled cell with peripheral nucleus	Signet ring (gastric carcinoma)
Narrowing of bowel lumen on barium radiograph	"String sign" (Crohn's disease)
Needle-shaped, negatively birefringent crystals	Gout (hyperuricemia)
Nodular hyaline deposits in glomeruli	Kimmelstiel-Wilson nodules (diabetic nephropathy)
"Nutmeg" appearance of liver	Chronic passive congestion of liver due to right heart failure
"Onion-skin" periosteal reaction	Ewing's sarcoma (malignant round-cell tumor)
Periosteum raised from bone, creating triangular area	Codman's triangle on x-ray (osteosarcoma, Ewing's sarcoma, pyogenic osteomyelitis)
Podocyte fusion on EM	Minimal change disease (child with nephrotic syndrome)
Polished, "ivory-like" appearance of bone at cartilage erosion	Eburnation (osteoarthritis resulting in bony sclerosis)
Protein aggregates in neurons from hyperphosphorylation of protein tau	Neurofibrillary tangles (Alzheimer's disease and CJD)
Pseudopalisading tumor cells on brain biopsy	Glioblastoma multiforme
RBC casts in urine	Acute glomerulonephritis

Rectangular, crystal-like, cytoplasmic inclusions in Leydig cells	Reinke crystals (Leydig cell tumor)
Renal epithelial casts in urine	Acute toxic/viral nephrosis
Rhomboid crystals, positively birefringent	Pseudogout (calcium pyrophosphate dihydrate)
Rib notching	Coarctation of the aorta
Sheets of medium-sized lymphoid cells ("starry sky" appearance on histology)	Burkitt's lymphoma (t[8:14] c-*myc* activation, associated with EBV)
Silver-staining spherical aggregation of tau proteins in neurons	Pick bodies (Pick's disease: progressive dementia, similar to Alzheimer's)
"Soap bubble" in femur or tibia on x-ray	Giant cell tumor of bone (generally benign)
"Spikes" on basement membrane, "dome-like" endothelial deposits	Membranous glomerulonephritis (may progress to nephrotic syndrome)
Stacks of red blood cells	Rouleaux formation (high ESR, multiple myeloma)
Stippled vaginal epithelial cells	"Clue cells" (*Gardnerella vaginalis*)
"Tennis-racket"-shaped cytoplasmic organelles (EM) in Langerhans cells	Birbeck granules (histiocytosis X: eosinophilic granuloma)
Thrombi made of white/red layers	Lines of Zahn (arterial thrombus, layers of platelets/RBCs)
"Thumb sign" on lateral x-ray	Epiglottitis (*Haemophilus influenzae*)
Thyroid-like appearance of kidney	Chronic bacterial pyelonephritis
"Tram-track" appearance on LM	Membranoproliferative glomerulonephritis
Triglyceride accumulation in liver cell vacuoles	Fatty liver disease (alcoholic or metabolic syndrome)
WBCs that look "smudged"	CLL (almost always B cell; affects the elderly)
"Wire loop" glomerular appearance on LM	Lupus nephropathy
Yellow CSF	Xanthochromia (subarachnoid hemorrhage)

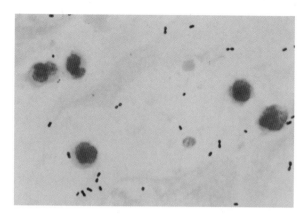

Image 1. *Streptococcus pneumoniae.* Sputum sample from a patient with pneumonia shows gram-positive diplococci.

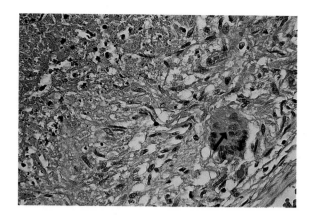

Image 2A. *Mycobacterium tuberculosis* is characterized by caseating granulomas containing Langhans' giant cells, which have a "horseshoe" pattern of nuclei (see arrow).*

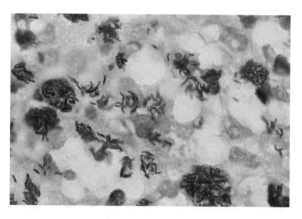

Image 2B. *Mycobacterium tuberculosis* organisms are identified by their red color on acid-fast staining ("red snappers").*

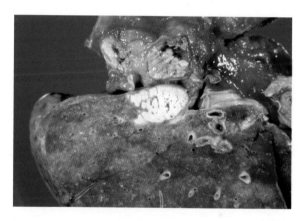

Image 2C. Miliary tuberculosis is seen here with large caseous lesions at the left medial upper lobe and miliary lesions in the surrounding hilar node. This life-threatening infection is caused by blood-borne dissemination of *Mycobacterium tuberculosis* to many organs from a quiescent site of infection.*

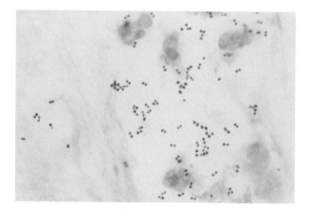

Image 3. *Staphylococcus aureus.* Sputum sample from another patient with pneumonia shows gram-positive cocci in clusters.

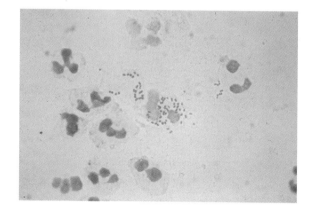

Image 4. *Neisseria gonorrhoeae.* Gram stain shows multiple gram-negative diplococci within polymorphonuclear leukocytes as well as in the extracellular areas of a smear from a urethral discharge. (Reproduced, with permission, from Wolff K et al. *Fitzpatrick's Color Atlas and Synopsis of Clinical Dermatology,* 5th ed. New York: McGraw-Hill, 2005: 906.)

*Images reproduced courtesy of the Pathology Education Instructional Resource Digital Library (http://peir.net) at the University of Alabama, Birmingham.

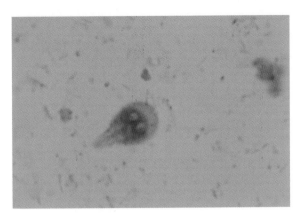

Image 5. *Giardia lamblia*, small intestine, microscopic. The trophozoite has a classic pear shape, with double nuclei giving an "owl's-eye" appearance.

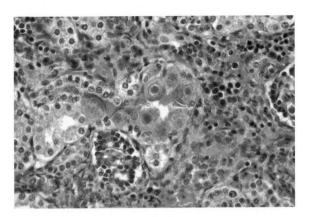

Image 6. Cytomegalovirus (CMV). Renal tubular cells in a neonate with congenital CMV infection show prominent Cowdry type A nuclear inclusions resembling owls' eyes. (Reproduced, with permission, from USMLERx.com.)

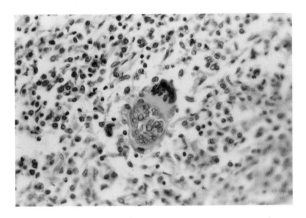

Image 7. Coccidioidomycosis. Endospores within a spherule in infected lung parenchyma. Initial infection usually resolves spontaneously, but when immunity is compromised, dissemination to almost any organ can occur. Endemic in the southwestern United States.

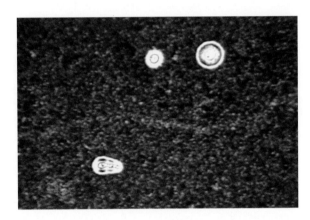

Image 8. *Cryptococcus neoformans*. The polysaccharide capsule is visible by India ink preparation in CSF from an AIDS patient with meningoencephalitis.*

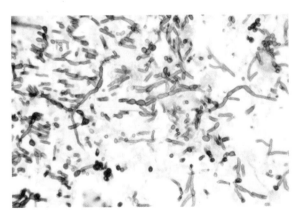

Image 9. *Candida albicans*. Silver stain preparation. Note the branched budding and pseudohyphae.*

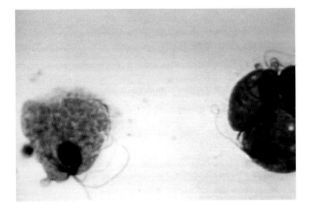

Image 10. *Trichomonas vaginalis* demonstrating trophozoites with flagellae.*

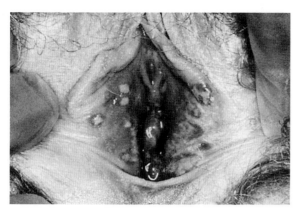

Image 11. Herpes genitalis. Ulcerating vesicles associated with HSV-2. (Reproduced, with permission, from De-Cherney AH. *Current Obstetric and Gynecologic Diagnosis and Treatment*, 9th ed. New York: McGraw-Hill, 2003: 664.)

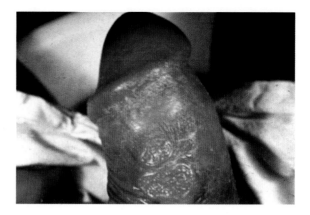

Image 12A. Syphilis. Chancre associated with primary syphilis. These ulcerative lesions are painless.*

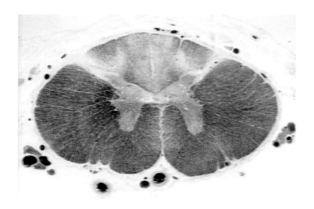

Image 12B. Syphilis. Tabes dorsalis resulting from progressive syphilis infection, thoracic spinal cord. Note degeneration of the dorsal columns and dorsal roots.*

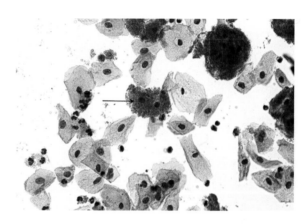

Image 13. Bacterial vaginosis. Arrow points to a clue cell. (Reproduced, with permission, from USMLERx.com.)

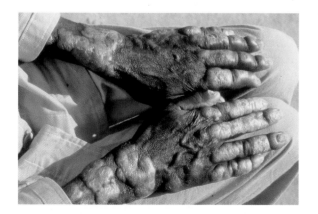

Image 14. Leprosy, lepromatous type. Note the nodules and thick plaques on the dorsa of the fingers, wrists, and forearms, with hypopigmentation of the overlying skin. Also note the symmetry of involvement and loss of tissue of several fingertips. (Reproduced, with permission, from Wolff K et al. *Fitzpatrick's Color Atlas and Synopsis of Clinical Dermatology*, 5th ed. New York: McGraw-Hill, Fig. 22-52.)

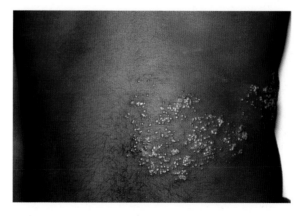

Image 15. Herpes zoster. Reactivation of virus spreads along the dermatomal distribution of infected nerves and can occur many years after initial infection. It is considered benign unless it affects an immunocompromised host or is a reinfection of the V_1 branch of the trigeminal nerve with eye/cornea involvement.*

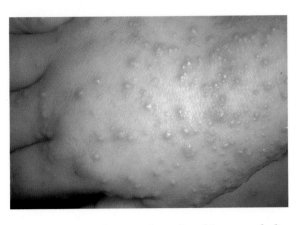

Image 16. Coxsackie exanthem (hand-foot-mouth disease). Diffuse eruptive vesiculopapules are seen on the hand of a three-year-old child. (Reproduced, with permission, from Hurwitz RM et al. *Pathology of the Skin: Atlas of Clinical-Pathological Correlation*, 2nd ed. Stamford, CT: Appleton & Lange, 1998.)

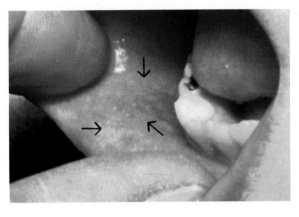

Image 17. Koplik spots. Pathognomonic for measles, Koplik spots appear as tiny white lesions with an erythematous halo, like "grains of sand." They precede the generalized rash by 1–2 days. (Reproduced, with permission, from Wolff K et al. *Fitzpatrick's Dermatology in General Medicine*, 7th ed. New York: McGraw-Hill, 2007, Fig. 192-1.)

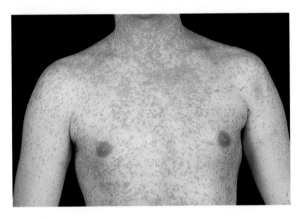

Image 18A. Rash of measles. Discrete erythematous lesions become confluent as the rash spreads downward. (Reproduced, with permission, from Fitzpatrick TB et al. *Fitzpatrick's Color Atlas and Synopsis of Clinical Dermatology*, 5th ed. New York: McGraw-Hill, 2001: 788.)

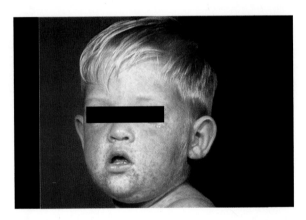

Image 18B. Rash of measles. In measles, rash often begins in the head and neck area.

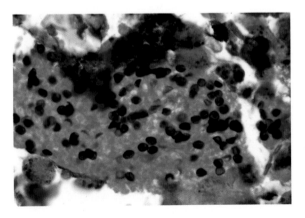

Image 19A. *Pneumocystis jiroveci* (formerly *carinii*). Special silver stain of lung epithelium shows numerous small, disk-shaped organisms. (Reproduced, with permission, from USMLERx.com.)

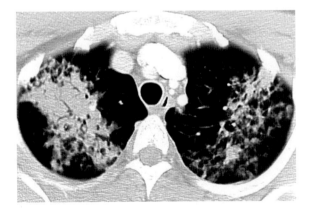

Image 19B. *Pneumocystis* pulmonary infection seen on CT chest image. Note the bilateral confluent air-space opacities in a central distribution.

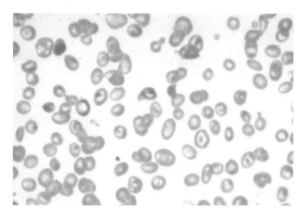

Image 20A. Target cells. Due to an increase in surface area–to-volume ratio from iron deficiency anemia (decreased cell volume) or in obstructive liver disease (increased cell membrane).*

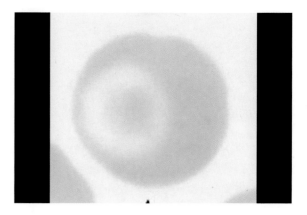

Image 20B. Target cell, solitary. Note the classic target-shaped appearance.

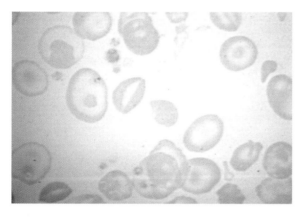

Image 21. Thalassemia major. A blood dyscrasia caused by a defect in β-chain synthesis in hemoglobin. Note the presence of target cells.*

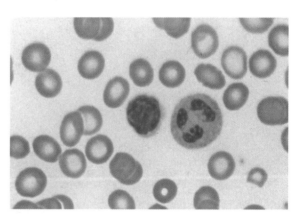

Image 22. Iron deficiency anemia. Microcytosis and hypochromia can be seen.

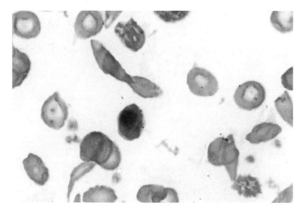

Image 23A. Sickle cell anemia. Sickle cell peripheral blood smear. Note the sickled cells as well as anisocytosis, poikilocytosis, and nucleated RBCs.*

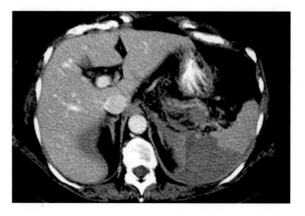

Image 23B. Sickle cell anemia. Splenic infarction. The splenic artery lacks collateral supply, making the spleen particularly susceptible to ischemic damage. Coagulative necrosis has occurred in a wedge shape. Individual sickle cells cause generalized splenic infarcts that result in autosplenectomy by adolescence.*

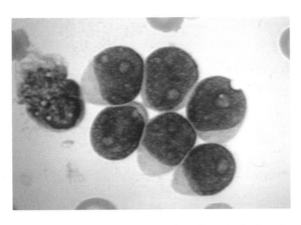

Image 24A. Leukemia. Acute lymphocytic leukemia, peripheral blood smear. Affects children less than 10 years of age.*

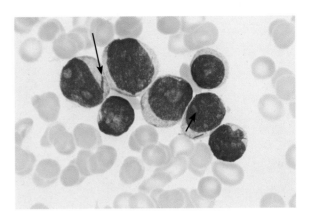

Image 24B. Leukemia. Acute myelocytic leukemia with Auer rods (long arrow), peripheral blood smear. Affects adolescents to young adults, but most commonly diagnosed in older adults.*

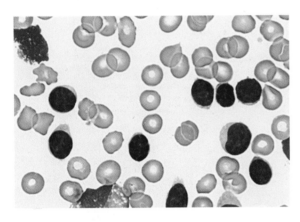

Image 24C. Leukemia. Chronic lymphocytic leukemia, peripheral blood smear. In CLL, the lymphocytes are excessively fragile. These lymphocytes are easily destroyed during slide preparation, forming "smudge cells." Affects individuals older than 60 years of age.*

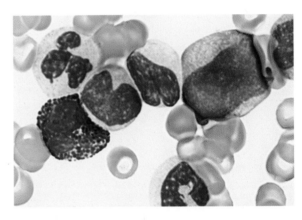

Image 24D. Leukemia. Chronic myeloid leukemia, peripheral blood smear. Promyelocytes and myelocytes are seen adjacent to a vascular structure. Affects individuals from 30 to 60 years of age.*

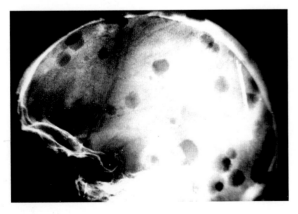

Image 25A. Multiple myeloma. Classic bone lytic lesions seen in multiple myeloma.*

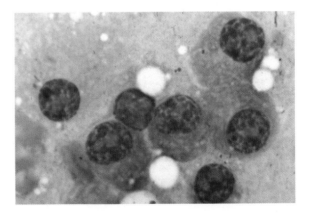

Image 25B. Multiple myeloma. Smears from a patient with multiple myeloma display an abundance of plasma cells. RBCs will often be seen in rouleaux formation, stacked like poker chips.*

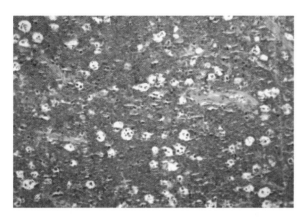

Image 26A. Burkitt's lymphoma. The classic "starry-sky" appearance from macrophage ingestion of tumor cells can be seen.*

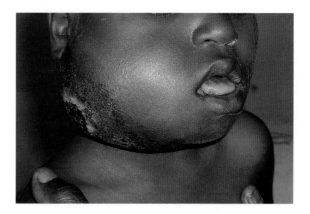

Image 26B. Burkitt's lymphoma. Young Nigerian boy with history of jaw swelling unresponsive to antibiotics.

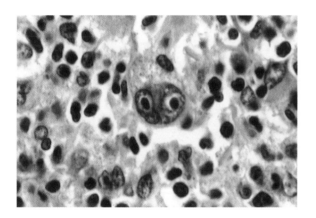

Image 27. Hodgkin's disease (Reed-Sternberg cells). Binucleate RS cells displaying prominent inclusion-like nucleoli surrounded by lymphocytes and other reacting inflammatory cells. The RS cell is a necessary but insufficient pathologic finding for the diagnosis of Hodgkin's disease.

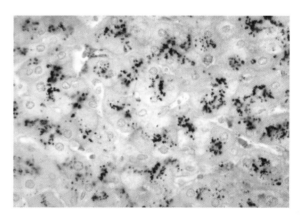

Image 28. Hemochromatosis with cirrhosis. Prussian blue iron stain shows hemosiderin in the liver parenchyma. Such deposition occurs throughout the body, causing organ damage and the characteristic darkening of the skin.*

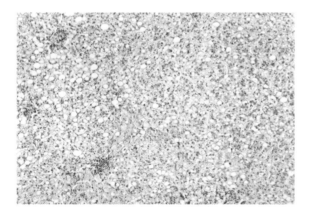

Image 29A. Fatty metamorphosis (macrovesicular steatosis) of the liver, microscopic. Early reversible change associated with alcohol consumption can be seen; there are abundant fat-filled vacuoles, but as yet there is no inflammation due to fibrosis of more serious alcoholic liver damage.*

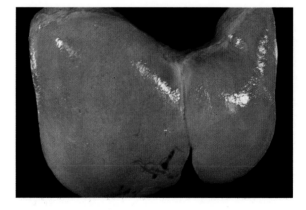

Image 29B. Fatty liver. Gross specimen showing enlarged yellow appearance.

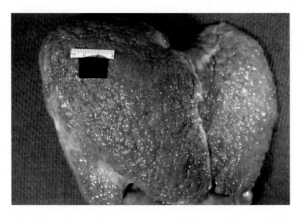

Image 30A. Cirrhosis. Micronodular cirrhosis of the liver, gross, from an alcoholic patient. The liver is approximately normal in size with a fine, granular appearance. Later stages of disease result in an irregularly shrunken liver with larger nodules, giving it a "hobnail" appearance.*

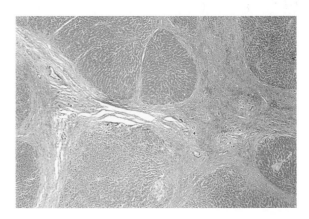

Image 30B. Cirrhosis, microscopic. Regenerative lesions are surrounded by fibrotic bands of collagen ("bridging fibrosis"), forming the characteristic nodularity.*

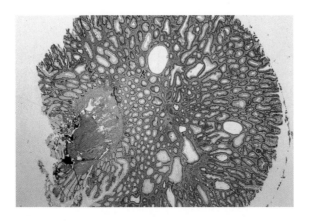

Image 31A. Colonic polyps. Tubular adenomas are smaller and rounded in morphology and have less malignant potential than do **villous adenomas**.

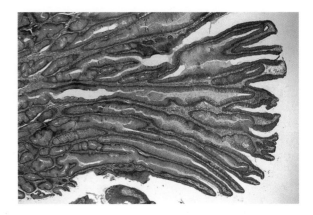

Image 31B. Villous adenomas are composed of long, fingerlike projections.

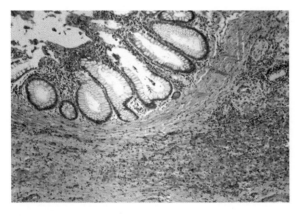

Image 32. Diverticulitis. Inflammation of the diverticula typically causes LLQ pain and can progress to perforation, peritonitis, abscess formation, or bowel stenosis. Note the presence of macrophages. Gut lumen is seen at the top of the photo.*

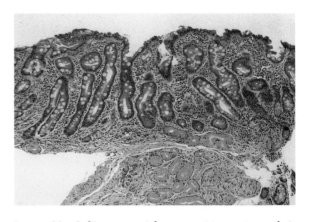

Image 33. Celiac sprue (gluten-sensitive enteropathy). Histology shows blunting of villi and crypt hyperplasia.

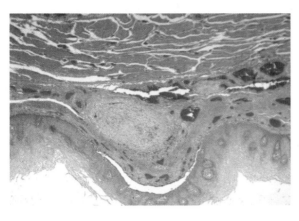

Image 34. Sclerosed **esophageal varix**. Overlying esophageal mucosa is generally normal.*

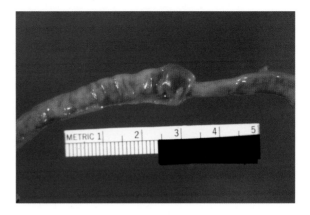

Image 35. **Intussusception** of infant gut, gross.*

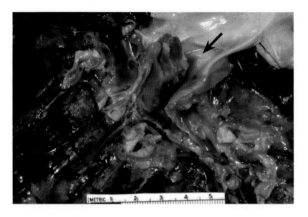

Image 36A. Pulmonary emboli. Pulmonary thromboembolus (arrow), gross. Most often arises from deep venous thrombosis.*

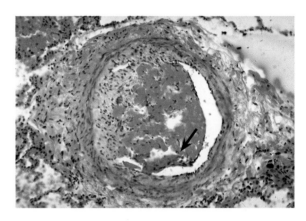

Image 36B. **Pulmonary thromboembolus** in a small muscular pulmonary artery. The interdigitating areas of pale pink and red within the organizing embolus form the "lines of Zahn" (arrow) characteristic of a thrombus. These lines represent layers of red cells, platelets, and fibrin that are laid down in the vessel as the thrombus forms.*

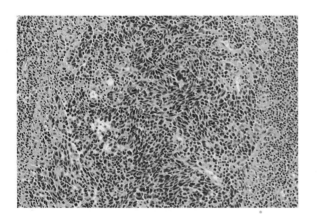

Image 37. **Small (oat) cell carcinoma** in a pulmonary hilar lymph node. Almost all of these tumors are related to tobacco smoking. They can arise anywhere in the lung, most often near the hilum, and quickly spread along the bronchi.*

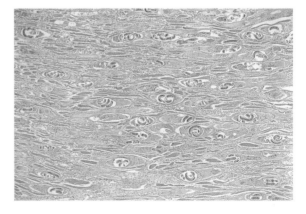

Image 38. *Taenia solium*, the pig tapeworm, infesting porcine myocardium. When humans ingest this meat, the larvae attach to the wall of the small intestine and mature to adult worms.

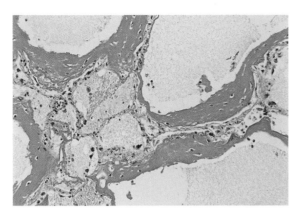

Image 39. Acute respiratory distress syndrome (ARDS). Persistent inflammation leads to poor pulmonary compliance and edema; note both alveolar fluid and hyaline membranes.

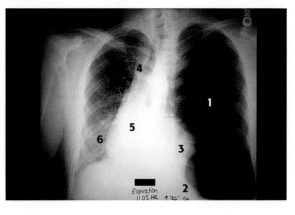

Image 40. Tension pneumothorax. Note these features: 1—Hyperlucent lung field; 2—Hyperexpansion lowers diaphragm; 3—Collapsed lung; 4—Deviation of trachea; 5—Mediastinal shift; 6—Compression of opposite lung.

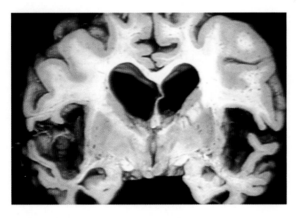

Image 41A. Alzheimer's disease. Key histologic features include "senile plaques" (not pictured); a coronal section showing atrophy, especially of the temporal lobes.*

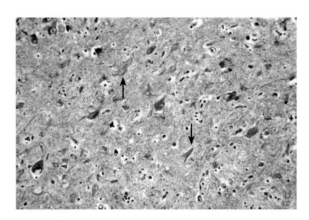

Image 41B. Focal masses of interwoven neuronal processes around an amyloid core; arrows mark neurofibrillary tangles).*

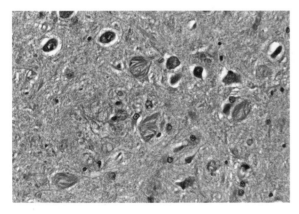

Image 41C. The remnants of neuronal degeneration are also associated with Alzheimer's disease, the most common cause of dementia in older persons.*

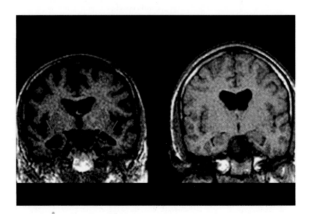

Image 41D. Alzheimer's disease. The T1-weighted coronal brain MRI image on the left demonstrates bilateral temporal lobe atrophy (arrows) as compared with normal appearance on the right.

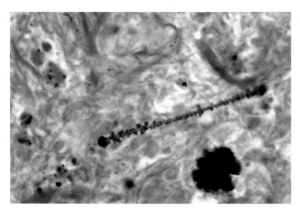

Image 42. Asbestosis. Ferruginous bodies (asbestos bodies with Prussian blue iron stain) in the lung, microscopic. Inhaled asbestos fibers are ingested by macrophages.*

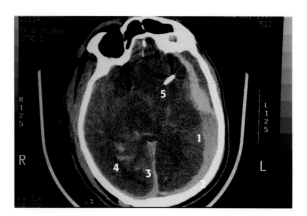

Image 43. Subdural hemorrhage. Note the hyperdense extra-axial blood on the left side. Concomitant subarachnoid hemorrhage. 1—subdural blood, layering; 2—skull; 3—falx; 4—subarachnoid blood; 5—shunt catheter; 6—frontal sinus.

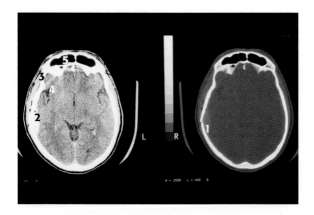

Image 44. Epidural hematoma from skull fracture. Note the lens-shaped (biconvex) dense blood next to the fracture. 1—skull fracture; 2—hematoma in epidural space; 3—temporalis muscle; 4—Sylvian fissure; 5—frontal sinus.

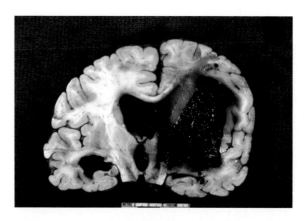

Image 45. Brain with **hypertensive hemorrhage** in the region of the left basal ganglia, gross.*

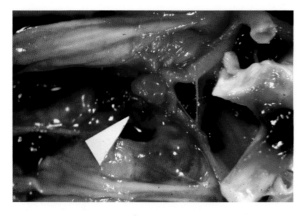

Image 46A. Berry aneurysm located on the anterior cerebral artery. The small, saclike structure can easily rupture during periods of hypertension or stress.*

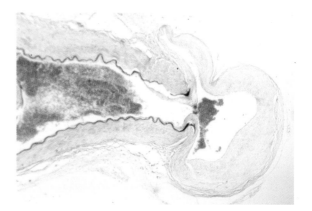

Image 46B. Berry aneurysm histologic section at the origin of the aneurysm shows lack of internal elastic lamina.*

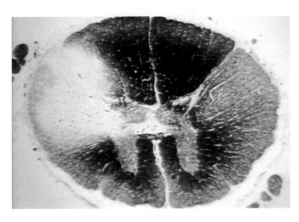

Image 47A. Multiple sclerosis. Lumbar spinal cord with mostly random and asymmetric white-matter lesions.*

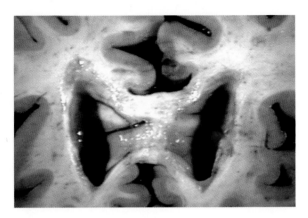

Image 47B. Multiple sclerosis. Brain with periventricular white-matter plaques of demyelination, gross. Demyelination occurs in a bilateral asymmetric distribution. Classic clinical findings are nystagmus, scanning speech, and intention tremor.*

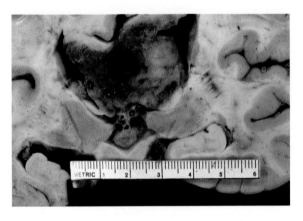

Image 48A. Glioblastoma multiforme extending across the midline of the cerebral cortex, gross.*

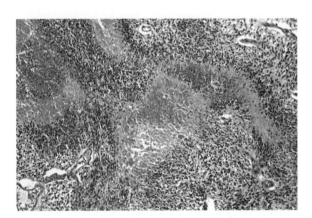

Image 48B. Glioblastoma multiforme. Histology shows necrosis with surrounding pseudopalisading of malignant tumor cells. (Reproduced, with permission, from USMLERx.com.)

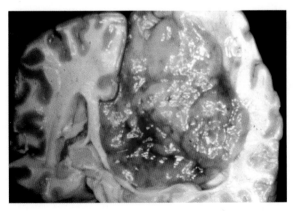

Image 49A. Oligodendroglioma. Gross natural-color coronal section of cerebral hemisphere with a large lesion of the left parieto-occipital white matter.*

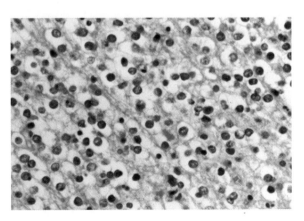

Image 49B. Oligodendroglioma. Classic "fried egg" appearance with perinuclear halos and "chicken-wire" capillary pattern.*

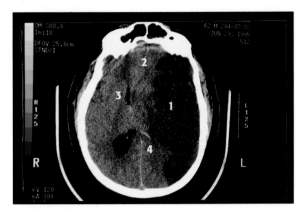

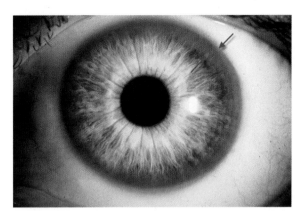

Image 50. Left middle cerebral artery stroke. Large left MCA territory stroke with edema and mass effect but no visible hemorrhage. The patient experienced deficits in speech and in the right side of the face and upper extremities. 1—ischemic brain parenchyma; 2—subtle midline shift to the right; 3—the right frontal horn of the lateral ventricle; 4—the left lateral ventricles obliterated by edema.

Image 51. Kayser-Fleischer ring in Wilson's disease. This corneal ring (between arrows) was golden brown and contrasted clearly against a gray-blue iris. Note that the darkness of the ring increases as the outer border (limbus) of the cornea is approached (right arrow).

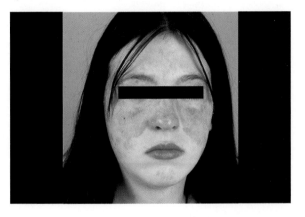

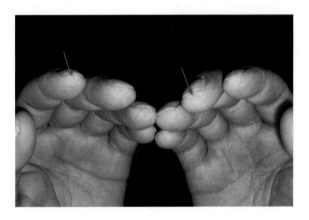

Image 52. Acute systemic lupus erythematosus. Bright red, sharply defined erythema is seen with slight edema and minimal scaling in a "butterfly pattern" on the face (the typical "malar rash"). Note also that the patient is female and young. (Reproduced, with permission, from Wolff K et al. *Fitzpatrick's Color Atlas and Synopsis of Clinical Dermatology*, 5th ed. New York: McGraw-Hill, 2005: 385.)

Image 53. Scleroderma. The progressive "tightening" of the skin has contracted the fingers. Also note ulceration of fingertips. Fibrosis is widespread and may also involve the esophagus (dysphagia), lung (restrictive disease), and small vessels of the kidney (hypertension).

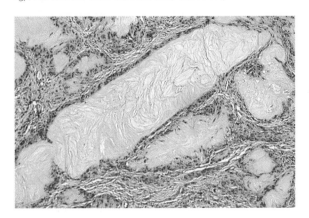

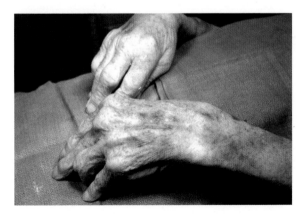

Image 54A. Gout. Tophi within joints consist of aggregates of urate crystals surrounded by an inflammatory reaction consisting of macrophages, lymphocytes, and giant cells. (Reproduced, with permission, from USMLERx.com.)

Image 54B. Gout. Tophi affect the proximal interphalangeal (PIP) joints, knees, and elbows, growing like tubers from the bones.*

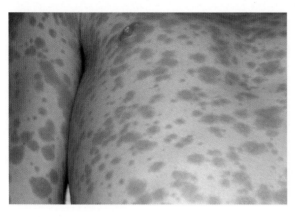

Image 55. Erythema multiforme. Erythematous macules and papules are seen. (Reproduced, with permission, from USMLERx.com.)

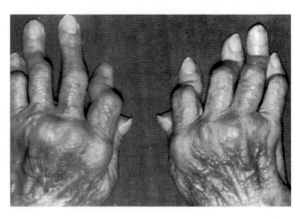

Image 56. Rheumatoid arthritis. Note the swan-neck deformities of the digits and severe, symmetric involvement of the PIP joints.

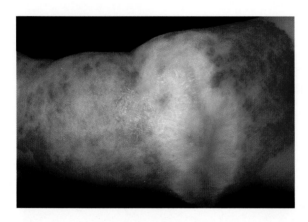

Image 57. Arteriovenous malformation. The markedly enlarged and distorted arm of a six-month-old boy with confluent erythematous papules and nodules. (Reproduced, with permission, from Hurwitz RM et al. *Pathology of the Skin: Atlas of Clinical-Pathological Correlation*, 2nd ed. Stamford, CT: Appleton & Lange, 1998.)

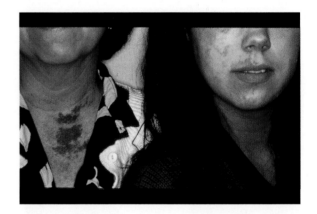

Image 58. Capillary malformation, port-wine type. Irregular purple patches and plaques are seen on the neck and chest of the mother, and pink patches are seen on the cheek, lip, chin, neck, and chest of the daughter. Both lesions were present at birth. (Reproduced, with permission, from Hurwitz RM et al. *Pathology of the Skin: Atlas of Clinical-Pathological Correlation*, 2nd ed. Stamford, CT: Appleton & Lange, 1998.)

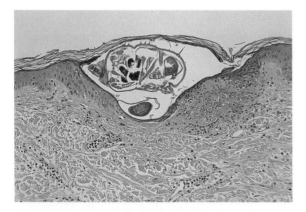

Image 59. Scabies. Adult female mite with egg containing embryo within the epidermis. (Reproduced, with permission, from Hurwitz RM et al. *Pathology of the Skin: Atlas of Clinical-Pathological Correlation*, 2nd ed. Stamford, CT: Appleton & Lange, 1998.)

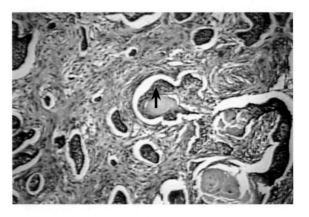

Image 60. Squamous cell carcinoma. Malignant skin tumor involving the epidermal skin layer. Note the presence of keratin pearls (arrows).*

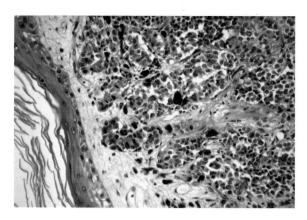

Image 61A. Malignant melanoma. Lesion just beneath the epidermis with pigmented and nonpigmented cells. The tumor cells are usually polyhedral but may be spindle shaped, dendritic, or ballooned or may resemble oat cells. Many but by no means all melanomas make melanin. Large nucleoli are common.*

Image 61B. Malignant melanoma. A multicolored tan, red, and dark brown irregular plaque. Note the "hazy," indefinite border and pigmentary variation. The depth of the lesion is a prognostic indicator.*

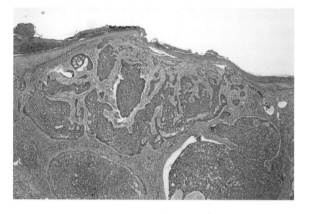

Image 62A. Basal cell carcinoma. Nests of basaloid cells are present within the dermis with peripheral palisading and prominent retraction artifacts. (Reproduced, with permission, from USMLERx.com.)

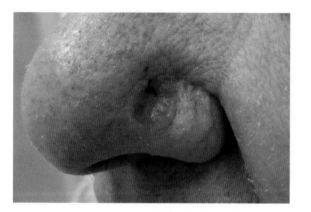

Image 62B. Basal cell carcinoma. Note the appearance of the small lesion on the nose.

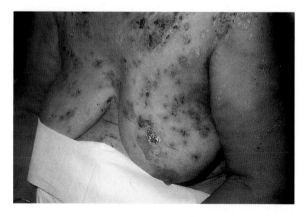

Image 63A. Pemphigus vulgaris. Numerous crusted, denuded, and weepy erythematous plaques are seen on the chest, breast, abdomen, and arms. (Reproduced, with permission, from Hurwitz RM et al. *Pathology of the Skin: Atlas of Clinical-Pathological Correlation*, 2nd ed. Stamford, CT: Appleton & Lange, 1998.)

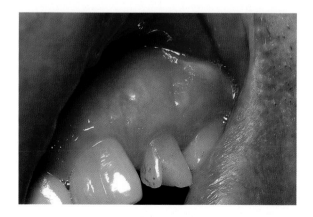

Image 63B. Pemphigus vulgaris. Vesicles on the gingiva. (Reproduced, with permission, from Hurwitz RM et al. *Pathology of the Skin: Atlas of Clinical-Pathological Correlation*, 2nd ed. Stamford, CT: Appleton & Lange, 1998.)

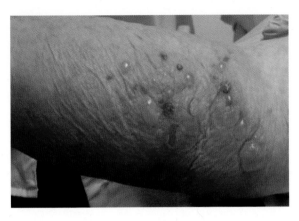

Image 64. Bullous pemphigoid. Note the tense bullae and urticarial plaques. (Reproduced, with permission, from USMLERx.com.)

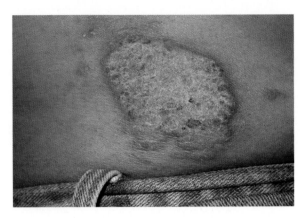

Image 65. Psoriasis. Note the well-demarcated, erythematous plaque with scale. (Reproduced, with permission, from USMLERx.com.)

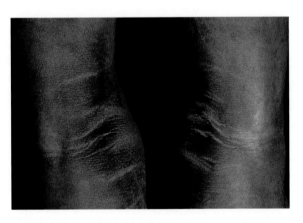

Image 66A. Acanthosis nigricans. Extensive hyperpigmented plaques on the arms in a patient with congenital lipodystrophy. This is an unusual distribution for acanthosis nigricans. (Reproduced, with permission, from Hurwitz RM et al. *Pathology of the Skin: Atlas of Clinical-Pathological Correlation*, 2nd ed. Stamford, CT: Appleton & Lange, 1998.)

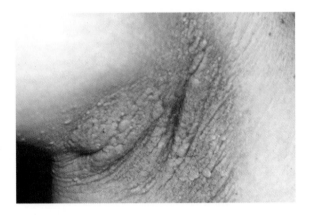

Image 66B. Acanthosis nigricans. Typical distribution at the underarm.

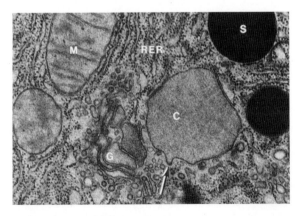

Image 67A. Pancreas. Pancreatic acinar cell (EM). A condensing vacuole (C) is receiving secretory product (arrow) from the Golgi complex (G). M—mitochondrion; RER—rough endoplasmic reticulum; S—mature condensed secretory zymogen granules.

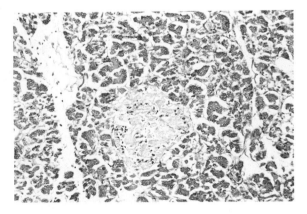

Image 67B. Pancreas. Pancreatic islet cells in **diabetes mellitus type 1.** In patients with diabetes mellitus type 1, autoantibodies against β cells cause a chronic inflammation until, over time, islet cells are entirely replaced by fibrosis.

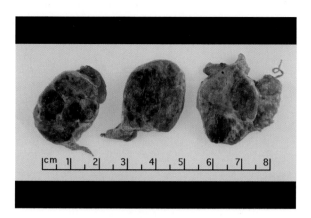

Image 68. Adrenocortical adenoma, gross. Cause of hypercortisolism (Cushing's syndrome) or hyperaldosteronism (Conn's syndrome).*

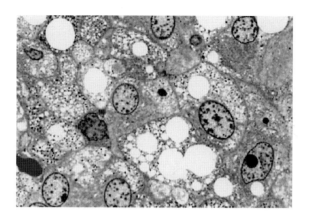

Image 69. Pheochromocytoma. The tumor cells have numerous vacuolar spaces within the cytoplasm (pseudoacini). Most of the punctate blue-black granules of variable density are dense-core neurosecretory granules.*

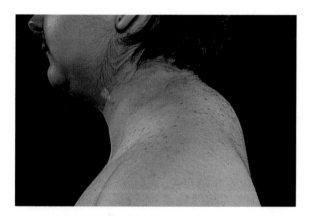

Image 70A. Cushing's disease. The clinical picture includes moon facies and buffalo hump.

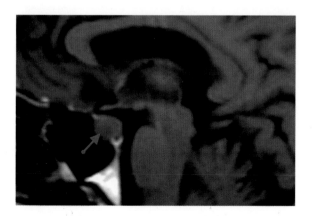

Image 70C. Cushing's disease. Sagittal T1-weighted MRI image showing a small pituitary mass (hormone-secreting). Note the accessibility to a transsphenoidal surgical approach.

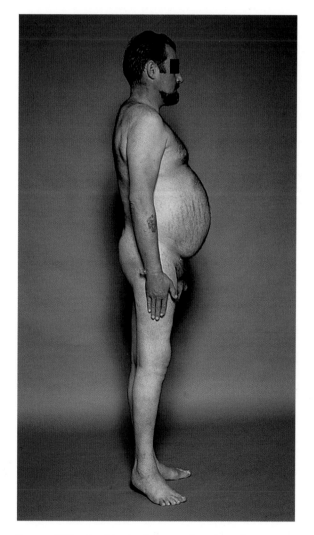

Image 70B. Cushing's disease. The clinical picture includes truncal obesity and abdominal striae.

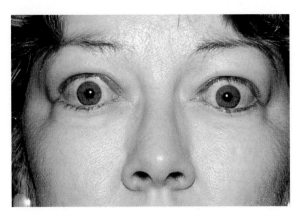

Image 71A. Graves' disease. Exophthalmos in a patient with proptosis and periorbital edema.*

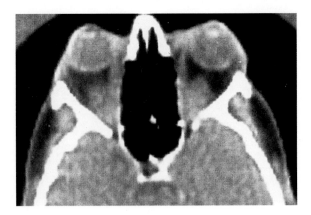

Image 71B. Graves' disease. CT shows extraocular muscle enlargement at the orbital apex.*

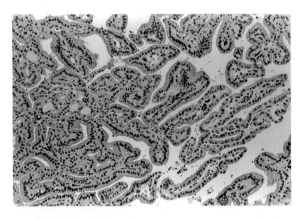

Image 71C. Graves' disease. Stimulation of follicular cells by autoantibodies that stimulate TSH receptors causes the normal uniform architecture to be replaced by hyperplastic papillary, involuted borders, and decreased colloid. Typical medical therapy is propylthiouracil, which inhibits the production of thyroid hormone as well as peripheral conversion of T_4 to T_3.*

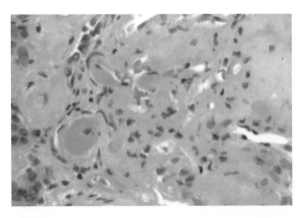

Image 72. Arteriolar sclerosis showing masses of hyaline material in glomerular afferent and efferent arterioles and in the glomerulus. From a type 1 diabetic patient.*

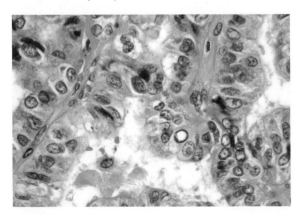

Image 73A. Papillary carcinoma. The image shows the papillary architecture and classic nuclear features that are key in making the diagnosis, including ground-glass or "Orphan Annie eye" chromatin, nuclear grooves, and intranuclear pseudoinclusions. Psammoma bodies are not seen here but are often present. (Reproduced, with permission, from USMLERx.com.)

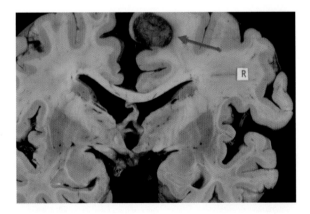

Image 73B. Papillary carcinoma. Metastatic solitary lesion seen on gross specimen in the coronal plane.

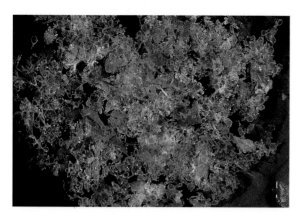

Image 74. Hydatidiform mole. The characteristic gross appearance is a "bunch of grapes." Hydatidiform moles are the most common precursors of choriocarcinoma. Complete moles usually display a 46,XX diploid pattern with all the chromosomes derived from the sperm. In partial moles, the karyotype is triploid or tetraploid, and fetal parts may be present.

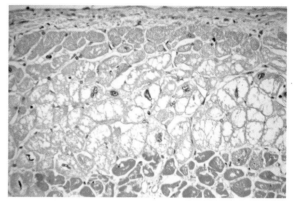

Image 75. Endocardial chronic ischemia. Microscopic example of myocytolysis and coagulation necrosis beneath the endocardium.*

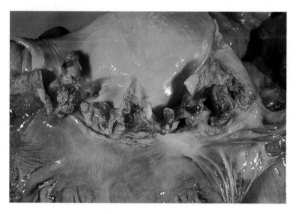

Image 76. Acute bacterial endocarditis. Virulent organisms (e.g., *Staphylococcus aureus*) infect previously normal valves, causing vegetations (here, in the aortic valve) and potentially giving rise to septic emboli.

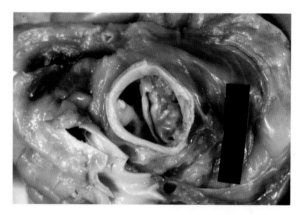

Image 77. Calcified **bicuspid aortic valve** showing false raphe. The abnormal architecture of the valve makes its leaflets susceptible to otherwise ordinary hemodynamic stresses, which ultimately leads to valvular thickening, calcification, increased rigidity, and stenosis.*

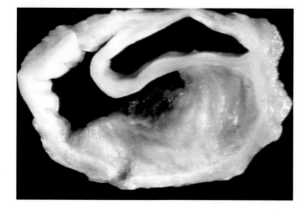

Image 78. Aortic dissection with a blood clot compressing the aortic lumen. A tear in the intima allowed blood to surge through the muscular layer to the adventitia (may lead to sudden death from hemothorax). Risk factors are hypertension, Marfan's syndrome, pregnancy, Ehlers-Danlos syndrome, and trauma.*

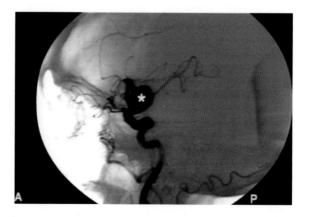

Image 79. Carotid angiogram showing aneurysm. Note the path of the internal carotid artery through the neck and its major branches (ophthalmic artery, anterior cerebral artery, middle cerebral artery). The aneurysm is inferior to the terminal branches in this angiogram.*

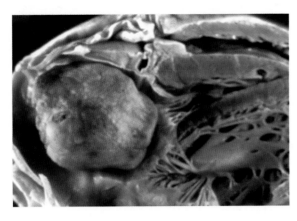

Image 80A. Left atrial myxoma. The most common primary cardiac tumor; known to produce VEGF (vascular endothelial growth factor).*

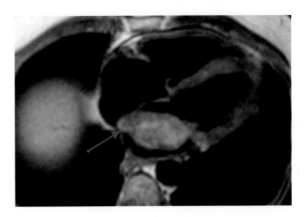

Image 80B. Left atrial myxoma. Axial T1-weighted cardiac MRI demonstrates ovoid mass attached to the interatrial septum.

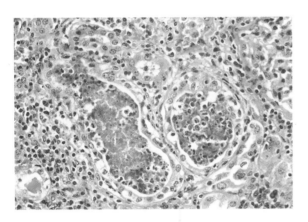

Image 81A. Acute pyelonephritis is characterized by neutrophilic infiltration and abscess formation within the renal interstitium. Abscesses may rupture, introducing collections of white cells to the tubular lumen.

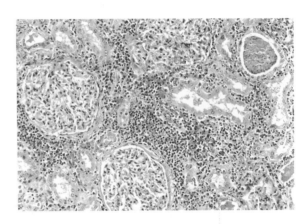

Image 81B. Chronic pyelonephritis has a lymphocytic invasion with fibrosis.

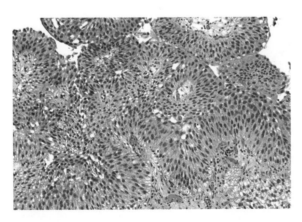

Image 82. Transitional cell carcinoma. The image shows a papillary growth lined by transitional epithelium with mild nuclear atypia and pleomorphism. (Reproduced, with permission, from USMLERx.com.)

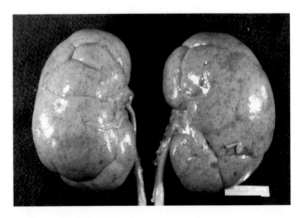

Image 83. Lupus erythematosus, kidneys. Enlarged, very pale kidneys with "flea bite" or ectasia from a patient with nephrotic syndrome or subacute glomerulonephritis as a result of lupus erythematosus.*

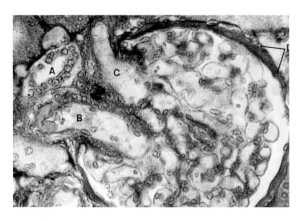

Image 84. Normal glomerulus, microscopic, with (A) macula densa and (B) afferent and (C) efferent arterioles.

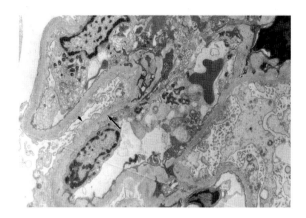

Image 85. Minimal change disease (lipoid nephrosis) shows normal glomeruli on light microscopy but effacement of foot processes on EM (arrowhead). The full arrow points to a normal foot process. Treatment consists of corticosteroids.

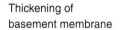

Thickening of basement membrane

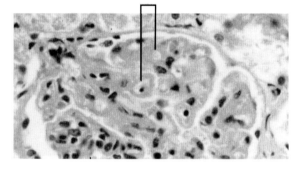

Image 86A. Systemic lupus erythematosus, kidney pathology. In the membranous glomerulonephritic pattern, "wire-loop" thickening occurs as a result of immune complex deposition. Associated with subendothelial deposits and mesangial hyercellularity.

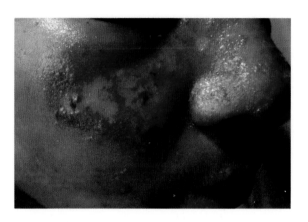

Image 86B. Systemic lupus erythematosus. Typical facial malar rash.

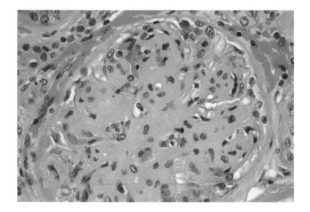

Image 87A. Diabetic glomerulosclerosis. Nodular diabetic glomerulosclerosis is also known as Kimmelstiel-Wilson syndrome and is characterized by acellular ovoid nodules in the periphery of the glomerulus. (Reproduced, with permission, from USMLERx.com.)

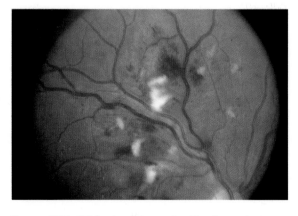

Image 87B. Diabetic retinopathy. Funduscopic image showing cotton wool spots and macular edema.

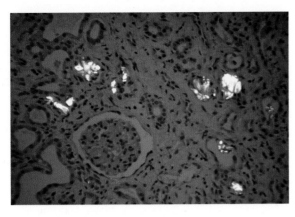

Image 88A. Calcium oxalate crystals in the kidney, viewed with partially crossed polarizers. Tubular failure in oxalate nephropathy can result from vitamin C or antifreeze abuse.*

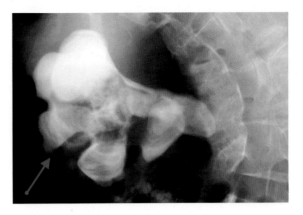

Image 88B. Calcium oxalate outlining a large right renal collecting system creating a "staghorn" calculus.

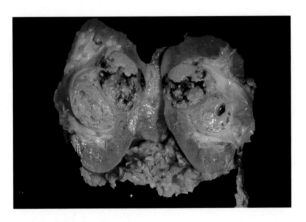

Image 89A. Renal cell carcinoma. Gross. The kidney has been bivalved, revealing a nodular, golden-yellow tumor in the midkidney with areas of hemorrhage and necrosis. (Reproduced, with permission, from USMLERx.com.)

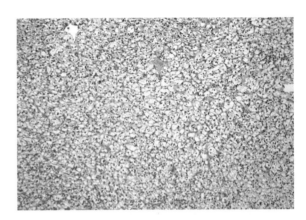

Image 89B. Renal cell carcinoma. Histology shows polygonal cells with small nuclei and abundant clear cytoplasm with a rich, delicate branching vasculature. (Reproduced, with permission, from USMLERx.com.)

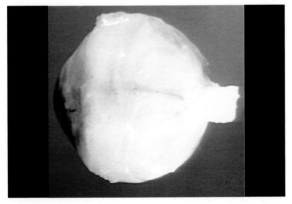

Image 90A. Osteogenesis imperfecta. Blue sclera caused by translucency of connective tissue over the choroid. The optic nerve is on the right side of the image.*

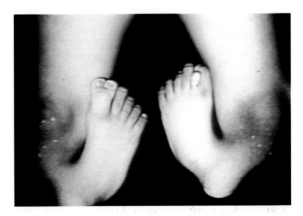

Image 90B. Osteogenesis imperfecta. Abnormal collagen synthesis results from a variety of gene mutations and causes brittle bones and connective tissue malformations.*

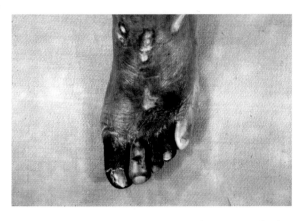

Image 91. Foot gangrene. The first four toes and adjacent skin are dry, shrunken, and blackened with superficial necrosis and peeling of the skin. A well-defined line of demarcation separates the black region from the viable skin.*

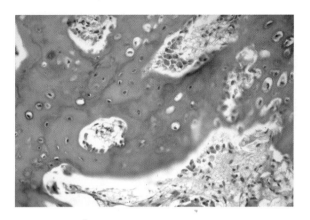

Image 92. Bone fracture. New bone formation with osteoblasts.*

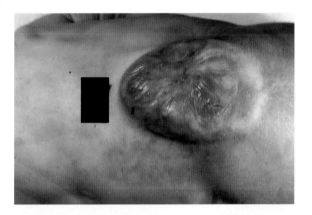

Image 93. Meningomyelocele. A neural tube defect in which the meninges and spinal cord herniate through the spinal canal; gross image of infant's lower back.*

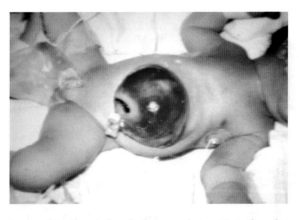

Image 94. Omphalocele in a newborn. Note that the defect is midline and is covered by peritoneum, as opposed to gastroschisis, which is not covered by peritoneum and is often not midline.*

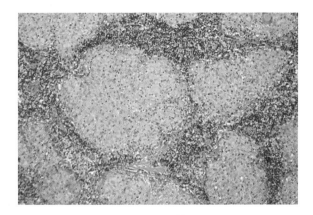

Image 95. Sarcoidosis. Numerous tightly formed granulomas are seen on histology of a lymph node in a patient with sarcoidosis. (Reproduced, with permission, from USMLERx.com.)

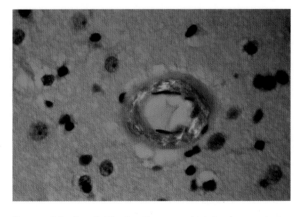

Image 96. Amyloidosis. Congo red stain demonstrates amyloid deposits in the artery wall that show apple-green birefringence under polarized light. (Reproduced, with permission, from USMLERx.com.)

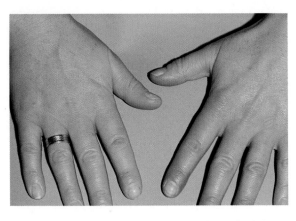

Image 97A. Raynaud's disease. The left hand exhibits a distal cyanosis compared to the right hand; it is seen especially well in the nail beds. Unilateral episodes such as this one may occur after contact with a cold object. (Reproduced, with permission, from Wolff K et al. *Fitzpatrick's Color Atlas and Synopsis of Clinical Dermatology*, 5th ed. New York: McGraw-Hill, 2005: 403.)

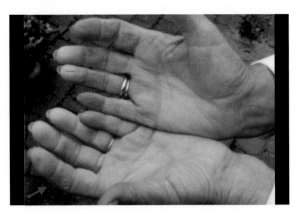

Image 97B. Raynaud's disease. Note the bilateral distal distribution of cyanosis.

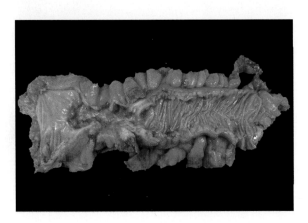

Image 98A. Colon cancer. Note the circumferential tumor with heaped-up edges and central ulceration. (Reproduced, with permission, from USMLERx.com.)

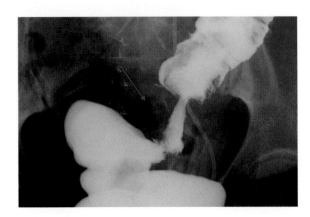

Image 98B. Colon cancer. Classic "apple-core" lesion of the sigmoid colon seen on barium enema. (Reproduced, with permission, from USMLERx.com.)

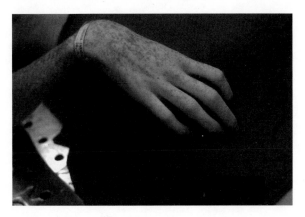

Image 99. Marfan's syndrome. Patients are tall with very long extremities. The joints are hyperextensible, with slim bone structure and wiry muscles.*

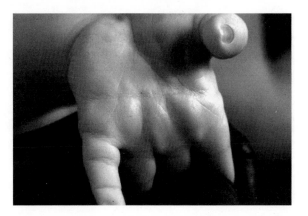

Image 100. Simian crease. A characteristic feature of Down syndrome (trisomy 21). The palm has a single transverse crease instead of the normal two creases.*

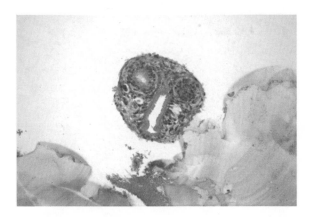

Image 101. Hydatid cyst. *Echinococcus* eggs develop into larvae in the intestine, penetrate the intestinal wall, and disseminate throughout the body. The larvae form hydatid cysts in the liver and, less commonly, in the lungs, kidney, and brain. (Reproduced, with permission, from USMLERx.com.)

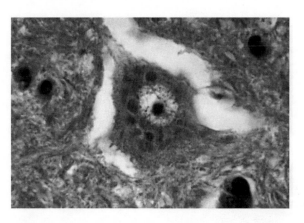

Image 102. Negri bodies are pathognomonic inclusions in the cytoplasm of neurons infected by the rabies virus. (Reproduced, with permission, from the Centers for Disease Control and Prevention, Atlanta, GA.)

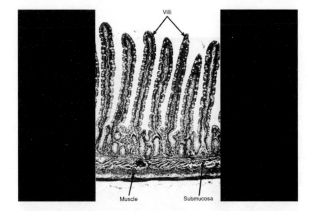

Image 103. Photomicrograph of the **small intestine.**

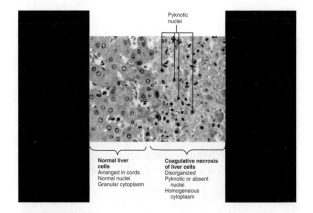

Image 104. Coagulative necrosis of hepatocytes.

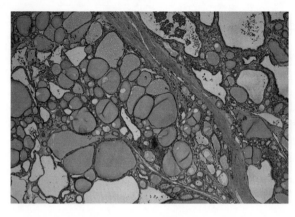

Image 105. Multinodular goiter with hyperplasia and subsequent involution of the thyroid gland. The image shows follicles distended with colloid and lined by a flattened epithelium with areas of fibrosis and hemorrhage. (Reproduced, with permission, from USMLERx.com.)

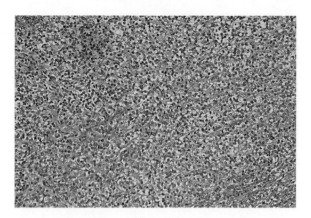

Image 106. Ewing's sarcoma. This malignant tumor of bone occurs in children and is characterized by the (11;22) translocation that results in the fusion gene EWS-FLI1. The tumor is composed of sheets of uniform small, round cells. (Reproduced, with permission, from USMLERx.com.)

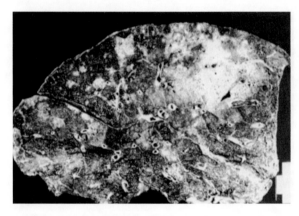

Image 107A. Pneumonia. Gross. Note the large area of consolidation at the base plus multiple small areas of consolidation (pale) involving bronchioles and surrounding alveolar sacs throughout the lung.

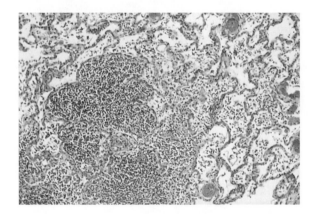

Image 107B. Pneumonia. "Bronchopneumonia" with neutrophils in alveolar spaces, microscopic.

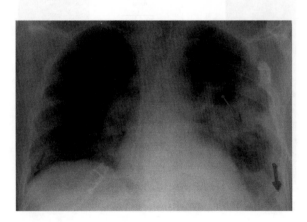

Image 107C. Cavitary pneumonia. Chest x-ray showing left-sided pneumonia with cavitation and bilateral pleural effusions. (Adapted, with permission, from A. Christaras.)

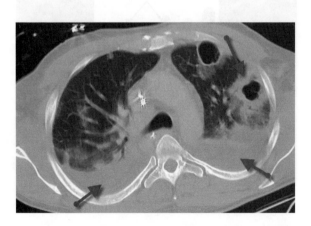

Image 107D. Cavitary pneumonia. Chest CT scan showing cavitary lesions with bilateral pleural effusions.

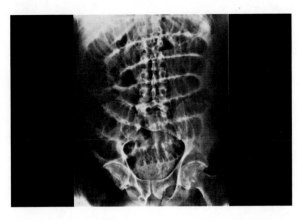

Image 108A. Small bowel obstruction on supine abdominal x-ray. Note dilated loops of small bowel in a ladder-like pattern. Air-fluid levels may be seen if an upright x-ray is done. (Reproduced, with permission, from Way L, Doherty G. *Current Surgical Diagnosis & Treatment*, 11th ed. New York: McGraw-Hill, 2003.)

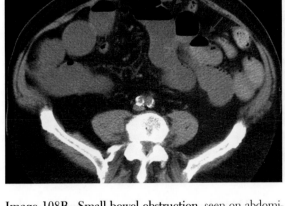

Image 108B. Small bowel obstruction, seen on abdominal CT scan showing multiple dilated loops of small bowel with air-fluid levels.

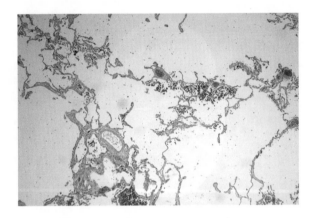

Image 109A. Emphysema. Note the abnormal permanent enlargement of the airspaces distal to the terminal bronchiole. On microscopy, enlarged alveoli are seen separated by thin septa, some of which appear to float within the alveolar spaces. (Reproduced, with permission, from USMLERx.com.)

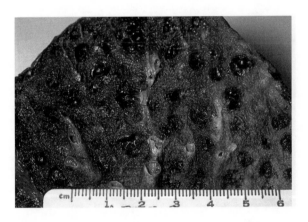

Image 109B. Emphysema. Gross specimen showing multiple cavities lined by heavy black carbon deposits, typical of smoking.

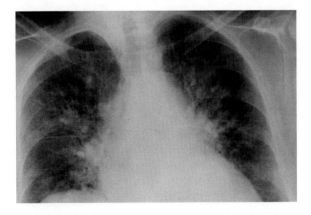

Image 110. Pulmonary edema. Posteroanterior chest x-ray in a man with acute pulmonary edema due to left ventricular failure. Note the bat's-wing density, cardiac enlargement, increased size of upper lobe vessels, and pulmonary venous congestion. (Reproduced, with permission, from McPhee SJ et al. *Pathophysiology of Disease: An Introduction to Clinical Medicine*, 4th ed. New York: McGraw-Hill, 2002.)

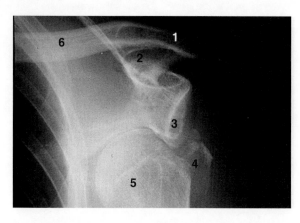

Image 111A. Anterior shoulder dislocation. Note the humeral head inferior and medial to the glenoid fossa and fracture fragments from the greater tuberosity. 1—Acromion; 2—Coracoid; 3—Glenoid fossa; 4—Fracture fragments; 5—Humeral head; 6—Clavicle

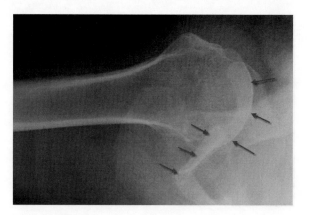

Image 111B. Anterior shoulder dislocation. Axillary view showing humeral head dislocated anteriorly with respect to the glenoid fossa.

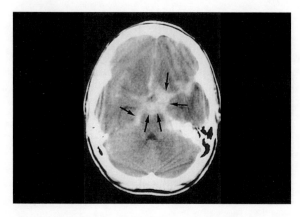

Image 112A. Subarachnoid hemorrhage. CT scan without contrast reveals blood in the subarachnoid space at the base of the brain.

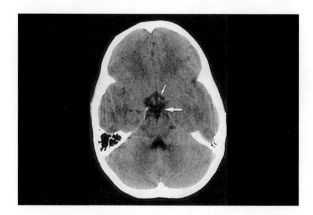

Image 112B. Subarachnoid hemorrhage. Normal comparison study at the same level.

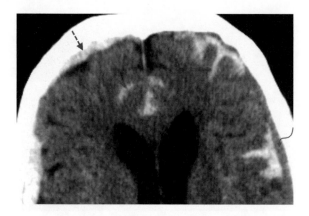

Image 112C. Subarachnoid hemorrhage. CT scan showing subarachnoid hemorrhage (straight arrow), acute subdural hemorrhage (dotted arrow), and chronic isodense subdural hemorrhage (curved arrow).

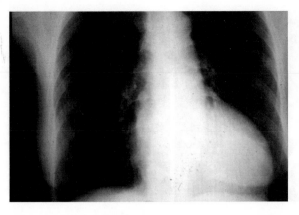

Image 113. Left ventricular hypertrophy (mediastinum wider than 50% of the width of the chest) from aortic valve stenosis, a borderline case.*

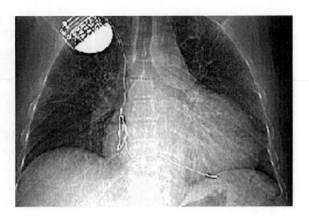

Image 114. Amiodarone toxicity. Diffuse interstitial bilateral pulmonary markings in a reticular nodular pattern, most prominent in the lung bases and posteriorly, are evidence of pulmonary fibrosis.*

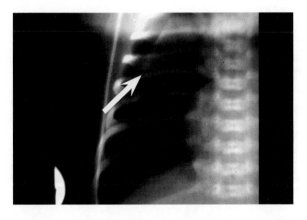

Image 115A. Pneumothorax. The right lung is collapsed; the apparent straight line off the rightmost edge of the pleural space indicated by the arrow shows the edge of the collapsed lung.*

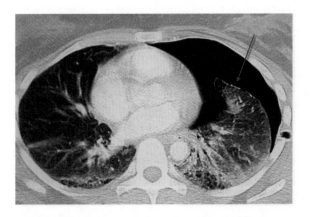

Image 115B. Pneumothorax. CT chest image showing collapsed left lung with ipsilateral increased density of the lung parenchyma.

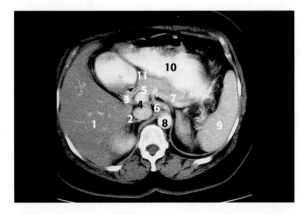

Image 116. CT of the abdomen with contrast—normal anatomy. 1—Liver; 2—IVC; 3—Portal vein; 4—Hepatic artery; 5—Gastroduodenal artery; 6—Celiac trunk; 7—Splenic vein; 8—Aorta; 9—Spleen; 10—Stomach; 11—Pancreas

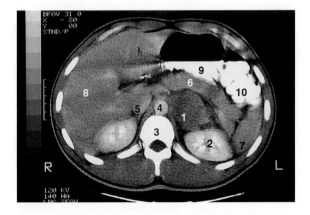

Image 117. Left adrenal mass. 1—Large left adrenal mass; 2—Kidney; 3—Vertebral body; 4—Aorta; 5—IVC; 6—Pancreas; 7—Spleen; 8—Liver; 9—Stomach with air and contrast; 10—Colon–splenic flexure

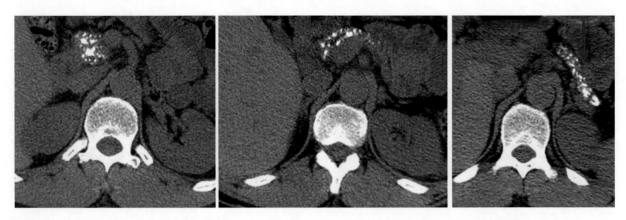

Image 118. Chronic pancreatitis seen on three consecutive non-contrast CT scan images showing punctate calcifications in the head, body, and tail of the pancreas.

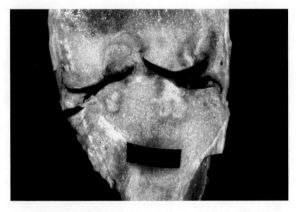

Image 119A. Osteoarthritis. Increased fibrosis of the joint and a decreased amount of cartilage are apparent.*

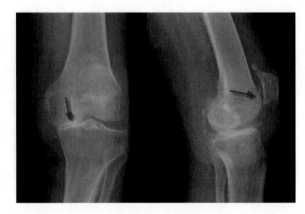

Image 119B. Osteoarthritis. X-ray of the knee, frontal and lateral views, showing medial and patello femoral join space narrowing and sclerosis.

Disease/finding	Most common/important associations
Actinic (solar) keratosis	Precursor to squamous cell carcinoma
Acute gastric ulcer associated with CNS injury	Cushing's ulcer ($\uparrow$ ICP stimulates vagal gastric secretion)
Acute gastric ulcer associated with severe burns	Curling's ulcer (greatly reduced plasma volume results in sloughing of gastric mucosa)
Alternating areas of transmural inflammation and normal colon	Skip lesions (Crohn's disease)
Aneurysm, dissecting	Hypertension
Aortic aneurysm, abdominal and descending aorta	Atherosclerosis
Aortic aneurysm, ascending	3° syphilis, Marfan's syndrome
Atrophy of the mammillary bodies	Wernicke's encephalopathy (thiamine deficiency causing ataxia, ophthalmoplegia, and confusion)
Autosplenectomy (fibrosis and shrinkage)	Sickle cell anemia (HbS)
Bacteria associated with stomach cancer	*H. pylori*
Bacterial meningitis (adults and elderly)	*Neisseria meningitidis*
Bacterial meningitis (newborns and kids)	Group B streptococcus (newborns), *S. pneumoniae/Neisseria meningitidis* (kids)
Benign melanocytic nevus	Spitz nevus (most common in first two decades)
Bleeding disorder with GpIb deficiency	Bernard-Soulier disease (defect in platelet adhesion to von Willebrand's factor)
Brain tumor (adults)	Supratentorial: mets > astrocytoma (including glioblastoma multiforme) > meningioma > schwannoma
Brain tumor (kids)	Infratentorial: medulloblastoma (cerebellum) or supratentorial: craniopharyngioma (cerebrum)
Breast cancer	Infiltrating ductal carcinoma (in the United States, 1 in 9 women will develop breast cancer)
Breast mass	1. Fibrocystic change 2. Carcinoma (in postmenopausal women)
Breast tumor (benign)	Fibroadenoma
Cardiac 1° tumor (kids)	Rhabdomyoma
Cardiac manifestation of lupus	Libman-Sacks endocarditis (nonbacterial, affecting mitral)
Cardiac tumor (adults)	1. Metastasis 2. 1° myxoma (4:1 left to right atrium; "ball and valve")
Cerebellar tonsillar herniation	Chiari malformation (often presents with progressive hydrocephalus or syringomyelia)
Chronic arrhythmia	Atrial fibrillation (associated with high risk of emboli)
Chronic atrophic gastritis (autoimmune)	Predisposition to gastric carcinoma (can also cause pernicious anemia)

Clear cell adenocarcinoma of the vagina	DES exposure in utero
Congenital adrenal hyperplasia, hypotension	21-hydroxylase deficiency
Congenital cardiac anomaly	VSD
Congenital conjugated hyperbilirubinemia (black liver)	Dubin-Johnson syndrome (inability of hepatocytes to secrete conjugated bilirubin into bile)
Constrictive pericarditis in developing world	Tuberculosis
Coronary artery involved in thrombosis	LAD > RCA > LCA
Cretinism	Iodine deficit/hypothyroidism
Cushing's syndrome	1. Corticosteroid therapy 2. Excess ACTH secretion by pituitary
Cyanosis (early; less common)	Tetralogy of Fallot, transposition of great vessels, truncus arteriosus
Cyanosis (late; more common)	VSD, ASD, PDA
Death in CML	Blast crisis
Death in SLE	Lupus nephropathy
Dementia	1. Alzheimer's disease 2. Multiple infarcts
Demyelinating disease in young women	Multiple sclerosis
DIC	Gram-negative sepsis, obstetric complications, cancer, burn trauma
Dietary deficit	Iron
Diverticulum in pharynx	Zenker's diverticulum (diagnosed by barium swallow)
Ejection click	Aortic /pulmonic stenosis
Esophageal cancer	Squamous cell carcinoma (worldwide); adenocarcinoma (U.S.)
Food poisoning (exotoxin mediated)	*S. aureus, B. cereus*
Glomerulonephritis (adults)	Berger's disease (IgA nephropathy)
Gynecologic malignancy	Endometrial carcinoma (most common)
Heart murmur, congenital	Mitral valve prolapse
Heart valve in bacterial endocarditis	Mitral (rheumatic fever), tricuspid (IV drug abuse), aortic (2nd affected in rheumatic fever)
Helminth infection (U.S.)	1. *Enterobius vermicularis* 2. *Ascaris lumbricoides*
Hematoma—epidural	Rupture of middle meningeal artery (crescent shaped)
Hematoma—subdural	Rupture of bridging veins (trauma; lentiform shaped)
Hemochromatosis	Multiple blood transfusions or hereditary HFE mutation (can result in CHF, "bronze diabetes," and ↑ risk of hepatocellular carcinoma)
Hepatocellular carcinoma	Cirrhotic liver (often associated with hepatitis B and C)

Hereditary bleeding disorder	von Willebrand's disease
Hereditary harmless jaundice	Gilbert's syndrome (benign congenital unconjugated hyperbilirubinemia)
HLA-B27	Ankylosing spondylitis, Reiter's syndrome, ulcerative colitis, psoriasis
HLA-DR3 or -DR4	Diabetes mellitus type 1, rheumatoid arthritis, SLE
Holosystolic murmur	VSD, tricuspid regurgitation, mitral regurgitation
Hypercoagulability, endothelial damage, blood stasis	Virchow's triad (results in venous thrombosis)
Hypertension, 2°	Renal disease
Hypoparathyroidism	Thyroidectomy
Hypopituitarism	Pituitary adenoma (usually benign tumor)
Infection 2° to blood transfusion	Hepatitis C
Kidney stones	1. Calcium = radiopaque 2. Struvite (ammonium) = radiopaque (formed by urease-positive organisms such as *Proteus vulgaris* or *Staphylococcus*) 3. Uric acid = radiolucent
Late cyanotic shunt (uncorrected L → R becomes R → L)	Eisenmenger's syndrome (caused by ASD, VSD, PDA; results in pulmonary hypertension/polycythemia)
Liver disease	Alcoholic cirrhosis
Lysosomal storage disease	Gaucher's disease
Male cancer	Prostatic carcinoma
Malignancy associated with noninfectious fever	Hodgkin's lymphoma
Malignant skin tumor	Basal cell carcinoma (rarely metastasizes)
Mental retardation	1. Down syndrome 2. Fragile X syndrome
Metastases to bone	Breast, lung, thyroid, testes, prostate, kidney
Metastases to brain	Lung, breast, skin (melanoma), kidney (renal cell carcinoma), GI
Metastases to liver	Colon, gastric, pancreatic, breast, and lung carcinomas
Mitral valve stenosis	Rheumatic heart disease
Mixed (UMN and LMN) motor neuron disease	ALS
Myocarditis	Coxsackie B
Neoplasm (kids)	1. ALL 2. Cerebellar medulloblastoma
Nephrotic syndrome (adults)	Membranous glomerulonephritis
Nephrotic syndrome (kids)	Minimal change disease (associated with infections/vaccinations; treat with corticosteroids)
Nosocomial pneumonia	*Klebsiella, E. coli, Pseudomonas aeruginosa*
Obstruction of male urinary tract	BPH

Opening snap	Mitral stenosis
Opportunistic infection in AIDS	*Pneumocystis jiroveci* (formerly *carinii*) pneumonia
Osteomyelitis	*S. aureus*
Osteomyelitis in sickle cell disease patients	*Salmonella*
Osteomyelitis with IV drug use	*Pseudomonas, S. aureus*
Ovarian metastasis from gastric carcinoma or breast cancer	Krukenberg tumor (mucin-secreting signet-ring cells)
Ovarian tumor (benign)	Serous cystadenoma
Ovarian tumor (malignant)	Serous cystadenocarcinoma
Pancreatitis (acute)	Gallstones, alcohol
Pancreatitis (chronic)	Alcohol (adults), cystic fibrosis (kids)
Patient with ALL /CLL /AML /CML	ALL: child, CLL: adult > 60, AML: adult > 60, CML: adult 35–50
Pelvic inflammatory disease	*Neisseria gonorrhoeae* (monoarticular arthritis)
Philadelphia chromosome t(9;22) (*bcr-abl*)	CML (may sometimes be associated with ALL/AML)
Pituitary tumor	1. Prolactinoma 2. Somatotropic "acidophilic" adenoma
Primary amenorrhea	Turner syndrome (XO)
Primary bone tumor (adults)	Multiple myeloma
Primary hyperaldosteronism	Adenoma of adrenal cortex
Primary hyperparathyroidism	1. Adenomas 2. Hyperplasia 3. Carcinoma
Primary liver cancer	Hepatocellular carcinoma (chronic hepatitis, cirrhosis, hemochromatosis, α-1 antitrypsin)
Pulmonary hypertension	COPD
Recurrent inflammation/thrombosis of small/medium vessels in extremities	Buerger's disease (strongly associated with tobacco)
Renal tumor	Renal cell carcinoma: associated with von Hippel–Lindau and adult polycystic kidney disease; paraneoplastic syndromes (erythropoietin, renin, PTH, ACTH)
Right heart failure due to a pulmonary cause	Cor pulmonale
S3 (protodiastolic gallop)	$\uparrow$ ventricular filling (L $\rightarrow$ R shunt, mitral regurgitation, LV failure [CHF])
S4 (presystolic gallop)	Stiff/hypertrophic ventricle (aortic stenosis, restrictive cardiomyopathy)
Secondary hyperparathyroidism	Hypocalcemia of chronic kidney disease
Sexually transmitted disease	Chlamydia (usually coinfected with gonorrhea)
SIADH	Small cell carcinoma of the lung

Site of diverticula	Sigmoid colon
Sites of atherosclerosis	Abdominal aorta > coronary > popliteal > carotid
Stomach cancer	Adenocarcinoma
Stomach ulcerations and high gastrin levels	Zollinger-Ellison syndrome (gastrinoma of duodenum or pancreas)
t(14;18)	Follicular lymphomas (*bcl*-2 activation)
t(8;14)	Burkitt's lymphoma (*c-myc* activation)
t(9;22)	Philadelphia chromosome, CML (*bcr-abl* hybrid)
Temporal arteritis	Risk of ipsilateral blindness due to thrombosis of ophthalmic artery; polymyalgia rheumatica
Testicular tumor	Seminoma
Thyroid cancer	Papillary carcinoma
Tumor in women	Leiomyoma (estrogen dependent)
Tumor of infancy	Hemangioma (usually regresses spontaneously by childhood)
Tumor of the adrenal medulla (adults)	Pheochromocytoma (usually benign)
Tumor of the adrenal medulla (kids)	Neuroblastoma (malignant)
Type of Hodgkin's	Nodular sclerosis (vs. mixed cellularity, lymphocytic predominance, lymphocytic depletion)
Type of non-Hodgkin's	Diffuse large cell
UTI	*E. coli, Staphylococcus saprophyticus* (young women)
Viral encephalitis affecting temporal lobe	HSV
Vitamin deficiency (U.S.)	Folic acid (pregnant women are at high risk; body stores only 3- to 4-month supply; prevents neural tube defects)

Topic	Equation	Page
Sensitivity	$\text{Sensitivity} = TP / (TP + FN)$	51
Specificity	$\text{Specificity} = TN / (TN + FP)$	51
Positive predictive value	$PPV = TP / (TP + FP)$	51
Negative predictive value	$NPV = TN / (TN + FN)$	51
Relative risk	$RR = \dfrac{\left[\dfrac{a}{a+b}\right]}{\left[\dfrac{c}{c+d}\right]}$	52
Attributable risk	$AR = \left[\dfrac{a}{a+b}\right] - \left[\dfrac{c}{c+d}\right]$	52
Number needed to treat	1/absolute risk reduction	52
Number needed to harm	1/attributable risk	52
Hardy-Weinberg equilibrium	$p^2 + 2pq + q^2 = 1$ $p + q = 1$	84
Henderson-Hasselbalch equation	$pH = pKa + \log \dfrac{[HCO_3^-]}{0.03\ P_{CO_2}}$	465
Volume of distribution	$V_d = \dfrac{\text{amount of drug in the body}}{\text{plasma drug concentration}}$	232
Clearance	$CL = \dfrac{\text{rate of elimination of drug}}{\text{plasma drug concentration}}$	232
Half-life	$t_{1/2} = \dfrac{0.7 \times V_d}{CL}$	232
Loading dose	$LD = C_p \times \dfrac{V_d}{F}$	233
Maintenance dose	$MD = C_p \times \dfrac{CL}{F}$	233
Cardiac output	$CO = \dfrac{\text{rate of } O_2 \text{ consumption}}{\text{arterial } O_2 \text{ content} - \text{venous } O_2 \text{ content}}$	254
Cardiac output	$CO = \text{stroke volume} \times \text{heart rate}$	254
Mean arterial pressure	$MAP = \text{cardiac output} \times \text{total peripheral resistance}$ $MAP = \frac{1}{3} \text{ systolic} + \frac{2}{3} \text{ diastolic}$	254 254
Stroke volume	$SV = \text{end diastolic volume} - \text{end systolic volume}$	254
Ejection fraction	$EF = \dfrac{\text{stroke volume}}{\text{end diastolic volume}} \times 100$	255
Resistance	$R = \dfrac{\text{driving pressure}}{\text{flow}} = \dfrac{8\eta \text{ (viscosity)} \times \text{length}}{\pi\ r^4}$	256
Net filtration pressure	$P_{net} = \left[(P_c - P_i) - (\pi_c - \pi_i)\right]$	266
Glomerular filtration rate	$GFR = U_{inulin} \times \dfrac{V}{P_{inulin}} = C_{inulin}$	459

Glomerular filtration rate	$GFR = K_f \, [(P_{GC} - P_{BS}) - (\pi_{GC} - \pi_{BS})]$	459
Effective renal plasma flow	$ERPF = U_{PAH} \times \dfrac{V}{P_{PAH}} = C_{PAH}$	459
Renal blood flow	$RBF = \dfrac{RPF}{1 - Hct}$	459
Filtration fraction	$FF = \dfrac{GFR}{RPF}$	460
Physiologic dead space	$V_D = V_T \times \dfrac{(Paco_2 - Peco_2)}{Paco_2}$	505

Top-Rated Review Resources

This section is a database of top-rated basic science review books, sample examination books, software, Web sites, and commercial review courses that have been marketed to medical students studying for the USMLE Step 1. At the end of the section is a list of publishers and independent bookstores with addresses and phone numbers. For each recommended resource, we list the **Title** of the book, the **First Author** (or editor), the **Series Name** (where applicable), the **Current Publisher**, the **Copyright Year**, the **Number of Pages**, the **ISBN Code**, the **Approximate List Price**, the **Format** of the resource, and the **Number of Test Questions**. The entries for most books also include **Summary Comments** that describe their style and overall utility for studying. Finally, each recommended resource receives a **Rating**. Within each section, books are arranged first by Rating and then alphabetically by First Author within each Rating group.

A letter rating scale with six different grades reflects the detailed student evaluations for **Rated Resources.** Each rated resource receives a rating as follows:

A+	Excellent for boards review.
A A–	Very good for boards review; choose among the group.
B+ B	Good, but use only after exhausting better sources.
B–	Fair, but there are many better books in the discipline; or low-yield subject material.

The Rating is meant to reflect the overall usefulness of the resource in helping medical students prepare for the USMLE Step 1 examination. This is based on a number of factors, including:

- The cost
- The readability of the text
- The appropriateness and accuracy of the material
- The quality and number of sample questions
- The quality of written answers to sample questions
- The quality and appropriateness of the illustrations (e.g., graphs, diagrams, photographs)
- The length of the text (longer is not necessarily better)
- The quality and number of other resources available in the same discipline
- The importance of the discipline for the USMLE Step 1 examination

Please note that ratings do not reflect the quality of the resources for purposes other than reviewing for the USMLE Step 1 examination. Many books with lower ratings are well written and informative but are not ideal for boards preparation. We have not listed or commented on general textbooks available in the basic sciences.

Evaluations are based on the cumulative results of formal and informal surveys of thousands of medical students at many medical schools across the country. The summary comments and overall ratings represent a consensus opinion, but there may have been a broad range of opinion or limited student feedback on any particular resource.

Please note that the data listed are subject to change in that:

- Publishers' prices change frequently.
- Bookstores often charge an additional markup.
- New editions come out frequently, and the quality of updating varies.
- The same book may be reissued through another publisher.

We actively encourage medical students and faculty to submit their opinions and ratings of these basic science review materials so that we may update our database. (See p. xv, How to Contribute.) In addition, we ask that publishers and authors submit for evaluation review copies of basic science review books, including new editions and books not included in our database. We also solicit reviews of new books or suggestions for alternate modes of study that may be useful in preparing for the examination, such as flash cards, computer software, commercial review courses, and Web sites.

Disclaimer/Conflict of Interest Statement

No material in this book, including the ratings, reflects the opinion or influence of the publisher. All errors and omissions will gladly be corrected if brought to the attention of the authors through our blog at www.firstaidteam.com. Please note that *USMLERx* and the entire *First Aid for the USMLE* series are publications by the senior authors of this book; their ratings are based solely on recommendations from the student authors of this book as well as data from the student survey and feedback forms.

A⁺

USMLEWorld Qbank
USMLEWORLD
www.usmleworld.com

$99 for 1 month;
$185 for 3 months

Test/2000 q

An excellent bank of well-constructed questions that closely mirror those found on Step 1. Questions demand multistep reasoning and are often more difficult than those on the actual exam. Offers excellent, detailed explanations with figures and tables. Features a number of test customization and analysis options. Unfortunately, the program does not allow other application windows to be open for reference. Users can see cumulative results both over time and compared to other test takers.

A

Kaplan Qbank
KAPLAN
www.kaplanmedical.com

$109 for 1 month;
$189 for 3 months

Test/2400 q

A high-quality question bank that covers most content found on Step 1, but sometimes emphasizes recall of overly specific details rather than integrative problem-solving skills. Test content and performance feedback can be organized by both organ system and discipline. Includes detailed explanations of all answer choices with references to *First Aid*. Users can see cumulative results both over time and compared to other test takers.

A

USMLERx Qmax
MEDIQ LEARNING
www.usmlerx.com

$89 for 1 month;
$169 for 3 months

Test/3000 q

A well-priced question bank that offers Step 1–style questions accompanied by thorough explanations. Some obscure material is omitted, making it more straightforward than other question banks. Each explanation includes high-yield facts and references from *First Aid*. However, the proportion of questions covering a given subject area does not always reflect the actual exam's relative emphasis. Question stems occasionally rely on "buzzwords." Most useful to help memorize *First Aid* facts. Provides detailed performance analyses.

USMLE Consult
ELSEVIER

$75 for 1 month;
$135 for 3 months

Test/2500 q

www.usmleconsult.com

A solid question bank that can be divided according to discipline and subject area. Questions are more straightforward than those on actual exam. Offers concise explanations with links to Student Consult and First Consult content. Users can see cumulative results both over time and compared to other test takers. Student Consult also offers a Robbins Pathology Test Bank ($35 for 1 month, $49 for 3 months) featuring 500 USMLE-style questions as well as the Scorrelator ($35), a 3-hour, 150-question mock exam that predicts your USMLE Step 1 score. Limited student feedback on Student Consult products.

USMLEasy
McGRAW-HILL

$79 for 1 month;
$169 for 3 months

Test/2000 q

www.usmleasy.com

A question bank based on the PreTest series. Many questions are shorter and more obscure than those on the actual Step 1 exam. Users can track questions completed as well as customize tests. Useful as a supplemental review after other resources have been exhausted.

B+

Kaplan USMLE Step 1 Qbook
KAPLAN

$44.95   Test/850 q

Kaplan, 2008, 480 pages, ISBN 9781419553158

A resource consisting of seventeen 50-question exams organized by the traditional basic science disciplines. Similar to the Kaplan Qbank, and offers good USMLE-style questions with clear, detailed explanations; however, lacks the classic images typically seen on the exam. Also includes a guide on test-taking strategies.

B+

First Aid Q&A for the USMLE Step 1
LE

$44.95   Test/1000 q

McGraw-Hill, 2009, 676 pages, ISBN 9780071597944

A great source of more than 1000 questions drawn from the USMLE Step 1 Qmax test bank, organized according to subject. Also features one full-length exam of 350 questions. Questions are slightly easier than those found on Step 1, but provide representative coverage of the concepts typically tested. Includes brief but adequate explanations of both correct and incorrect answer choices.

B+

PreTest Clinical Vignettes for the USMLE Step 1
MCGRAW-HILL

$29.95   Test/336 q

McGraw-Hill, 2010, 336 pages, ISBN 9780071668064

Clinical vignette–style questions with detailed explanations, divided into seven blocks of 46 questions covering basic sciences. In general, questions are representative of the length and complexity of those on Step 1. One of the better books in the PreTest series.

B

Blueprints Q&A Step 1
CLEMENT

$36.95   Test/350 q

Lippincott Williams & Wilkins, 2003, 184 pages,
ISBN 9781405103237

Contains one full-length exam of 350 questions written by students. Good for practicing the multistep questions common on Step 1, but questions are easier than those on the actual test.

B

Lange Practice Tests: USMLE Step 1
GOLDBERG

$45.95   Test/650 q

McGraw-Hill, 2005, 240 pages, ISBN 9780071446150

A good resource for review questions consisting of 13 blocks of 50 questions with explanations. In general, questions are not as lengthy or challenging as those on the actual Step 1 exam. Includes explanations of correct answer choices only.

Lange Q&A: USMLE Step 1   ***$45.95***   Test/1200 q

KING

McGraw-Hill, 2008, 528 pages, ISBN 9780071492195

Offers many questions organized by subject area along with three comprehensive practice exams. Questions are often challenging and are not always representative of Step 1 style. Includes detailed explanations of both correct and incorrect answer choices. Black-and-white images only.

NMS Review for USMLE Step 1   ***$48.95***   Test/850 q

LAZO

Lippincott Williams & Wilkins, 2005, 480 pages + CD-ROM, ISBN 9780781779210

A text and CD-ROM that offers 17 practice exams with answers. Some questions are too picky or difficult. Annotated explanations are well written but are sometimes unnecessarily detailed. The six pages of color plates are helpful. The CD-ROM attempts to simulate the computer-based testing format but is disorganized.

A

WebPath: The Internet Pathology Laboratory

Free   Review/Test/1100 q

http://library.med.utah.edu/WebPath/

Features more than 2000 outstanding gross and microscopic images, clinical vignette questions, and case studies. Includes eight general pathology exams and 11 system-based exams with approximately 1000 questions. Also features 170 questions associated with images. Questions are useful for reviewing boards content but are typically easier and shorter. No multimedia practice questions.

B

The Pathology Guy

FRIEDLANDER

Free   Review

www.pathguy.com

A free Web site containing extensive but poorly organized information on a variety of fundamental concepts in pathology. A high-yield summary intended for USMLE review can be found at www.pathguy.com/meltdown.txt, but the information given is limited by a lack of images and frequent digressions.

B

Lippincott's 350-Question Practice Test for USMLE Step 1

LIPPINCOTT WILLIAMS & WILKINS

Free   Test/350 q

www.lww.com/medstudent/usmle

A free, full-length, seven-block, 350-question practice exam in a format similar to that of the real Step 1. Questions are easier than those on the actual exam, and the explanations provided are sparse. Users can bookmark questions and can choose between taking the test all at once or by section.

B

Radiopaedia.org

Free   Cases/test

www.radiopaedia.org

A user-friendly Web site with thousands of well-organized radiology cases and articles. Encyclopedia entries contain high-yield bullet points of anatomy and pathology. Images contain detailed descriptions but no arrows to demarcate findings. Quiz mode allows students to make a diagnosis based on radiographic findings. Content may be too broad for boards review but is a good complement to classes and clerkships.

B⁻

The Whole Brain Atlas

JOHNSON

Free   Review

www.med.harvard.edu/AANLIB/home.html

A collection of high-quality brain MR and CT images with views of normal and diseased brains. The interface is technologically impressive but complex, and many images are without explanations. Subject matter is overly specific, limiting its use as a boards review study tool.

Digital Anatomist Interactive Atlases

UNIVERSITY OF WASHINGTON

Free   Review

www9.biostr.washington.edu/da.html

A good site containing an interactive neuroanatomy course along with
a three-dimensional atlas of the brain, thorax, and knee. Atlases have
computer-generated images and cadaver sections. Each atlas also has
a quiz in which users identify structures in the slide images; however,
questions do not focus on high-yield anatomy for Step 1.

REVIEW RESOURCES

COMPREHENSIVE

First Aid Cases for the USMLE Step 1
LE

$44.95   Review

McGraw-Hill, 2009, 497 pages, ISBN 9780071601351

A series of more than 400 high-yield cases divided into sections by organ system. Each case features a paragraph-long clinical vignette with relevant images, followed by questions and short explanations. Offers great coverage of many frequently tested concepts, and integrates subject matter in the discussion of a single vignette. A good source of questions to review material outlined in *First Aid for the USMLE Step 1*.

USMLE Step 1 Secrets
BROWN

$39.95   Review

Elsevier, 2008, 740 pages, ISBN 9780323054393

Clarifies difficult concepts in a concise, easy-to-read manner. Employs a case-based format and integrates information well. Complements other boards study resources, with a focus on understanding preclinical fundamentals rather than on rote memorization. Slightly long for last-minute board cramming.

First Aid for the Basic Sciences: General Principles
LE

$69.95   Review

McGraw-Hill, 2008, 561 pages, ISBN 9780071545457

Excellent comprehensive review of the basic sciences covered in year 1 of medical school. Organized by discipline, and includes hundreds of full-color images and tables. Can be started with coursework and then used as a review/reference during boards preparation.

First Aid for the Basic Sciences: Organ Systems
LE

$89.95   Review

McGraw-Hill, 2008, 938 pages, ISBN 9780071545433

A comprehensive review of the basic sciences covered in year 2 of medical school. Organized by organ system, and includes hundreds of full-color images and tables. Can be started with coursework and then used as a review/reference during boards preparation. Each organ system contains discussion of embryology and anatomy, physiology, pathology, pharmacology, and a high-yield rapid review section. Limited student feedback.

Déjà Review: USMLE Step 1 $24.95   Review
NAHEEDY
McGraw-Hill, 2010, 412 pages, ISBN 9780071627184
A resource featuring questions and answers in a two-column, quiz-yourself format similar to that of the Recall series, divided according to discipline. Features a section of high-yield clinical vignettes along with useful mnemonics throughout. Contains a few mistakes, but remains a good alternative to flash cards as a last-minute review before the exam.

Cases & Concepts Step 1: Basic Science Review $42.95   Review
CAUGHEY
Lippincott Williams & Wilkins, 2009, 400 pages,
ISBN 9780781793919
One hundred sixteen clinical cases integrating basic science with clinical data, followed by USMLE-style questions with answers and rationales. Thumbnail and key-concept boxes highlight key facts. Limited student feedback.

Kaplan's USMLE Step 1 Home Study Program $499.00   Review
KAPLAN
Kaplan, 2008, 1900 pages, ISBN 0S4005C
A resource consisting of two general principle and two organ system review books. All are highly comprehensive, but can be overwhelmingly lengthy if they are not started very early. Although costly, the program can serve as an excellent reference for studying by virtue of its detail. Books can be purchased at www.kaptest.com.

medEssentials for the USMLE Step 1 $49.95   Review
MANLEY
Kaplan, 2009, 576 pages, ISBN 9781607144823
A comprehensive review divided into general principles and organ systems, and organized using high-yield tables and figures. Excellent for visual learners, but can be overly detailed and time consuming. Also includes color images in the back along with a monthly subscription to online interactive exercises, although these are of limited value for Step 1 preparation.

B+

Step-Up to USMLE Step 1
MEHTA
Lippincott Williams & Wilkins, 2009, 424 pages,
ISBN 9781605474700

An organ system–based review text with clinical vignettes that is useful for integrating the basic sciences covered in Step 1. The text is composed primarily of outlines, charts, tables, and diagrams, making the depth of material covered somewhat limited. Includes access to a sample online question bank.

$46.95   Review

B+

USMLE Step 1 Recall: Buzzwords for the Boards
REINHEIMER
Lippincott Williams & Wilkins, 2007, 480 pages,
ISBN 9780781770705

A review of core Step 1 topics presented in a two-column, quiz-yourself format. Best for a quick last-minute review before the exam. Covers many important subjects, but not comprehensive or tightly organized. Sometimes focuses on obscure details. Compare with the Déjà Review series. Includes all questions and answers in downloadable MP3 files so that files can be used on any digital audio playback device.

$46.95   Review

B+

Underground Clinical Vignettes: Step 1 Bundle
SWANSON
Lippincott Williams & Wilkins, 2007, 9 volumes,
ISBN 9780781763622

A bundle that includes nine books. Designed for easy quizzing with a group. Case-based vignettes provide a good review supplement. Best when started early with coursework or when used in conjunction with another primary review resource.

$189.95   Review

B

USMLE Step 1 Made Ridiculously Simple
CARL
MedMaster, 2010, 400 pages, ISBN 9780940780910

A quick and easy read. Uses a table and chart format organized by subject, but some charts are poorly labeled. Consider as an adjunct to more comprehensive sources.

$29.95   Review

A⁻   ***High-Yield Embryology***   **$32.95**   Review

DUDEK

Lippincott Williams & Wilkins, 2009, 176 pages,
ISBN 9781605473161

A good review of a relatively low-yield subject. Offers excellent organization with clinical correlations. Includes a high-yield list of embryologic origins of tissues.

A⁻   ***High-Yield Neuroanatomy***   **$28.95**   Review/Test/50

FIX   Q&A provided

Lippincott Williams & Wilkins, 2008, 160 pages,   online
ISBN 9780781779463

An easy-to-read, straightforward format with excellent diagrams and illustrations. Features a useful atlas of brain section images, a glossary of important terms, an appendicized table of neurologic lesions, and an expanded index. Overall, a great resource, but more detailed than what is required for Step 1.

A⁻   ***Underground Clinical Vignettes: Anatomy***   **$27.95**   Review/Test/20 q

SWANSON

Lippincott Williams & Wilkins, 2007, 256 pages,
ISBN 9780781764759

Concise clinical cases illustrating approximately 100 frequently tested diseases with an anatomic basis. Cardinal signs, symptoms, and buzzwords are highlighted. Also includes 20 additional boards-style questions. A useful source for isolating important anatomy concepts tested on Step 1.

A⁻   ***USMLE Road Map: Gross Anatomy***   **$31.95**   Review/Test/150 q

WHITE

McGraw-Hill, 2005, 240 pages, ISBN 9780071445160

An overview of high-yield gross anatomy with clinical correlations throughout. Also features numerous effective charts and clinical problems with explanations at the end of each chapter. Features good integration of facts, but may be overly detailed and offers few illustrations. May require an anatomy reference text.

High-Yield Gross Anatomy

$29.95   Review

DUDEK

Lippincott Williams & Wilkins, 2010, 320 pages,
ISBN 9781605477633

A good review of gross anatomy with some clinical correlations. Contains well-labeled, high-yield radiographic images, but often goes into excessive detail that is beyond the scope of the boards.

Atlas of Anatomy

$74.95   Review

GILROY

Thieme, 2008, 672 pages, ISBN 9781604060621

A good atlas with more than 2200 high-quality, uncluttered illustrations. Includes clinical correlates and a brief introduction to new topics. Radiographs, MRIs, CT scans, and endoscopic views of the organs also included. Best if used as a reference or during coursework. Access to accompanying Web site with more than 600 illustrations, label on/off function, and timed self-tests also provided.

Clinical Anatomy Made Ridiculously Simple

$29.95   Review

GOLDBERG

MedMaster, 2010, 175 pages, ISBN 9780940780972

An easy-to-read text offering simple diagrams along with numerous mnemonics and amusing associations. The humorous style has variable appeal for students, so browse before buying. Offers good coverage of selected topics. Best if used during coursework. Includes more detail than typically tested on Step 1.

Crash Course: Anatomy

$30.95   Review

GRANGER

Elsevier, 2007, 264 pages, ISBN 9780323043199

Part of the Crash Course review series for basic sciences, integrating clinical topics. Offers two-color illustrations, handy study tools, and Step 1 review questions. Includes online access. Provides a solid review of anatomy for Step 1. Best if started early.

Rapid Review: Gross and Developmental Anatomy

$39.95   Review/Test/450 q

MOORE

Elsevier, 2010, 304 pages, ISBN 9780323072946

A detailed treatment of basic anatomy and embryology, presented in an outline format similar to that of other books in the series. More detailed than necessary for boards review. Contains high-yield charts and figures throughout, in color. Includes two 50-question tests with extensive explanations, with an additional 350 questions available online.

Case Files: Gross Anatomy
TOY

$33.95 Review/Test/150 q

McGraw-Hill, 2008, 384 pages, ISBN 9780071489805
Review text that includes 53 well-chosen cases with discussion, comprehension questions, and a box of take-home pearls. Tables are good, but the images are black and white and of poor quality. A reasonable book to work through for those who benefit from problem-based learning.

Déjà Review: Neuroscience
TREMBLAY

$19.95 Review

McGraw-Hill, 2010, 272 pages, ISBN 9780071627276
A resource that features questions and answers in a two-column, quiz-yourself format similar to that of the Recall series. Includes several useful diagrams and CT images. A perfect length for Step 1 neurophysiology and anatomy review.

Elsevier's Integrated Anatomy and Embryology
BOGART

$37.95 Review

Elsevier, 2007, 448 pages, ISBN 9781416031659
Part of the Integrated series that seeks to link basic science concepts across disciplines. Case-based and Step 1–style questions at the end of each chapter allow readers to gauge their comprehension of the material. Includes online access. Best if used during coursework. Limited student feedback.

BRS Embryology
DUDEK

$39.95 Review/Test

Lippincott Williams & Wilkins, 2010, 320 pages,
ISBN 9781605479019
An outline-based review of embryology that is typical of the BRS series. Offers a good review, but has limited illustrations and includes much more detail than is required for Step 1. A discussion of congenital malformations is included at the end of each chapter along with relevant questions. The comprehensive exam at the end of the book is high yield.

Anatomy Flash Cards
GILROY

$34.95 Flash cards

Thieme, 2009, 376 flash cards, ISBN 9781604060720
High-quality illustrations with numbered labels on one side and answers on the other for self-testing. Occasional radiographic image. Best if used with coursework; too long for boards preparation. Limited student feedback.

B ***Clinical Neuroanatomy Made Ridiculously Simple***   **$22.95**   Review/Test/Few q
GOLDBERG
MedMaster, 2007, 96 pages + CD-ROM, ISBN 9780940780576
An easy-to-read, memorable, and simplified format with clever diagrams. Offers a quick, high-yield review of clinical neuroanatomy, but does not serve as a comprehensive resource for boards review. Places good emphasis on clinically relevant pathways, cranial nerves, and neurologic diseases. Includes a CD-ROM with CT and MR images as well as a tutorial on neurologic localization. Compare with *High-Yield Neuroanatomy*.

B ***Netter's Anatomy Flash Cards***   **$33.25**   Flash cards
HANSEN
Saunders, 2010, 324 pages, ISBN 9781437716757
Netter's illustrations with numbered labels on one side and answers on the other for self-testing. Each card includes a commentary on the structures and a clinical correlation. Best if used with coursework, but much too detailed for boards preparation. Includes online access with additional bonus cards and more than 300 multiple-choice questions.

B ***PreTest Neuroscience***   **$29.95**   Test/500 q
SIEGEL
McGraw-Hill, 2010, 399 pages, ISBN 9780071623476
A high-yield introduction followed by 500 questions with detailed explanations. The question format differs significantly from that typically found on Step 1. Sparse, poor-quality images.

B ***BRS Gross Anatomy Flash Cards***   **$34.95**   Flash cards
SWANSON
Lippincott Williams & Wilkins, 2004, 250 pages,
ISBN 9780781756549
Clinical anatomy cases presented in flash-card format. Cases are too specific for boards preparation, and anatomy basics and radiographic images are generally excluded. Best suited to students who are already relatively well versed in anatomy.

B ***Case Files: Neuroscience***   **$33.95**   Review
TOY
McGraw-Hill, 2008, 408 pages, ISBN 9780071489218
Includes 48 clinical cases with lengthy discussion and 3–5 multiple-choice questions at the end of each case. Cases are well chosen, but the discussion is too lengthy. Questions are not the most representative of those seen on boards.

B

Rapid Review: Neuroscience
WEYHENMEYER

$38.95   Review

Elsevier, 2006, 320 pages, ISBN 9780323022613

A detailed treatment of neuroscience, presented in an outline format similar to that of other books in the series. Should be started early given its extensive treatment of a relatively narrow topic. Contains high-yield charts and figures throughout. Includes two 50-question tests with extensive explanations as well as 250 additional questions online

B

USMLE Road Map: Neuroscience
WHITE

$31.95   Review/Test/300 q

McGraw-Hill, 2008, 224 pages, ISBN 9780071496230

An outline review of basic neuroanatomy and physiology with clinical correlations throughout. Also features high-yield facts in boldface along with numerous charts and figures. Clinical problems with explanations are given at the end of each chapter. May be overly detailed for Step 1 review, but a good tool to use as a reference.

B⁻

Gray's Anatomy for Students Flash Cards
DRAKE

$36.95   Flash cards

Elsevier, 2010, 748 pages, ISBN 9780702031784

These flash cards feature renowned Gray's illustrations on the front and labels on the back for self-testing. Notes on clinical importance and reference to accompanying textbook given on back. Much too detailed information on a relatively low-yield subject for effective boards studying. Limited student feedback.

B⁻

Medical Imaging of Normal and Pathologic Anatomy
VILENSKY

$39.95   Review

Saunders, 2010, 192 pages, ISBN 9781437706345

High-quality radiographic images, but much too advanced for boards. Useful as a reference only. Limited student feedback.

BRS Behavioral Science

FADEM

Lippincott Williams & Wilkins, 2008, 216 pages,
ISBN 9780781782579

An easy-to-read outline-format review of behavioral science. Offers good, detailed coverage of essential topics, but at a level of depth that often exceeds what is tested on Step 1. Incorporates excellent tables and charts as well as a short but complete statistics chapter. Features high-quality review questions, including a 100-question comprehensive exam.

$39.95 Review/Test/500 q

High-Yield Behavioral Science

FADEM

Lippincott Williams & Wilkins, 2008, 160 pages,
ISBN 9780781782586

An extremely concise yet comprehensive review of behavioral science for Step 1. Offers a logical presentation with charts, graphs, and tables, but lacks questions. Features brief but adequate coverage of statistics. Overall, an excellent, high-yield resource.

$28.95 Review

High-Yield Biostatistics

GLASER

Lippincott Williams & Wilkins, 2005, 128 pages,
ISBN 9780781796446

A well-written, easy-to-read text that offers extensive coverage of epidemiology and biostatistics. Includes good review questions and tables, but somewhat lengthy given the low-yield nature of the subject matter on Step 1.

$28.95 Review

Underground Clinical Vignettes: Behavioral Science

SWANSON

Lippincott Williams & Wilkins, 2007, 256 pages,
ISBN 9780781764643

Concise clinical cases illustrating commonly tested diseases in behavioral science. Cardinal signs, symptoms, and buzzwords are highlighted. Useful for picking out important points in this very broad subject, but requires supplementation from other review sources. Also includes 20 Step 1–style questions.

$27.95 Review/Test/20 q

B+

High-Yield Brain & Behavior

FADEM

Lippincott Williams & Wilkins, 2007, 256 pages,
ISBN 9780781792288

$34.95   Review

Part of the new High-Yield Systems series that covers embryology, gross anatomy, radiology, histology, physiology, microbiology, and pharmacology as they relate to the nervous system. Written by the same author as the *High-Yield Behavioral Science* and *BRS Behavioral Science* texts. Overall, provides a good review of neuroscience and behavioral science.

B+

Déjà Review: Behavioral Science

QUINN

McGraw-Hill, 2010, 240 pages, ISBN 9780071627283

$19.95   Review

Features questions and answers in a two-column, quiz-yourself format similar to that of the Recall series. Coverage of some topics is too lengthy for Step 1 review purposes. Limited student feedback.

B

PreTest Behavioral Sciences

EBERT

McGraw-Hill, 2001, 300 pages, ISBN 9780071374705

$26.95   Test/500 q

Contains good questions and detailed answers cross-referenced with other resources. Some questions test material beyond the scope of Step 1. Requires time commitment.

B

Kaplan USMLE Medical Ethics

FISCHER

Kaplan, 2009, 216 pages, ISBN 9781419553141

$39.00   Review

Includes 100 cases, each followed by a single question and a detailed explanation. Also offers guidelines on how Step 1 requires test takers to think about ethics and medicolegal questions. Unfortunately, a lengthy review for such a low-yield subject.

B

Blueprints Notes & Cases: Behavioral Science and Epidemiology

NEUGROSCHL

Lippincott Williams & Wilkins, 2003, 224 pages,
ISBN 9781405103558

$32.95   Review/Test/184 q

A case-oriented approach to behavioral science. Each case includes a clinical history, a basic science review and discussion, key points, and questions. The 8.5″ × 11″ layout may feel overwhelming to some, but the font size is conducive to easy review. A good way to master the intangibles of behavioral science, but more detailed than necessary for Step 1 review.

REVIEW RESOURCES

BEHAVIORAL SCIENCE

Rapid Review: Behavioral Science $39.95   Review/Test/350 q

STEVENS

Elsevier, 2006, 320 pages, ISBN 9780323045711

Similar in style to other books in the Rapid Review series. Provides a good but low-yield review of a broad subject. Includes 100 questions and explanations along with an additional 250 questions online. Limited student feedback.

Lange Flash Cards Biochemistry and Genetics
BARON

$34.95   Flash cards

McGraw-Hill Medical, 2005, 300 flash cards,
ISBN 9780071447362

Great flash cards featuring a clinical vignette on one side and concise discussion on the other. Each section contains 2–3 cards on biochemistry principles. Excellent resource for boards studying.

Déjà Review: Biochemistry
MANZOUL

$19.95   Review

McGraw-Hill, 2010, 224 pages, ISBN 9780071627177

Features questions and answers in a two-column, quiz-yourself format similar to that of the Recall series. Includes a helpful chapter on molecular biology and many good diagrams. More detailed than is usually tested on Step 1.

Rapid Review: Biochemistry
PELLEY

$39.95   Review/Test/350 q

Elsevier, 2010, 208 pages, ISBN 9780323068871

A review of basic topics in biochemistry. Presented in outline format, but often goes beyond the level of detail tested on Step 1. High-yield disease correlation boxes are especially useful. Excellent tables and helpful figures are included throughout the text. Best if used as a reference to clarify topics. Offers 350 questions online.

BRS Biochemistry, Molecular Biology, and Genetics
SWANSON

$42.95   Review/Test

Lippincott Williams & Wilkins, 2009, 432 pages,
ISBN 9780781798754

A highly detailed review featuring many excellent figures and clinical correlations highlighted in colored boxes. The biochemistry portion includes much more detail than required for Step 1, but may be useful for students without a strong biochemistry background or as a reference text. The molecular biology section is more focused and high yield. Also offers a chapter on laboratory techniques and a comprehensive, 120-question exam. Questions are clinically oriented.

A⁻ *Underground Clinical Vignettes: Biochemistry*   **$27.95**   Review/Test/20 q

SWANSON

Lippincott Williams & Wilkins, 2007, 256 pages,
ISBN 9780781764728

Concise clinical cases illustrating approximately 100 frequently tested
diseases with a biochemical basis. Cardinal signs, symptoms, and
buzzwords are highlighted. Also includes 20 additional boards-style
questions. A nice review of "take-home" points for biochemistry and a
useful supplement to other sources of review.

B⁺ *Lippincott's Illustrated Reviews: Biochemistry*   **$54.95**   Review/Test/250 q

CHAMPE

Lippincott Williams & Wilkins, 2010, 544 pages,
ISBN 9781608314126

An excellent, integrative, comprehensive review of biochemistry that
includes good clinical correlations and highly effective color diagrams. Extremely detailed and requires significant time commitment,
so it should be started with coursework. High-yield summaries at the
end of each chapter. Comes with access to the companion Web site
with USMLE-style questions.

B⁺ *USMLE Road Map: Biochemistry*   **$31.95**   Review

MACDONALD

McGraw-Hill, 2007, 223 pages, ISBN 9780071442053

A clear, readable outline review of biochemistry. High-yield references to important diseases of metabolism are scattered throughout,
but coverage of clinical correlations is not comprehensive. Includes
brief review questions at the end of each chapter. Lacks "big picture"
integration of related pathways. Limited student feedback.

B *Clinical Biochemistry Made Ridiculously Simple*   **$22.95**   Review

GOLDBERG

MedMaster, 2004, 93 pages + foldout, ISBN 9780940780309

A conceptual approach to clinical biochemistry, presented with humor. The casual style does not appeal to all students. Offers a good
overview and integration of all metabolic pathways. Includes a 23-
page clinical review that is very high yield and crammable. Also contains a unique foldout "road map" of metabolism. For students who
already have a solid grasp of biochemistry.

B

BRS Biochemistry and Molecular Biology Flash Cards

SWANSON

Lippincott Williams & Wilkins, 2007, 512 pages,
ISBN 9780781779029

Quick-review flash cards covering a range of topics in biochemistry and molecular biology. Inadequate for learning purposes, as cards provide only snippets of isolated information and contain some inaccuracies.

$39.95 Flash cards

B

High-Yield Biochemistry

WILCOX

Lippincott Williams & Wilkins, 2009, 128 pages,
ISBN 9780781799249

A concise and crammable text in outline format with good clinical correlations at the end of each chapter. Features many diagrams and tables. Best used as a supplemental review, as explanations are scarce and details are limited.

$29.95 Review

B–

Case Files: Biochemistry

TOY

McGraw-Hill, 2008, 456 pages, ISBN 9780071486651

Includes 51 clinical cases with comprehensive discussion and summary box, but too much depth and not enough breadth for boards. Some cases will almost certainly *not* be tested. Questions at the end of each case are not representative of those seen on boards.

$33.95 Review

B–

PreTest Biochemistry and Genetics

WILSON

McGraw-Hill, 2010, 545 pages, ISBN 9780071623483

Difficult questions with detailed, referenced explanations. Features a high-yield appendix, but overall is an overly detailed review of a relatively low-yield subject.

$29.95 Test/500 q

High-Yield Cell and Molecular Biology

DUDEK

Lippincott Williams & Wilkins, 2010, 272 pages,
ISBN 9781609135737

Cellular and molecular biology presented in an outline format, with
good diagrams and clinical correlations. Includes subjects that other
review resources do not cover in detail, such as laboratory techniques
and second-messenger systems. Not all sections are equally useful;
many students skim or read select chapters. Contains no questions or
vignettes.

$29.95   Review

Rapid Review: Histology and Cell Biology

BURNS

Elsevier, 2006, 336 pages, ISBN 9780323044257

A resource whose format is similar to that of other books in the Rapid
Review series. Features an outline of basic concepts with numerous
charts, but histology images are limited. Two 50-question multiple-
choice tests are presented with explanations, along with 250 more
questions online.

$39.95   Review/Test/350 q

High-Yield Genetics

DUDEK

Lippincott Williams & Wilkins, 2008, 134 pages,
ISBN 9780781768771

A concise, clinically oriented summary of genetics in the popular outline format. Illustrated with schematic line drawings and photographs
of the most clinically relevant diseases. Limited student feedback.

$28.95   Review

Déjà Review: Histology & Medical Cell Biology

GRISSON

McGraw-Hill, 2010, 304 pages, ISBN 9780071627269

Features questions and answers in a two-column, quiz-yourself format
similar to that of the Recall series. Sections are divided by organ system and vary in quality. Histology images are few and are printed in
black and white. Good for a quick review.

$19.95   Review

Crash Course: Cell Biology and Genetics

LAMB

Elsevier, 2006, 224 pages, ISBN 9780323044943

Part of the Crash Course review series for basic sciences, integrating
clinical topics. Offers two-color illustrations, handy study tools, and
Step 1 review questions. Includes online access. Too much coverage
for a low-yield subject.

$49.95   Review

REVIEW RESOURCES

CELL BIOLOGY AND HISTOLOGY

B+

USMLE Road Map: Histology
SHEEDLO

$31.95   Review

McGraw-Hill, 2005, 224 pages, ISBN 9780071440127

A concise review book with many clinical correlations. Questions at the end of each chapter are not in clinical vignette format but are suitable for testing comprehension. Black-and-white images. Good for a quick review of a low-yield subject.

B

Elsevier's Integrated Genetics
ADKISON

$37.95   Review

Elsevier, 2007, 272 pages, ISBN 9780323043298

Part of the Integrated series that seeks to link basic science concepts across disciplines. Case-based and Step 1–style questions at the end of each chapter allow readers to gauge their comprehension of the material. Includes online access. Best if used during coursework. Limited student feedback.

B

High-Yield Histology
DUDEK

$26.95   Review

Lippincott Williams & Wilkins, 2004, 288 pages,
ISBN 9780781747639

A quick and easy review of a relatively low-yield subject. Tables include some high-yield information. Contains good pictures. The appendix features classic electron micrographs. Too lengthy for Step 1 review.

B

BRS Cell Biology and Histology
GARTNER

$39.95   Review/Test/500 q

Lippincott Williams & Wilkins, 2010, 384 pages,
ISBN 9781608313211

Covers concepts in cell biology and histology in an outline format. Can be used alone for cell biology study, but does not include enough histology images to be considered comprehensive on that subject. Includes more detail than is required for Step 1, and information is less high yield than that of other books in the BRS series.

B

USMLE Road Map: Genetics
SACK

$31.95   Review

McGraw-Hill, 2008, 224 pages, ISBN 9780071498203

Efficient review of genetics with an emphasis on clinical correlations. Includes a few questions at the end of each chapter that are best suited to test comprehension and are not representative of boards. Use only if genetics is a weak subject; otherwise, too much depth for a quick review.

B⁻ *PreTest Anatomy, Histology, and Cell Biology*   **$29.95**   Test/500 q

KLEIN

McGraw-Hill, 2010, 654 pages, ISBN 9780071623438

A resource containing difficult questions with detailed answers as well as some illustrations. Requires extensive time commitment, and much of the material is beyond what is required for Step 1. The most useful part of the book is the high-yield facts section at the beginning, which is divided according to discipline.

B⁻ *Wheater's Functional Histology*   **$79.95**   Review

YOUNG

Elsevier, 2006, 448 pages, ISBN 9780443068508

A color atlas with illustrations of normal histology with image captions and accompanying text. Far too detailed to use for boards studying given the low-yield nature of the material, but useful as a coursework text or boards reference.

A⁻

The Big Picture: Medical Microbiology

CHAMBERLAIN

McGraw-Hill, 2008, 456 pages, ISBN 9780071476614

Excellent atlas of pathogens and clinical signs of infection. Discussion targets quick boards review. Especially good for visual learners. High-yield appendix. Includes 100 practice questions with discussion.

$49.95   Review

A⁻

Déjà Review: Microbiology & Immunology

CHEN

McGraw-Hill, 2010, 432 pages, ISBN 9780071627153

Features questions and answers in a two-column, quiz-yourself format similar to that of the Recall series. Provides an excellent review of high-yield facts. Good mnemonics, but only a few images of pathogens in black and white. Good review text on a high-yield topic.

$19.95   Review

A⁻

Clinical Microbiology Made Ridiculously Simple

GLADWIN

MedMaster, 2007, 392 pages, ISBN 9780940780811

An excellent, easy-to-read, detailed review of microbiology that includes clever and memorable mnemonics. The style of the series does not appeal to everyone. The sections on bacterial disease are most high yield, whereas the pharmacology chapters lack sufficient detail. Recommended to read during coursework and review the concise charts at the end of each chapter during boards review. All images are cartoons; no microscopy images that appear on boards. Requires a supplemental source for immunology.

$32.95   Review

A⁻

Microcards Flash Cards

HARPAVAT

Lippincott Williams & Wilkins, 2007, 300 pages, ISBN 9780781769242

A well-organized and complete resource for students who like to use flash cards for review. Cards feature the clinical presentation, pathobiology, diagnosis, treatment, and high-yield facts for a particular organism. Some cards also include excellent flow charts organizing important classes of bacteria or viruses. Overall, a good review resource, but at times it is overly detailed, requiring a significant time commitment.

$36.95   Flash cards

REVIEW RESOURCES

MICROBIOLOGY AND IMMUNOLOGY

High-Yield Microbiology and Infectious Diseases
HAWLEY
Lippincott Williams & Wilkins, 2006, 240 pages,
ISBN 9780781760324

A very concise review of central concepts and keywords, with chapters organized by microorganism. The last few sections contain brief questions and answers organized by organ system. Also offers a useful chapter on "microbial comparisons" that groups organisms by shared virulence factors, lab results, and the like. Some students may prefer alternative resources with more explanations.

$28.95   Review/Test/200 q

High-Yield Immunology
JOHNSON
Lippincott Williams & Wilkins, 2006, 112 pages,
ISBN 9780781774697

Accurately covers high-yield immunology concepts, although at times it includes more detail than necessary for Step 1 preparation. Good for quick review. The newest edition includes many improvements.

$28.95   Review

Review of Medical Microbiology
MURRAY
Elsevier, 2005, 176 pages, ISBN 9780323033251

A resource that features Step 1–style questions divided into bacteriology, virology, mycology, and parasitology. All questions are accompanied by detailed explanations, and some are paired with high-quality images. Questions are similar to those on Step 1 and provide a nice review. Supplements Murray's *Medical Microbiology*.

$39.95   Test/550 q

Medical Microbiology and Immunology Flash Cards
ROSENTHAL
Elsevier, 2008, 414 pages, ISBN 9780323065337

Flash cards covering the microorganisms most commonly found on Step 1. Each card features full-color microscopic images and clinical presentations on one side and relevant bug information in conjunction with a short case on the other side. Also includes Student Consult online access for extra features. Overemphasizes "trigger words" related to each bug. Not a comprehensive resource.

$35.95   Flash cards

Lange Microbiology & Infectious Diseases Flash Cards
SOMERS
McGraw-HIll, 2010, 200 flash cards, ISBN 9780071628792

Contains a clinical vignette on one side and discussion on the other. Excellent condensed summaries of pathogens, but limited by lack of images that will be tested on boards.

$31.45   Flash cards

BRS Microbiology Flash Cards
SWANSON
Lippincott Williams & Wilkins, 2003, 500 pages,
ISBN 9780781744270
A concise series of flash cards featuring high-yield microbiology facts with an emphasis on virulence factors. A good last-second microbiology review after study of a more comprehensive text.

$39.95   Flash cards

Underground Clinical Vignettes: Microbiology Vol. I: Virology, Immunology, Parasitology, Mycology
SWANSON
Lippincott Williams & Wilkins, 2007, 256 pages,
ISBN 9780781764704
A resource containing 100 concise clinical cases that illustrate frequently tested diseases in microbiology and immunology. Cardinal signs, symptoms, and buzzwords are highlighted. Also includes 20 additional boards-style questions. Best if used as a supplement to other review resources.

$22.95   Review/Test/20 q

Underground Clinical Vignettes: Microbiology Vol. II: Bacteriology
SWANSON
Lippincott Williams & Wilkins, 2007, 256 pages,
ISBN 9780781764711
A resource containing 100 concise clinical cases that illustrate frequently tested diseases in microbiology and immunology. Cardinal signs, symptoms, and buzzwords are highlighted. Also includes 20 additional boards-style questions. Best if used as a supplement to other review resources.

$22.95   Review/Test/20 q

Basic Immunology
ABBAS
Elsevier, 2010, 312 pages, ISBN 9781416055693
A useful text that offers clear explanations of complex topics in immunology. Best if used during the year in conjunction with coursework and later skimmed for quick Step 1 review. Includes colorful diagrams, images, tables, and a lengthy glossary for further study. Features online access.

$64.95   Review

Elsevier's Integrated Immunology and Microbiology

ACTOR

Elsevier, 2006, 192 pages, ISBN 9780323033893

$40.95   Review

Part of the Integrated series that seeks to link basic science concepts across disciplines. Case-based and Step 1–style questions at the end of each chapter allow users to gauge their comprehension of the material. Includes online access. Best if used during coursework. Limited student feedback.

Concise Medical Immunology

DOAN

Lippincott Williams & Wilkins, 2005, 256 pages, ISBN 9780781757416

$39.95   Review

Lives up to its name as a concise text with useful diagrams, illustrations, and tables. Good for students who need extra immunology review or for those who wish to study the subject thoroughly for the boards. End-of-chapter multiple-choice questions help reinforce key concepts.

Case Studies in Immunology: Clinical Companion

GEHA

Garland Science, 2007, 328 pages, ISBN 9780815341451

$49.95   Review

A text that was originally designed as a clinical companion to *Janeway's Immunobiology*. Provides a great synopsis of the major disorders of immunity in a clinical vignette format. Integrates basic and clinical sciences. Features excellent images and illustrations from Janeway, as well as questions and discussions.

Review of Medical Microbiology and Immunology

LEVINSON

McGraw-Hill, 2010, 640 pages, ISBN 9780071700283

$49.95   Review/Test/654 q

A clear, comprehensive text with outstanding diagrams and tables. Includes an excellent immunology section. The "Summary of Medically Important Organisms" is highly crammable. Can be detailed and dense at points, so best if started early. Features comprehensive coverage of material. Includes practice questions of mixed quality and does not provide detailed explanation of answers. Compare with *Lippincott's Illustrated Reviews: Microbiology*; both require time commitment.

Review of Immunology
LICHTMAN

$33.95   Test/500 q

Elsevier, 2005, 192 pages, ISBN 9780721603438

Complements Abbas's *Cellular and Molecular Immunology* and *Basic Immunology* textbooks. Contains 500 boards-style questions featuring full-color illustrations along with explanations of all answer choices. A good resource for questions in a lower-yield topic. Limited student feedback.

Crash Course: Immunology
NOVAK

$49.95   Review

Elsevier, 2006, 144 pages, ISBN 9781416030072

Part of the Crash Course review series for basic sciences, integrating clinical topics. Offers two-color illustrations, handy study tools, and Step 1 review questions. Includes online access. Good length and detail for boards review.

Rapid Review: Microbiology and Immunology
ROSENTHAL

$39.95   Review/Test/400 q

Elsevier, 2010, 240 pages, ISBN 9780323069380

A resource presented in a format similar to that of other books in the Rapid Review series. Contains many excellent tables and figures, but requires significant time commitment and is not as high yield as comparable review books. Includes access to companion Web site with more than 400 questions.

Case Files: Microbiology
TOY

$33.95   Review

McGraw-Hill, 2008, 432 pages, ISBN 9780071492584

Fifty clinical microbiology cases followed by a clinical correlation, a discussion with boldfaced buzzwords, and questions. Cases are well chosen, but the text lacks the high-yield charts and tables found in comparable review resources. Images are sparse and of poor black-and-white quality.

USMLE Road Map: Microbiology and Infectious Diseases
BOS

$31.95   Review

McGraw-Hill, 2004, 240 pages, ISBN 9780071435079

A concise review of microbiology in outline format. Includes several questions at the end of each chapter for comprehension testing. Good tables but few images of pathogens or symptoms. Limited student feedback.

Lippincott's Illustrated Reviews: Immunology
DOAN

$54.95   Review/Test/Few q

Lippincott Williams & Wilkins, 2007, 384 pages,
ISBN 9780781795432

A clearly written, highly detailed review of basic concepts in immunology. Features many useful tables and review questions at the end of each chapter. Offers abbreviated coverage of immune deficiencies and autoimmune disorders. Best if started with initial coursework and used as a reference during Step 1 study.

Lippincott's Illustrated Reviews: Microbiology
HARVEY

$54.95   Review/Test/Few q

Lippincott Williams & Wilkins, 2006, 432 pages,
ISBN 9780781782159

A comprehensive, highly illustrated review of microbiology that is similar in style to other titles in the Illustrated Reviews series. Includes a 50-page color section with more than 150 clinical and laboratory photographs. Compare with Levinson's *Review of Medical Microbiology and Immunology.*

Pretest: Microbiology
KETTERING

$29.95   Review/Test/500 q

McGraw-Hill, 2010, 400 pages, ISBN 97800716233530

Includes a short section on high-yield facts followed by 500 questions in a clinical vignette format. Questions are more difficult than encountered on the boards and some topics discussed are not likely to be tested. A reasonable book to work through with coursework but too low yield for review purposes.

USMLE Road Map: Immunology
PARMELY

$31.95   Review

McGraw-Hill, 2006, 223 pages, ISBN 9780071452984

An outline review of immunology with a special focus on molecular mechanisms and laboratory techniques. Features abbreviated coverage of immunologic deficiency and autoimmune diseases that are emphasized on Step 1. Offers a collection of brief review questions at the end of each chapter. Limited student feedback.

A   ***Rapid Review: Pathology***   **$44.95**   Review/Test/350 q

GOLJAN

Elsevier, 2009, 656 pages, ISBN 9780323068628

A comprehensive source for key concepts in pathology, presented in a bulleted outline format with many high-yield tables and color figures. Features detailed explanations of disease mechanisms. Integrates concepts across disciplines with a strong clinical orientation. Lengthy, so best if started early with coursework. Includes access to online Qbank.

A   ***The Big Picture: Pathology***   **$49.95**   Review/Test/130 q

KEMP

McGraw-Hill, 2007, 512 pages, ISBN 9780071477482

Excellent atlas of pathologic images with distilled notes on pathophysiology and treatment. Good for quick review and especially good for visual learners. The 130 questions included at the end are more straightforward than those seen on boards, but they emphasize important and tricky concepts.

A   ***Robbins and Cotran Review of Pathology***   **$49.95**   Review/Test/1100 q

KLATT

Elsevier, 2009, 464 pages, ISBN 9781416049302

A review question book that follows the main Robbins textbooks. Questions are more detailed and difficult than those on the actual Step 1 exam, but the text offers a great review of pathology integrated with excellent images. Thorough answer explanations reinforce key points. Requires significant time commitment, so best if started with coursework.

A   ***BRS Pathology***   **$39.95**   Review/Test/450 q

SCHNEIDER

Lippincott Williams & Wilkins, 2009, 464 pages, ISBN 9780781779418

An excellent, concise review with appropriate content emphasis. Chapters are organized by organ system and feature an outline format with boldfacing of key facts. Includes good questions with explanations at the end of each chapter plus a comprehensive exam at the end of the book. Offers well-organized tables and diagrams as well as photographs representative of classic pathology. Contains a chapter on laboratory testing and "key associations" with each disease. The new edition contains excellent color images and access to an online test and interactive question bank. Most effective if started early in conjunction with coursework, as it does not discuss detailed mechanisms of disease pathology.

REVIEW RESOURCES

PATHOLOGY

Pathophysiology for the Boards and Wards
AYALA

Lippincott Williams & Wilkins, 2006, 430 pages,
ISBN 9781405105101

$39.95   Review/Test/75 q

A systems-based outline with a focus on pathology. Well organized with glossy color plates of relevant pathology and excellent, concise tables. The appendix includes a helpful overview of neurology, immunology, unusual "zebra" syndromes, and high-yield pearls. Features good integration of Step 1–relevant material from various subject areas. Compare with *Rapid Review: Pathology*.

Lange Pathology Flash Cards
BARON

McGraw-Hill, 2009, 277 flash cards, ISBN 9780071613057

$34.95   Flash cards

Flash cards with clinical vignette on one side and discussion including etiology, pathology, clinical manifestations, and treatment on the other. Good tables to help organize diseases, but lack of images limits its utility. Best if used in conjunction with another resource.

Déjà Review: Pathology
DAVIS

McGraw-Hill, 2010, 480 pages, ISBN 9780071627146

$19.95   Review

Features questions and answers in a two-column, quiz-yourself format similar to that of the Recall series. A great review that integrates pathophysiology and pathology. Includes many vignette-style questions, but only a few images in black and white. Limited student feedback.

Lippincott's Illustrated Q&A Review of Rubin's Pathology
FENDERSON

Lippincott Williams & Wilkins, 2010, 336 pages,
ISBN 9781608316403

$48.95   Review/Test/1100 q

A review book featuring more than 1100 multiple-choice questions that follow the Step 1 template. Questions frequently require multi-step reasoning, probing the student's ability to integrate basic science knowledge in a clinical situation. Detailed rationales are linked to clinical vignettes and address incorrect answer choices. More than 300 full-color images link clinical and pathologic findings, with normal lab values provided for reference. Questions are presented both online and in print. Students can work through the online questions either in "quiz mode," which provides instant feedback, or in "test mode," which simulates the Step 1 experience. Overall, a resource that is similar in quality to *Robbins and Cotran Review of Pathology*.

Underground Clinical Vignettes: Pathophysiology Vol. I: Pulmonary, Ob/Gyn, ENT, Hem/Onc   **$27.95**   Review/Test/20 q

SWANSON

Lippincott Williams & Wilkins, 2007, 228 pages,
ISBN 9780781764650

Concise clinical cases illustrating 100 frequently tested pathology and physiology concepts. Cardinal signs, symptoms, and buzzwords are highlighted. Also includes 20 additional boards-style questions. Best if used as a supplement to other sources of review.

Underground Clinical Vignettes: Pathophysiology Vol. II: GI, Neurology, Rheumatology, Endocrinology   **$27.95**   Review/Test/20 q

SWANSON

Lippincott Williams & Wilkins, 2007, 256 pages,
ISBN 9780781764667

Concise clinical cases illustrating 100 frequently tested pathology and physiology concepts. Cardinal signs, symptoms, and buzzwords are highlighted. Also includes 20 additional boards-style questions. Best if used as a supplement to other sources of review.

Underground Clinical Vignettes: Pathophysiology Vol. III: CV, Dermatology, GU, Orthopedics, General Surgery, Peds   **$27.95**   Review/Test/20 q

SWANSON

Lippincott Williams & Wilkins, 2007, 256 pages,
ISBN 9780781764681

Concise clinical cases illustrating 100 frequently tested pathology and physiology concepts. Cardinal signs, symptoms, and buzzwords are highlighted. Also includes 20 additional boards-style questions. Best if used as a supplement to other sources of review.

MedMaps for Pathophysiology   **$39.95**   Review

AGOSTI

Lippincott Williams & Wilkins, 2007, 259 pages,
ISBN 9780781777551

A rapid review that contains 102 concept maps of disease processes and mechanisms organized by organ system, as well as classic diseases. Useful for both coursework and Step 1 preparation. Ample room is provided for notes. A good resource for looking up specific mechanisms, especially when used in conjunction with other primary review sources.

Cases & Concepts Step 1: Pathophysiology Review   **$42.95**   Review/Test/150 q

CAUGHEY
Lippincott Williams & Wilkins, 2009, 376 pages,
ISBN 9780781782548

Eighty-eight clinical cases integrating basic science concepts with
clinical data, followed by USMLE-style questions with answers and
rationales. Thumbnail and key-concept boxes highlight key facts.
Limited student feedback.

B+ Case Files: Pathology   **$33.95**   Review

TOY
McGraw-Hill, 2008, 456 pages, ISBN 9780071486668

Includes 50 clinical cases followed by discussion, comprehension
questions, and a pathology pearls box. Cases are well chosen and
good for those who prefer problem-based learning; however, utility is
limited by scarce and poor-quality black-and-white images.

B+ USMLE Road Map: Pathology   **$31.95**   Test/500 q

WETTACH
McGraw-Hill, 2009, 412 pages, ISBN 9780071482677

A concise yet thorough outline-format review of diseases that are
tested on boards. Text is easy to read and includes a glossary of commonly used terms. Questions at the end of each chapter are useful
only for testing comprehension. Black-and-white images.

B PreTest Pathology   **$29.95**   Test/500 q

BROWN
McGraw-Hill, 2010, 612 pages, ISBN 9780071623490

Difficult questions with detailed, complete answers. High-yield facts
at the beginning are useful for concept summaries, but information
can easily be obtained in better review books. Features high-quality
black-and-white photographs but no color illustrations. Best used as a
supplement to other review books.

**B Blueprints Notes & Cases—Pathophysiology: Renal,
Hematology, and Oncology**   **$34.95**   Review

CAUGHEY
Lippincott Williams & Wilkins, 2003, 208 pages,
ISBN 9781405103527

A review book that follows the format of the Blueprints series, in
which each case takes the form of a discussion followed by key points
and a series of questions. The pathophysiology volumes would be a
good companion to organ-based teaching modules, but the content is
not always representative of what will be tested on the boards.

REVIEW RESOURCES

PATHOLOGY

Colour Atlas of Anatomical Pathology
COOKE

$103.95   Review

Elsevier, 2003, 300 pages, ISBN 9780443073601

An impressive color atlas of gross pathology. Photographs are clinically relevant and have concise captions that include relevant pathologic details. Limited student feedback.

High-Yield Histopathology
DUDEK

$27.95   Review

Lippincott Williams & Wilkins, 2007, 336 pages,
ISBN 9780781769594

A new book that reviews the relationship of basic histology to the pathology, physiology, and pharmacology of clinical conditions that are tested on Step 1. Includes case studies, numerous light and electron micrographs, and pathology photographs. Given its considerable length, should be started with coursework. Limited student feedback.

Crash Course: Pathology
FISHBACK

$49.95   Review

Elsevier, 2005, 384 pages, ISBN 9780323033084

Part of the Crash Course review series for basic sciences, integrating clinical topics. Offers two-color illustrations, handy study tools, and Step 1 review questions. Includes online access. Best if started during coursework.

Blueprints Notes & Cases—Pathophysiology: Cardiovascular, Endocrine, and Reproduction
LEUNG

$32.00   Review

Lippincott Williams & Wilkins, 2003, 208 pages,
ISBN 9781405103503

A review book that follows the format of the Blueprints series, in which each case takes the form of a discussion followed by key points and a series of questions. The pathophysiology volumes would be a good companion to organ-based teaching modules, but the content is not always representative of what will be tested on the boards.

Pathcards
MARCUCCI

$39.95   Flash cards

Lippincott Williams & Wilkins, 2003, 553 pages,
ISBN 9780781743990

Flash cards that offer comprehensive and detailed information instead of a bulleted, high-yield facts format. Appropriate level of depth for Step 1 pathology. Lacks clinical vignettes and color images found in other review resources. Compare with *Lange Flash Cards*.

Pathophysiology of Disease: Introduction to Clinical Medicine
McPHEE

$69.95   Review/Test/Few q

McGraw-Hill, 2009, 752 pages, ISBN 9780071621670
An interdisciplinary text useful for understanding the pathophysiology of clinical symptoms. Effectively integrates the basic sciences with mechanisms of disease. Features great graphs, diagrams, and tables. In view of its length, most useful if started during coursework. Includes a few non–boards-style questions. The text's clinical emphasis nicely complements *BRS Pathology*.

Haematology at a Glance
MEHTA

$40.95   Review

Blackwell Science, 2009, 128 pages, ISBN 9781405179706
A resource that covers common hematologic issues. Includes color illustrations. Presented in a logical sequence that is easy to read. Good for use with coursework.

Pocket Companion to Robbins and Cotran Pathologic Basis of Disease
MITCHELL

$42.95   Review

Elsevier, 2006, 816 pages, ISBN 9780721602653
A resource that is good for reviewing keywords associated with most important diseases. Presented in a highly condensed format, but the text is complete and easy to understand. Contains no photographs or illustrations. Useful as a quick reference.

PreTest Pathophysiology
MUFSON

$28.95   Test/500 q

McGraw-Hill, 2004, 480 pages, ISBN 9780071434928
Includes 500 questions and answers with explanations. Questions are often overly specific, and explanations vary in quality. Features a brief section of high-yield topics. Good economic value.

Color Atlas of Physiology
SILBERNAGL

$44.95   Review

Thieme, 2009, 456 pages, ISBN 9783135450063
A text containing more than 180 high-quality illustrations of disturbed physiologic processes that lead to dysfunction. An alternative to standard texts, but not high yield for boards review.

BRS Pathology Flash Cards

$39.95   Flash cards

SWANSON

Lippincott Williams & Wilkins, 2002, 250 flash cards,
ISBN 9780781737104

A series of 250 pathology flash cards categorized by organ system. Effective when used in combination with the *BRS Pathology* textbook or another pathology review text, but not comprehensive enough when used alone.

Kaplan Medical USMLE Pharmacology and Treatment Flashcards
FISCHER
Kaplan, 2008, 200 flash cards, ISBN 9781427797063
Excellent, easy-to-read flash cards with drug and questions on one side and discussion on the other, offering just the right amount of detail for the boards. Alternative to more traditional pharmacology textbooks.

$44.95   Flash cards

Déjà Review: Pharmacology
GLEASON
McGraw-Hill, 2010, 224 pages, ISBN 9780071627290
Features questions and answers in a two-column, quiz-yourself format similar to that of the Recall series. Covers most of the drugs needed for Step 1 pithily and directly. Includes clinical vignettes at the end of chapters for review.

$19.95   Review

Lange Pharmacology Flash Cards
BARON
McGraw-Hill, 2009, 189 pages, ISBN 9780071622417
A total of 189 pocket-sized flash cards featuring clinical vignettes involving relevant drugs, with high-yield information highlighted in bold. Limited student feedback.

$34.95   Flash cards

BRS Pharmacology Flash Cards
KIM
Lippincott Williams & Wilkins, 2004, 640 pages,
ISBN 9780781747967
A series of flash cards that facilitate memorization of the appropriate clinical use of drugs rather than describing mechanisms and toxicities in detail. Not a comprehensive review resource, but may be useful for those who find other pharm cards overwhelming. Considered by many to be an excellent resource for quick, last-minute review.

$32.95   Flash cards

Pharmacology for the Boards and Wards
AYALA
Lippincott Williams & Wilkins, 2006, 256 pages,
ISBN 9781405105118
Like other books in the Boards and Wards series, the pharmacology volume is presented primarily in tabular format with bulleted key points. Review questions are in Step 1 style. At times can be too dense, but does a great job of focusing on the clinical aspects of drugs.

$39.95   Review/Test/150 q

REVIEW RESOURCES

PHARMACOLOGY

Crash Course: Pharmacology

BARNES

$49.95   Review

Elsevier, 2006, 248 pages, ISBN 9781416029595

Part of the Crash Course review series for basic sciences, integrating clinical topics. Offers two-color illustrations, handy study tools, and Step 1–style review questions. Includes online access. Gives a solid, easy-to-follow overview of pharmacology. Limited student feedback.

Pharmacology Flash Cards

BRENNER

$36.95   Flash cards

Elsevier, 2009, 640 pages, ISBN 9781437703115

Flash cards for more than 200 of the most commonly tested drugs. Cards include the name of the drug (both generic and brand) on the front and basic drug information on the back. Divided and color coded by class, and comes with a compact carrying case. Lacks figures and clinical vignettes.

Lippincott's Illustrated Reviews: Pharmacology

HARVEY

$59.95   Review/Test/200 q

Lippincott Williams & Wilkins, 2009, 564 pages, ISBN 9780781771559

A resource presented in outline format with practice questions, many excellent illustrations, and comparison tables. Effectively integrates pharmacology and pathophysiology. The new edition has been updated to cover recent changes in pharmacotherapy. Best started with coursework, as it is highly detailed and requires significant time commitment.

Pharm Cards: Review Cards for Medical Students

JOHANNSEN

$37.95   Flash cards

Lippincott Williams & Wilkins, 2010, 240 flash cards, ISBN 9780781787413

A series of flash cards that cover the mechanisms and side effects of major drugs and drug classes. Good for class review, but the level of detail is beyond what is necessary for Step 1. Lacks pharmacokinetics, but features good charts and diagrams. Well liked by students who enjoy flash card–based review. Compare with *BRS Pharmacology Flash Cards.*

B⁺

Elsevier's Integrated Pharmacology
KESTER

Elsevier, 2007, 336 pages, ISBN 9780323034081

Part of the Integrated series that seeks to link basic science concepts across disciplines. Case-based and Step 1–style questions at the end of each chapter allow readers to gauge their comprehension of the material. Includes online access. Best if used during coursework. Limited student feedback.

$39.95   Review

B⁺

Rapid Review: Pharmacology
PAZDERNIK

Elsevier, 2010, 360 pages, ISBN 9780323068123

A detailed treatment of pharmacology, presented in an outline format similar to that of other books in the series. More detailed than necessary for Step 1 review. Contains high-yield charts and figures. Includes access to the companion Web site with 450 USMLE-style questions.

$39.95   Review

B⁺

Pharmacology Recall
RAMACHANDRAN

Lippincott Williams & Wilkins, 2008, 592 pages + audio, ISBN 9780781787307

A resource presented in the two-column, question-and-answer format typical of the Recall series. At times questions delve into more clinical detail than required for Step 1, but overall the breadth of coverage is appropriate. Includes a high-yield drug summary. Includes questions and answers that are recorded in MP3 format so that they can be used on any audio player.

$42.95   Review

B⁺

Underground Clinical Vignettes Step 1: Pharmacology
SWANSON

Lippincott Williams & Wilkins, 2007, 256 pages, ISBN 9780781764858

Concise clinical cases illustrating approximately 100 frequently tested pharmacology concepts. Cardinal signs, symptoms, and buzzwords are highlighted. Also includes 20 additional boards-style questions. Omits some important drugs and lacks detail on mechanisms, so best used as a supplement to other sources of review.

$27.95   Review/Test/20 q

Katzung & Trevor's Pharmacology: Examination and Board Review
TREVOR

$49.95   Review/Test/1000 q

McGraw-Hill, 2010, 640 pages, ISBN 9780071701586

A well-organized text in narrative format with concise explanations. Features good charts and tables; the crammable list of "top boards drugs" is especially high yield. Also good for drug interactions and toxicities. Offers two practice exams but no explanations of the answers. Includes many low-yield/obscure drugs. Compare with *Lippincott's Illustrated Reviews: Pharmacology*, both of which are better suited to complementing coursework than last-minute studying for boards.

USMLE Road Map: Pharmacology
KATZUNG

$31.95   Review

McGraw-Hill, 2006, 178 pages, ISBN 9780071445818

An outline review of pharmacology divided either by organ system or by disease process. Includes a collection of brief review questions at the end of each chapter. The appendix has a useful table of common side effects. Does not contain enough detail to serve as a comprehensive review. Limited student feedback.

BRS Pharmacology
ROSENFELD

$39.95   Review/Test/200 q

Lippincott Williams & Wilkins, 2009, 368 pages, ISBN 9780781789134

Features two-color tables and figures that summarize essential information for quick recall. A list of drugs organized by drug family is included in each chapter. Too detailed for boards review; best used as a reference. Also offers end-of-chapter review tests with Step 1–style questions and a comprehensive exam with explanations of answers. An additional question bank is available online.

PreTest Pharmacology
SHLAFER

$29.95   Test/500 q

McGraw-Hill, 2010, 558 pages, ISBN 9780071623421

Good questions divided into sections by organ system and accompanied by detailed answers. Sections on general principles and autonomics are especially useful. Best used as a resource for additional questions after other sources have been exhausted.

REVIEW RESOURCES

PHARMACOLOGY

Case Files: Pharmacology
TOY

$33.95   Review/Test/150 q

McGraw-Hill, 2008, 440 pages, ISBN 9780071488587
Includes 53 cases with detailed discussion, comprehension questions, and a box of clinical pearls. An appealing text for students who prefer problem-based learning, but lacks the level of detail typically tested on Step 1.

High-Yield Pharmacology
WEISS

$27.95   Review

Lippincott Williams & Wilkins, 2009, 160 pages,
ISBN 9780781792738
A succinct pharmacology review presented in an easy-to-follow outline format. Features a drug index, key points in bold, and summary tables of high-yield facts. Lacks details on mechanisms or drug specifics, so best used with a more comprehensive resource.

A

BRS Physiology
COSTANZO

$39.95   Review/Test/400 q

Lippincott Williams & Wilkins, 2010, 384 pages,
ISBN 9780781798761

A clear, concise review of physiology that is both comprehensive and efficient, making for fast, easy reading. Includes excellent high-yield charts and tables, but lacks some figures from Costanzo's *Physiology*. Features high-quality practice questions with explanations in each chapter along with a clinically oriented final exam. An excellent boards review resource, but best if started early in combination with coursework. Respiratory and acid-base sections are comparatively weak.

A⁻

Physiology
COSTANZO

$59.95   Text

Elsevier, 2009, 512 pages, ISBN 9781416062165

A comprehensive, clearly written text that covers concepts outlined in *BRS Physiology* in greater detail. Offers excellent color diagrams and charts. Each systems-based chapter features a detailed summary of objectives and a Step 1–relevant clinical case. Includes access to on-line interactive extras. Requires time commitment; best started with coursework.

A⁻

The Big Picture: Medical Physiology
KIBBLE

$46.95   Review/Text/108 q

McGraw-Hill, 2009, 448 pages, ISBN 9780071485678

Well-written text supplemented by 450 illustrations. Chapters conclude with approximately 10 study questions/answers. Viable alternative to Costanzo's Physiology, with more clinical correlations. Includes a 108-question practice exam with answers. Best if started early with coursework.

B⁺

Rapid Review: Physiology
BROWN

$39.95   Review

Elsevier, 2006, 352 pages, ISBN 9780323019910

A resource that offers a good review of physiology in a format typical of the Rapid Review series. Features 100 questions with explanations. Includes online access to an additional 250 questions along with other extras. Limited student feedback.

REVIEW RESOURCES

PHYSIOLOGY

BRS Physiology Cases and Problems
COSTANZO
Lippincott Williams & Wilkins, 2008, 352 pages,
ISBN 9780781788717
Sixty classic cases presented in vignette format with several questions
per case. Includes exceptionally detailed explanations of answers. For
students interested in an in-depth discussion of physiology concepts.
May be useful for group review.

$39.95   Review/Test/Many q

High-Yield Physiology
DUDEK
Lippincott Williams & Wilkins, 2008, 240 pages,
ISBN 9780781745871
An outline review of major concepts written at an appropriate level
of depth for Step 1; includes especially detailed coverage of cardiovascular, respiratory, and renal physiology. Features many excellent
diagrams and boxes highlighting important equations. Large blocks of
dense text make it a slow and disorienting read at times. Limited student feedback.

$28.95   Review

Déjà Review: Physiology
GOULD
McGraw-Hill, 2010, 288 pages, ISBN 9780071627252
Features questions and answers in a two-column, quiz-yourself format similar to that of the Recall series. Includes helpful graphs and
diagrams. Contains clinical vignettes at the end of each organ system
similar to those seen on the Step 1 exam. Limited student feedback.

$19.95   Review

High-Yield Acid-Base Review
LONGENECKER
Lippincott Williams & Wilkins, 2006, 128 pages,
ISBN 9780781796552
A concise and well-written description of acid-base disorders. Includes
chapters discussing differential diagnoses and 12 clinical cases. Intro-
duces a multistep approach to the material. A bookmark with useful
factoids is included with the text. No index or questions.

$26.95   Review

Appleton & Lange Review: Physiology
PENNEY
McGraw-Hill, 2005, 224 pages, ISBN 9780071445177
Step 1–style questions divided into subcategories under physiology.
Good if subject-specific questions are desired, but may be too detailed
for many students. Some diagrams are used to explain answers. A
good way to test knowledge after coursework.

$39.95   Test/700 q

B   *Elsevier's Integrated Physiology*   ***$37.95***   Review

CARROLL

Elsevier, 2006, 256 pages, ISBN 9780323043182

Part of the Integrated series that seeks to link basic science concepts across disciplines. A good text for initial coursework, but too long for Step 1 review. Case-based and Step 1–style questions are included at the end of each chapter. Limited student feedback.

B   *PreTest Physiology*   ***$29.95***   Test/500 q

METTING

McGraw-Hill, 2010, 448 pages, ISBN 9780071623506

Contains questions with detailed, well-written explanations. One of the best of the PreTest series. Best for use by the motivated student after extensive review of other sources. Includes a high-yield facts section with useful diagrams.

B   *Netter's Physiology Flash Cards*   ***$35.95***   Flash cards

MULRONEY

Saunders, 2010, 200+ flash cards, ISBN 9781416046288

Flash cards contain a high-quality illustration on one side with question and commentary on the other. Good for self-testing, but too fragmented for learning purposes and not comprehensive enough for boards. Limited student feedback.

B   *USMLE Road Map: Physiology*   ***$26.95***   Review/Test/50 q

PASLEY

McGraw-Hill, 2006, 219 pages, ISBN 9780071445177

A text in outline format incorporating useful comparison charts and clear diagrams. Provides a concise approach to physiology. Clinical correlations are referenced to the text. Questions build on basic concepts and include detailed explanations. Limited student feedback.

B   *Acid-Base, Fluids, and Electrolytes Made Ridiculously Simple*   ***$22.95***   Review

PRESTON

MedMaster, 2010, 156 pages, ISBN 9780940780989

A resource that covers major acid-base and renal physiology concepts. Provides information beyond the scope of Step 1, but remains a useful companion for studying kidney function, electrolyte disturbances, and fluid management. Includes scattered diagrams and questions at the end of each chapter. Consider using after exhausting more high-yield physiology review resources.

REVIEW RESOURCES

PHYSIOLOGY

Case Files: Physiology
TOY

$33.95   Review

McGraw-Hill, 2009, 456 pages, ISBN 9780071493741

A review text divided into 51 clinical cases followed by clinical correlations, a discussion, and take-home pearls, presented in a format similar to that of other texts in the Case Files series. A few questions accompany each case. Too lengthy for rapid review; best for students who enjoy problem-based learning.

Vander's Renal Physiology
EATON

$39.95   Text

McGraw-Hill, 2009, 240 pages, ISBN 9780071613033

Well-written text on renal physiology, with helpful diagrams and questions at the end of each chapter. Far too detailed for Step 1 review, however. Best if used with coursework to understand the principles of renal physiology.

Clinical Physiology Made Ridiculously Simple
GOLDBERG

$19.95   Review

MedMaster, 2007, 160 pages, ISBN 9780940780217

An easy-to-read text with many amusing associations and memorable mnemonics. The style does not work for everyone. Not as well illustrated as the rest of the series, and lacks some important concepts. Best used as a supplement to other review books.

Endocrine Physiology
MOLINA

$42.95   Text

McGraw-Hill, 2009, 312 pages, ISBN 9780071613019

Good but lengthy text on endocrine physiology. Questions at the end of each chapter are helpful to work through, but most are not representative of Step 1 questions. Provides more detailed explanations of endocrine physiology than Costanzo offers, so is good for use with coursework, but much too lengthy for Step 1 review.

Pulmonary Pathophysiology: The Essentials
WEST

$42.95   Review/Test/50 q

Lippincott Williams & Wilkins, 2007, 224 pages,
ISBN 9780781764148

A volume offering comprehensive coverage of respiratory physiology. Clearly organized with useful charts and diagrams. Review questions at the end of each chapter have letter answers only and no explanations. Best used as a course supplement.

Commercial Review Courses

- ▶ Falcon Physician Reviews
- ▶ Kaplan Medical
- ▶ Northwestern Medical Review
- ▶ The Princeton Review
- ▶ Doctor Youel's™ Prep, Inc.

Commercial preparation courses can be helpful for some students, but such courses are expensive and may leave limited time for independent study. They are usually an effective tool for students who feel overwhelmed by the volume of material they must review in preparation for the boards. Also note that while some commercial courses are designed for first-time test takers, others are geared toward students who are repeating the examination. Still other courses have been created for IMGs who want to take all three Steps in a limited amount of time. Finally, student experience and satisfaction with review courses are highly variable, and course content and structure can evolve rapidly. We thus suggest that you discuss options with recent graduates of review courses you are considering. Some student opinions can be found in discussion groups on the World Wide Web.

Falcon Physician Reviews

Established in 2002, Falcon Physician Reviews provides intensive and comprehensive live reviews for students preparing for the USMLE and COMLEX. The seven-week Step 1 reviews are held throughout the year with small class sizes in order to increase student involvement and instructor accessibility. Falcon Physician Reviews uses an active learning system that focuses on comprehension, retention, and application of concepts. Falcon Online program components include:

- A full set of color Falcon textbooks
- Hundreds of hours of lectures optimized into high-yield streaming video
- On-screen PowerPoint slides
- A three-month USMLEWorld or six-month USMLE Consult Question Bank subscription
- Diagnostic exam
- Available as an iPhone application

Falcon Live programs are currently offered in Dallas, Texas; Pittsburgh, Pennsylvania; and New York City, New York. The fee is $4950. The all-inclusive program tuition fee includes:

- Lodging
- Complimentary daily breakfast and lunch
- A full set of color Falcon textbooks
- Daily clinical vignettes
- Daily tutoring
- High-speed Internet service
- Local hotel shuttle service
- A three-month USMLEWorld or six-month USMLE Consult Question Bank subscription

For more information, contact:

Falcon Physician Reviews
440 Wrangler Drive, Suite 100
Coppell, TX 75019
Phone: (888) 516-9991
Fax: (214) 292-8568
www.falconreviews.com

Kaplan Medical

Kaplan Medical offers a wide range of options for USMLE preparation, including live lectures, center-based study, and online products. All of its courses and products focus on providing the most exam-relevant information available.

Live Lectures. Kaplan's LivePrep offers a highly structured, interactive live lecture series led by expert faculty as 7-, 14-, or 16-week courses. This course's advantages include interaction with faculty and peers.

Kaplan also offers LivePrep Retreat, a seven-week course during which students stay and study in high-end hotel accommodations.

Center Study. Kaplan's CenterPrep, a center-based lecture course, is designed for medical students seeking flexibility. Essentially an independent study course, it is offered at more than 150 Kaplan Centers across the United States in three-, six-, or nine-month periods. Students have access to more than 160 hours of video lecture review. CenterPrep features seven volumes of lecture notes; a question book that includes 850 practice questions with answers and explanations; and a full-length simulated exam with a complete performance analysis and detailed explanations. The course also includes a Personalized Learning System (PLS), which allows students to create a customized study schedule and track their performance.

Online Resources. Kaplan Medical provides online content- and question-based review. WebPrep offers 100 hours of video-streamed lectures, seven volumes of lecture notes, a full online Step 1 simulated exam, and access to Kaplan Medical's popular online question bank, Qbank, which contains more than 2150 USMLE-style practice questions with detailed explanations. WebPrep is designed to provide students with the most flexible content- and question-based review available.

Kaplan's popular Qbank allows students to create practice tests by discipline and organ system, receive instant on-screen feedback, and track their cumulative performance. Qbank demos are available at www.kaplanmedical.com.

More information can be obtained at (800) 533-8850 or by visiting www.kaplanmedical.com.

Northwestern Medical Review

Northwestern Medical Review offers live-lecture review courses, videotaped lectures, and home-study plans in preparation for both the COMLEX Level I and USMLE Step 1 examinations. Four review plans are available for each exam: NBI 100, a three-day course; NBI 150, a four-day course; NBI 200, a five-day course; and NBI 300, from 8 to 21 days. All courses are in live-lecture format, and most are taught by the authors of the Northwestern Review Books. In addition to organized lecture notes and books for each subject, courses include Web-based question bank access, audio CDs, and a large pool of practice questions and simulated exams. All plans are available in a customized, onsite format for groups of second-year students from individual U.S. medical schools. Additionally, public sites are frequently offered in East Lansing, Detroit, Philadelphia, San Antonio, Los Angeles, Chicago, New York City, Las Vegas, and San Juan. Live courses and Center preparations are also globally available in India, China, the Persian Gulf area, Eastern Europe, and select Caribbean islands.

Tuition ranges from $395 for the three-day to $1495 for the 15-day course. Tuition includes all study materials and Web usage services, and it is based on group size, program duration, and early-enrollment discounts. Home-study materials, CBT question-bank access, and DVD materials are also available for purchase independent of the live-lecture plans. Northwestern offers a retake option as well as a liberal cancellation policy.

For more information, contact:

Northwestern Medical Review
P.O. Box 22174
Lansing, MI 48909-2174
Phone: (866) MedPass
Fax: (517) 347-7005
E-mail: contactus@northwesternmedicalreview.com
www.northwesternmedicalreview.com

The Princeton Review

The Princeton Review offers three flexible preparation options for the USMLE Step 1: the USMLE Online Course, the USMLE Classroom Course, and the USMLE Online Workout. In selected cities, The Princeton Review also offers a more intensive preparation course for IMGs.

USMLE Step 1 Classroom Courses for Medical Students. The USMLE Classroom Courses offer comprehensive preparation that includes the following:

- Seven hours of classroom review
- Seventy-five hours of online review, including lessons, vignettes, and drills
- Three full-length diagnostic tests with detailed score reports
- Seven comprehensive review manuals consisting of more than 1500 pages
- Seven minitests to gauge students' knowledge in each subject
- Twenty-four-hour e-mail support from The Princeton Review Online instructors
- Three months of online access

USMLE Online Courses. The USMLE Online Courses offer the following:

- Seventy-five hours of online review, including lessons, vignettes, and drills
- Complete review of all USMLE Step 1 subjects
- Three full-length CBTs
- Seven one-hour subject-based tests
- Complete set of print materials
- E-mail support from expert instructors
- 24/7 real-time support from The Princeton Review Online Coach
- Three months of access to tests, drills, and lessons

More information can be found on The Princeton Review's Web site at www.princetonreview.com.

Doctor Youel's™ Prep, Inc.

Doctor Youel's™ Prep, Inc., has specialized in medical board preparation for 30 years. The company provides DVDs, audiotapes, videotapes, a CD (Pre-Prep™, Quick Start™), books, live lectures, and tutorials for small groups as well as for individuals (TutorialPrep™). All DVDs, videotapes, audiotapes, live lectures, and tutorials are correlated with a three-book set of Prep Notes© consisting of two textbooks, *Youel's Jewels I*© and *Youel's Jewels II*© (984 pages), and *Case Studies*©, a question-and-answer book (1854 questions, answers, and explanations).

The Comprehensive DVD program consists of 56 hours of lectures by the systems with a three-book set: *Youel's Jewels I and II* and *Case Studies*. Integrated with these programs are pre-tests and post-tests.

All Doctor Youel's Prep courses are taught and written by physicians, reflecting the clinical slant of the boards. All programs are systems based. In addition, all programs are updated continuously. Accordingly, books are not printed until the order is received.

Delivery in the United States or overseas is usually within one week. Optional express delivery is also available. Doctor Youel's Prep Home Study Program™ allows students to own their materials and to use them for repetitive study in the convenience of their homes. Purchasers of any of Doctor Youel's Prep materials, programs, or services are enrolled as members of the Doctor Youel's Prep Family of Students™, which affords them access to free telephone tutoring at (800) 645-3985. Students may call 24/7. Doctor Youel's Prep live lectures are held at select medical schools at the invitation of the school and students.

Programs are custom-designed for content, number of hours, and scheduling to fit students' needs. First-year students are urged to call early to arrange live-lecture programs at their schools for next year.

For more information, contact:

Youel's Prep, Inc.
P.O. Box 31479
Palm Beach Gardens, FL 33420
Phone: (800) 645-3985
Fax: (561) 622-4858
E-mail: info@youelsprep.com
www.youelsprep.net

REVIEW RESOURCES

COMMERCIAL COURSES

587

Publisher Contacts

ASM Press
P.O. Box 605
Herndon, VA 20172
(800) 546-2416
Fax: (703) 661-1501
asmmail@presswarehouse.com
www.asmpress.org

Biotest Publishing Company, Inc.
5850 Thille Street, Suite 103
Ventura, CA 93003
SkeletonDude@BiotestOnline.com
www.biotestonline.com

Churchill Livingstone
(see Elsevier Science)

Elsevier Science
Order Fulfillment
3251 Riverport Lane
Maryland Heights, MO 63043
(800) 545-2522
Fax: (800) 535-9935
www.us.elsevierhealth.com

Exam Master
500 Ethel Court
Middletown, DE 19709-9410
(800) 572-3627
Fax: (302) 378-1153
customer_service@exammaster.com
www.exammaster.com

Garland Science Publishing
Taylor & Francis Group Ltd
2 Park Square
Milton Park, Abingdon
Oxford
OX14 4RN
UK
Tel: +44 (0) 20 7017 6000
Fax: +44 (0) 20 7017 6699
www.garlandscience.co.uk

Gold Standard Board Prep
3204 30th Street
Lubbock, TX 79410
(806) 773-3197
www.boardprep.net

Icon Learning Systems
(see Elsevier Science)

John Wiley & Sons
10475 Crosspoint Blvd.
Indianapolis, IN 46256
(877) 762-2974
Fax: (800) 597-3299
consumers@wiley.com
www.wiley.com

Kaplan, Inc.
888 Seventh Avenue
New York, NY 10106
(212) 492-5800
www.kaplan.com

Lippincott Williams & Wilkins
P.O. Box 1620
Hagerstown, MD 21741
(800) 638-3030
Fax: (301) 223-2400
orders@lww.com
www.lww.com

MedMaster, Inc.
P.O. Box 640028
Miami, FL 33164
(800) 335-3480
Fax: (954) 962-4508
mmbks@aol.com
www.medmaster.net

McGraw-Hill Companies
Order Services
P.O. Box 182604
Columbus, OH 43272-3031
(877) 833-5524
Fax: (614) 759-3749
customer.service@mcgraw-hill.com
www.mhprofessional.com

Mosby-Year Book
(see Elsevier Science)

Parthenon Publishing/CRC Press
Taylor & Francis Group
6000 Broken Sound Parkway, NW, Suite 300
Boca Raton, FL 33487
(800) 272-7737
Fax: (800) 374-3401
orders@crcpress.com
www.crcpress.com

Princeton Review
2315 Broadway
New York, NY 10024
(212) 874-8282
Fax: (212) 874-0775
www.princetonreview.com

Thieme New York
333 Seventh Avenue
New York, NY 10001
(800) 782-3488
Fax: (212) 947-1112
www.thieme.com
customerservice@thieme.com

W. B. Saunders
(see Elsevier Science)

Abbreviations and Symbols

Abbreviation	Meaning
1°	primary
2°	secondary
3°	tertiary
AA	amino acid
AAMC	Association of American Medical Colleges
aa-tRNA	aminoacyl-tRNA
Ab	antibody
ABP	androgen-binding protein
ACA	anterior cerebral artery
ACC	acetyl-CoA carboxylase
Ac-CoA	acetylcoenzyme A
ACD	anemia of chronic disease
ACE	angiotensin-converting enzyme
ACh	acetylcholine
AChE	acetylcholinesterase
AChR	acetylcholine receptor
ACL	anterior cruciate ligament
ACTH	adrenocorticotropic hormone
ADA	adenosine deaminase, Americans with Disabilities Act
ADH	antidiuretic hormone
ADHD	attention-deficit hyperactivity disorder
ADP	adenosine diphosphate
ADPKD	autosomal-dominant polycystic kidney disease
AFP	α-fetoprotein
Ag	antigen
AICA	anterior inferior cerebellar artery
AIDS	acquired immunodeficiency syndrome
AL	Amyloid Light [Chain]
ALA	aminolevulinic acid
ALL	acute lymphocytic leukemia
ALP	alkaline phosphatase
ALS	amyotrophic lateral sclerosis
ALT	alanine transaminase
AMA	antimitochondrial antibody
AML	acute myelocytic leukemia
AMP	adenosine monophosphate
ANA	antinuclear antibody
ANCA	antineutrophil cytoplasmic antibody
ANOVA	analysis of variance

Abbreviation	Meaning
ANP	atrial natriuretic peptide
ANS	autonomic nervous system
AOA	American Osteopathic Association
AP	action potential
APC	antigen-presenting cell
APP	amyloid precursor protein
APRT	adenine phosphoribosyltransferase
APSAC	anistreplase
aPTT	activated partial thromboplastin time
AR	autosomal recessive, aortic regurgitation
ARB	angiotensin receptor blocker
ARDS	acute respiratory distress syndrome
Arg	arginine
ARMD	age-related macular degeneration
ARPKD	autosomal-recessive polycystic kidney disease
ASA	acetylsalicylic acid, anterior spinal artery
ASD	atrial septal defect
ASO	antistreptolysin O
Asp	aspartic acid
AST	aspartate transaminase
AT	angiotensin, antithrombin
ATCase	aspartate transcarbamoylase
ATP	adenosine triphosphate
ATPase	adenosine triphosphatase
AV	atrioventricular, azygous vein
AVM	arteriovenous malformation
AZT	azidothymidine
BAL	British anti-Lewisite [dimercaprol]
BCG	bacille Calmette-Guérin
BIMS	Biometric Identity Management System
BM	basement membrane
BMI	body-mass index
BMR	basal metabolic rate
BP	bisphosphate, blood pressure
BPG	bisphosphoglycerate
BPH	benign prostatic hyperplasia
BUN	blood urea nitrogen
CAD	coronary artery disease

Abbreviation	Meaning
CAF	common application form
CALLA	common acute lymphoblastic leukemia antigen
cAMP	cyclic adenosine monophosphate
c-ANCA	cytoplasmic antineutrophil cytoplasmic antibody
CBG	corticosteroid-binding globulin
Cbl	cobalamin
CBSSA	Comprehensive Basic Science Self-Assessment
CBT	computer-based test, cognitive-behavioral therapy
CCK	cholecystokinin
CCl_4	carbon tetrachloride
CCS	computer-based case simulation
CCT	cortical collecting tubule
CD	cluster of differentiation
CDK	cyclin-dependent kinase
CE	cholesterol ester
CEA	carcinoembryonic antigen
CETP	cholesterol-ester transfer protein
CF	cystic fibrosis
CFTR	cystic fibrosis transmembrane conductance regulator
CFX	circumflex [artery]
CGD	chronic granulomatous disease
cGMP	cyclic guanosine monophosphate
CGN	cis-Golgi network
CGRP	calcitonin gene–related peptide
ChAT	choline acetyltransferase
CHF	congestive heart failure
CI	confidence interval
CIN	candidate identification number, cervical intraepithelial neoplasia
CIS	Communication and Interpersonal Skills
CJD	Creutzfeldt-Jakob disease
CK	clinical knowledge
CK-MB	creatine kinase, MB fraction
CL	clearance
CLL	chronic lymphocytic leukemia
CML	chronic myeloid leukemia
CMV	cytomegalovirus
CN	cranial nerve, cyanide
CNS	central nervous system
CO	cardiac output
CoA	coenzyme A
COMLEX	Comprehensive Osteopathic Medical Licensing Examination
COMSAE	Comprehensive Osteopathic Medical Self-Assessment Examination
COMT	catechol-O-methyltransferase
COP	coat protein
COPD	chronic obstructive pulmonary disease
CoQ	coenzyme Q

Abbreviation	Meaning
COX	cyclooxygenase
C_p	plasma concentration
CPAP	continuous positive airway pressure
CPK	creatine phosphokinase
CRC	colorectal cancer
CRH	corticotropin-releasing hormone
CRP	C-reactive protein
CS	clinical skills
CSF	cerebrospinal fluid, colony-stimulating factor
CT	computed tomography
CTL	cytotoxic T lymphocyte
CTP	cytidine triphosphate
CV	cardiovascular
CVA	cerebrovascular accident, costovertebral angle
CVID	common variable immune deficiency
Cx	complication
CXR	chest x-ray
Cys	cysteine
d4T	didehydrodeoxythymidine [stavudine]
DAF	decay-accelerating factor
DAG	diacylglycerol
dATP	deoxyadenosine triphosphate
DCIS	ductal carcinoma in situ
DCT	distal convoluted tubule
ddC	dideoxycytidine [zalcitabine]
ddI	didanosine
DES	diethylstilbestrol
DHAP	dihydroxyacetone phosphate
DHB	dihydrobiopterin
DHEA	dehydroepiandrosterone
DHF	dihydrofolic acid
DHS	Department of Homeland Security
DHT	dihydrotestosterone
DI	diabetes insipidus
DIC	disseminated intravascular coagulation
DIP	distal interphalangeal [joint]
DIT	diiodotyrosine
DKA	diabetic ketoacidosis
DM	diabetes mellitus
DNA	deoxyribonucleic acid
2,4-DNP	2,4-dinitrophenol
DO	doctor of osteopathy
2,3-DPG	2,3-diphosphoglycerate
DPM	doctor of podiatric medicine
dsDNA	double-stranded deoxyribonucleic acid
dsRNA	double-stranded ribonucleic acid
dTMP	deoxythymidine monophosphate
DTR	deep tendon reflex
DTs	delirium tremens
dUDP	deoxyuridine diphosphate
dUMP	deoxyuridine monophosphate
DVT	deep venous thrombosis

Abbreviation	Meaning
EBV	Epstein-Barr virus
EC	ejection click
EC_{50}	median effective concentration
ECF	extracellular fluid
ECFMG	Educational Commission for Foreign Medical Graduates
ECG	electrocardiogram
ECL	enterochromaffin-like [cell]
ECM	extracellular matrix
ECT	electroconvulsive therapy
ED_{50}	median effective dose
EDRF	endothelium-derived relaxing factor
EDTA	ethylenediamine tetra-acetic acid
EDV	end-diastolic volume
EEG	electroencephalogram
EF	ejection fraction, elongation factor
EGF	epidermal growth factor
eIF	eukaryotic initiation factor
ELISA	enzyme-linked immunosorbent assay
EM	electron micrograph/microscopy
EMB	eosin–methylene blue
EOM	extraocular muscle
epi	epinephrine
EPO	erythropoietin
EPS	extrapyramidal system
ER	endoplasmic reticulum, estrogen receptor
ERAS	Electronic Residency Application Service
ERCP	endoscopic retrograde cholangiopancreatography
ERP	effective refractory period
ERPF	effective renal plasma flow
ERT	estrogen replacement therapy
ERV	expiratory reserve volume
ESR	erythrocyte sedimentation rate
ESRD	end-stage renal disease
ESV	end-systolic volume
EtOH	ethyl alcohol
EV	esophageal vein
F1,6BP	fructose-1,6-bisphosphate
F2,6BP	fructose-2,6-bisphosphate
F6P	fructose-6-phosphate
FA	fatty acid
FAD	oxidized flavin adenine dinucleotide
$FADH_2$	reduced flavin adenine dinucleotide
FAP	familial adenomatous polyposis
FBPase	fructose bisphosphatase
FcR	Fc receptor
5f-dUMP	5-fluorodeoxyuridine monophosphate
Fe_{Na}	excreted fraction of filtered sodium
FEV_1	forced expiratory volume in 1 second
FF	filtration fraction
FFA	free fatty acid
FGF	fibroblast growth factor
FGFR	fibroblast growth factor receptor

Abbreviation	Meaning
FISH	fluorescence in situ hybridization
f-met	formylmethionine
FMG	foreign medical graduate
FMN	flavin mononucleotide
FN	false negative
FP	false positive
FRC	functional residual capacity
FSH	follicle-stimulating hormone
FSMB	Federation of State Medical Boards
FTA-ABS	fluorescent treponemal antibody—absorbed
5-FU	5-fluorouracil
FVC	forced vital capacity
G3P	glucose-3-phosphate
G6P	glucose-6-phosphate
G6PD	glucose-6-phospate dehydrogenase
GABA	γ-aminobutyric acid
GBM	glomerular basement membrane
G-CSF	granulocyte colony-stimulating factor
GDP	guanosine diphosphate
GE	gastroesophageal
GERD	gastroesophageal reflux disease
GFAP	glial fibrillary acid protein
GFR	glomerular filtration rate
GGT	γ-glutamyl transpeptidase
GH	growth hormone
GHRH	growth hormone–releasing hormone
GI	gastrointestinal
GIP	gastric inhibitory peptide
GIST	gastrointestinal stromal tumor
Glu	glutamic acid
GLUT	glucose transporter
GM-CSF	granulocyte-macrophage colony-stimulating factor
GMP	guanosine monophosphate
GN	glomerulonephritis
GnRH	gonadotropin-releasing hormone
GP	glycogen phosphorylase, glycoprotein
GPe	globus pallidus externa
GPi	globus pallidus interna
GPI	glycosyl phosphatidylinositol
GPP	glycogen phosphorylase phosphatase
GRP	gastrin-releasing peptide
GS	glycogen synthase
GSH	reduced glutathione
GS-P	glycogen synthase phosphatase
GSSG	oxidized glutathione
GTP	guanosine triphosphate
GU	genitourinary
HAART	highly active antiretroviral therapy
HAV	hepatitis A virus
HAVAb	hepatitis A antibody
Hb	hemoglobin
HBcAb	hepatitis B core antibody
HBcAg	hepatitis B core antigen
HBeAb	hepatitis B early antibody

Abbreviation	Meaning
HBeAg	hepatitis B early antigen
HBsAb	hepatitis B surface antibody
HBsAg	hepatitis B surface antigen
HBV	hepatitis B virus
hCG	human chorionic gonadotropin
Hct	hematocrit
HCV	hepatitis C virus
HDL	high-density lipoprotein
HDV	hepatitis D virus
H&E	hematoxylin and eosin
HEV	hepatitis E virus
HGPRT	hypoxanthine-guanine phosphoribosyltransferase
HHS	[Department of] Health and Human Services
HHV	human herpesvirus
5-HIAA	5-hydroxyindoleacetic acid
His	histidine
HIT	heparin-induced thrombocytopenia
HIV	human immunodeficiency virus
HL	hepatic lipase
HLA	human leukocyte antigen
HMG-CoA	hydroxymethylglutaryl-coenzyme A
HMP	hexose monophosphate
HMSN	hereditary motor and sensory neuropathy
HMWK	high-molecular-weight kininogen
HNPCC	hereditary nonpolyposis colorectal cancer
hnRNA	heterogeneous nuclear ribonucleic acid
HPA	hypothalamic-pituitary-adrenal [axis]
HPG	hypothalamic-pituitary-gonadal [axis]
HPO	hypothalamic-pituitary-ovarian [axis]
HPSA	Health Professional Shortage Area
HPV	human papillomavirus
HR	heart rate
HRT	hormone replacement therapy
HSV	herpes simplex virus
HSV-1	herpes simplex virus 1
HSV-2	herpes simplex virus 2
5-HT	5-hydroxytryptamine (serotonin)
HTLV	human T-cell leukemia virus
HUS	hemolytic-uremic syndrome
HVA	homovanillic acid
IBD	inflammatory bowel disease
IBS	irritable bowel syndrome
IC	inspiratory capacity, immune complex
ICA	internal carotid artery
ICAM	intracellular adhesion molecule
ICE	Integrated Clinical Encounter
ICF	intracellular fluid
ICP	intracranial pressure, inferior cerebellar peduncle
IDDM	insulin-dependent diabetes mellitus
IDL	intermediate-density lipoprotein
I/E	inspiratory/expiratory [ratio]

Abbreviation	Meaning
IEV	inferior epigastric vein
IF	immunofluorescence
IFN	interferon
Ig	immunoglobulin
IGF	insulin-like growth factor
IL	interleukin
Ile	isoleucine
IMA	inferior mesenteric artery
IMED	International Medical Education Directory
IMG	international medical graduate
IMP	inosine monophosphate
IMV	inferior mesenteric vein
INH	isonicotine hydrazine [isoniazid]
INR	International Normalized Ratio
IO	inferior orbital [muscle]
IP_3	inositol triphosphate
IPV	inactivated polio vaccine
IR	inferior rectus [muscle]
IRV	inferior rectal vein, inspiratory reserve volume
ITP	idiopathic thrombocytopenic purpura
IUGR	intrauterine growth retardation
IV	intravenous
IVC	inferior vena cava
JG	juxtaglomerular [cells]
JGA	juxtaglomerular apparatus
JVD	jugular venous distention
JVP	jugular venous pulse
K_f	filtration constant
KOH	potassium hydroxide
KSHV	Kaposi's sarcoma–associated herpesvirus
LA	left atrial, left atrium
LAD	left anterior descending [artery]
LAF	left anterior fascicle
LCA	left coronary artery
LCAT	lecithin-cholesterol acyltransferase
LCFA	long-chain fatty acid
LCL	lateral collateral ligament
LCME	Liaison Committee on Medical Education
LCMV	lymphocytic choriomeningitis virus
LCX	left circumflex artery
LD_{50}	median lethal dose
LDH	lactate dehydrogenase
LDL	low-density lipoprotein
LES	lower esophageal sphincter
Leu	leucine
LFA-1	leukocyte function–associated antigen 1
LFT	liver function test
LGN	lateral geniculate nucleus
LGV	left gastric vein
LH	luteinizing hormone
LLQ	left lower quadrant

Abbreviation	Meaning
LM	light microscopy
LMN	lower motor neuron
LP	lumbar puncture
LPL	lipoprotein lipase
LPS	lipopolysaccharide
LR	lateral rectus [muscle]
LSE	Libman-Sacks endocarditis
LT	leukotriene
LV	left ventricle, left ventricular
Lys	lysine
MAC	membrane attack complex, minimal alveolar concentration
MALT	mucosa-associated lymphoid tissue
MAO	monoamine oxidase
MAOI	monoamine oxidase inhibitor
MAP	mean arterial pressure
MC	midsystolic click
MCA	middle cerebral artery
MCHC	mean corpuscular hemoglobin concentration
MCL	medial collateral ligament
MCP	metacarpophalangeal [joint], middle cerebellar peduncle
M-CSF	macrophage colony-stimulating factor
MCV	mean corpuscular volume
MD	macula densa
MEN	multiple endocrine neoplasia
MEOS	microsomal ethanol oxidizing system
Met	methionine
MGN	medial geniculate nucleus
MGUS	monoclonal gammopathy of undetermined significance
MHC	major histocompatibility complex
MHPSA	Mental Health Professional Shortage Area
MI	myocardial infarction
MIF	müllerian inhibiting factor
MIT	monoiodotyrosine
MLCK	myosin light-chain kinase
MLF	medial longitudinal fasciculus
MMC	migrating motor complex
MMR	measles, mumps, rubella [vaccine]
6-MP	6-mercaptopurine
MPGN	membranoproliferative glomerulonephritis
MPO	myeloperoxidase
MPTP	1-methyl-4-phenyl-1,2,3,6-tetrahydropyridine
MR	medial rectus [muscle], mental retardation, mitral regurgitation
MRI	magnetic resonance imaging
mRNA	messenger ribonucleic acid
MRSA	methicillin-resistant S. aureus
MS	multiple sclerosis, mitral stenosis
MSH	melanocyte-stimulating hormone
mtDNA	mitochondrial DNA

Abbreviation	Meaning
mTOR	mammalian target of rapamycin
MTP	metatarsophalangeal [joint]
MTX	methotrexate
MUA/P	Medically Underserved Area and Population
MVO_2	myocardial oxygen consumption
NAD^+	oxidized nicotinamide adenine dinucleotide
NADH	reduced nicotinamide adenine dinucleotide
$NADP^+$	oxidized nicotinamide adenine dinucleotide phosphate
NADPH	reduced nicotinamide adenine dinucleotide phosphate
NBME	National Board of Medical Examiners
NBOME	National Board of Osteopathic Medical Examiners
NBPME	National Board of Podiatric Medical Examiners
NC	no change
NE	norepinephrine
NEG	nonenzymatic glycosylation
NF	neurofibromatosis
NH_3	ammonia
NHL	non-Hodgkin's lymphoma
NIDDM	non-insulin-dependent diabetes mellitus
NK	natural killer [cells]
NMDA	N-methyl D-aspartate
NMJ	neuromuscular junction
NMS	neuroleptic malignant syndrome
NNRTI	non-nucleoside reverse transcriptase inhibitor
NO	nitric oxide
NPV	negative predictive value
NRTI	nucleoside reverse transcriptase inhibitor
NSAID	nonsteroidal anti-inflammatory drug
OAA	oxaloacetic acid
OCD	obsessive-compulsive disorder
OCP	oral contraceptive pill
OMT	osteopathic manipulative technique
OPV	oral polio vaccine
OR	odds ratio
OS	opening snap
OTC	ornithine transcarbamoylase
OVLT	organum vasculosum of the lamina terminalis
PA	posteroanterior
PABA	para-aminobenzoic acid
PAH	para-aminohippuric acid
PALS	periarterial lymphatic sheath
PAN	polyarteritis nodosa
p-ANCA	perinuclear antineutrophil cytoplasmic antibody

Abbreviation	Meaning
PAP	prostatic acid phosphatase
PAS	periodic acid Schiff
PBP	penicillin-binding protein
P_c	capillary pressure
PC	pyruvate carboxylase
PCL	posterior cruciate ligament
P_{CO_2}	partial pressure of carbon dioxide
PCOS	polycystic ovarian syndrome
PCP	phencyclidine hydrochloride, *Pneumocystis carinii* (now *jiroveci*) pneumonia
PCR	polymerase chain reaction
PCT	proximal convoluted tubule
PCWP	pulmonary capillary wedge pressure
PD	posterior descending [artery]
PDA	patent ductus arteriosus
PDE	phosphodiesterase
PDGF	platelet-derived growth factor
PDH	pyruvate dehydrogenase
PE	pulmonary embolism
PECAM	platelet–endothelial cell adhesion molecule
PEP	phosphoenolpyruvate
PF	platelet factor
PFK	phosphofructokinase
PFT	pulmonary function test
PG	phosphoglycerate, prostaglandin
Phe	phenylalanine
P_i	interstitial fluid pressure, inorganic phosphate
PICA	posterior inferior cerebellar artery
PID	pelvic inflammatory disease
PIP	proximal interphalangeal [joint]
PIP_2	phosphatidylinositol 4,5-bisphosphate
PK	pyruvate kinase
PKD	polycystic kidney disease
PKU	phenylketonuria
PLP	pyridoxal phosphate
PML	progressive multifocal leukoencephalopathy
PMN	polymorphonuclear [leukocyte]
P_{net}	net filtration pressure
PNET	primitive neuroectodermal tumor
PNH	paroxysmal nocturnal hemoglobinuria
PNS	peripheral nervous system
P_{O_2}	partial pressure of oxygen
POMC	pro-opiomelanocortin
PPAR	peroxisome proliferator-activated receptor
PPD	purified protein derivative
PPI	proton pump inhibitor
PPRF	paramedian pontine reticular formation
PPV	positive predictive value
PrP	prion protein
PRPP	phosphoribosylpyrophosphate

Abbreviation	Meaning
PSA	prostate-specific antigen
PSS	progressive systemic sclerosis
PT	prothrombin time
PTH	parathyroid hormone
PTHrP	parathyroid hormone–related protein
PTSD	post-traumatic stress disorder
PTT	partial thromboplastin time
PUV	paraumbilical vein
PV	plasma volume, portal vein
RA	rheumatoid arthritis, right atrium
RAAS	renin-angiotensin-aldosterone system
RANK-L	receptor activator of nuclear factor-κ B ligand
RBC	red blood cell
RBF	renal blood flow
RCA	right coronary artery
RDS	respiratory distress syndrome
REM	rapid eye movement
RER	rough endoplasmic reticulum
RNA	ribonucleic acid
RNP	ribonucleoprotein
ROI	reactive oxygen intermediate
RPF	renal plasma flow
RPR	rapid plasma reagin
RR	relative risk, respiratory rate
rRNA	ribosomal ribonucleic acid
RS	Reed-Sternberg [cells]
RSV	respiratory syncytial virus
RTA	renal tubular acidosis
RUQ	right upper quadrant
RV	renal vein, residual volume, right ventricle, right ventricular
RVH	right ventricular hypertrophy
SA	sinoatrial, subarachnoid
SAA	serum amyloid–associated [protein]
SAM	S-adenosylmethionine
SARS	severe acute respiratory syndrome
SC	subcutaneous
SCC	squamous cell carcinoma
SCID	severe combined immunodeficiency disease
SCJ	squamocolumnar junction
SCN	suprachiasmatic nucleus
SCP	superior cerebellar peduncle
SD	standard deviation, subdural
SEM	standard error of the mean
SEP	Spoken English Proficiency
SER	smooth endoplasmic reticulum
SERM	selective estrogen receptor modulator
SEV	superficial epigastric vein
SEVIS	Student and Exchange Visitor Information System
SEVP	Student and Exchange Visitor Program
SGOT	serum glutamic oxaloacetic transaminase

Abbreviation	Meaning
SGPT	serum glutamic pyruvate transaminase
SHBG	sex hormone–binding globulin
SIADH	syndrome of inappropriate [secretion of] antidiuretic hormone
SLE	systemic lupus erythematosus
SLL	small lymphocytic lymphoma
SMA	superior mesenteric artery
SMV	superior mesenteric vein
SMX	sulfamethoxazole
SNc	substantia nigra compacta
SNP	single nucleotide polymorphism
SNr	substantia nigra pars reticulata
SNRI	selective norepinephrine receptor inhibitor
snRMP	small nuclear ribonucleoprotein
SO	superior oblique [muscle]
SOD	superoxide dismutase
SR	sarcoplasmic reticulum, superior rectus [muscle]
SRP	sponsoring residency program
SRV	superior rectal vein
SS	single stranded
SSB	single-stranded binding
ssDNA	single-stranded deoxyribonucleic acid
SSPE	subacute sclerosing panencephalitis
SSRI	selective serotonin reuptake inhibitor
ssRNA	single-stranded ribonucleic acid
SSSS	staphylococcal scalded-skin syndrome
STD	sexually transmitted disease
STN	subthalamic nucleus
SV	sinus venosus, splenic vein, stroke volume
SVC	superior vena cava
SVT	supraventricular tachycardia
$t_{1/2}$	half-life
T_3	triiodothyronine
T_4	thyroxine
TA	truncus arteriosus
TAPVR	total anomalous pulmonary venous return
TB	tuberculosis
TBG	thyroxine-binding globulin
TBW	total body weight
3TC	dideoxythiacytidine [lamivudine]
TCA	tricarboxylic acid [cycle], tricyclic antidepressant
Tc cell	cytotoxic T cell
TCR	T-cell receptor
TdT	terminal deoxynucleotidyl transferase
TFT	thyroid function test
6-TG	6-thioguanine
TG	triglyceride
TGA	trans-Golgi apparatus
TGF	transforming growth factor
THB	tetrahydrobiopterin

Abbreviation	Meaning
Th cell	helper T cell
THF	tetrahydrofolate
Thr	threonine
TI	therapeutic index
TIA	transient ischemic attack
TIBC	total iron-binding capacity
TIPS	transjugular intrahepatic portosystemic shunt
TLC	total lung capacity
TMP-SMX	trimethoprim-sulfamethoxazole
TN	true negative
TNF	tumor necrosis factor
TNM	tumor, node, metastases [staging]
TOEFL	Test of English as a Foreign Language
TP	true positive
tPA	tissue plasminogen activator
TPP	thiamine pyrophosphate
TPR	total peripheral resistance
TR	tricuspid regurgitation
TRAP	tartrate-resistant acid phosphatase
TRH	thyrotropin-releasing hormone
tRNA	transfer ribonucleic acid
Trp	tryptophan
TSH	thyroid-stimulating hormone
TSI	thyroid-stimulating immunoglobulin
TSS	toxic shock syndrome
TSST	toxic shock syndrome toxin
TTP	thrombotic thrombocytopenic purpura
TV	tidal volume
TxA	thromboxane
UA	urinalysis
UCB	unconjugated bilirubin
UCV	Underground Clinical Vignettes
UDP	uridine diphosphate
UMN	upper motor neuron
UMP	uridine monophosphate
URI	upper respiratory infection
USDA	United States Department of Agriculture
USIA	United States Information Agency
USMLE	United States Medical Licensing Examination
UTI	urinary tract infection
UV	ultraviolet
VA	ventral anterior [nucleus], Veterans Administration
Val	valine
VC	vital capacity
V_d	volume of distribution
VDRL	Venereal Disease Research Laboratory
VF	ventricular fibrillation
VHL	von Hippel–Lindau [disease]
VIP	vasoactive intestinal peptide

Abbreviation	Meaning
VIPoma	vasoactive intestinal polypeptide-secreting tumor
VL	ventral lateral [nucleus]
VLDL	very low density lipoprotein
VMA	vanillylmandelic acid
VPL	ventral posterior nucleus, lateral
VPM	ventral posterior nucleus, medial
VPN	ventral posterior nucleus

Abbreviation	Meaning
V/Q	ventilation/perfusion [ratio]
VRE	vancomycin-resistant enterococcus
VSD	ventricular septal defect
vWF	von Willebrand factor
VZV	varicella-zoster virus
WBC	white blood cell
XR	X-linked recessive
ZDV	zidovudine [formerly AZT]

Index

Aspergillosis, 158

Aspergillus fumigatus, 158

Aspirin, 363, 391

Asthma, 510, 515

Astrocytes, 396

Ataxia-telangiectasia, 214

Atheromas, 269

Atherosclerosis, 407

Athetosis, 401

ATIII deficiency, 356

Atopic dermatitis (eczema), 388

Atorvastatin, 282

ATP production, 97

Atrial fibrillation, 263

Atrial flutter, 263

"Atrial kick," 257

Atrial natriuretic peptide (ANP), 265, 464

Atrial repolarization, 262

Atrial septal defect (ASD), 258, 267

Atrophy, 221

Atropine, 239

Attention-deficit hyperactivity disorder (ADHD), 442, 452

Attributable risk, 532

Atypical depression, 446

Auer bodies (rods), 360, I-6

Auscultation, heart, 257, **258–259**

Auspitz sign, 388

Autistic disorder, 442

Autoantibodies, 212

Autoimmune hemolytic anemia, 353

Autonomic drugs, 235–242

  ACh receptors for, 235

  α-blockers, 241

  atropine, 239

  β-blockers, 242

  cholinergic vs. noradrenergic, 237

  cholinomimetic agents, 238

  G-protein-linked 2nd messengers, 236

  hexamethonium, 239

  muscarinic antagonists, 239

  sympathomimetics, 240

  sympathoplegics, 241

Autonomic regulation, 398

Autonomy, 57

Autoregulation, blood pressure, 266

Autosomal-dominant diseases, 86

Autosomal dominant inheritance, 85

Autosomal-recessive diseases, 87

Autosomal recessive inheritance, 85

Autosomal trisomies, 88

AV block, 263

AV nodes, 254, 261

Avoidant disorder, 448

A wave, 257

Axillary n., 374

Azathioprine, 216

Azithromycin, 188

Azole antimicrobials, 193

Aztreonam, 186

B

Babesia, 153, 161

Bacillary angiomatosis, 154, 279

Bacillus

  cultivation, 138

  morphology, 137

Bacillus anthracis

  profile, 147

  virulence factors, 141

Bacillus cereus, 147

Bacteria

  antimicrobial therapies, 184–191

  cell-wall deficient, 156

  fungi-like bacteria, 148

  genetics, 143

  gram-negative lab algorithm, 149

  gram-positive lab algorithm, 144

  growth curves, 142

  lab characteristics, 138–139

  normal flora, 175

  oncogenic, 229

  organ systems affected, 175–183

  profiles by organism, 145–156

  spore-forming, 147

  structure and composition, 136

  taxonomy, 137

  virulence factors, 140–142

  zoonotic, 154

Bacterial endocarditis, 275, I-19

Bacterial vaginosis, 154, I-3

Bacteriostatic vs. bactericidal, 185

Bacteroides

  cultivation, 139

  morphology, 137

Baker's cyst, 383

Barbiturates, 432, 434, 450

Baroreceptors, 265

Barrett's esophagus, 322

Bartonella

  bacillary angiomatosis, 279

  morphology, 137

  transmission, 154

Basal cell carcinoma, I-15

Basal electric rhythm, 310

Basal ganglia, 400

Basophilic stippling, 348

Basophils, 343

B cells. *See* Lymphocytes

BCG vaccination, 148

B-complex vitamins, 90, 91–92, 350

Becker's muscular dystrophy, 87

Beclomethasone, 305

Behavioral science, 49–63

  development, 60–61

  epidemiology/biostatistics, 50–56

  ethics, 57–59

  physiology, 61–63

Bell-shaped curves, 53

Bell's palsy, 419

Beneficence, 57

Benign prostatic hyperplasia (BPH), 495

Benign tumors, 226

Benzodiazepines, 431, 432, 433, 434, 450

Berger's disease, 467

Beriberi, 91, 273

Bernard-Soulier disease, 355

β-agonists, 515

β-blocker drugs, 242, 280, 285, 430

β cells, pancreas, 289

β-hCG, 484

β-hydroxybutyrate, 112

β-lactam antimicrobials, 185

β-thalassemia, 349

Betaxolol, 430

Bezafibrate, 282

Bias, 53

Bicarbonate, 318, 509

Bicornuate uterus, 133
Biguanides, 304
Bile, 320
Bile acid resins, 282
Biliary tract, 314, 334–335
Bilirubin, 321, 332
Bimodal curves, 53
Biochemistry, 65–115
    cellular, 76–80
    genetics, 83–89
    laboratory techniques, 81–82
    metabolism, 95–115
    molecular, 66–75
    nutrition, 90–94
Biofilms, 145
Biostatistics. *See* Epidemiology/
    biostatistics
Biotin, 93
Bipolar disorder, 445, 452
Bismuth, 338
Bisphosphonates, 392
Bite cells, 102, 348
Bivalirudin, 362
Blastomycosis, 157
Bleomycin, 366, 511
Blood-brain barrier, 396, 398
Blood cell differentiation, 342–
    344
Blood cultures, contamination of,
    145
Blood groups, 83, 345
Blood, oxygen content of, 508
Blotting procedures, 81
"Blue babies," 267
"Blue bloater" bronchitis, 510
"Blue kids," 267
Body dysmorphic disorder, 447
Body-mass index (BMI), 61
Boerhaave syndrome, 322
Bone formation, 379
Bone fracture, I-23
Bone/joint disorders
    achondroplasia, 379
    gout, 384
    infectious arthritis, 384
    lab values in, 380
    osteitis deformans, 380
    osteoarthritis, 382
    osteomalacia, 379
    osteopetrosis, 379
    osteoporosis, 379

polyostotic fibrous dysplasia,
    380
pseudogout, 384
rheumatoid arthritis, 383
seronegative spondylo-
    arthropathies, 385
Sjögren's syndrome, 383
tumors, 381
Borderline disorder, 448
Bordetella
    cultivation, 138
    morphology, 137
Bordetella pertussis
    virulence factors, 141
Bordet-Gengou agar, 138
Borrelia
    morphology, 137
    profile, 152
    staining, 138
Borrelia burgdorferi
    profile, 153
    transmission, 154
Borrelia recurrentis
    transmission, 154
Bosentan, 516
Botulism, 140
Bouchard's nodes, 382
Bowenoid papulosis, 496
Bowen's disease, 496
Bowman capsule, 460, 461
Brachial plexus
    conditions involving, 375
    lesions, 373
Brain
    berry aneurysm, I-11
    blood circulation to, 266
    cerebral arteries, 404–405
    cerebral cortex functions, 402
    dural venous sinuses, 407
    epidural hematoma, I-11
    glucose uptake, 289
    herniation syndromes, 429
    hydrocephalus, 408
    hypertensive hemorrhage, I-11
    ischemic brain disease, 407
    lesions, 403, 429
    multiple sclerosis, I-12
    subarachnoid hemorrhage, I-28
    subdural hemorrhage, I-11
    tumors of, 428
    ventricular system, 408

Brain stem, anatomy of, 415
Branched-chain AA
    dehydrogenase, 91
Branchial development, 127–129
Breasts
    benign tumors, 492
    malignant tumors, 493
    other pathologies, 494
Brenner tumor, 492
Brief psychotic disorder, 444
Brimonidine, 430
Broca's aphasia, 404
Bronchiectasis, 510
Bronchitis, 510
Bronchopulmonary segments, 503
"Bronze" diabetes, 334
Brown-Séquard syndrome, 412
Brucella
    cultivation, 139
    morphology, 137
    transmission, 154
Brucellosis, 154
Brudzinski's sign, 177
Brunner's glands, 320
Bruton's agammaglobulinemia,
    213
Budd-Chiari syndrome, 331, 332
Buerger's disease, 278
"Bug hints" (study aid), 183
Bulimia nervosa, 449, 452
Bullous pemphigoid, 389, I-16
Bundle of His, 260
Bundle of Kent, 263
Bupropion, 456
Burkitt's lymphoma, 358, 360, I-7
Burton's lines, 350
Buspirone, 454
Busulfan, 366, 511
Butorphanol, 430
"Butterfly glioma," 428

C

"Café-au-lait" spots, 380, 427
Caffeine, 450
Calcitonin, 294
Calcium
    cardiac contraction and, 260
    homeostasis of, 293
Calcium carbonate, 338
Calcium channel blockers, 280,
    286

steroid/thyroid hormone
  mechanism, 295
  vitamin D/calcitonin, 294
Endoderm, 119
Endodermal sinus tumor, 491, 496
Endometrial proliferation, 489
Endometriosis, 489
Endoneurium, 397
Endotoxins, 140, 142
Enoxacin, 190
Entamoeba histolytica, 160
Enteric gram-negative bacilli. *See*
  also individual organism
  names
  cultivation, 138
  endotoxins, 142
  lactose-fermenting, 150
  morphology, 137
Enterobacter, 137
Enterobius vermicularis, 162
Enterococci, 146
Enterotoxins, immune response
  and, 209
Enzyme-linked immunosorbent
  assay (ELISA), 81
Enzymes
  liver disease markers, 331
  pancreatic, 320
  in pharmacology, 232
  terminology, 95
  vitamin cofactors, 91
Eosin-methylene blue (EMB) agar,
  138
Eosinophilic granuloma, 511
Eosinophils, 343
EPEC (enteropathogenic *E. coli*),
  151
Ependymoma, 428
Ephelis, 388
Epidemiology/biostatistics, 50–56
  ANOVA analysis, 55
  bias, 53
  clinical trials, 50
  confidence intervals, 55
  correlation coefficient, 55
  deaths, leading causes of, 56
  diagnostic test evaluation, 51
  disease prevention, 55
  error types, 54
  Medicare and Medicaid, 56
  meta-analysis, 50

odds ratio vs. relative risk, 52
power $(1 - \beta)$, 54
precision vs. accuracy, 52
prevalence vs. incidence, 52
reportable diseases, 56
standard deviation vs. standard
  error, 54
statistical distribution, 53
statistical hypotheses, 54
study types and designs, 50
Epidermis layers, 370
Epidermophyton, 158
Epiglottitis, 150
Epilepsy drugs, 431, 432
Epinephrine, 109, 430
Epineurium, 397
Epispadias, 134
Epithelial cell junctions, 370
Equations, rapid review, 532
Erb-Duchenne palsy, 375
Ergocalciferol (Vitamin D$_2$), 93
Error types, 54
Erythema chronicum migrans, 153
Erythema multiforme, 389, I-14
Erythema nodosum, 389
Erythroblastosis fetalis, 353
Erythrocyte sedimentation rate
  (ESR), 223
Erythrocytes (RBCs), 342, 348–
  354
Erythromycin, 188
Erythroplasia of Queyrat, 496
Erythropoietin, 463
"Escape from aldosterone"
  mechanism, 265
Eschars
  cutaneous, 147
  nasal, 158
Esophagus
  anatomy, 310
  pathologies, 322–323, I-9
ESR. *See* Erythrocyte
  sedimentation rate (ESR)
Essential hypertension, therapy for,
  280
Essential thrombocytosis, 361
Estrogen, 482, 498
Etanercept, 393
Ethacrynic acid, 474
Ethanol metabolism, 94
Ethics, 57–59

advance directives, 57
confidentiality, 58
consent for minors, 57
core ethical principles, 57
decision-making capacity, 57
ethical vignettes, 59
informed consent, 57
malpractice, 58
Ethinyl estradiol, 498
Ethosuximide, 431, 432
Etoposide (VP-16), 366
Eukaryotes, RNA in, 72–73, 74
Ewing's sarcoma, 360, 381, I-26
Exam preparation. *See* USMLE
  Step 1 exam
Excitatory pathway, 400
Exemestane, 498
Exenatide, 304
Exercise, response to, 509
Exotoxins, 140–141, 143, 147,
  151, 209
Expectorants, 516
Expiratory reserve volume (ERV),
  504
Extracellular volume, 459
Extraocular muscles/nerves,
  421–422
Extrinsic pathway, 220
Eyes, 420–424
Ezetimibe, 282

F

Fabry's disease, 111
Facial lesions, 419
Facial n., 416
Factitious disorder, 447
Factor V Leiden disease, 356
Falciform ligament, 309
Fallopian tubes, 478
Familial adenomatous polyposis
  (FAP), 86, 329
Familial dyslipidemias, 115
Famotidine, 337
Fat necrosis, 494
Fat soluble vitamins, 90
Fatty acid metabolism, 95, 112
Femoral hernias, 316
Femoral n., 376
Femoral sheath, 314
Femoral triangle, 314
Fenofibrate, 282

Niemann-Pick disease, 111
Nikolsky's sign, 389
Nissl substance, 396
Nitric oxide, 317
Nitroglycerin, 280
Nitrosoureas, 365
Nizatidine, 337
NNRTIs (HIV therapy), 197
Nocardia
    cultivation, 138
    morphology, 137
Nocardia asteroides, 148
Nonbenzodiazepine hypnotics,
    433
Noncompetitive inhibitors, 232
Non–germ cell tumors
    ovarian, 492
    testicular, 496
Nongonococcal urethritis (NGU),
    156
Non-Hodgkin's lymphoma,
    357–358
Nonmaleficence, 57
Nonmegaloblastic macrocytic
    anemias, 350
Norfloxacin, 190
Normal bacterial flora, 175
Normal splitting, 258
Northern blot, 81
Nosocomial infections, 181
NPH, 304
NPV. *See* Negative predictive value
    (NPV)
NRTIs (HIV therapy), 197
NSAIDs, 391
Nucleotides
    DNA and RNA synthesis, 92
    structure, 67
Number needed to harm, 532
Number needed to treat, 532
"Nutmeg" liver, 331
NutraSweet, 107
Nutrition, 90–94
Nystatin, 192

O

Obligate aerobic bacteria, 138
Obligate anaerobic bacteria, 139
Obsessive-compulsive disorder
    (OCD), 447, 448, 452
Obstructive lung disease
    (COPD), 510, 512
Obturator n., 376

Ochronosis. *See* Alkaptonuria
    (ochronosis)
Octreotide, 338
Odds ratio vs. relative risk, 52
Ofloxacin, 190
Olanzapine, 453
Olfactory n., 416
Oligodendroglia, 396
Oligodendroglioma, 428, I-12
Oligohydramnios, 488
Oligomenorrhea, 483
Oligosaccharide hydrolases, 320
Omphalocele, 130, I-23
Onchocerca volvulus, 162
Oncogenes, 227
Oncology drugs, 364–368
Ondansetron, 339
Oogenesis, 484
Operant conditioning, 438
Opiates, 434
Opioid analgesics, 430
Opioids, 450
Opponens digiti minimi m., 376
Opponens pollicis m., 376
Oppositional defiant disorder,
    442
Opsonization, 140
Optic n., 416
Oral contraceptives, 91, 499
Organ morphogenesis errors,
    119–121
Orientation, loss of, 443
Ornithine transcarbamoylase
    (OTC), 105
Orotic aciduria, 68
Oseltamivir, 195
Osler's nodes, 275
Osler-Weber-Rendu syndrome, 86
Osteitis deformans, 380
Osteoarthritis, 382, I-30
Osteoblastoma, 381
Osteochondroma (exostosis), 381
Osteogenesis imperfecta, 80, I-22
Osteoid osteoma, 381
Osteoma, 381
Osteomalacia, 379
Osteomyelitis, 177
Osteoporosis, 379
Osteosarcoma, 381
Otitis externa, 151
Otitis media, 145, 150

Ovaries
    cysts, 490
    histology, 478
    ovulation, 484
    premature failure, 489
    tumors, 491–492
"Owl's eyes" tumor cells, 357
Oxidative phosphorylation, 100
Oxygen deprivation, 508–509
Oxygen-hemoglobin dissociation
    curve, 506
Oxytocin, 305, 484

P

P-450 interactions, 245
Pacemakers, 261
Pacinian corpuscles, 397
Paclitaxel, 78, 367
Paget's disease, 380, 493
Pain disorder, 447
Palmar interosseous m.'s, 376
Pancoast's tumor, 513
Pancreas
    acinar cells, I-16
    acute pancreatitis, 335
    adenocarcinoma, 336
    cell types, 289
    chronic pancreatitis, I-30
    embryonic development, 131
    insufficiency, 323
    islet cells, I-16
Panic disorder, 446
Pantothenate (Vitamin B₅), 91
Papillary carcinoma, I-18
Papilledema, 421
Pap smears, 488
Paracoccidioidomycosis, 157
Paradoxical splitting, 258
Paragonimus westermani, 163
Paramyxoviruses, 170
Paranoid disorder, 448
Parasites
    antimicrobial therapies, 194
    clinical diagnosis, 163
    helminths, 162–163
    oncogenic, 229
    protozoa, 160–161
Parathyroid hormone (PTH), 293,
    464
Parietal cells, 319
Parinaud syndrome, 415

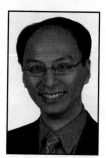

Tao Le, MD, MHS

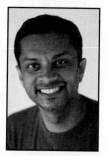

Vikas Bhushan, MD

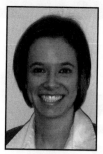

Juliana Tolles

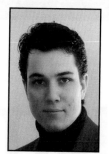

Jeffrey Hofmann

Tao Le, MD, MHS

Tao has pursued his passion for medical education for the past 18 years. As senior editor, he has led the expansion of *First Aid* into a global educational series. In addition, he is the founder of the *USMLERx* online learning system as well as a cofounder of the *Underground Clinical Vignettes* series. As a medical student, he was editor-in-chief of the University of California, San Francisco *Synapse,* a university newspaper with a weekly circulation of 9000. Tao earned his medical degree from the University of California, San Francisco in 1996 and completed his residency training in internal medicine at Yale University and allergy and immunology fellowship training at Johns Hopkins University. At Yale, he was a regular guest lecturer on USMLE review and an adviser to the Yale University School of Medicine curriculum committee. Tao subsequently went on to cofound Medsn, a medical e-learning company, and served as its chief medical officer. He is currently section chief of adult allergy and immunology at the University of Louisville. He enjoys travel, movies, good food, and spending time with his family.

Vikas Bhushan, MD

Vikas is an author, editor, entrepreneur, and teleradiologist. In 1990 he conceived and authored the original *First Aid for the USMLE Step 1*. His entrepreneurial adventures include a successful software company, a medical publishing enterprise (S2S), an e-learning company (Medsn), and an ER teleradiology service (24/7 Radiology). His eclectic interests include medical informatics, independent film, humanism, Urdu poetry, world music, South Asian diasporic culture, and avoiding a day job. A dilettante at heart, he coproduced a music documentary on qawwali music and coproduced and edited *Shabash 2.0: The Hip Guide to All Things South Asian in North America*. Vikas completed a bachelor's degree in biochemistry from the University of California, Berkeley; an MD with thesis from the University of California, San Francisco; and a radiology residency from the University of California, Los Angeles.

Juliana Tolles

Juliana is a fifth-year medical student at the Yale University School of Medicine, and this is her second year on the *First Aid* team. Raised in Edina, Minnesota, she graduated from Harvard University in 2005 with a degree in biochemical sciences. At Harvard, she was an editor for the *Let's Go* travel guide series. After a year conducting research in the application of statistical models to tumor markers, she will graduate in 2011 with a dual degree in medicine and master's of health science. In her free time, she enjoys running and hiking in New England's beautiful parks.

Jeffrey Hofmann

Jeff grew up in Barrington, Rhode Island, and graduated from Brown University in 2008 with an ScB in computational biology. As an undergraduate, he rowed on the men's crew for four years and spent several years researching mitochondrial evolution and aging. Jeff is currently in his third year of Brown's MD/PhD program, where he has served as a student representative on the curriculum committee and as a co-president of the medical school's Aging Interest Group. For his PhD, he is studying the role of cellular signaling pathways in aging, for which he is funded by the NIH. Jeff also enjoys hiking, swimming, cycling, and playing the guitar.

ABOUT THE AUTHORS

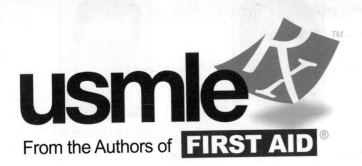
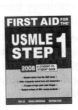
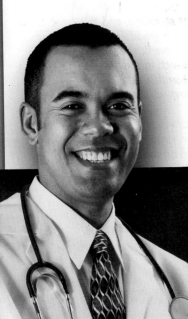